EAI/Springer Innovations in Communication and Computing

The impact of information technologies is creating a new world yet not fully understood. The extent and speed of economic, life style and social changes already perceived in everyday life is hard to estimate without understanding the technological driving forces behind it. This series presents contributed volumes featuring the latest research and development in the various information engineering technologies that play a key role in this process. The range of topics, focusing primarily on communications and computing engineering include, but are not limited to, wireless networks; mobile communication; design and learning; gaming; interaction; e-health and pervasive healthcare; energy management; smart grids; internet of things; cognitive radio networks; computation; cloud computing; ubiquitous connectivity, and in mode general smart living, smart cities, Internet of Things and more. The series publishes a combination of expanded papers selected from hosted and sponsored European Alliance for Innovation (EAI) conferences that present cutting edge, global research as well as provide new perspectives on traditional related engineering fields. This content, complemented with open calls for contribution of book titles and individual chapters, together maintain Springer's and EAI's high standards of academic excellence. The audience for the books consists of researchers, industry professionals, advanced level students as well as practitioners in related fields of activity include information and communication specialists, security experts, economists, urban planners, doctors, and in general representatives in all those walks of life affected ad contributing to the information revolution.

Indexing: This series is indexed in Scopus, Ei Compendex, and zbMATH.

About EAI - EAI is a grassroots member organization initiated through cooperation between businesses, public, private and government organizations to address the global challenges of Europe's future competitiveness and link the European Research community with its counterparts around the globe. EAI reaches out to hundreds of thousands of individual subscribers on all continents and collaborates with an institutional member base including Fortune 500 companies, government organizations, and educational institutions, provide a free research and innovation platform. Through its open free membership model EAI promotes a new research and innovation culture based on collaboration, connectivity and recognition of excellence by community.

Ferdin Joe John Joseph • Valentina Emilia Balas
S. Suman Rajest • R. Regin
Editors

Computational Intelligence for Clinical Diagnosis

Springer

EAI
RESEARCH MEETS INNOVATION

Editors
Ferdin Joe John Joseph
Thai-Nichi Institute of Technology
Bangkok, Thailand

S. Suman Rajest
Department of Research, Arts and Humanities
Bharath Institute of Higher Education and Research
Chennai, Tamil Nadu, India

Valentina Emilia Balas
Department of Automation and Applied Informatics
Aurel Vlaicu University of Arad
Arad, Arad, Romania

R. Regin
Department of Computer Science and Engineering
SRM Institute of Science and Technology
Chennai, Tamil Nadu, India

ISSN 2522-8595 ISSN 2522-8609 (electronic)
EAI/Springer Innovations in Communication and Computing
ISBN 978-3-031-23682-2 ISBN 978-3-031-23683-9 (eBook)
https://doi.org/10.1007/978-3-031-23683-9

This Springer imprint is published by the registered company Springer Nature Switzerland AG
The registered company address is: Gewerbestrasse 11, 6330 Cham, Switzerland

To Our Family, Scholars, Students, and Dear Friends

Preface

Computational medicine has emerged as an outcome of the advancement of medical science and the scientific field's ushering in of the big data era, which is supported by and powered by artificial intelligence software. In order to further the evolution of precision medicine, people must be able to extract useful information from this vast biological data. Traditionally, machine learning techniques are used to extract biomedical data and identify features from the data. These techniques typically rely on feature engineering and subject-matter expertise of specialists, which takes a lot of time and resources. Deep learning, a trimming computational branch, can detect and classify strong, complex features from raw data in contrast to conventional methods without the necessity of classifier. It is suggested that deep learning has clear advantages in maximizing the use of data sources and enhancing medical health level in the areas of research in medical images, genomics, and medication discovery. Deep learning is becoming more and more significant in the realm of medicine and has a wide range of potential applications. Deep learning in computerized medical health still faces a number of issues, including variance, interpretability, and a lack of sufficient data. These issues are examined and discussed in order to better the use of deep education in the context of medicine. Deep learning increases time and energy efficiency since it eliminates the need for manual feature extraction, in contrast to typical machine learning techniques. Neural networks made up of neurons carry out deep learning. The input of the subsequent layer is considered to be the output of the upper layer in neural networks, which have many neurons in each layer. The neuron can transform the initial input to the output by connections among layers and nonlinear processing. More crucially, the high-level network avoids the drawback that machine learning requires manual feature extraction by automatically recognizing more abstractions and generalized features from the input. Deep learning, the much more sophisticated AI technique, offers a mechanism for computerized medicine; hence, it is fashionable to use deep learning to analyze biomedical data. To fully utilize supervised learning in digital medicine, biomedical data must be cleaned, processed, and obtained more easily than data from other domains.

This book contains 42 transdisciplinary advancements in healthcare and technology through artificial intelligence. The topics are crafted in such a way as to cover all the areas of healthcare that require AI for further development. Some of the topics which contain algorithms and techniques are explained with the help of source code developed by the chapter contributors. The healthcare sector witnessed a surge of growth in terms of technology during the COVID-19 pandemic. This book covers most of the advancements from the COVID-19 pandemic. This also encompasses the readiness and need for advancements in managing yet another pandemic in the future. This results in the self-sustainability goals in healthcare across the globe. Most of the technologies addressed in this book are added with a concept of encapsulation to obtain a cookbook for anyone who needs to reskill or upskill themselves in order to contribute to an advancement in the field. This book benefits students, professionals, and anyone from any background to learn about digital disruptions in healthcare.

Bangkok, Thailand — Ferdin Joe John Joseph
Arad, Romania — Valentina Emilia Balas
Chennai, Tamil Nadu, India — S. Suman Rajest
Chennai, Tamil Nadu, India — R. Regin

Acknowledgments

We appreciate the Almighty, our parents, our wives, and our children for their unending love, guidance, and support throughout our lives. We are grateful to our cherished family members for supporting us throughout our career and allowing us to advance it by editing this book.

We would like to express our gratitude to Dr. R. Venkatesh Babu, Pro Vice-Chancellor, and Dr. A Muthukumaravel, Dean of Arts and Science, Bharath Institute of Higher Education and Research (BIHER), Tamil Nadu, India, for their ongoing support and encouragement in the creation of this book. We dedicate this book to them, as well as our collaborators and family members. Our heartfelt gratitude goes to our students who have given their time and effort to help and contribute in any way. We want to thank everyone who helped, shared, talked things over, read, wrote, made opinions, let us quote them, and helped with editing, proofreading, and design during this book journey.

We feel that the team of authors provides the ideal combination of knowledge and skills for authoring this book. We would like to thank all of the writers for committing their time, patience, dedication, and work to this book; we believe it will be a valuable resource for all researchers in this subject! We are grateful to the EAI and Springer Publishing teams for guiding us through the process of writing this book. We would not have started or created this book without their encouragement and knowledge. Their faith in us and their advice, as well as their provision of the required time and resources, enabled us the flexibility to manage this book. Last but not least, we appreciate our readers for their confidence in us; we hope our work inspires and guides them.

Bangkok, Thailand — Ferdin Joe John Joseph
Arad, Romania — Valentina Emilia Balas
Chennai, Tamil Nadu, India — S. Suman Rajest
Chennai, Tamil Nadu, India — R. Regin

Contents

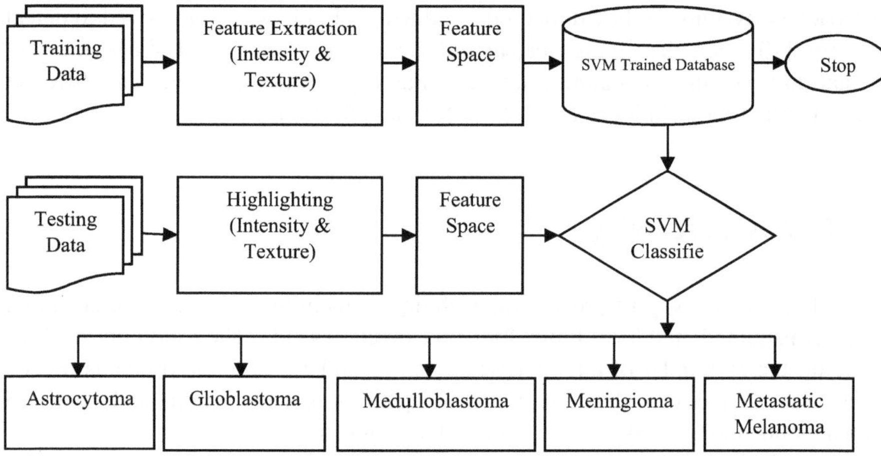

Fig. 1.5 Tumour cataloguing [16]

1.2.1 Proposed Algorithm

The suggested approach was created, and it is helpful to the radiologist for classifying the brain tumour with the MR images. The approach divides tumour types into primary and secondary categories based on their severity. Figure 1.5 shows the proposed system's architecture. The method consists of three basic types that are used to classify the five kinds of tumours. (i) Approaches for extracting features for tumour cataloguing. (ii) The creation of a training database and the creation of a feature space. (iii) The five main forms of brain tumours are classified using a multiclass SVM classifier [15]. A dataset of 394 brain tumour MR images donated by the National Cancer Society was used in this investigation. MRI scans of astrocytoma, Glioblastoma, medulloblastoma, meningioma, and metastatic melanoma total 80. The training dataset was extracted using Colormens, the Gabor filter, and the wavelet transform. A total of 94 features are used in this study, 44 of which are features of Gabor; colour moments are 6, and 44 are wavelet features. These features are transformed into a three-dimensional feature space.

This feature space is fed into the SVM classifier as an input. For a multiclass classification, the SVM classifier uses a one-against-one strategy. Following the classification, tumour region segmentation is used to decide the strict area of the tumour. As a result, these will also produce a variety of brain tumours.

1.2.2 Feature Extraction Methods

This describes the characteristics that are useful in identifying whether the brain MRI pictures are normal or abnormal. Because tumours differ according to their classes, the outcomes have a wide range of entrance. The features employed for segmentation of brain tumours are highly dependent on the kind of tumour and its grade. For the classification of the five types of tumours described below, we primarily used texture and intensity parameters.

1.2.3 Gray-level Co-occurrence Matrix (GLCM) (Texture)

Only power distribution-based criteria are insufficient for brain tumour separation because they lack spatial information. These elements are created by the combined chance delivery of pel sets. The co-occurrence matrix has a size identical to the amount of grey levels in the brain MRI. It is described as the incidence of intensity levels at another location that is altered by an off-established direction [17]. Fourteen well-known coefficients were employed as GLCM-based characteristics, but only six of them are the most important, as indicated below.

$$\text{Angular second moment (energy)}: \sum_{l=0}^{G-1}\sum_{l=0}^{G-1}[p(a,b)]^2 \tag{1.1}$$

$$\text{Correlation}: \sum_{l=0}^{G-1}\sum_{l=0}^{G-1}\frac{ab\,p(a,b)-\mu_x\mu_y}{\sigma_x\sigma_y} \tag{1.2}$$

$$\text{Inertia}: \sum_{l=0}^{G-1}\sum_{l=0}^{G-1}(a-b)^2p(a,b) \tag{1.3}$$

$$\text{Absolute value}: \sum_{l=0}^{G-1}\sum_{l=0}^{G-1}|a-b|p(a,b) \tag{1.4}$$

$$\text{Inverse difference}: \sum_{l=0}^{G-1}\sum_{l=0}^{G-1}\frac{p(a,b)}{1+(a-b)^2} \tag{1.5}$$

$$\text{Entropy}: -\sum_{l=0}^{G-1}\sum_{l=0}^{G-1}p(a,b)\log_2[p(a)] \tag{1.6}$$

$$\text{Max probability}: \max_{a,b}\ p(a,b) \tag{1.7}$$

1.2.4 Gabor Transform (Texture)

Gabor was the first to develop Gabor texture descriptors in 1946. It is used to extract texture information from images that have been analysed in the frequency domain. In

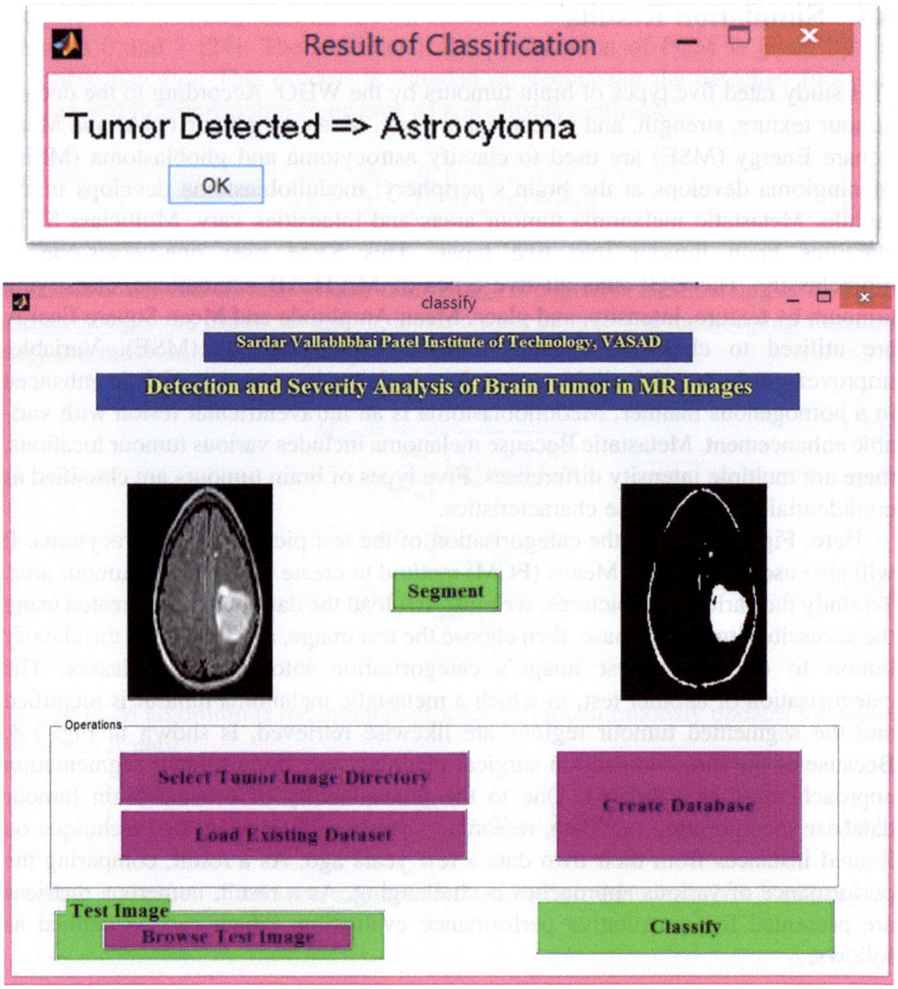

Fig. 1.7 Correct classification of astrocytoma tumour [25]

individual class accuracy, that is, 80% for astrocytoma, 82.5% for glioblastoma, 92.5 for medulloblastoma, 90% for meningioma, and 91.89% for metastatic melanoma. The overall system accuracy is 86.29%.

Based on the characteristics identified, we calculate the classification accuracy for each class, and the specific region of the brain affected by the tumour is segmented using the Fuzzy Means (FCM) method, as shown in Table 1.2.

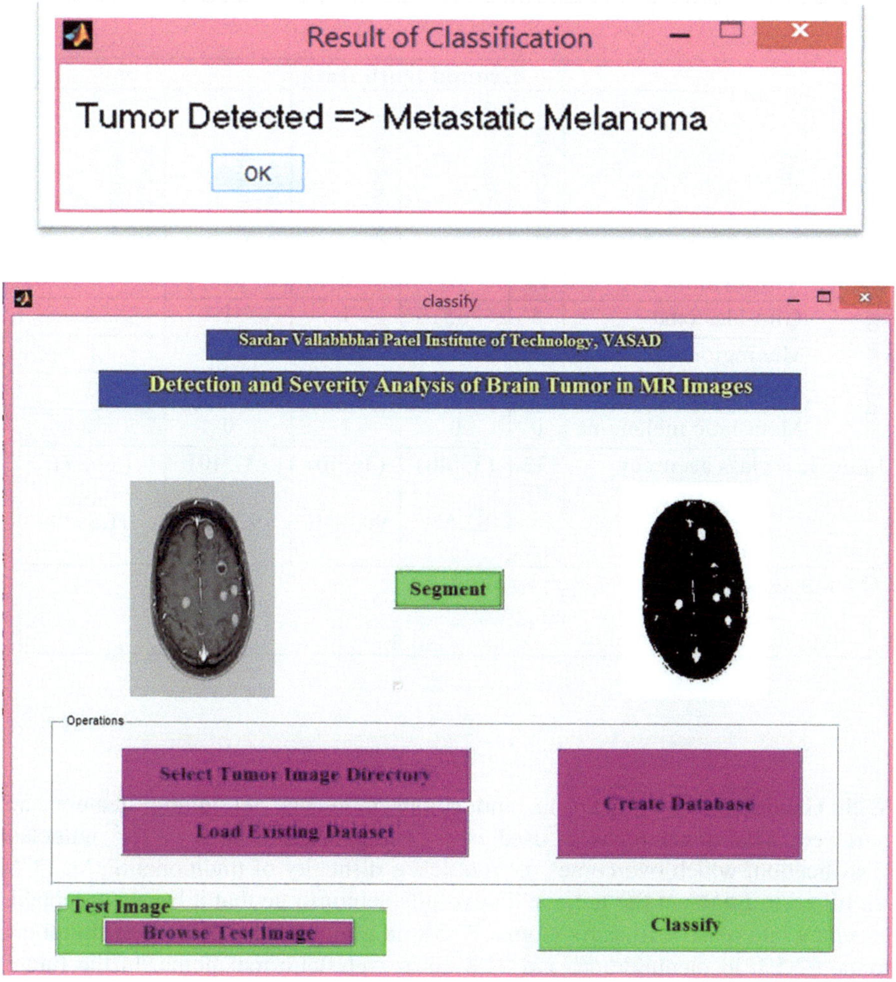

Fig. 1.8 Correct classification of metastatic melanoma tumour [25]

1.5 Conclusion and Future Work

The primary tool for diagnosing brain tumours is MRI, which is extensively utilised by doctors for manual segmentation. Doctors' burden is reduced through computer-assisted analysis. Normally, doctors perform a biopsy to determine the kind of tumour and its grade. The concept classifies tumours into five groups according on the WHO grading system: astrocytoma (Grade I), glioblastoma multiforme (Grade IV), meningioma (Grade II), medulloblastoma (Child tumour) (Grade IV), and metastatic melanoma (Grade IV). Each stage of the automated brain tumour abstraction technique has been rigorously studied and analysed using MATLAB.

Table 1.1 Confusion matrix

		Ground truth Data				
	Class	Astrocytoma	Glio-blastoma	Meningioma	Medullo blastoma	Metastatic melanoma
Predicted class	Astrocytoma	32	4	2	1	1
	Glio-blastoma	5	33	1	1	1
	Meningioma	3	3	36	1	1
	Medullo-blastoma	0	0	0	37	0
	Metastatic melanoma	0	0	1	0	32
Individual class accuracy		(32/40) 80%	(33/40) 82.5%	(36/40) 90.00%	(37/40) 92.5%	(34/37) 91.89%
Overall system accuracy		(170/197) 86.29%				

With Gabor, wavelet transform, and colour moments, 94 tumour features are retrieved. Traditional SVM is used in a one-against-one strategy for multiclass classification, which overcomes the multiclass difficulty of traditional SVM. FCM is utilised to fragment the tumour. The results demonstrate that it has an acceptable accuracy rate of 80% in astrocytoma, 82.5% in glioblastoma, 90% in medulloblastoma, 92.5% in meningioma, and 91.89% in metastatic melanoma. In the future, more information will be extracted and a more accurate multiclass technique will be used to differentiate between low-and high-grade brain tumours. We can also separate different areas of the tumour, such as oedema, which can have an impact on the patient's health. If possible, we'll apply machine-learning algorithms and customised datasets to complete the process.

Acknowledgement Dr. Sushil Mansingani (Radiologist) helped the writers grasp medical terms related to brain tumours and provided encouragement and support throughout the dissertation process.

Table 1.2 Outcomes of tumour cataloguing for five different classes [26]

Tumour Type	Accuracy (%)	Tumour image	Segmented tumour
Astrocytoma	80	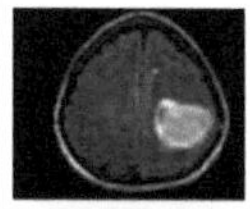	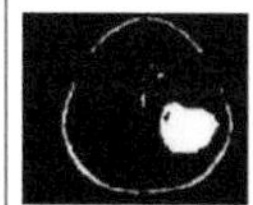
		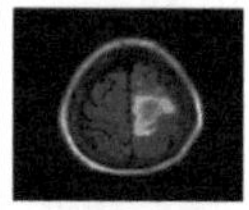	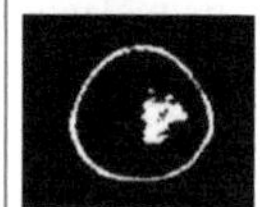
		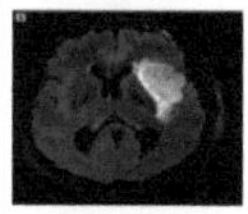	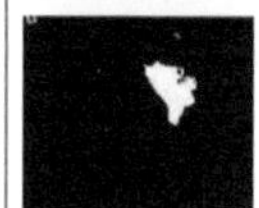
Glioblastoma	82.5	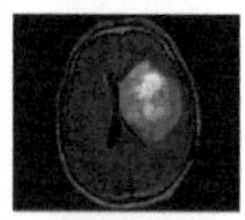	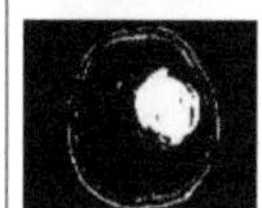
		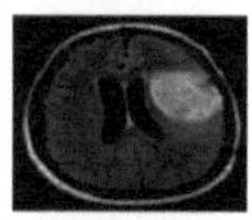	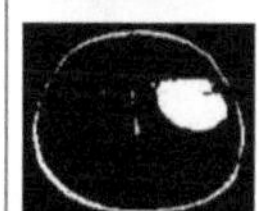
		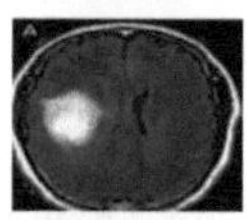	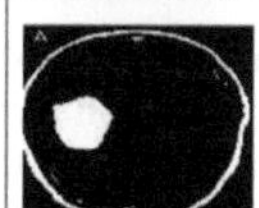
Medulloblastoma	92.5	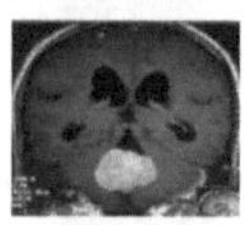	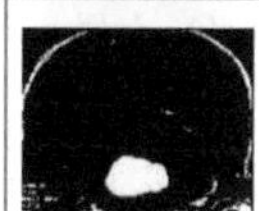
		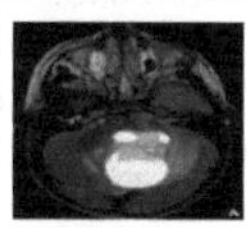	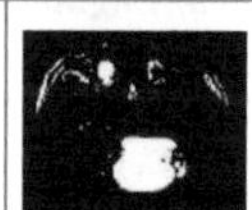
		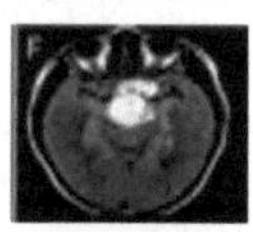	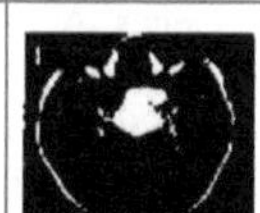
Meningioma	90.00	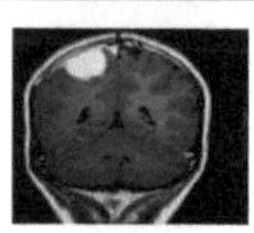	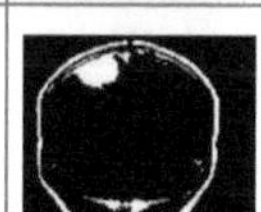
		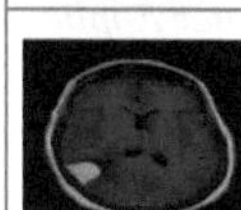	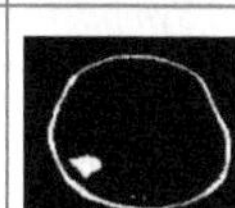

(continued)

Table 1.2 (continued)

Tumour Type	Accuracy (%)	Tumour image	Segmented tumour
		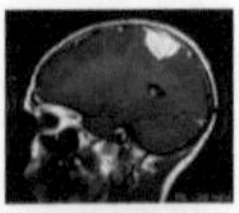	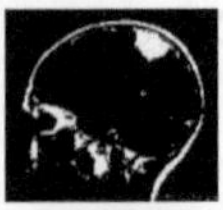
Metastatic melanoma	91.89	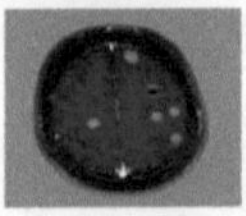	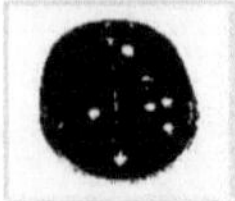
		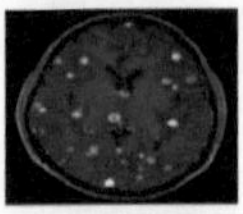	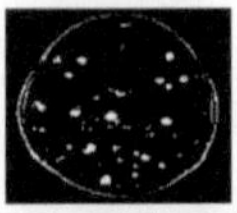
		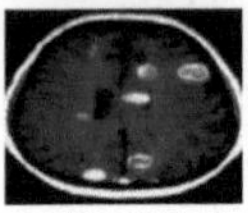	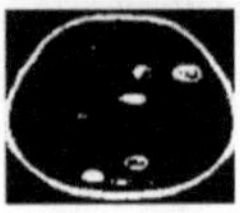

References

1. Liu, J., Li, M., Wang, J., Wu, F., Liu, T., & Pan, Y. (2014). A survey of MRI-based brain tumor segmentation methods. *Tsinghua Science and Technology, 19*, 578–595.
2. Bauer, S., Wiest, R., Nolte, L., & Reyes, M. (2013). A survey of MRI-based medical image analysis for brain tumor studies. *Physics in Medicine and Biology, 58*, R97–R129.
3. Ain, Q., Jaffar, M., & Choi, T. (2014). Fuzzy anisotropic diffusion based segmentation and texture based ensemble classification of brain tumor. *Applied Soft Computing, 21*, 330–340.
4. Huang, M., Yang, W., Wu, Y., Jiang, J., Chen, W., & Feng, Q. (2014). Brain tumor segmentation based on local independent projection-based classification. *IEEE Transactions on Biomedical Engineering, 61*, 2633–2645.
5. Nandpuru, S. S., & Bora, V. (2014). MRI brain cancer classification using support vector machine. In *IEEE Students' Conference on Electrical, Electronics and Computer Science.*
6. Ratan, R., Sharma, S., & Sharma, S. K. (2009). Brain tumor detection based on multi-parameter MRI image analysis. *International Journal on Graphics, Vision and Image Processing, 9*, 9–11.
7. Drevelegas, A., & Papanikolaou, N. (2011). Imaging modalities in brain tumors. In *Imaging of brain tumors with histological correlations* (pp. 13–33). Springer.
8. Singh, P. (2015). Detection of brain tumor in MRI images, using combination of fuzzy C-means and SVM. In *IEEE 2nd International Conference on Signal Processing and Integrated Networks (SPIN)* (pp. 98–102).
9. Ahmad, W., & Fauzi, M. (2008). Comparison of different feature extraction techniques in content-based image retrieval for CT brain images. In *IEEE 10th Workshop on Multimedia Signal Processing* (pp. 503–508).
10. Roslan, R., & Jamil, N. (2012). Texture feature extraction using 2-D gabor filters. In *International Symposium on Computer Applications and Industrial Electronics (ISCAIE), Kota Kinabalu Malaysia* (pp. 173–178).
11. Manjunath, B. S., & Ma, W. Y. (1996). Texture features for browsing and retrieval of image data. *IEEE Transactions on Pattern Analysis and Machine Intelligence, 18*, 837–842.

12. Kumar, G., & Bhatia, P. (2014). A Detailed review of feature extraction in image processing systems. In *IEEE Fourth International Conference on Advanced Computing & Communication Technologies* (pp. 5–12).
13. Demirhan, M. T., & Guler, I. (2015). Segmentation of tumor and edema along with healthy tissues of brain using wavelets and neural networks. *IEEE Journal of Biomedical and Health Informatics, 19*, 1451–1458.
14. Bauer, S., Fejes, T., Slotboom, J., Wiest, R., Nolte, L.-P., & Reyes, M. (2012). *Segmentation of brain tumor images based on integrated hierarchical classification and regularization.* Presented at the Med. ImageComput. Comput.-Assisted Intervention Conf.–Brain Tumor Segmentation Challenge, Nice, France.
15. Bauer, S., Nolte, L. P., & Reyes, M. (2011). Fully automatic segmentation of brain tumor images using support vector machine classification in combination with hierarchical conditional random field regularization. In *Proceedings of Medical Image Computing and Computer-Assisted Intervention* (pp. 354–361).
16. Alahmer, H., & Ahmed, A. (2016). Computer-aided classification of liver lesions from CT images based on multiple ROI. *Procedia Computer Science, 90*, 80–86., ISSN 1877-0509. https://doi.org/10.1016/j.procs.2016.07.027
17. Cao, G., Shi, P., & Hu, B. (2005). Liver fibrosis identification based on ultrasound images. *Conference Proceedings: Annual International Conference of the IEEE Engineering in Medicine and Biology Society, 2005*, 6317–6320. https://doi.org/10.1109/IEMBS.2005.1615942
18. Santos-Bustos, D. F., Nguyen, B. M., & Espitia, H. E. (2022). Towards automated eye cancer classification via VGG and ResNet networks using transfer learning. *Engineering Science and Technology, an International Journal*, 101214., ISSN 2215-0986. https://doi.org/10.1016/j.jestch.2022.101214
19. Mohsen, H., El-Dahshan, E.-S., El-Horbarty, E.-S., Salem, M., & Abdel-Badeeh. (2017). *Brain tumor type classification based on support vector machine in magnetic resonance images.* Annals of Dunarea de Jos University of Galati. Fascicle II, Year IX.
20. Platt, J. C., Cristianini, N., & Shawe-Taylor, J. (2000). Large margin DAGs for multiclass classification. *Advances in Neural Information Processing Systems*, MIT Press,, *12*, 547–553.
21. Hsu, C.-W., & Lin, C.-J. (2002). A comparison of methods for multiclass support vector machines. *IEEE Transactions on Neural Networks, 13*, 415–425.
22. Thao, P. T. X., Tri, T. Q., Dien, D., & Collier, N. (2008). Named entity recognition in Vietnamese using classifier voting. *ACM Transactions on Asian Language Information Processing, 6*(4) Article 3 (December 2007), 18 pages. https://doi.org/10.1145/1316457.1316460
23. Mehmood, I., Ejaz, N., Sajjad, M., & Baik, S. (2013). Prioritization of brain MRI volumes using medical image perception model and tumor region segmentation. *Computers in Biology and Medicine, 43*, 1471–1483. https://doi.org/10.1016/j.compbiomed.2013.07.001
24. Mehmood, I., et al. (2013). Prioritization of brain MRI volumes using medical image perception model and tumor region segmentation. *Computers in Biology and Medicine, 43*(10), 1471–1483.
25. Hassan, E., & Aboshgifa, A. (2015). Detecting brain tumour from Mri image using Matlab GUI programme. *International Journal of Computer Science & Engineering Survey, 6*, 47–60. https://doi.org/10.5121/ijcses.2015.6604
26. http://radiopaedia.org/cases/

Chapter 2
Chicken Swarm-Based Feature Selection with Optimal Deep Belief Network for Thyroid Cancer Detection and Classification

M. Gokilavani, Sriram, S. P. Vijayaragavan, and V. Nirmalrani

2.1 Introduction

Goswami et al. [1] proposed that the number of thyroid cancer survivors is increasing day by day. Cancer survivors' quality of life (QOL) was predicted to be considerably impacted by increased intensity of treatment and its concomitant side effects. According to the National Cancer Institute, more than 760,000 Americans have survived thyroid cancer (NCI). Many individuals in the United States have been able to live with thyroid cancer because of a threefold rise in incidence and high survival rates in recent decades. HRQOL is equivalent to or worse for individuals with thyroid cancer than those with malignancies with a worse prognosis, according to self-reported data. This population's reasons for low HRQOL ratings are not fully understood. When a cancer patient is diagnosed and treated, they may have physical, emotional, or psychological changes as a result. After therapy, these effects may continue to affect HRQOL for years to come. Thyroid cancer surgery and radioactive iodine (RAI) ablation, for example, are well-documented as having various possible side effects. Scarring, hypocalcemia, discomfort, infection, dysphonia, and dysphagia are all possible complications of surgery.

M. Gokilavani · Sriram
CSE, Bharath Institute of Higher Education and Research, Chennai, Tamil Nadu, India
e-mail: sriramm.cse@bharathuniv.ac.in

S. P. Vijayaragavan (✉)
EEE, Bharath Institute of Higher Education and Research, Chennai, Tamil Nadu, India
e-mail: vijayaragavan.eee@bharathuniv.ac.in

V. Nirmalrani
CSE, Sathyabama Institute of Science and Technology, Chennai, Tamil Nadu, India
e-mail: nirmalrani.it@sathyabama.ac.in

F. J. Joseph et al. (eds.), *Computational Intelligence for Clinical Diagnosis*,
EAI/Springer Innovations in Communication and Computing,
https://doi.org/10.1007/978-3-031-23683-9_2

Qian et al. [2] proposed that the prevalence of thyroid cancer in the United States has grown in the recent times. There were 4.6 per 100,000 population growth between 1974 and 2013. Incidence rates increased by 3% per 100,000 person between 1974 and 1977, reaching 14.4 per 100,000 person between 2010 and 2013. Overdiagnosis has been blamed for this problem because of the increased ability to identify and diagnose slow-growing malignancies that would otherwise go unnoticed. Thyroid cancer fatality rates have risen steadily since the late 1980s, as much as the occurrences of large tumors and more advanced stages of the disease. The most frequent endocrine cancer in children is thyroid cancer. To lower the risk of cancer in kids, many initiatives were launched beginning in 2002 to limit kids' exposure to ionizing radiation. Thyroid cancer is the most common endocrine cancer in kids. According to one study, the incidence rate is rising at a 1.1% annual rate. As a result of this linear approach, this study failed to account for changes in incidence over time. Additionally, it is not clear whether there has been an increase in incidence rates since 2004.

Kim et al. [3] proposed that thyroid cancer incidence has gradually increased over the last half century worldwide. One reason for the seemingly wide range in prevalence is that different diagnostic procedures, environmental exposures, and individual risk factors have been identified. There is also a regional disparity in healthcare access, healthcare systems, and national databases that contributes to this difference. For instance, the incidence of breast cancer in women varies tenfold over the world. Compared to low- and middle-income nations, both women and men are more likely to be diagnosed with breast cancer in high-income countries. Over the past decade, thyroid cancer mortality has been the subject of discussion, as the general trend differs. In most high-income nations, mortality from thyroid cancer has decreased since the 1960s, except in the United States, where mortality increased in 1980. Traditional methods of geographic segmentation, such as countries or continents, are commonly used to characterize illness incidence in contemporary research. The screening and treatment of thyroid cancer in high- and middle- and low-income nations are comparable. Consequently, the use of income grouping to explain thyroid cancer incidence is advantageous. There are currently 189 member countries in the World Bank's four income tiers: low, medium, upper-middle, and high. It's crucial to keep in mind that the disparities between the various groups are measured in terms of US per capita gross national income.

Mirian et al. [5] proposed to the Western world that thyroid carcinoma is the most prevalent endocrine tumor. In most wealthy nations, it has been on the rise for over three decades, although overall mortality has fallen. A palpable nodule is a common clinical presentation for thyroid cancer, which affects 4–7% of the adult Western population. Women are roughly three times as likely to have malignant thyroid cancer as males. Thyroid cancer is divided into nine distinct subgroups by the World Health Organization (WHO). Most thyroid malignancies are differentiated and have a good prognosis, but anaplastic carcinomas are more difficult to treat and have a bad outlook. This is the most often increasing category of carcinomas, and the diagnosis is often made by chance. Thyroid cancer survival rates have risen in lockstep with the rise in cases. People with differentiated thyroid carcinoma benefit greatly from intravenous iodine therapy. Oncologists, pathologists, nuclear medicine specialists, endocrinologists, doctors, and radiologists work together at multidisciplinary university facilities in Denmark to treat thyroid cancer. To treat thyroid cancer, hemi thyroidectomy and neck dissection are the most common surgical options in Denmark, whereas radioactive iodine therapy is the most common treatment for high-risk individuals.

Gsior-Percza et al. [6] proposed that papillary thyroid carcinoma (PTC) has surpassed all other types of endocrine cancer around the globe in recent decades. Diagnostic imaging and biopsies have helped considerably to the increase in PTC diagnosis rates over the last decade. Thyroid cancers, no matter how large or small, are on the rise, according to several studies. The rise in DTC cases cannot be attributed only to better imaging techniques.

Prete et al. [7] proposed that thyroid cancer (TC) has been more common during the last four decades, according to the WHO. Papillary, follicular, and medullary T-cells are three unique forms of T-cell differentiation. Undifferentiated T-cells are the third type (poorly differentiated and anaplastic). The most widely recognized theory of follicular cell carcinogenesis holds that the transformation of thyroid follicular cells can lead to either differentiated or undifferentiated TC. The genome sequence has been available for the last 30 years, and this has allowed researchers to make significant progress in understanding the molecular processes driving TC. As a result, TC is considered to be a genetically simple disease.

Kovatch et al. [9] proposed that thyroid cancer is the most common endocrine cancer. Well-differentiated thyroid carcinoma has steadily increased in incidence over the last several decades, although fatality rates have not altered much. Treatment for well-differentiated thyroid cancer (DTC) has gained popularity as more thyroid nodules are found. Thyroid cancer cases are on the rise, and this is most likely owing to an increase in the number of people seeking medical attention and the use of imaging tests to detect small nodules that could otherwise go undetected. Diagnoses and treatment of illnesses that would not ordinarily cause symptoms or death are known as "overdiagnosis." It is possible that the incidence of histologically verifiable PTC in post-mortem tissues is significantly greater and may even exist as a "normal variation" that is not clinically relevant. Prostate, Thyroid, skin, and breast cancer overdiagnosis are only a few examples of overdiagnosis (mammogram).

A subgroup of these cancers appears to have indolent biology and may not necessitate therapy, even though they are generally linked with higher death rates [4]. The incidence of well-differentiated thyroid carcinoma is likely being overdiagnosed due to the extensive use of high-sensitivity screening methods (mostly ultrasonography). During the same time, disease-specific mortality did not vary. More and more nations are seeing similar trends [8]. As a result, the inclusion of imaging and biopsy recommendations based on imaging results and risk classification in revised treatment guidelines for differentiated thyroid carcinoma is not surprising. There is a very low recurrence rate of 2–6% for papillary thyroid microcarcinomas (PTMCs), which are PTCs with a diameter of less than 1 centimeter (1%). Since PTMC is the primary source of newly diagnosed malignancies, over-treating thyroid ailment at low risk of cancer is a significant problem [10].

2.5 Conclusion

In this study, the CSOFS-ODBN model was used to suggest an automated deep learning approach to the identification and classification of thyroid cancer. The existence of thyroid cancer is something that the CSOFS-ODBN model that has been suggested hopes to identify and classify. To begin, the CSOFS-ODBN model uses a min-max data normalization strategy to pre-process the input data. This step is performed right after the initialization phase. In addition to this, the CSOFS algorithm is run in order to select the best possible subset of features. In addition, the DBN model classifies thyroid cancer after receiving the features of choice and carrying out the process. The final step in the process is applying the Adam optimizer to the DBN model in order to do hyperparameter optimization. A comprehensive experimental investigation is carried out, and the results report the superiority of the CSOFS-ODBN model. This is done with the intention of reporting the improved performance of the CSOFS-ODBN model.

References

1. Goswami, S., Peipert, B. J., Mongelli, M. N., Kurumety, S. K., Helenowski, I. B., Yount, S. E., & Sturgeon, C. (2019). Clinical factors associated with worse quality-of-life scores in United States thyroid cancer survivors. *Surgery, 166*(1), 69–74.
2. Qian, Z. J., Jin, M. C., Meister, K. D., & Megwalu, U. C. (2019). Pediatric thyroid cancer incidence and mortality trends in the United States, 1973–2013. *JAMA Otolaryngology–Head & Neck Surgery, 145*(7), 617–623.
3. Kim, J., Gosnell, J. E., & Roman, S. A. (2020). Geographic influences in the global rise of thyroid cancer. *Nature Reviews Endocrinology, 16*(1), 17–29.
4. Kitahara, C. M., & Sosa, J. A. (2020). Understanding the ever-changing incidence of thyroid cancer. *Nature Reviews Endocrinology, 16*(11), 617–618.
5. Mirian, C., Grønhøj, C., Jensen, D. H., Jakobsen, K. K., Karnov, K., Jensen, J. S., & von Buchwald, C. (2018). Trends in thyroid cancer: Retrospective analysis of incidence and survival in Denmark 1980–2014. *Cancer Epidemiology, 55*, 81–87.
6. Gąsior-Perczak, D., Pałyga, I., Szymonek, M., Kowalik, A., Walczyk, A., Kopczyński, J., & Kowalska, A. (2018). The impact of BMI on clinical progress, response to treatment, and disease course in patients with differentiated thyroid cancer. *PLoS One, 13*(10), e0204668.
7. Prete, A., Borges de Souza, P., Censi, S., Muzza, M., Nucci, N., & Sponziello, M. (2020). Update on fundamental mechanisms of thyroid cancer. *Frontiers in Endocrinology, 11*, 102.
8. Laha, D., Nilubol, N., & Boufraqech, M. (2020). New therapies for advanced thyroid cancer. *Frontiers in Endocrinology, 11*, 82.
9. Kovatch, K. J., Hoban, C. W., & Shuman, A. G. (2018). Thyroid cancer surgery guidelines in an era of de-escalation. *European Journal of Surgical Oncology, 44*(3), 297–306.
10. Geron, Y., Benbassat, C., Shteinshneider, M., Koren, S., Or, K., Markus, E., & Muallem Kalmovich, L. (2019). Long-term outcome after hemi thyroidectomy for papillary thyroid cancer: A comparative study and review of the literature. *Cancers, 11*(1), 26.
11. Chen, D. W., Reyes Gastelum, D., Wallner, L. P., Papaleontiou, M., Hamilton, A. S., Ward, K. C., & Haymart, M. R. (2020). Disparities in risk perception of thyroid cancer recurrence and death. *Cancer, 126*(7), 1512–1521.

12. Stefan, A. I., Piciu, A., Mester, A., Apostu, D., Badan, M., & Badulescu, C. I. (2020). Paediatric thyroid cancer in Europe: An over diagnosed condition? A literature review. *Diagnostics, 10*(2), 112.
13. Lee, K. A., Sharabiani, M. T. A., Tumino, D., Wadsley, J., Gill, V., Gerrard, G., & Newbold, K. (2019). Differentiated thyroid cancer in children: A UK multicentre review and review of the literature. *Clinical Oncology, 31*(6), 385–390.
14. Gonçalves Filho, J., Zafereo, M. E., Ahmad, F. I., Nixon, I. J., Shaha, A. R., Vander Poorten, V., & Kowalski, L. P. (2018). Decision making for the central compartment in differentiated thyroid cancer. *European Journal of Surgical Oncology, 44*(11), 1671–1678.
15. Lima, M. J., Soares, V., Koch, P., Silva, A., & Taveira-Gomes, A. (2018). Autonomously hyper functioning cystic nodule harbouring thyroid carcinoma–case report and literature review. *International Journal of Surgery Case Reports, 42*, 287–289.
16. Vargas-Pinto, S., & Arenas, M. A. R. (2019). Lobectomy compared to total thyroidectomy for low-risk papillary thyroid cancer: A systematic review. *Journal of Surgical Research, 242*, 244–251.
17. Goswami, S., Mongelli, M., Peipert, B. J., Helenowski, I., Yount, S. E., & Sturgeon, C. (2018). Benchmarking health-related quality of life in thyroid cancer versus other cancers and United States normative data. *Surgery, 164*(5), 986–992.
18. Saeed, M. I., Hassan, A. A., Butt, M. E., Baniyaseen, K. A., Siddiqui, M. I., Bogari, N. M., & Taher, M. M. (2018). Pattern of thyroid lesions in western region of Saudi Arabia: A retrospective analysis and literature review. *Journal of Clinical Medicine Research, 10*(2), 106.
19. Peng, C., Li, Z., Gao, H., Zou, X., Wang, X., Zhou, C., & Niu, J. (2019). Synchronous primary sigmoid colon cancer and primary thyroid cancer followed by a malignant tumor of the kidney: Case report of multiple primary cancer and review of the literature. *Oncology Letters, 17*(2), 2479–2484.
20. Ma, B., Wei, W., Xu, W., Wang, Y., Guan, H., Fan, J., & Ji, Q. (2018). Surgical confirmation of incomplete treatment for primary papillary thyroid carcinoma by percutaneous thermal ablation: A retrospective case review and literature review. *Thyroid, 28*(9), 1134–1142.
21. Sawka, A. M., Gagliardi, A. R., Haymart, M. R., Sturgeon, C., Bernet, V., Hoff, K., & Jonklaas, J. (2020). A survey of American Thyroid Association members regarding the 2015 adult thyroid nodule and differentiated thyroid cancer clinical practice guidelines. *Thyroid, 30*(1), 25–33.
22. Roth, E. M., Lubitz, C. C., Swan, J. S., & James, B. C. (2020). Patient-reported quality-of-life outcome measures in the thyroid cancer population. *Thyroid, 30*(10), 1414–1431.
23. Verburg, F. A., Flux, G., Giovanella, L., van Nostrand, D., Muylle, K., & Luster, M. (2020). Differentiated thyroid cancer patients potentially benefitting from postoperative I-131 therapy: A review of the literature of the past decade. *European Journal of Nuclear Medicine and Molecular Imaging, 47*(1), 78–83.

where S_i is a space vector with K dimensions while C_i denotes the vector class to which it belongs. The hyper plane divides training data, and the general form represents that division.

$$MS + B = 0 \tag{3.2}$$

M stands for the K-dimensional space vector orthogonal to the hyperplane, and B is a scalar. The following equations show two hyperplanes that belong to two different classes.

$$MS + B = 1 \tag{3.3}$$

$$MS + B = -1 \tag{3.4}$$

Advantages of SVM:

- It prevents data from being overfitted and improves prediction accuracy.
- As it uses only a subset of the training data, it uses less memory.

Logistic Regression:

This is a regression analysis procedure that describes the link between one dependent binary variable and one or more independent ratio-point variables. Discrete predictions here are those that are assigned to specific values or categories. They can also see the probability ratings that underpin the classifications of the model. The logistic function can be defined as follows:

$$\text{Prob(event)} = P\left(\vec{m}\right) = \frac{1}{1 + e^{-g\left(\vec{m}\right)}} = \frac{e^{g\left(\vec{m}\right)}}{1 + e^{g\left(\vec{m}\right)}} \tag{3.5}$$

where $P\left(\vec{m}\right)$ denotes the probability of a given output event, $\vec{m}$ denotes the input vector relating to the independent variables (predictors), and $g\left(\vec{m}\right)$ denotes the logit model.

This approach is best suited for variables that are continuous. Logistic regression has the advantage of being simpler to implement and train.

3.4 Results and Discussions

The following metrics are used to evaluate the predicted classification effectiveness of the algorithm:

Table 3.1 Accuracy by Logistic Regression and Support Vector Machine

No of iterations	Logistic Regression accuracy %	Support Vector Machine accuracy %
10	76.99	86.19
20	77.06	86.59
30	77.56	87.96
40	77.97	88.02
50	78.97	88.64

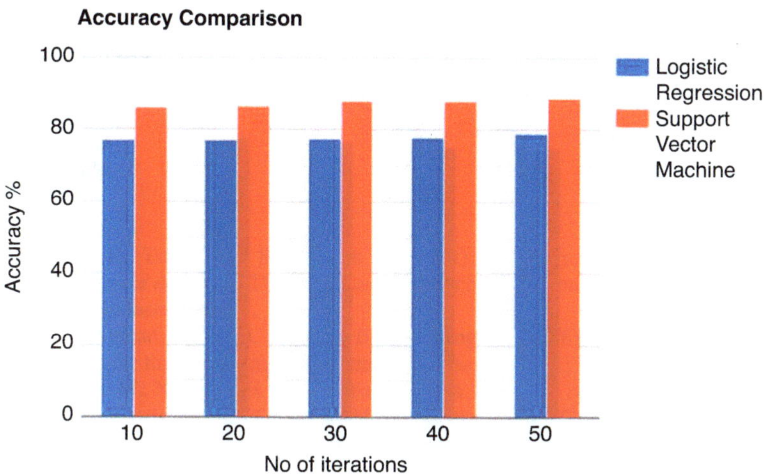

Fig. 3.1 Accuracy by logistic regression and support vector machine graph

Accuracy:

The system's accuracy is measured by its ability to correctly distinguish between healthy and sick cases. The fraction of true positive and true negative should be estimated in all studied cases to estimate the accuracy of the result. This can be demonstrated as follows:

$$\text{Accuracy} = \frac{\text{True Positive} + \text{True Negative}}{\text{True Positive} + \text{False Positive} + \text{True Negative} + \text{False Negative}} \tag{3.6}$$

The following Table 3.1 and Fig 3.1 show the accuracy obtained from the dataset by Logistic Regression and Support Vector Machine. It clearly shows that, in terms of accuracy, Support Vector Machine outperforms Logistic Regression.

According to WHO, a Health Emergency and Disaster Risk Management Framework (EDRM) has been developed that aims to react to crises and disasters that have a significant impact on both people's health and healthcare systems throughout the world. It is the most recent framework and has been used in all the studies revolving around COVID-19 only [36, 37]. In the framework, prevention, preparation, and readiness are emphasized. There is an urgent need to react and recover from each tragedy or emergency that occurs. The discussion initiated by [38] indicates that the global health crises including climate change and extremes, the global rise of resistant antibiotics, and others have led to unprecedented mortality and morbidity, which is why the structured development of EDRM is necessary. The framework suggests that the strategic and operational requirements for not just the prevention but also the rehabilitation challenges associated with global public health crises are to be met. Furthermore, the work highlighted that there is a need to recognize the need for changing operational competencies, gaining expertise and knowledge, developing decision-making skill sets, and addressing healthcare management needs at all levels of governance. The framework given by WHO also indicates that emergencies and disasters affect all communities, requiring all agencies to work together. WHO did not discuss the financial implications of the integration of EDRM and no studies have evaluated the budget for the incorporation of the framework, particularly in the Indian context.

4.3.1 Proposed Conceptual Framework

According to the Indian Ministry of Health & Family Welfare, the Directorate General of Health Services has published instructions on how to minimize the transmission of airborne illnesses in healthcare institutions such as hospitals. Many of the recommendations apply to other respiratory illnesses that are transmitted by airborne means, even though tuberculosis is the prototypical disease that is the focus of the majority of the guidelines.

This chapter aims to develop a framework that can help management in controlling airborne infections at hospitals. The literature reveals that administrative controls, environmental controls, and engineering controls [39] are the three important factors that ensure management's commitment to providing the best healthcare facilities. Both administrative and environmental controls can be different for indoor and outdoor patient and staff settings. Engineering controls are used to prevent the transmission and limit the concentration of infectious aerosols in the process rooms, laboratories, etc.

Another crucial factor that can contribute toward the elimination of airborne infectious agents is the budget for maintenance of healthcare facilities to control airborne diseases. As a result of the SARS-CoV-2 pandemic, numerous organizations are considering policies such as enhanced ventilation and safety measures to limit the spread of acute respiratory infections such as Coronavirus 2 (SARS-CoV-2)

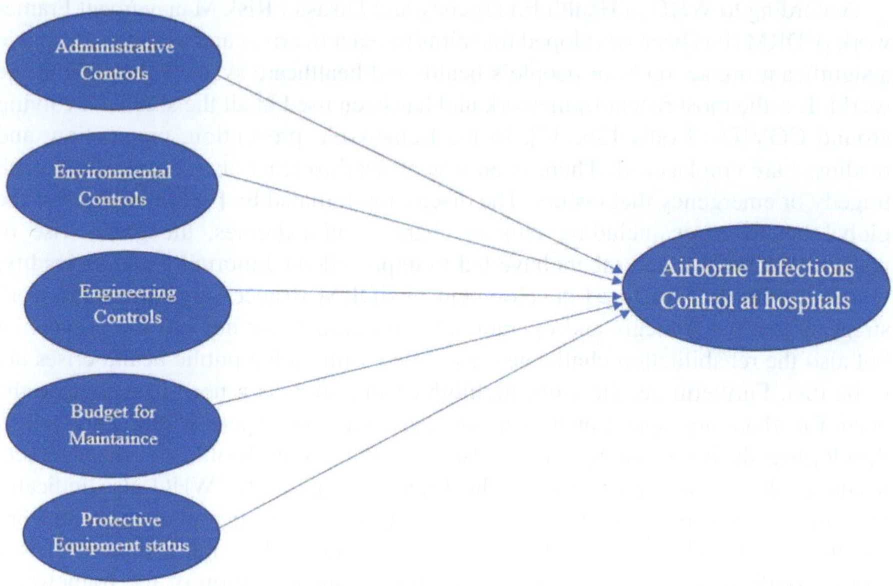

Fig. 4.2 Initial conceptual framework from literature review

(COVID-19) [40]. Improved ventilation, an increase in basic equipment, and safety measures (e.g., masks and PPE) will increase the cost, exacerbating financial challenges for the management (Fig. 4.2).

4.4 Conclusion

The healthcare administration bears the obligation of providing the patients with the highest quality of care that can be offered, with the goals of enhancing the patients' overall health and transforming their stay in the hospital into a beneficial one through a timely discharge. The majority of hospital-acquired infections are caused by airborne pathogens, which explains why the infection incidence in hospitals is so high. It will be able, as a result of the research that has been carried out, to identify the gaps in the hospital management system that exist in relation to the tactics that are utilized for controlling the spread of airborne illnesses. Following this, the development of methods and strategies for a better management of airborne illnesses can be offered, along with their explanation [41]. The findings of this research will also fill the theoretical void that now exists as a result of there being insufficient situationally relevant theoretical frameworks. In conclusion, the findings of the research will assist in the determination of enhancements that can be implemented in various crisis management systems and will assist in the achievement of three essential goals of sustainable development [42].

4.4.1 Future Directions

There is very little information on how to control the spread of various airborne diseases caused by COVID-19, SARS-CoV-2, influenza, Zika virus, etc. The consequences of such pandemics have been disastrous and have caused significant social and economic stress by making the workforce less productive [43]. Therefore, capacity-building efforts are required, and thus as a step toward supporting the notion, this chapter focuses on identifying the factors that can help in capacity building by controlling acute airborne infections. The WHO estimates that low- and middle-income countries require an extra USD 370 billion per year for primary healthcare to accomplish UHC SDG objectives. Development cooperation is critical in this area, with official development aid (ODA) to health reaching USD 26 billion in 2018. It accounted for 13% of total health expenditure in lower-middle-income nations and 29% in low-income countries. Hospitals and other healthcare facilities adhere to strict regulations for ventilation systems and other precautions to protect patients from particles that cause airborne illnesses and other health issues. Control banding and the NIOSH hierarchy of controls could be useful in developing risk management methods. These models were created with the goal of reducing chemical risks, but they can be modified to fit the needs of fighting highly contagious and lethal pathogens such as SARS-CoV-2.

References

1. Lewis, D. (2020). *Is the coronavirus airborne? Experts can't agree*. Nature News.
2. Morawska, L., Tang, J. W., Bahnfleth, W., Bluyssen, P. M., Boerstra, A., Buonanno, G., et al. (2020). How can airborne transmission of COVID-19 indoors be minimised? *Environment International, 142*, 105832.
3. Eames, I., Tang, J., Li, Y., & Wilson, P. (2009). Airborne transmission of disease in hospitals. *Journal of the Royal Society Interface, 6*(suppl_6), S697. https://doi.org/10.1098/rsif.2009.0407.focus
4. Memarzadeh, F., & Xu, W. (2012, March). Role of air changes per hour (ACH) in possible transmission of airborne infections. In *Building simulation* (Vol. 5, No. 1, pp. 15–28). Springer.
5. Wong, J., Goh, Q., Tan, Z., Lie, S., Tay, Y., Ng, S., & Soh, C. (2020). Preparing for a COVID-19 pandemic: A review of operating room outbreak response measures in a large tertiary hospital in Singapore. *Canadian Journal of Anesthesia/Journal CanadienD'anesthésie, 67*(6), 732–745. https://doi.org/10.1007/s12630-020-01620-9
6. Henderson, D. (2009). An apparatus for the study of airborne infection. *Journal of Hygiene, 50*(1), 53–68. https://doi.org/10.1017/s0022172400019422
7. Nicas, M., Nazaroff, W., & Hubbard, A. (2005). Toward understanding the risk of secondary airborne infection: Emission of respirable pathogens. *Journal of Occupational and Environmental Hygiene, 2*(3), 143–154. https://doi.org/10.1080/15459620590918466
8. Beggs, C. (2003). The airborne transmission of infection in hospital buildings: Fact or fiction? *Indoor and Built Environment, 12*(1–2), 9–18. https://doi.org/10.1177/1420326x03012001002
9. Qudiesat, K., Abu-Elteen, K., Elkarmi, A., Hamad, M., & Abussaud, M. (2009). Assessment of airborne pathogens in healthcare settings. *African Journal of Microbiology Research, 3*(2), 66–76. https://doi.org/10.5897/AJMR.9000102

Chapter 5
Adaptive Sailfish Optimization-Contrast Limited Adaptive Histogram Equalization (ASFO-CLAHE) for Hyperparameter Tuning in Image Enhancement

S. Surya and A. Muthukumaravel

5.1 Introduction

Breast tumours are the most common tumours found in women. Mammography has been shown to be one of the most powerful prognostic methods for identifying breast tumours earlier. A digital mammogram [1] has a limited range of grey tones. Digital mammograms' histogram structure is not well-defined. In mammographic films, non-tumorous and malignant breast lumps appear as white patches. The fatty tissues are seen as dark areas. On a digital mammogram, other elements of the breast, including glands, connective tissue, cancers, and calcium deposits, appear as shades of grey with a brighter intensity [2, 3]. Because of the various grey-level representations, digital mammograms are as challenging to interpret as traditional mammography. Each year, a considerable number of digital mammograms are produced, necessitating precise and quick image interpretation. Non-tumorous lesions may be mistaken for tumours (false-positive rate), whereas malignancies can go undetected (false-negative rate). Thus, 10–30% of breast malignancies go undetected by radiologists. Radiologists can use computer-aided diagnostic (CAD) tools to aid in the accurate interpretation of digital mammograms. Pre-processing of digital mammography pictures for CE while maintaining brightness is the initial stage in the CAD model for analysing the mammogram pictures [4–6]. IE is the practise of enhancing picture excellence in order to improve visual and computational analysis [7]. Because of its capacity to circumvent some of the limits imposed by image acquisition techniques, it is frequently employed in a variety of applications.

S. Surya (✉) · A. Muthukumaravel
Department of Computer Applications, Bharath Institute of Higher Education and Research, Chennai, Tamil Nadu, India
e-mail: surya.mca@bharathuniv.ac.in

F. J. Joseph et al. (eds.), *Computational Intelligence for Clinical Diagnosis*, EAI/Springer Innovations in Communication and Computing,
https://doi.org/10.1007/978-3-031-23683-9_5

For rapid and correct analysis of mammograms, contrast augmentation and brightness preservation procedures must not erode or lose the details in the picture. As a result, digital mammography contrast augmentation and brightness preservation are critical for premature recognition and diagnosis of breast tumours. A recent study [8] provides a complete assessment of histogram-based approaches. These strategies are frequently divided into global and local categories. For photographs requiring local details or images with fluctuating lighting, the utilization of global CE conditions might not be appropriate. Nonetheless, when the procedure is employed in the vicinity, those constraints can be circumvented [9]. CLAHE is a prominent scheme for local CE, which has proven to be effective and beneficial in a variety of settings [10–12]. CLAHE has been widely employed in image processing and object detection purposes to improve visual contrast. In the medical field, it has been used to improve breast ultrasound and mammography images [12, 13], cell image segmentation [14], fundus examination [15, 16], and bone fracture picture improvement.

Several studies were presented in the previous centuries to improve image contrast based on the HE [11, 12, 14]. HE, in general, increases the contrast of large histogram parts while decreasing the contrast of small histogram parts [17]. They generate level saturation effects by pushing the intensities to the extreme right or left of the histogram, and if the Region-Of-Interest (ROI) has a low percentage of the picture, then it cannot be appropriately boosted. The primary idea behind CLAHE is to use interpolation to recover randomness across boundaries when applying HE to non-overlapping sub-parts of the image. CLAHE aided in the reduction of picture restoration algorithm complexity while also providing good CE. Apart from its prominence in the work, CLAHE is mostly dependent on two variables: NT and CL. The initial variable NT specifies how the picture is partitioned into tiles and is comprised of two values: m and n. As a result, the picture is broken down into $m \times n$ local parts. The CL, the second variable, affects how much noise is amplified in the picture. The CL keeps the intensity ranges of each tile's histogram from exceeding the chosen CL. This circumstance may result in poor image quality and noise when such variables are not chosen properly. Because the CLAHE's efficacy is mostly determined by the two variables listed above, more perfect ranges for these two variables will result in higher CE [18]. As a result, according to recent research [19], the fundamental flaw in CLAHE is poor hyper parameter selection, which leads to a reduction in picture quality. So, establishing the ideal parameters is a time-consuming operation, necessitating the use of an automatic parameter detection technique. Manually adjusting the hyperparameter values in such a trial-and-error manner is a time-consuming and inefficient approach. Artificial intelligence (AI) methods have recently been used to overcome these problems [18, 20, 21].

The NT and CL are the two variables used by CLAHE. These two criteria determine the CLAHE's efficiency. As a result, adjusting the CLAHE's parameters can alter the results. The appropriate parameters' value varies depending on the image type. In this research, Adaptive Sailfish Optimization (ASFO) is used to find the best CLAHE settings to improve image contrast. The suggested approach automates the CL selection, making it more versatile and adaptable to image data.

The mammograms derived from the Mammographic Image Analysis Society (MIAS) corpus are used in the experiments. Image quality measuring techniques such as the PSNR, SSIM, and MSE are contrasted with various HE approaches.

5.2 Literature Survey

More et al. [18] proposed a multi-objective meta-heuristic (SMPSO) for CLAHE parameter tuning, in which the fitness factors are both maximization of the quantity of data obtainable (by Entropy) and minimization of misrepresentation in the resultant pictures (by SSIM) simultaneously. The findings reveal that this method generates a Pareto group of non-dominated results that represent pictures with varying contrast ranges and a trade-off between entropy and SSIM. Such fitness factors, in particular, are incompatible. Such improved photos give specialists vital information for making decisions.

Ma et al. [20] introduced a CLAHE-based fusion technique for picture improvement in several colour schemes. The RGB colour space of the original colour image is first transformed into two distinct superior colour spaces: YIQ and HSI. The RGB to YIQ colour space conversion is linear, whereas the RGB to HSI colour space transformation is nonlinear. The programme then runs CLAHE in both the YIQ and HSI colour spaces to produce two distinct enhanced pictures. The CLAHE algorithm improves the luminance factor (Y) in the YIQ colour space and the intensity factor (I) in the HSI colour space. Block size and CL are two critical CLAHE settings that affect the excellence of the CLAHE-enhanced picture. Moreover, the YIQ and HSI enhanced pictures are transformed back to RGB colour, respectively. If the three elements of red, green, and blue in YIQ-RGB or HSI-RGB pictures are not coherent, the three elements must be harmonized in RGB space using the CLAHE algorithm. Finally, a self-dynamic weight choice non-linear IE is performed using a four direction Sobel boundary recognizer in the constrained general logarithm ratio operation to fuse YIQ-RGB and HSI-RGB pictures to obtain the absolute merged picture. The mean of the Sobel boundary recognizer and the merging coefficient are two crucial components in the enhanced fusion method, and these two factors define the procedure's results. The suggested enhancement approach is evaluated using a number of metrics, including average, variance, entropy, colourfulness measure (CM), MSE, and PSNR. According to the results of the testing, the suggested approach provides better IE and wider colour recovery ranges. The suggested technique effectively suppresses noise interference and improves image quality for underwater images.

Campos et al. [21] established a training-based hyperparameter choice method, or the CLAHE methodology to create a strong regression model that can estimate highly possible CLAHE's hyperparameter for adjusting a picture depending on its attributes. As a result, an appropriate learning collection for the system initiation was required. In studies, the following algorithms were used: CART (Classification and Regression Tree), MLP (Multilayer Perceptron), ANN (Artificial Neural Network),

SVM (Support Vector Machine), RF (Random Forest), and EGB (Extreme Gradient Boosting) (XGBoost). Contrast alterations from familiar picture quality valuation corpora were used to build and test the proposed supervised approach. In addition, a more difficult dataset encompassing approximately 6200 photos with a wide variety of contrast and intensity fluctuations is introduced. The findings reveal that the suggested method is effective in estimating CLAHE hyperparameters with an RMSE of 0.014 and an R2 of 0.935. Furthermore, by boosting visual contrast while maintaining its natural aspect, our technique outperforms both tested baselines.

Wu et al. [22] presented a novel scheme for mammographic image characteristics and CE. Multiscale transforms and mathematical morphologies are used. To begin, the mammography is decomposed into distinct multiscale sub-band sub-images using the Laplacian Gaussian pyramid transform. In addition, the CLAHE equalizes the information or high-frequency sub-pictures, while mathematical morphology processes the low-frequency sub-images. Finally, the improved picture of characteristics and contrast is restored by using CLAHE and statistical morphology to modify the Laplacian Gaussian pyramid coefficients at single or multiple layers. In order to achieve a natural outcome, the augmented picture is analysed by a global non-linear function. The findings of the experiments suggest that this scheme is successful for mammography features and CE. The contrast assessment measure for pictures, signal-noise-ratio (SNR), and CII are used to evaluate the suggested scheme's performance.

He et al. [23] proposed an automated IE method that used both cranial and mediolateral oblique perspectives. Predict the qualified breast density percentage at a considered projection site to improve mammographic picture quality by altering or correcting an inconsistent intensity distribution. A quantitative and qualitative evaluation was conducted using a dataset of 360 full-field digital mammographic pictures. Visual inspection revealed that the processed images had good and consistent intensity fluctuation, while texture data (breast parenchymal shapes) was kept and/or increased. This technique has shown a promising gain in density-based mammographic partitioning and risk analysis by enhancing the uniformity of the intensity distribution on mammographic pictures. This can then be used in computer-aided mammography, which is valuable in a medicinal context via assisting forecasting radiologists in their decision-making task.

Jenifer et al. [24] developed the Fuzzy Clipped CLAHE (FC-CLAHE) scheme that chooses the CL automatically and improves the local contrast of mammograms using fuzzy logic and histograms. Only a few control parameters are required by the fuzzy inference method developed to choose the CL. The fuzzy rules were created in order to provide the CL with a reliable and adaptable mammography picture with no need for labour involvement. The 322 digitized mammograms retrieved from the MIAS corpora are used in the experiments. The suggested strategy is compared to picture quality measuring tools such as CII, Discrete Entropy (DE), Absolute Mean Brightness Coefficient (AMBC), and PSNR, as well as other HE methods. According to experimental results, the suggested FC-CLAHE scheme outperforms various state-of-the-art schemes.

Al-Juboori [25] proposed that the contrast of mammography pictures be increased. For this objective, many improvement methods such as HE, CLAHE, morphological, and Retinex are applied. To boost its performance, the Retinex technique combines it once with HE and then with CLAHE. The results of the experiments suggest that utilizing Retinex with CLAHE can yield images with stronger CE than using it with HE and is better than other approaches.

Castro et al [26] proposed an algorithm for obtaining ROI in mammography to analyse parameters by regions, starting with IE via HE using the CLAHE method, with the goal of generating relevant information that could become a bio marker for breast radiologists in breast cancer detection. In addition, the use of different three-dimensional representations is proposed to provide the medical community with a new viewpoint on analysis. Gradient vectors are also employed on three-dimensional representations to demonstrate a link between the magnitude and direction of intensity values in mammography masses, which can help determine the direction of a growing anomaly. In terms of anomaly radii, the algorithm yields an average of 75 pixels.

Dabass et al. [27] proposed a CLAHE and an entropy-based intuitionistic fuzzy approach suggested to improve the contrast of digital mammography pictures. Subjective, quantitative, and visual evaluations are performed using the publicly available MIAS corpus to evaluate the efficacy of this approach compared with the type-II fuzzy set-based strategies. This approach produces superior visual quality, according to the findings of the experiments. It outperforms various classical approaches regarding subjective and numerical criteria.

Carneiro et al. [28] presented the CLAHE with various variables (window dimension) in 98 pictures for the purpose of photographic examination and evaluation with the corresponding actual picture. The PSNR, the variation, and SSIM were determined, along with a photographic examination of an experienced and dedicated radiologist. The numerical findings revealed the closeness of the mean PSNR for the group of windows validated. Based on the radiologist's evaluation, the window dimension of 15 × 15 offered a higher contrast between fibroglandular tissue and nearby patterns. This investigation donated to the CE in dense mammograms fitting for such patients who have a greater chance of breast tumours. It was promising to produce superior final pictures in contrast to the actual pictures using a basic mathematically and quickly computational processing technique, which could benefit radiologists in improving prognostic efficiency and premature detection of breast tumours.

Byra Reddy and Prasanna Kumar [29] proposed that non-local filtered images be used to enhance mammography pictures using an entropy improvement method. These techniques may aid in the accurate detection of masses and microcalcifications in mammography. A filtering approach with a high PSNR and a low MSE value is a good filtering technique. According to experimental results on a digital database using screening mammography pictures, the non-local mean filter by entropy improvement strategy is better for mammogram IE. Suradi and Abdullah [30] suggested FC-CLAHE with an Anisotropic Diffusion Filter as a new image enhancing solution for digital mammography pictures (FC-CLAHE-ADF). This scheme uses a fuzzy and histogram-based IE method to provide noiseless mammograms by preserving contrast and brightness. The MIAS open-source corpus yielded an overall of six mammograms. FC-CLAHE-ADF's performance was evaluated against RMSHE (Recursive Mean-Separate HE), FDCT-USFFT (Fast Discrete Curvelet Transform through Unequally Spaced Fast Fourier Transform), and FC-CLAHE alone. In conclusion, amongst other enhancement strategies, the innovative FC-CLAHE-ADF scheme has produced the best solutions. The resulting photos were able to better demonstrate breast lesions.

5.3 Proposed Methodology

The ASFO-CLAHE technique is a unique optimization and histogram-based algorithm for increasing the local contrast of mammograms. ASFO optimizes the local contrast of digital mammograms by automating the CL and NT that are relevant to the mammogram. As additional photos become available, the ASFO approach builds new members of the ensemble from mini-batches of images to make the CL flexible and the NT variable mammography data without the need for human involvement. Figure 5.1 depicts the entire flow of the presented method and tentative methodologies, including the CBIS-DDSM corpus, parameter optimization, and performance evaluation. it is worth noting that the proposed approach's eventual applicability is contingent on evaluation metrics. In other words, the hyperparameters predicted from the previously optimized model are used to alter a given new image.

5.3.1 *Histogram Equalization*

The probability density function, $p(X_k)$, for a considered picture $X = \{X(i,j)\}$ with L discrete grey points denoted as $\{X_0, X_1, \ldots, X_{L-1}\}$, is provided by Eq. (5.1),

$$p(X_k) = \frac{N_k}{N} \text{ for } k = 0, \ldots L - 1 \tag{5.1}$$

N_k is the number of times the point X_k seems in the given picture X, and N denotes the overall amount of examples in the picture. The amount of grey points in the provided picture is $L(L = 256)$. The Cumulative Density Factor (CDF), $c(x)$, is therefore determined by Eq. (5.2), which is

$$c(X_k) = \sum_{j=0}^{k} p(X_j) \text{for } k = 0, \ldots L - 1 \tag{5.2}$$

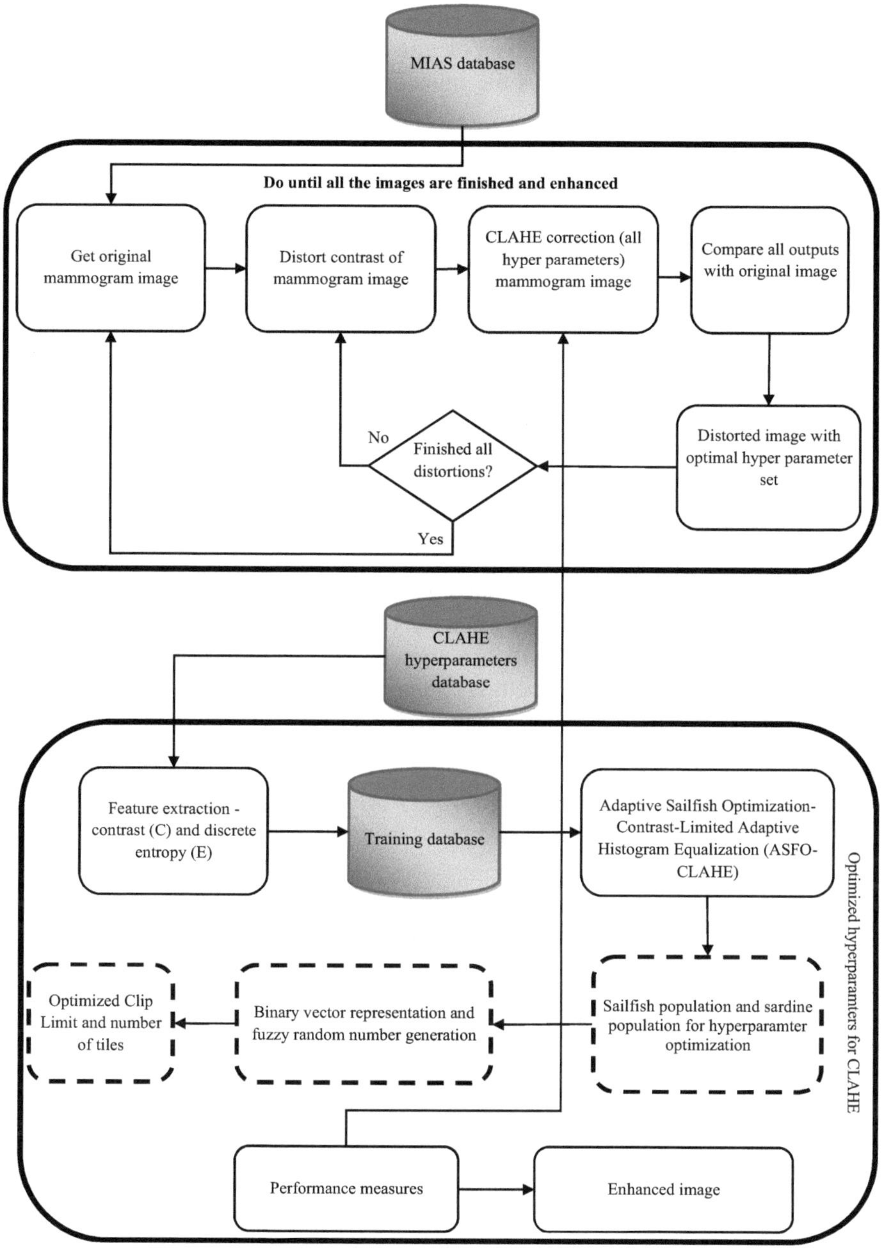

Fig. 5.1 Entire flow of the presented ASFO-CLAHE system

where x is equal to $x = 0, 1, \ldots, L - 1$. HE is an approach, which uses the CDF as a conversion factor to transfer the given picture into the complete dynamic collection (X_0, X_{L-1}). Equation (5.3) gives the transformation factor $f(x)$ depending on the CDF

$$f(x) = x_0 + (X_{L-1} - X_0).c(x) \tag{5.3}$$

In Eq. (5.3), (X_{L-1}) is the highest grey point. It expresses the resultant picture generated via HE, Eq. (5.4)

$$Y = f(x) = \{f(X(i,j)) \mid \forall X(i,j) \in X \tag{5.4}$$

In Eq. (5.4), (i, j) denotes the spatial coordinates of the pixel in the picture [31].

5.3.2 Clipped Histogram Equalization

The contrast of the larger histogram areas is stretched, while the contrast of the small histogram areas is compressed. So, when the ROI in a picture simply takes up a low percentage of the image, HE will not appropriately enhance it. By limiting the enhancement rate, clipped HE methods attempt to address these issues. The boost achieved using the HE technique is dependent on c, $c(x)$ as shown in Eq. (5.3).

$$\frac{d}{dX} c(x) = p(x) \tag{5.5}$$

As a result, by constraining the range of $p(x)$ or h, the enhancement rate can be limited (x). As a result, before the equalization procedure, the clipped histogram adjusts the form of the given histogram via lowering or raising the range in the histogram bins depending on a threshold bound. Clipping/CL is another name for this threshold limit. The CL is calculated using Eq. (5.6) to clip the histogram of the supplied image.

$$\text{Clip Limit} = \left[\frac{\varphi}{256}\right] + \left[\beta.\left(\varphi - \left[\frac{\varphi}{256}\right]\right)\right] \tag{5.6}$$

In Eq. (5.6), β = clipping improvement variable, [.] implies truncation to the nearest integer, and = block size product the number of bins (0–255) is represented by the integer 256. The histogram is then reallocated to include the cut portion. This modified histogram [32] is used for HE. The suggested ASFO-CLAHE improvement approach performs the choice of an appropriate CL for the image data. As a result, the technique is adaptable and suitable for real-world uses. The original image's histogram is created. The picture's contrast and entropy values are retrieved and sent into the ASFO as input.

5.3.3 Adaptive Sailfish Optimization (ASFO)-CLAHE Algorithm

The contrast of a mammographic picture refers to how well various prognostic characteristics like masses and micro calcifications may be clearly separated from the surrounding breast tissues. When compared to normal breast tissue, calcifications in mammograms are comparatively positive calcium patches. Calcifications found within dense masses may have a low contrast with the surrounding environment. The affluence of data in a mammographic picture later CE is measured by entropy.

$$\text{Contrast (C)} = \sum_{i,j=0}^{N-1} |i-j|^2 \, P(i,j) \tag{5.7}$$

$$\text{Entropy (E)} = \sum_{i,j=0}^{N-1} P(i,j)(-\ln P(i,j)) \tag{5.8}$$

$P(i,j)$ denotes the chance of a certain result. The summing value $(i,j=0)$ to $(N-1)$ essentially says that all elements in the matrix must be taken into account. The digital image of a mammogram's contrast and entropy are two crucial features for detecting abnormalities. To produce clipping improvement variable ($o\beta$), which is the ASFO's result value, ASFO takes into account two input values: contrast (C) and discrete entropy (E). The outcomes of clipping improvement techniques are worse than those of HE algorithms when a user sets incorrect settings. Experiments connecting image quality to blocksize and the clipping enhancement parameter have been conducted, revealing that image quality is mostly determined by the CL rather than blocksize. The ASFO-CLAHE algorithm calculates the new optimum CL using Eq. (5.9) which is a version based on the input image's contrast and entropy.

$$\text{Optimized Clip Limit} = \left\lceil \frac{\varphi}{256} \right\rceil + \left\lceil o\beta.\left(\varphi - \left\lceil \frac{\varphi}{256} \right\rceil\right) \right\rceil \tag{5.9}$$

In Eq. (5.9), $o\beta$ = optimized clipping improvement variable (values between 0 and 1), [.] implies truncating the range to the closest integer, φ = product of block size, and the number of bins is 256.

The hit-change tactic of a set of hunting sailfishes chasing a set of sardines inspired SFO, a populace-based meta-heuristic strategy [14]. This hunting strategy offers hunters the upper hand via permitting them to conserve their power. It takes into account two populaces: the sailfish and sardine populations. The issue variables (pixels of the image) are the sites of sailfishes in the hunt region, and the sailfishes are considered the optimal selection of CL and NT. This strategy intends to make the movement of hunt agents as random as possible (both sailfish and sardine). For the best selection of CL and NT, sailfishes are believed to be spread throughout the hunt region, whilst the placements of sardines aid in finding the optimum result in the hunt region. The 'elite' sailfish has the highest fitness, and its place in the iteration is determined by P^i_{SrdBest}. In the instance of sardines, the 'wounded' is the one having the finest fitness (CL and NT), and P^i_{SrdBest} determines its site at all iterations. The sites of sardines and sailfish are modified at all iterations. Using 'elite' sailfish and 'damaged' sardine, the new location P^{i+1}_{Slf} of a sailfish is updated at the i+1th iteration, as per Eq. (5.10).

$$P^{i+1}_{\text{Slf}} = P^{i+1}_{\text{SlfBest}} - \mu_i \left[F_{\text{rnd}} \times \frac{P^{i+1}_{\text{SlfBest}} + P^{i+1}_{\text{SlfInjured}}}{2} - P^i_{\text{Slf}} \right] \tag{5.10}$$

P^i_{Slf} is the earlier site of the Slfth sailfish, F_{rnd} is a fuzzy arbitrary value from 0 to 1, and I is a coefficient created according to Eq. (5.11)

$$\mu_i = 2 \times F_{\text{rnd}} \times \text{PrD} - \text{PrD} \tag{5.11}$$

PrD stands for quarry density that refers to the quantity of quarries present at all iterations. During group hunting, the range of PrD, determined by Eq. (5.12), drops with each repetition as the amount of quarry reduces.

$$\text{PrD} = 1 - \frac{\text{Num}_{\text{Slf}}}{\text{Num}_{\text{Slf}} + \text{Num}_{\text{Srd}}} \tag{5.12}$$

The amount of sailfish and sardines is Num_{Slf} and Num_{Srd}, correspondingly.

$$\text{Num}_{\text{Slf}} = \text{Num}_{\text{Srd}} \times \text{Prcnt} \tag{5.13}$$

In Eq. (5.13), Prcnt is the fraction of the initial sardine populace, which makes up the sailfish populace. The amount of sardines in the beginning is usually assumed to be more than the amount of sailfish. Each iteration updates the sardine sites according to Eq. (5.14),

$$P^{i+1}_{\text{Srd}} = F_{\text{rnd}}(0,1) \times \left(P^i_{\text{SLfBest}} - P^i_{\text{Srd}} + \text{ATK}\right) \tag{5.14}$$

$$\text{ATK} = A \times (1 - (2 \times \text{itr} \times k)) \tag{5.15}$$

where P^i_{Srd} and P^{i+1}_{Srd} describe the sardine's prior and updated sites (CL and NT), and ATK denotes the sailfish's hit strength at iteration itr. The amount of displacement and the amount of sardines, which modify their sites (CL and NT) are now determined by ATK. Convergence of hunt agents is aided by lowering the ATK. The amount of sardines, which change their site (CL and NT) and the number of variables of them Eq. (5.16) are computed using the parameter ATK as follows:

$$\gamma = \text{Num}_{\text{Srd}} \times \text{ATK} \times F_{\text{rnd}}(0,1) \tag{5.16}$$

$$\delta = v \times \text{ATK} \times F_{\text{rnd}}(0,1) \tag{5.17}$$

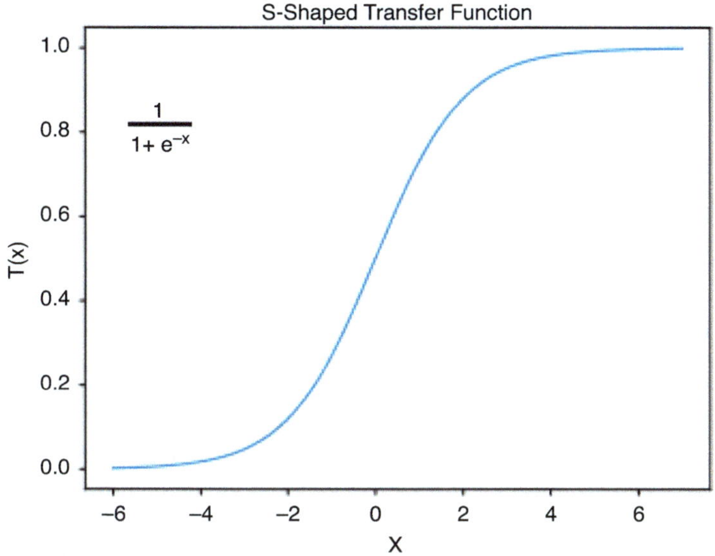

Fig. 5.2 Applied transfer factor for transforming continuous hunt region of SFO to binary

Num_{Srd} denotes the amount of sardines and v denotes the amount of parameters. The exploration of hunt region is ensured by the arbitrary choice of sailfish and sardines. ATK attempts to discover a trade-off between hunt and exploitation. In this chapter, a fuzzy distribution is created for balancing exploration and exploitation in order to pick the best CL and NT. Let the original picture set be $I = \{i_1, i_2, \ldots, i_N\}$, where N denotes the overall quantity of pictures in the dataset and the class tag be $C = \{c_1, \ldots, c_l\}$, where l denotes the amount of classes ($l = 3$). A solution is given here as a binary vector, with 1 indicating that the relevant CL and NT are picked and 0 indicating that the related CLAHE hyper-parameters are not selected. The number of hyper-parameters in the original CBIS-DDSM dataset is equal to the size of this vector. Use a transfer function [15] to convert the normal SFO's continuous hunt region to a binary one.

Figure 5.2 depicts the sigmoid transfer function, which is expressed by Eq. (5.18),

$$T(x) = \frac{1}{1 + e^{-x}} \tag{5.18}$$

Equation (5.19) will now be used to modify the current site of the sailfish employing the possibility values produced by Eqs. (5.18 and 5.19).

$$X^d(t) = \begin{cases} 1 \ \text{if} \ F_{\text{rnd}} < T\left(X^d(t)\right) \\ 0 \ \text{if} \ F_{\text{rnd}} \geq T\left(X^d(t)\right) \end{cases} \tag{5.19}$$

These two parameters are integrated using Eq. (5.20), and the IE issue is reduced to a single objective problem.

$$\text{Fitness} = \omega\gamma(C) + (1-\omega)\frac{|C|}{N} \tag{5.20}$$

In Eq. (5.20), C indicates the image contrast, $|C|$ is the cardinality of the image contrast, (C) is the picture quality in relation to the contrast, N is the original image, and $\omega \in [0, 1]$ is the weight. SFO now takes care of exploration [33, 34] via an arbitrary initiation of the sailfish and sardine populations, as well as an encircling strategy based on hyper-sphere neighbourhood. Exploitation is avoided by relying on the sardine population and mobility around the most excellent sailfish and sardine. The variable ATK (specified in Eq. 5.14) attempts to strike a trade-off between the algorithm's hunt and exploitation abilities. The traditional SFO, on the other hand, suffers from poor solution accuracy, slow convergence speed, early convergence, and an insufficient trade-off between global and local hunting capabilities. Second, to balance and enhance the hunt and exploitation abilities of algorithms, the adaptive fuzzy distribution is used to change individual sardines. Finally, genetic features are used to carry out natural inheritance of sailfish and sardines in order to increase the algorithm's solution accuracy and convergence speed. The worst-case scenario complexity of the ASFO strategy is $O(\max_{\text{Iter}} \times (N_{\text{Srd}} \times t_{\text{fitness}} + N))$, wherein $\max_{\text{Iter}}$ is the greatest amount of iteration, N_{Srd} is the amount of sardines, t_{fitness} denotes the duration required to calculate the fitness range of a specific agent by the considered classifier, and N denotes the overall quantity of images in the dataset. The standard approach for HE is to reallocate grey points in a given picture therefore that the histogram of the resultant picture approaches that of a regular distribution, leading to an enhancement in perceived quality. The probability density function X_{opt_k}, for an optimized clipped image is given by Eq. (5.21),

$$P_{\text{opt}}\left(X_{\text{opt}\_k}\right) = \frac{N_{\text{opt}\_k}}{N} \text{ for opt}\_k = 0, \ldots \text{L} - 1 \tag{5.21}$$

N_{opt_k} is the amount of times the point X_{opt_k} appears in the given picture X, and N denotes the overall quantity of examples in the picture. The amount of grey points $(L = 255)$ is represented by the letter L. The following is the conversion factor $f(x)$ depending on the CDF indicated in Eq. (5.2):

$$f(x) = X_0 + (X_{L-1} - X_0).c(x) \tag{5.22}$$

where (X_{L-1}) denotes the highest grey point. The following is the image obtained using optimal trimmed HE:

$$Y_{\text{opt}} = f(x) = \left\{f\left(X_{\text{opt}}(i,j)\right) | \forall X_{\text{opt}}(i,j) \in X_{\text{opt}}\right\} \tag{5.23}$$

The spatial coordinates of the pixel in the picture are (i,j)

5.4 Performance Measures

The results of the presented ASFO-CLAHE method and existing methods are evaluated against CLAHE, FC-CLAHE, and FC-CLAHE-ADF regarding picture quality measures such as PSNR, MSE, and SSIM.

The PSNR is utilized to assess the extent of relationship amongst an improved picture and its underlying picture.

$$\mathrm{PSNR} = 10\log_{10}\frac{R^2}{\mathrm{MSE}} \tag{5.24}$$

In Eq. (5.24), R indicates the utmost variation in the given picture and MSE is used to assess the dissimilarity amongst the improved picture and its underlying picture.

$$\mathrm{MSE} = \frac{1}{n}\sum_{i=1}^{n}\left(Y_i - \widehat{Y}_i\right)^2 \tag{5.25}$$

n = number of data points, Y_i = observed values, $\widehat{Y}_i$ = predicted values.

5.5 Performance Measures

MIAS database can be utilized for the experiment and validation of the IE methods. The test set includes 322 varied categories of mammographic pictures of dimension 1024 × 1024 pixels with 8 bits per pixel, the presented ASFO-CLAHE algorithm, FC-CLAHE-ADF, CLAHE, and FC-CLAHE were evaluated via various performance metrics. Various quantitative performance measures, such as PSNR MSE, RMSE, and SSIM as stated in the preceding section, were applied to demonstrate the enhanced efficacy of the suggested technique over conventional and advanced methods. Figure 5.3 displays a digital mammogram of a benign breast cancer sample from the MIAS database, which may be found at https://www.kaggle.com/datasets/awsaf49/cbis-ddsm-breast-cancer-image-dataset. This study was done on a MATLABR2021b with 4GB RAM and a 5th generation Intel Core i7 processor.

Figure 5.3 shows the results of various IE methods with respect to enhanced images and histogram of those algorithms. The left side of the Fig. 5.3a, c, e, g, i demonstrates the results of original low contrast image, IE by CLAHE, FC-CLAHE, FC-CLAHE-ADF, and proposed ASFO-CLAHE algorithm, respectively. The right side of the Fig. 5.3b, d, f, h, j demonstrates the histogram of original image, CLAHE, FC-CLAHE, FC-CLAHE-ADF, and proposed ASFO-CLAHE algorithm, respectively. Table 5.1 provides the relative analysis of various IE methods by pictures collected from MIAS corpus. Results analysis of PSNR reveals that the presented ASFO-CLAHE technique provides higher PSNR of 23.1823 dB which is improved

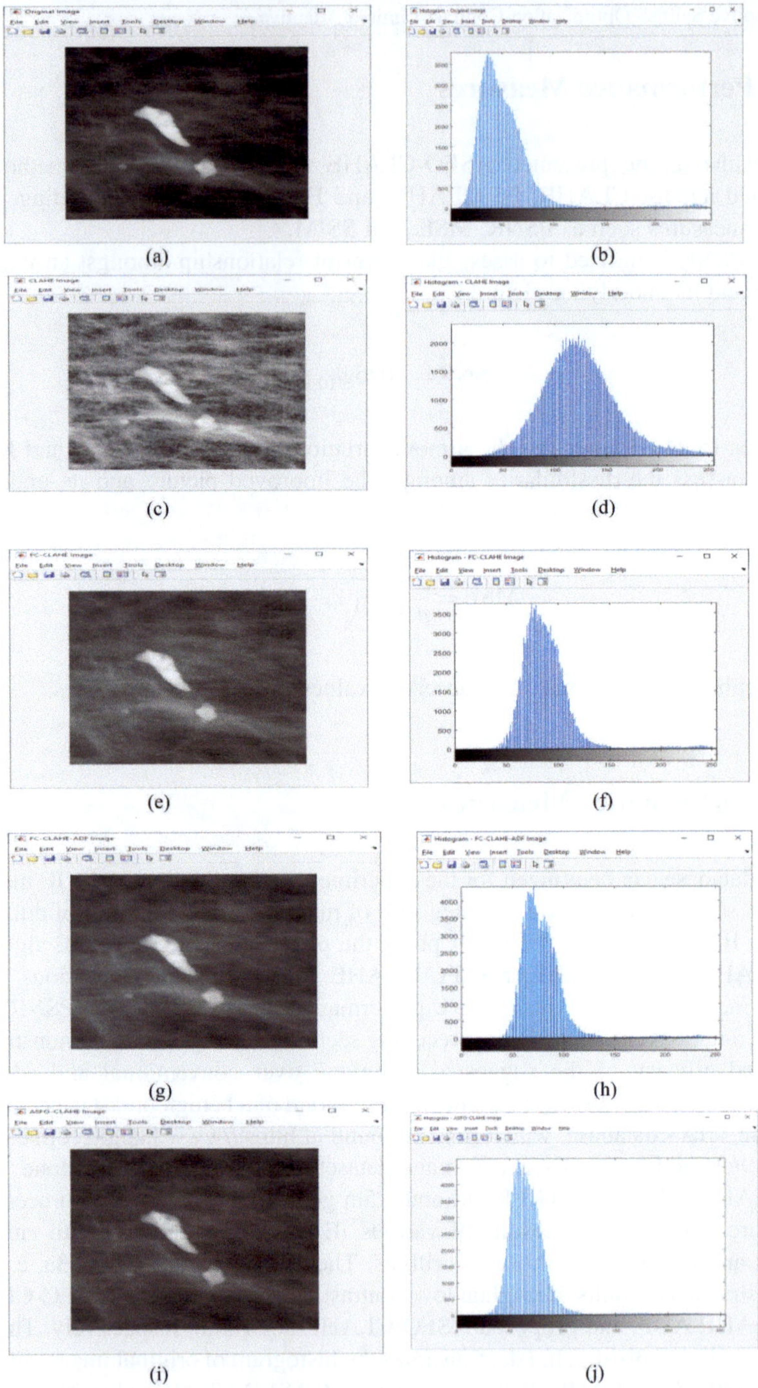

Fig. 5.3 Various image enhancement methods and histogram of benign-type digital mammogram. (**a**) Original low contrast image. (**b**) Histogram of low contrast image. (**c**) Image enhancement by CLAHE. (**d**) Histogram of image by CLAHE. (**e**) Image enhancement by FC-CLAHE. (**f**) Histogram of image by FC-CLAHE. (**g**) Image enhancement by FC-CLAHE-ADF. (**h**) Histogram of image by FC-CLAHE-ADF. (**i**) Image enhancement by ASFO-CLAHE. (**j**) Histogram of image by ASFO-CLAHE

than the other traditional IE methods. ASFO-CLAHE produces greater PSNR values while evaluated against the traditional IE techniques. This proves the enhancement is performed better than the other images. MSE is extremely less for ASFO-CLAHE (205.2463), higher for CLAHE (251.2517), FC-CLAHE (251.2517), and FC-CLAHE-ADF (249.8211). RMSE value of proposed ASFO-CLAHE system is 14.3267, CLAHE, FC-CLAHE, and FC-CLAHE-ADF methods produce higher RMSE results of 15.8509, 15.8057, and 15.6920, respectively. ASFO-CLAHE system gives less RMSE value when compared to other existing methods since the noisy backgrounds in the output picture that fairly interest a huge proportion of the picture part. SSIM is very higher for ASFO-CLAHE (0.9208), lower for CLAHE (0.4829), FC-CLAHE (0.7295), and FC-CLAHE-ADF (0.8322).

Figures 5.4, 5.5, 5.6, and 5.7 show the graphical evaluation of the metrics like PSNR, MSE, RMSE, and SSIM comparison for the enhanced results by CLAHE, FC-CLAHE, FC-CLAHE-ADF, and ASFO-CLAHE methods. From the results, it concludes that the presented method has considerably improved values of SSIM and PSNR.

Figure 5.4 exhibits the PSNR comparison of IE methods such as CLAHE, FC-CLAHE, FC-CLAHE-ADF, and proposed ASFO-CLAHE algorithm. Proposed ASFO-CLAHE algorithm gives improved PSNR (23.1823dB), traditional CLAHE (10.6513dB), FC-CLAHE (16.8773dB), and FC-CLAHE-ADF(19.1001 dB) has lesser PSNR, respectively (See Table 5.1).

Figures 5.5 and 5.6 show the overall error results of various IE algorithms. MSE and RMSE of the proposed technique are very low while evaluated against the existing IE techniques. Proposed algorithm gives lesser MSE (205.2463), other methods have higher MSE value of CLAHE (251.2517), FC-CLAHE (249.8211), and FC-CLAHE-ADF (246.2381). Proposed algorithm gives lesser RMSE (14.3267), other methods have higher RMSE value of CLAHE (15.8509), FC-CLAHE (15.8057), and FC-CLAHE-ADF (15.6920).

Figure 5.7, SSIM results of the proposed system is higher, i.e. 0.9208 and other methods, such as CLAHE, FC-CLAHE, FC-CLAHE-ADF give lower SSIM value

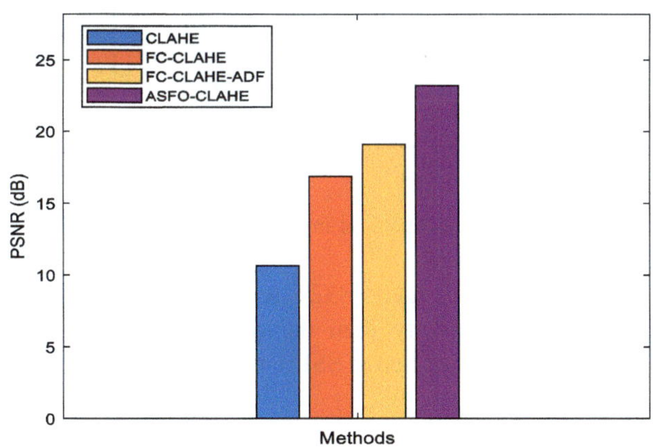

Fig. 5.4 PSNR comparison of image enhancement methods via Mias database

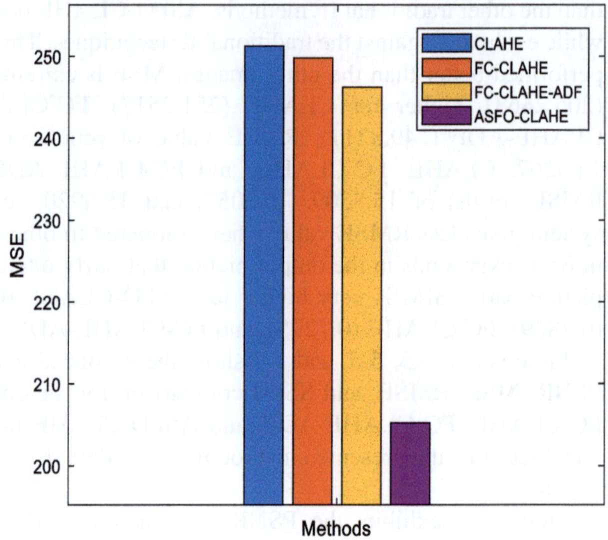

Fig. 5.5 MSE comparison of image enhancement methods via Mias database

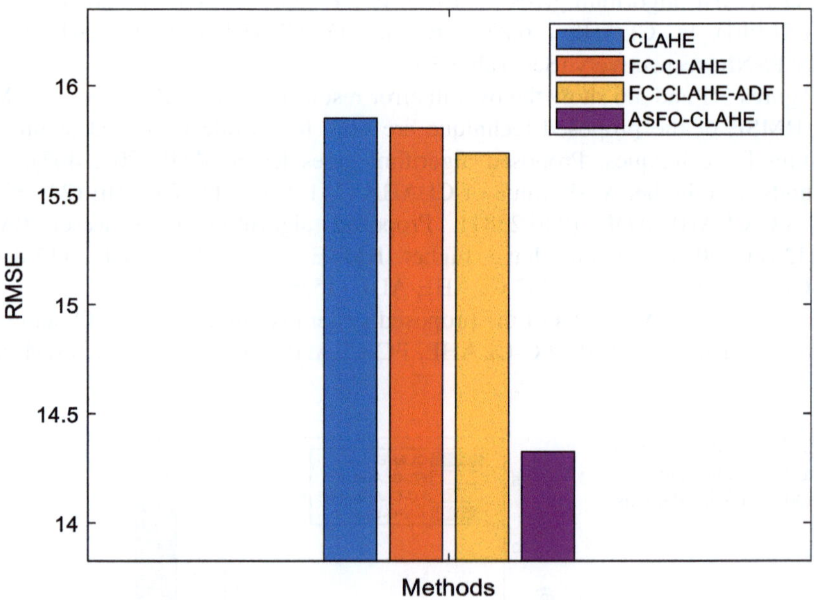

Fig. 5.6 RMSE comparison of image enhancement methods via Mias database

of 0.4829, 0.7295, and 0.8322, respectively. Proposed system optimizes the hyper-parameters efficiently than the other methods, which shows that the presented technique provides better SSIM range between original and contrast enhancement images.

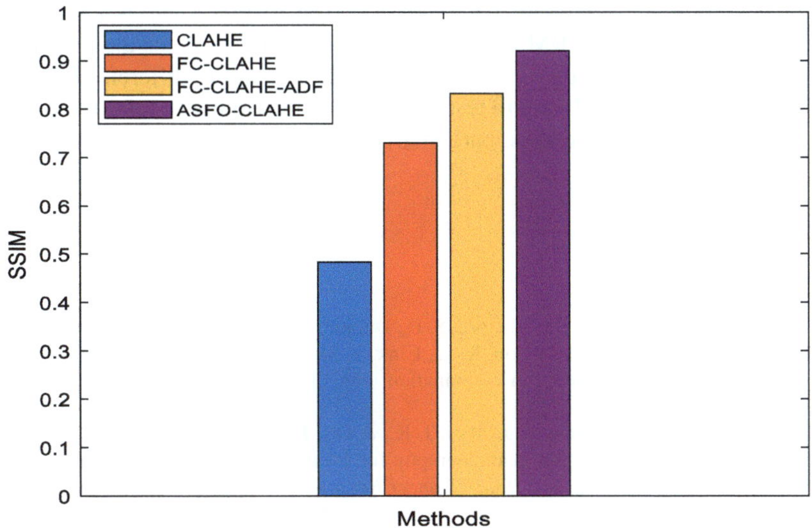

Fig. 5.7 SSIM comparison of image enhancement methods via Mias database

Table 5.1 Comparative analysis of various image enhancement algorithms (Mias Database)

Performance measures	CLAHE	FC-CLAHE	FC-CLAHE-ADF	ASFO-CLAHE
PSNR	10.6513	16.8773	19.1001	23.1823
MSE	251.2517	249.8211	246.2381	205.2463
RMSE	15.8509	15.8057	15.6920	14.3267
SSIM	0.4829	0.7295	0.8322	0.9208

5.6 Conclusion and Future Work

CLAHE, hyperparameter tuning which leads to reduction in image quality. ASFO-CLAHE algorithm is presented for detecting abnormalities in digital mammogram. In the proposed ASFO-CLAHE algorithm, CL, and NT of CLAHE technique is automatically selected using the ASFO algorithm. The quality of the improved picture is majorly depending on two parameters such as CL and NT. ASFO-CLAHE algorithm is capable of repeatedly computing hyperparameters of CLAHE's for pictures through varied contrast irregularities in the MIAS database. Experimental results demonstrate that the purpose of the proposed ASFO-CLAHE method is successful and gives better improvement for different mammogram images. It is obvious that the purpose of the presented technique has improve the identification capability of micro calcifications present in mammogram images and it is appropriate for each and every one category of breast images together with fatty, fatty glandular, and dense-glandular mammograms. The metrics such as PSNR, MSE, Root Mean Square Error (RMSE), and SSIM values are used for the performance analysis. These measures play a significant role in comparing different IE methods. The scope of the work will aim to test this system's capability to raise the results of following computer vision tasks, particularly object detection.

References

1. Friedewald, S. M., Rafferty, E. A., Rose, S. L., Durand, M. A., Plecha, D. M., Greenberg, J. S., Hayes, M. K., Copit, D. S., Carlson, K. L., Cink, T. M., & Barke, L. D. (2014). Breast cancer screening using tomosynthesis in combination with digital mammography. *JAMA, 311*(24), 2499–2507.
2. Yun, S. J., Ryu, C. W., Rhee, S. J., Ryu, J. K., & Oh, J. Y. (2017). Benefit of adding digital breast tomosynthesis to digital mammography for breast cancer screening focused on cancer characteristics: A meta-analysis. *Breast Cancer Research and Treatment, 164*(3), 557–569.
3. Li, H., Mendel, K. R., Lan, L., Sheth, D., & Giger, M. L. (2019). Digital mammography in breast cancer: Additive value of radiomics of breast parenchyma. *Radiology, 291*(1), 15–20.
4. Salama, M. S., Eltrass, A. S., & Elkamchouchi, H. M. (2018). An improved approach for computer-aided diagnosis of breast cancer in digital mammography. In *2018 IEEE international symposium on medical measurements and applications (MeMeA)* (pp. 1–5).
5. Henriksen, E. L., Carlsen, J. F., Vejborg, I. M., Nielsen, M. B., & Lauridsen, C. A. (2019). The efficacy of using computer-aided detection (CAD) for detection of breast cancer in mammography screening: A systematic review. *Acta Radiologica, 60*(1), 13–18.
6. Al-Antari, M. A., Al-Masni, M. A., Park, S. U., Park, J., Metwally, M. K., Kadah, Y. M., Han, S. M., & Kim, T. S. (2018). An automatic computer-aided diagnosis system for breast cancer in digital mammograms via deep belief network. *Journal of Medical and Biological Engineering, 38*(3), 443–456.
7. Asmare, M. H., Asirvadam, V. S., & Hani, A. F. M. (2015). Image enhancement based on contourlet transform. *Signal, Image and Video Processing, 9*(7), 1679–1690.
8. Gupta, S., & Kaur, Y. (2014). Review of different local and global contrast enhancement techniques for a digital image. *International Journal of Computers and Applications, 100*(18), 18–23.
9. Laksmi, T. V. H., Madhu, T., Kavya, K. C. S., & Basha, S. E. (2016). Novel image enhancement technique using CLAHE and wavelet transforms. *International Journal of Engineering, Science and Technology, 5*(11), 507–511.
10. Chang, Y., Jung, C., Ke, P., Song, H., & Hwang, J. (2018). Automatic contrast-limited adaptive histogram equalization with dual gamma correction. *IEEE Access, 6*, 11782–11792.
11. Stimper, V., Bauer, S., Ernstorfer, R., Schölkopf, B., & Xian, R. P. (2019). Multidimensional contrast limited adaptive histogram equalization. *IEEE Access, 7*, 165437–165447.
12. Mohan, S., & Ravishankar, M. (2012). Modified contrast limited adaptive histogram equalization based on local contrast enhancement for mammogram images. In *International conference on advances in information technology and mobile communication* (pp. 397–403). Springer.
13. Flores, W. G., & de Albuquerque Pereira, W. C. (2017). A contrast enhancement method for improving the segmentation of breast lesions on ultrasonography. *Computers in Biology and Medicine, 80*, 14–23.
14. Tareef, A., Song, Y., Cai, W., Huang, H., Chang, H., Wang, Y., Fulham, M., Feng, D., & Chen, M. (2017). Automatic segmentation of overlapping cervical smear cells based on local distinctive features and guided shape deformation. *Neurocomputing, 221*, 94–107.

15. Singh, N. P., & Srivastava, R. (2016). Retinal blood vessels segmentation by using Gumbel probability distribution function based matched filter. *Computer Methods and Programs in Biomedicine, 129*, 40–50.
16. Aslani, S., & Sarnel, H. (2016). A new supervised retinal vessel segmentation method based on robust hybrid features. *Biomedical Signal Processing and Control, 30*, 1–12.
17. Huang, S.-C., & Yeh, C.-H. (2013). Image contrast enhancement for preserving mean brightness without losing image features. *Engineering Applications of Artificial Intelligence, 26*, 1487–1492.
18. More, L. G., Brizuela, M. A., Ayala, H. L., Pinto-Roa, D. P., & Noguera, J. L. V. (2015). Parameter tuning of CLAHE based on multi-objective optimization to achieve different contrast levels in medical images. In *2015 IEEE International Conference on Image Processing (ICIP)* (pp. 4644–4648).
19. Hiary, H., Zaghloul, R., Al-Adwan, A., & Al-Zoubi, M. D. B. (2017). Image contrast enhancement using geometric mean filter. *Signal, Image and Video Processing, 11*(5), 833–840.
20. Ma, J., Fan, X., Yang, S. X., Zhang, X., & Zhu, X. (2018). Contrast limited adaptive histogram equalization-based fusion in YIQ and HSI color spaces for underwater image enhancement. *International Journal of Pattern Recognition and Artificial Intelligence, 32*(07), 1854018.
21. Campos, G. F. C., Mastelini, S. M., Aguiar, G. J., Mantovani, R. G., Melo, L. F. D., & Barbon, S. (2019). Machine learning hyperparameter selection for contrast limited adaptive histogram equalization. *EURASIP Journal on Image and Video Processing, 1*, 1–18.
22. Wu, S., Zhu, Q., Yang, Y., & Xie, Y. (2013). Feature and contrast enhancement of mammographic image based on multiscale analysis and morphology. In *2013 IEEE International Conference on Information and Automation (ICIA)* (pp. 521–526).
23. He, W., Kibiro, M., Juette, A., Denton, E. R., Hogg, P., & Zwiggelaar, R. (2014). A novel image enhancement methodology for full field digital mammography. In *International workshop on digital mammography* (pp. 650–657). Springer.
24. Jenifer, S., Parasuraman, S., & Kadirvelu, A. (2016). Contrast enhancement and brightness preserving of digital mammograms using fuzzy clipped contrast-limited adaptive histogram equalization algorithm. *Applied Soft Computing, 42*, 167–177.
25. Al-Juboori, R. A. L. (2017). Contrast enhancement of the mammographic image using retinex with CLAHE methods. *Iraqi Journal of Science, 58*(1B), 327–336.
26. Castro, T. S., Moreno, L. M., Martinez, B. M. R., Castaneda, M. R., Castaneda, M. C. L., Guerrero, O. H. A., Ortiz, R. J. M., Solis, S. L. O., & Vega, C. H. R. (2018). Breast cancer mass detection in mammograms and tridimensional representation. *Proceedings of the ISSSD, 2*, 115–134.
27. Dabass, J., Arora, S., Vig, R., & Hanmandlu, M. (2019). Mammogram image enhancement using entropy and CLAHE based intuitionistic fuzzy method. In *2019 6th International Conference on Signal Processing and Integrated Networks (SPIN)* (pp. 24–29).
28. Carneiro, P. C., Debs, C. L., Andrade, A. O., & Patrocinio, A. C. (2019). CLAHE parameters effects on the quantitative and visual assessment of dense breast mammograms. *IEEE Latin America Transactions, 17*(05), 851–857.
29. Byra Reddy, G. R., & Prasanna Kumar, H. (2019). Enhancement of mammogram images by using entropy improvement approach. *SN Applied Sciences, 1*(12), 1–5.
30. Suradi, S. H., & Abdullah, K. A. (2021). Using FC-CLAHE-ADF to enhance digital mammograms for detecting breast lesions. In *IOP Conference Series: Materials Science and Engineering* (Vol. 1173, no. 1, pp. 1–7).

31. Liang, K., Ma, Y., Xie, Y., Zhou, B., & Wang, R. (2021). A new adaptive contrast enhancement algorithm for infrared images based on double plateaus histogram equalization. *Infrared Physics and Technology, 55*, 309–315.
32. Shadravan, S., Naji, H. R., & Bardsiri, V. K. (2019). The sailfish optimizer: A novel nature-inspired metaheuristic algorithm for solving constrained engineering optimization problems. *Engineering Applications of Artificial Intelligence, 80*, 20–34.
33. Mafarja, M. M., & Mirjalili, S. (2017, October). Hybrid whale optimization algorithm with simulated annealing for feature selection. *Neurocomputing, 260*, 302–312.
34. Mirjalili, S., & Lewis, A. (2013, April). S-shaped versus V-shaped transfer functions for binary particle swarm optimization. *Swarm and Evolutionary Computation, 9*, 1–14.

Chapter 6
Efficient Method for Predicting Thyroid Disease Classification using Convolutional Neural Network with Support Vector Machine

V. Brindha and A. Muthukumaravel

6.1 Introduction

Thyroid disease is the most common ailment in the world. Thyroid hormones influence nearly all the organ in the body, especially heartbeat and brain function, since they govern the distribution of energy in the body. The thyroid gland generates the hormones levothyroxine (T4) and triiodothyronine (T3), and thyroid stimulating hormone (TSH) regulates the quantity of T3 and T4 in the blood. TSH and T4 levels if normal indicate that the thyroid gland is functioning correctly, whereas TSH levels that are low and T4 levels if high indicate hyperthyroidism. T3 tests are used to detect hyperthyroidism or to determine the severity of the condition. Secondary hypothyroidism is identified by a low TSH and lower T4, while primary hypothyroidism is noted by a higher TSH and lower T4.

The main goal of saving lives of many people is to diagnose thyroid disorders early using Thyroid disorder prediction techniques. AI is a cutting-edge technology that aids in thyroid disorder prediction. Machine learning (ML) is a subclass of AI in which data mining is used to train a function that translates an input to an output using various approaches. Labelled data on training is a feature of supervised machine learning that consists of a set of training samples. Unsupervised machine learning focuses on data analysis and can track numerous abnormalities by

V. Brindha (✉)
Department of Computer Applications, Bharath Institute of Higher Education and Research, Chennai, Tamil Nadu, India

A. Muthukumaravel
Arts & Science, Bharath Institute of Higher Education and Research, Chennai, Tamil Nadu, India
e-mail: dean.arts@bharathuniv.ac.in

F. J. Joseph et al. (eds.), *Computational Intelligence for Clinical Diagnosis*, EAI/Springer Innovations in Communication and Computing,
https://doi.org/10.1007/978-3-031-23683-9_6

understanding the behaviour of distinct entities. Despite the efficiency of ML algorithms, the traditional methodologies are confined to handling raw data. Deep learning (DL) is a subset of machine learning (ML) that includes a variety of representation learning approaches or methodologies. They can create data representations at several levels. The different layers in a deep neural network convert raw data representation at a lower level or input level into a higher level or abstraction level presentation.

Thyroid disease is becoming more difficult for medical researchers and doctors to understand. As a result, a deep learning algorithm is utilised in this study to detect the presence of many forms of thyroid diseases without the need for multiple physician consultations. The proposed Convolutional Neural Network (CNN) is compared to the Support Vector Machine (SVM) classifier for predicting thyroid disorders and classifying them as either hyperthyroidism or hypothyroidism from the given dataset. The following is how the rest of the chapter is organised: Through a study of the literature, Sect. 6.2 provides the relevant background knowledge. Section 6.3 contains the dataset and application of classification methods utilised in this experiment to diagnose thyroid disease. Section 6.4 summarises the research findings and discussion. Section 6.5 finishes with conclusions and recommendations for future research.

6.2 Literature Review

Chen et al. [1] present an expert model with three phases for identifying and treating thyroid issues, focusing on a hybrid SVM technique in this research. The first phase, which focuses on feature selection, tries to create a variety of feature subsets with varying discriminative capabilities. The generated feature groups are loaded into the specified SVM classifier in the second phase for training an optimum prediction system, whose parameters are tuned via particle swarm optimisation (PSO). Finally, utilising the best discriminative feature subset and ideal criteria, the resulting perfect SVM model accomplishes thyroid illness diagnosis assignments. The suggested expert model (FS-PSO-SVM) was thoroughly tested on the thyroid disease database, which is commonly used to detect thyroid problems. The suggested scheme was compared against two other equivalent systems in respect of classification accuracy: an SVM built on grid search methodology and an SVM built on grid search plus principal component analysis. The results demonstrate that FS-PSO-SVM performs much better than the others.

Nageswari et al.'s [2] work aims to identify and detect the existence of five different thyroid illnesses, including both hyper and hypothyroidism, thyroid carcinoma, thyroid gland, thyroiditis, and regular thyroid monitoring, without requiring numerous consultations. This results in predicted illness progression, allowing us to take quick action to avoid further repercussions in a cost-effective and efficient manner, reducing the rate of human error. The more time-consuming thyroid variety and patient expenditure will be removed using an internet tool that uses an image file of the inclusion.

The major purpose of this study by Borzouei et al. [3] was to use multivariate logistic regression and neural network (NN) schemes to diagnose the two most frequent thyroid diseases. In particular, the study looked at how well laboratory testing predicted specific clinical symptom scores. Individuals with thyroid problems who were directed to Hamadan's Hospitals provided the data for this study. The study included 310 patients who were classified as euthyroid, hyperthyroid, or hypothyroid. The characteristics collected included characteristics, indications of the disorders of concern, and laboratory tests. Various multinomial logistic regression and classifiers were validated experimentally to examine the predictive abilities of the clinical symptoms and laboratory findings. The accuracy average and the area under the curve of these models were compared. In every case, the neural network model outperformed the multinomial logistic regression model.

Bini et al. [4] introduce the main principles and process characteristics of machine learning, deep learning, and radiomics in their article. Data requirements, distinctions between these approaches, and their limitations are discussed. Following that, a brief description of the use of AI algorithms for the evaluation of thyroid pictures is offered. Before AI systems are developed for widespread clinical application, there should be a serious discussion about their limitations and open difficulties. Clarification of the drawbacks of AI-based solutions is critical for ensuring the best possible application for each patient.

Vasile et al. [5] devised an ensemble technique to discover new methods for improving the diagnosis process of thyroid problems. This strategy used two deep learning models: one using CNN architecture and the other using transfer learning. For the first model, 5-CNN, an effective, completely trained model with five convolution layers was created. The second model repurposed, refined, and trained the previously trained VGG-19 architecture. The other two models were surpassed by the proposed ensemble approach, which produced excellent results.

Makas et al. [6] used seven different kinds of NN to develop extremely stable and trustworthy models for thyroid evaluation in this study. The PSO and artificial bee colony methods are quite popular optimisation methods, while the migratory bird's optimisation technique, built on swarm intelligence, is a newer optimisation method. These evolutionary algorithms were then used to retrain the established feed-forward multilayer neural network. The dataset was found on the UCI machine learning repository website. The accuracy scores beat those of similar studies, according to the findings.

ThyNet, a deep learning AI network developed by Sui Peng et al. [7], can discriminate between cancerous and benign thyroid nodules. This model was tested to determine if it could help radiographers enhance diagnostic efficiency and prevent tiny needle extraction. ThyNet was created and provided with training on datasets from two hospitals in three stages before being tested on datasets from seven Chinese hospitals. Every lump in the training and overall test sets had its pathology verified. ThyNet's diagnosis results were compared to those of 12 radiologists in the first place (test set A). Then, to increase radiologists' diagnostic performance using images, a ThyNet-aided technique was devised, in which ThyNet helped diagnoses made by radiologists (test set B). After that, the ThyNet-assisted technique was put to the test in a real-life clinical scenario (test set C). The number of unwanted fine needle aspirations prevented by the ThyNet-assisted method was determined in a simulated situation.

In their paper, Yunjun Wang et al. [8] showed how DCNN models may be used in clinical situations to help differentiate thyroid nodules from each other using histology data. The DCNN models, particularly VGG-19, demonstrated outstanding diagnostic efficiency after being trained with a huge database. Pathologists' workloads might be reduced and their ability to determine the histology of thyroid cancers improved with the use of DCCN models.

If congenital hypothyroidism (CH) is identified early enough, infants with the illness can have normal or fairly normal cognitive ability. Zarin Mousavi et al. [9] chose to add many famous classification techniques to the new-born screening scheme after studying their efficacy in the detection of thyroid conditions. Using data from the Healthcare Department of Alborz Province, Iran, the effectiveness of these methods in diagnosing CH was assessed. Because the dataset was unbalanced, the base classifiers were coupled with the Bagging and AdaBoost algorithms to increase model performance. The SVM-Bagging could distinguish children with CH from healthy children with 99.58% accuracy, according to the findings.

The purpose of this study, according to Namdeo et al. [10], is to develop a unique thyroid detection system that includes two aspects: feature extraction and classification. Using Principal Component Analysis, two types of features are extracted: neighbourhood-based and gradient-based features, followed by CNN and NN classification techniques. While CNN is used to categorise images by pulling deep attributes, NN is used to classify diseases by combining image and data information. Finally, the two categorised findings are integrated to improve diagnosis accuracy. This research also seeks to stimulate the optimisation concept in order to improve the accuracy rate. The CNN convolutional layer is chosen optimally, and the given features should be the best when classifying under NN. For these improvements, a new modified method called Worst Fitness-based Cuckoo Search (WF-CS) is presented. Finally, the performance of the suggested WF-CS is compared to that of other traditional approaches, demonstrating that the proposed work is superior in detecting thyroid existence.

6.3 Materials and Methods

The proposed approach can help doctors achieve a definitive diagnosis by finding features that include significant detail, extracting key correlations between features, and concluding a diagnostic state. Data collection and preparation, classification, and evaluation are the three logical processes in the implementation technique. Cleaning, normalisation, transformation, feature extraction, and selection are all part of the initial phase of data pre-processing. A uniform format for the data model is defined at this stage, which handles missed values, duplicate values, and poor data filtering. After the dataset has been cleaned, data related to the evaluation is chosen and extracted. The chosen data is translated into data mining-friendly formats. To minimise the influence of scale on the data, the datasets are normalised and stored in the comma separated value file format. Feature selection (FS), also known as attributes selection, is the process of selecting the most essential attributes in a dataset for predictive analysis. The dataset is then subjected to two classification techniques: CNN and SVM. Finally, the models' performances are compared using several classification evaluation methods.

6.3.1 Dataset Description

This study's database originates from the UCI archive and includes 7200 cases with 21 features: 15 of those will be categories and six of which are numeric. The cases in the dataset are divided into three groups: hyper, hypo, and normal individuals. The subject groups are divided into 166 hyperthyroidism, 368 hypothyroidism, and 6666 normal occurrences. As indicated by the distribution of cases amongst the three classes, the dataset is considerably skewed. In addition, for analytical purposes, the full dataset was split into a train and test dataset in an 80:20 ratio. As a result, there are 5760 occurrences in the testing set and 1440 in the test sample. In the assessment, only five of the 21 criteria are employed. These are a few of the various thyroid activity examinations that reveal the amount of thyroid hormones present in the blood and are symptomatic of thyroid malfunction.

6.3.2 Convolutional Neural Network

CNN is a deep learning model that consists of numerous layers and is connected end-to-end. Convolutional layer, pooling layer, and fully connected layer are the three primary layers of a CNN. The CNN goes through two levels of training: forward and backward. The image is depicted in every layer with the existing parameters (weight and bias) in the forward stage of CNN training. Internal network parameters (weights) are modified during the backward propagation phase in order to compute the following forward stage. A standard CNN model is structured in a series of stages. Two types of layers make up the initial stages: convolutional layers and pooling layers. The convolutional layer is made up of a series of different feature maps with neurons placed inside. This layer's learnable parameters are filters or kernels. Each convolutional layer's feature map includes ReLU activated elements of the dot product of weights and the local input region to which the layer's neurons are attached. The raw pixel values of the image are stored in the input, which is an array. The output volume is produced by convolving filters or kernels on this input array. In equation (6.1), the mathematical term for convolution is provided.

$$G[x,y] = (j * k)[x,y] = \sum_{a}\sum_{b} k[a,b] j[x-a, y-b] \tag{6.1}$$

where $j$represents the input array; k represents the kernel or filter of size (a, b); and x and y indicate the row and column indexes in the output matrix.

The role of the pooling layer is to merge semantically related features into a single entity. The features hierarchy created by CNN's two interleaved main layers is passed to other fully connected layers for the network's ultimate output. This fully connected layer comes after the softmax function in the classification layer. The loss layer is the final layer of a completely linked network, and it calculates the error that occurs when the desired and real values disagree. This loss layer is frequently associated with the softmax function, which works on the basis of probability distribution.

6.3.3 *Support Vector Machine*

The SVM is a supervised learning classification algorithm that has been demonstrated to be effective for a variety of classification issues. Both regression and classification issues are solved using SVM. Support vectors are the data points on the boundary. It tries to find the best hyperplane across classes by counting the number of points on the class descriptors' edge. The space between two classes is measured by the margin. The accuracy of categorisation improves by a larger margin. This approach works well for situations with both linear and nonlinear datasets.

6.4 Results and Discussions

For the classification of thyroid illnesses, two AI algorithms, SVM and CNN, were used to distinguish between hyper and hypothyroid datasets from normal datasets. The results of this research are compared in terms of two parameters: precision and accuracy.

Accuracy:

$$\text{Accuracy} = \frac{\text{TP} + \text{TN}}{\text{TP} + \text{FP} + \text{TN} + \text{FN}} * 100\% \tag{6.2}$$

Table 6.1 and Fig. 6.1 show the accuracy obtained from the dataset by Support Vector Machine and Convolution Neural Network. It clearly shows that in terms of accuracy, convolution neural networks outperform support vector machines.

Precision:

$$\text{Precision} = \frac{\text{TP}}{\text{TP} + \text{FP}} * 100\% \tag{6.3}$$

Table 6.1 Accuracy by Support Vector Machine and Convolution Neural Network

No of iterations	Support Vector Machine accuracy %	Convolution Neural Network accuracy %
10	86.19	88.74
20	86.59	88.92
30	87.96	89.12
40	88.02	89.54
50	88.64	89.93

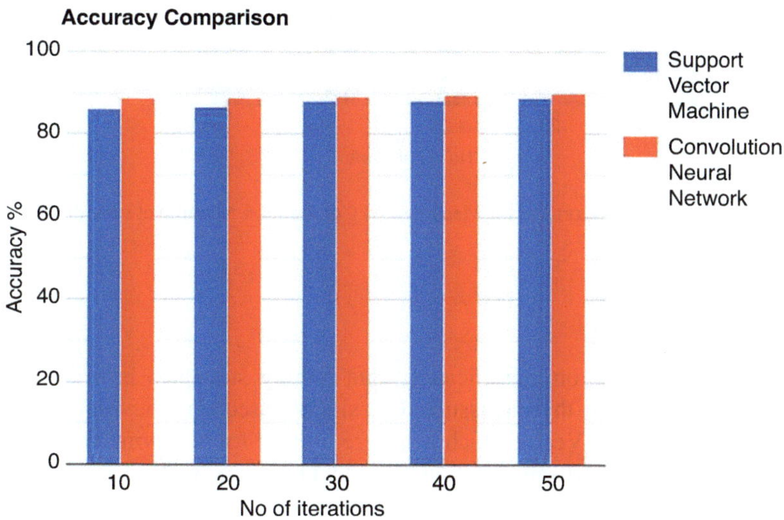

Fig. 6.1 Accuracy by Support Vector Machine and Convolution Neural Network graph

Table 6.2 Precision by Support Vector Machine and Convolution Neural Network

No of iterations	Support Vector Machine precision %	Convolution Neural Network precision %
10	84.92	86.94
20	85.33	87.19
30	85.72	87.46
40	86.12	88.02
50	86.70	88.54

Table 6.2 and Fig 6.2 show the precision obtained from the dataset by Support Vector Machine and Convolution Neural Network. It clearly shows that convolution neural networks perform better than support vector machines in terms of precision.

Here are the outcomes of research comparing the diagnostic ability of feature-based ML and DL algorithms. In comparison to the SVM classifier, the CNN classifier showed an improvement in precision and accuracy.

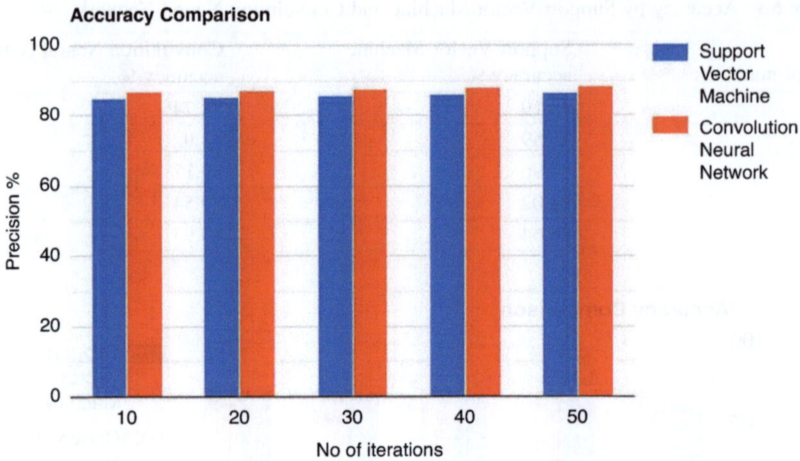

Fig. 6.2 Precision by Support Vector Machine and Convolution Neural Network graph

6.5 Conclusion

The researchers relied on classification data mining strategies in order to locate patients suffering from thyroid issues. Classifiers based on Convolutional Neural Networks and Support Vector Machines were utilised for achieving this. The CNN classifier had a better performance than the other classifiers, with an accuracy of 89% and a precision of 87%. We were able to make an early diagnosis of the disease, which allowed us to implement preventative measures that were both timely and cost-effective, thereby lowering the likelihood of making a mistake due to human error. The accuracy with which cancer is detected might also be improved through the application of this research. As a consequence, this line of work has a promising future ahead of it because the manual prediction process can be simply and inexpensively changed into computerised manufacturing.

References

1. Chen, H., Yang, B., Liu, J., Chen, Y.-D., & Liu, D.-Y. (2011). A three-stage expert system based on support vector machines for thyroid disease diagnosis. *Journal of Medical Systems, 36*, 1953–1963.
2. Nageswari, S., Vimal, M. N., Raveena, C., Sharma, J., & Yasodha, M. (2004). An identification and classification of thyroid diseases using deep learning methodology. *RevistaGestãoInovaçãoe Tecnologias., 11*, 10.47059/revistageintec.v11i2.1820.
3. Borzouei, S., Mahjub, H., Sajadi, N. A., & Farhadian, M. (2020). Diagnosing thyroid disorders: Comparison of logistic regression and neural network models. *Journal of Family Medicine and Primary Care, 9*, 1470. https://doi.org/10.4103/jfmpc.jfmpc_910_19

4. Bini, F., Pica, A., Azzimonti, L., Giusti, A., Ruinelli, L., Marinozzi, F., & Trimboli, P. (2021). Artificial intelligence in thyroid field. A comprehensive review. *Cancers, 13*, 4740. https://doi.org/10.3390/cancers13194740
5. Vasile, C., (Ion) Udristoiu, A., Ghenea, A., Popescu, M., Udristoiu, S., Gruionu, G., Gruionu, L., Iacob, A., & Alexandru, D. (2021). Intelligent diagnosis of thyroid ultrasound imaging using an ensemble of deep learning methods. *Medicina, 57*(4), 395. https://doi.org/10.3390/medicina57040395
6. Makas, H., & Yumusak, N. (2013). A comprehensive study on thyroid diagnosis by neural networks and swarm intelligence. In *2013 International Conference on Electronics, Computer and Computation, ICECCO* (pp. 180–183). https://doi.org/10.1109/ICECCO.2013.6718258.
7. Peng, S., Liu, Y., Lv, W., Liu, L., Zhou, Q., Yang, H., Ren, J., Liu, G., Wang, X., Zhang, X., Du, Q., Nie, F., Huang, G., Guo, Y., Li, J., Liang, J., Hu, H., Xiao, H., Liu, Z.-L., & Xiao, H. (2021). Deep learning-based artificial intelligence model to assist thyroid nodule diagnosis and management: A multicentre diagnostic study. *The Lancet Digital Health, 3*, e250–e259. https://doi.org/10.1016/S2589-7500(21)00041-8
8. Wang, Y., Guan, Q., Lao, I., Wang, L., Wu, Y., Li, D., Ji, Q., Wang, Y., Zhu, Y., Lu, H., & Xiang, J. (2019). Using deep convolutional neural networks for multi-classification of thyroid tumor by histopathology: A large-scale pilot study. *Annals of Translational Medicine., 7*, 468–468.
9. Mousavi, Z., Mohammadi Zanjireh, M., & Oghbaie, M. (2020). Applying computational classification methods to diagnose Congenital Hypothyroidism: A comparative study. *Informatics in Medicine Unlocked, 18*. https://doi.org/10.1016/j.imu.2019.100281
10. Namdeo, R., & Janardan, G. (2021). Thyroid disorder diagnosis by optimal convolutional neuron based CNN architecture. *Journal of Experimental & Theoretical Artificial Intelligence, 1–20*. https://doi.org/10.1080/0952813X.2021.1938694

Chapter 7
Deep Learning in Healthcare Informatics

Brijeshkumar Y. Panchal, Maharshi Joshi, Riya Kalpit Shah, Jesal Desai, Mohini Darji, and Arkesha Shah

7.1 Introduction

Any system that generates, saves, processes, and displays information is considered to be an informatics system. This field examines the relationship between information systems and their users, as well as the design of the interfaces that connect the two. It uses technology to solve problems in various fields such as storage, retrieval, classification of information, and facilitation of needs of humans. It employs computing as a general purpose tool for resolving issues in different domains, communicating, and expressing ideas.

7.1.1 Healthcare Informatics

In the health sector, health informatics [1] is a critical file because it provides methods and tools for processing and analyzing patient data from various health

B. Y. Panchal (✉)
Computer Engineering Department, Sardar Vallabhbhai Patel Institute of Technology (SVIT), Vasad, Gujarat Technological University (GTU), Ahmedabad, Gujarat, India

M. Joshi · R. K. Shah · J. Desai · M. Darji
Department of Computer Science and Engineering, Devang Patel Institute of Advance Technology and Research (DEPSTAR), Faculty of Technology and Engineering (FTE), Charotar University of Science and Technology (CHARUSAT), Anand, Gujarat, India

A. Shah
Department of Information Technology, Chandubhai S Patel Institute of Technology (CSPIT), Faculty of Technology and Engineering (FTE), Charotar University of Science and Technology (CHARUSAT), Anand, Gujarat, India

F. J. J. Joseph et al. (eds.), *Computational Intelligence for Clinical Diagnosis*, EAI/Springer Innovations in Communication and Computing,
https://doi.org/10.1007/978-3-031-23683-9_7

records and diagnosis reports. There are an extremely wide variety of problems in this particular health domain that can be solved with the help of science and technology and computational techniques. In this field, computers and information sciences are used to assist and advance the medical sector, public health, and the treatment of individual patients. Emerging technology, epidemiology and health management, advanced statistics, and health systems are four important interdisciplinary components of health informatics.

7.1.2 History

Health informatics can be considered as a scientific discipline that has been dealing with information technology in medicine. The concept of health informatics arose in the early 1950s when computer technology was introduced. Earlier they used to tackle healthcare problems with their logic and probabilistic reasoning. For the purpose of reducing mistakes and gaining additional advantages, doctors Lee Lusted and Robert Ledley issued a paper back in 1959 advocating the formalization of statistical approaches for modeling medical decision-making. Professionals in the area quickly understood the need to coin a phrase that would be widely accepted to encompass the intersection of science, engineering, and technology, and this is how the concept of health informatics emerged.

7.1.3 Need of Healthcare Informatics

The role of healthcare informatics is vital in the health sector. The health records will help the healthcare professionals to understand the medical history of the patient so that they can easily diagnose the disease and improve the patient experiment. These will also help to build communication between two different fields that include healthcare professionals and policymakers. Overall, this knowledge will help the community to improve the health sector.

Healthcare informatics has helped to reduce the cost as it is the only means of reducing medical errors in medical history. Medical errors, such as duplicates, mismatches, and allergies in patient data, can be detected by technology, such as Computer Provider Order Entry Systems (CPOE) or Clinical Decision Support Systems (CDSS) [2], saving healthcare organizations a lot of money. With the help of specialization in this field, it has helped the patient to get treatment from different medical professionals regarding various health issues under one stay only as it makes it easy for a healthcare professional to coordinate medical history of the patient. However, the booming of information technology has helped the patients, health sector, insurance companies, and even the government to save time and money. It has helped patients to keep watch on their medical records so that they can follow up easily and plan their treatments accordingly. Encryption means that patients and doctors will no longer have to worry about the security of their personal information being compromised. This boosts patients' confidence in doctors and encourages them to open up more about their medical histories. Health informatics' privacy benefits powered by blockchain are in the verge of becoming a norm.

7.1.4 Growth of Health Informatics

Within the broader science of health informatics, public health informatics is emerging as a new and unique specialization area. Several reports from throughout the world have identified the potential significance of informatics in addressing health inequities in marginalized groups. As a result of India's National Health Policy-2017, healthcare has become more efficient and effective. It is stated in the Indian National Health Policy 2017 (NHP 2017) [3] that a National Digital Health Authority (NDHA) will be established to regulate, develop, and implement digital health across the continuum of care to recognize the critical role of technology in healthcare. In order to assist the wider adoption of digital health in India, the NDHA's first task would be to draft a comprehensive National Digital Health Strategy in conjunction with all relevant parties. However, there is a lack of health information strategy in African countries which will threaten the HIS (Health Information System) [3] governance. The US Bureau of Labor Statistics has consistently reported major growth of jobs in the field. The expected growth is considered to be 13% from 2016 to 2026 which is high compared to the average growth. However, the projects related to health informatics will increase to 17% from 2014 to 2024 which is much faster than all other professions. Despite the fact that a health information system (HIS) is a must for any healthcare system, many developing countries still struggle to obtain reliable health data. As a result, they fall well short of the public's expectations when it comes to achieving beneficial health outcomes.

7.2 Deep Learning in Healthcare Informetric

You may wonder what is deep learning and what does it do to healthcare? Deep learning is a subset of machine learning, which is a subset of AI. Following sections will shed light on all of this.

7.2.1 Artificial Intelligence

Artificial intelligence (AI) [4] is a type of program that can mimic human intelligence using neural networks. It is the power of computer to think and act like humans. Neural Network [5] is analogous to neurons in human brain. You do not need to program it explicitly for its functions, it can learn on its own like humans. Artificial intelligence works on its subsets such as machine learning and deep learning which we will discuss further. Not all AI applications are similar, there are seven types of artificial intelligence which are categorized into two types:

1. Type-1 on basis of functionality
2. Type-2 on basis of capabilities

Type-1

1. *Reactive machine:* It is the most basic type of AI system which is solely reactive. They do not possess the ability to learn from past experiences to predict future actions. Take, for example, IBM's Deep Blue chess computer, which in the late 1990s defeated world chess champion Garry Kasparov.
2. *Insufficient memory:* Systems that can see back in time are included in this category. The best illustration of this is self-driving cars, which can keep tab on the speed and direction of other cars on the road. Identifying and tracking certain entities over time is required; this is not something that can be done in a flash.
3. *Theory of mind:* It is a psychological term, which means understanding of humans and other creatures which possess thought and emotions that can change the behavior. This is about future machines which can understand humans and emotions.
4. *Self-awareness:* This is expansion of "theory of mind" which states that to build AI such that they have the power to form representations about itself. For example, let us take statements such as "I want this" and "I know I want this"; both statements mean the same thing but in the second statement one is aware of oneself. The goal is to create AI which knows about itself.

Type-2

1. *Artificial narrow intelligence (ANI):* Majority of all AI applications fall under this category. It includes the systems that can perform specific tasks for which it was designed. It cannot perform tasks for which it was not programmed. For example, AI application to predict Stock Price cannot predict other tasks such as predicting weather as it was specifically designed to predict stocks. ANI is a blend of all-reactive and limited-memory artificial intelligence.
2. *Artificial general intelligence (AGI):* Similar to how humans learn and complete tasks, AI with AGI can do so. These systems have multifunctional capabilities that span a variety of fields. Progress has been made in this area despite the fact that no specific application has yet been developed [6].
3. *Artificial super intelligence (ASI):* AI technology will reach its zenith with ASI [7]. One of the most advanced artificial intelligence systems ever created is yet to be produced. Due of its greater memory and decision-making powers, it will be able to outperform humans in every aspect of life. There is concern among some academics that ASI may lead to unchecked technological growth, which could be harmful to human society as a whole.

7.2.2 Machine Learning

Machine learning is a branch of AI and data science that focuses on simulating human learning with data and algorithms. The goal is to improve accuracy over time. It was first mentioned in a research paper by Arthur Samuel [8]. It learns from present data to predict future data, for instance, YouTube's recommendation algorithm, it recommends us videos based on our previous viewing. It has three methods for learning:

1. *Supervised Learning:* In this type of ML model, we provide data with labels to predict outcomes. As more data is introduced into the model, the weights are adjusted to properly fit. For instance, spam email can be detected from your inbox by learning from previous data. It has certain algorithms to learn from data, such as Linear Regression, Random Forest, and Support Vector Machine (SVM) (Fig. 7.1).
2. *Unsupervised Learning:* It is a given data without labels, it analyses data by discovering patterns in the data. As it analyses patterns, it is useful for data analysis and picture recognition. To decrease the number of features and dimensions, it uses two methods: singular value decomposition (SVD) and principal component analysis (PCA). Unsupervised learning employs neural networks, k-means clustering, probabilistic clustering techniques, and other algorithms (Fig. 7.2).
3. *Reinforcement Learning:* No samples are needed to train reinforcement machine learning, which is a form of behavioral learning technique similar to supervised learning. Iterative learning is how this model picks up new skills. It is only after a string of successful outcomes has been established that the most appropriate advice or strategy can be determined.

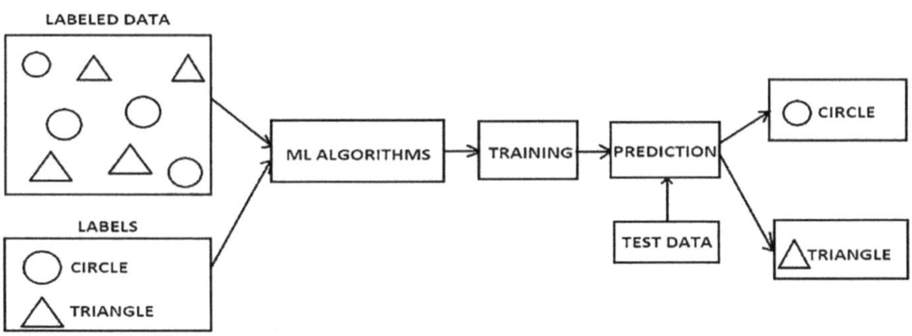

Fig. 7.1 Supervised machine learning [8]

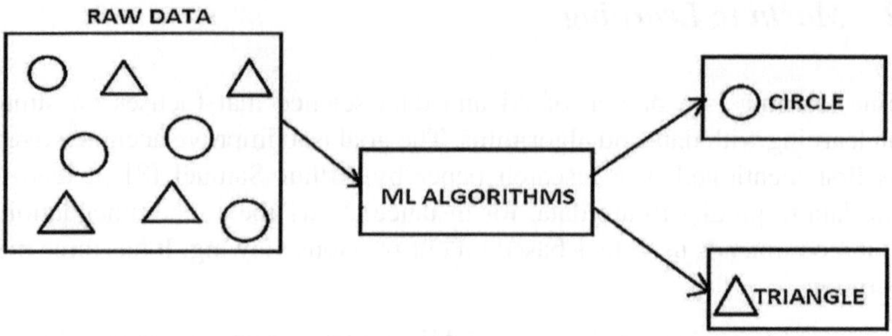

Fig. 7.2 Unsupervised machine learning [8]

7.2.3 Deep Learning

Deep learning is a technique of machine learning and artificial intelligence. Deep learning works with statistical and other mathematical algorithms. It requires processing enormous amount of data. It has certain methods for learning like machine learning. Inquiring minds may be wondering how deep learning differs from machine learning? In machine learning you have to pre-process data in deep learning while there is no need to pre-process data. The best example of deep learning is NVidia's Deep Learning Super Sampling (DLSS) [9] which uses deep learning to upscale image from lower resolution to higher resolution. This technique has been implemented in video games to improve performance.

7.2.3.1 Working of Deep Learning

There may be several layers of neurons in a deep learning module. There are three layers in a deep learning module: input layer, hidden layer, output layer. The hidden layer contains neurons which have some weight which determines the output. When you want to predict outcomes from your model, you need to train it with data following certain methods. It has two methods like ML: supervised and unsupervised. Any method can be used to train depending on your application. We use neural network to make the model work. In a neural network, there are many interconnected neurons just like a human brain. Each neuron carries some weight (values). This method was inspired by human brain where neurons send signals to each other. It works in a similar manner; the neurons pass some value and some function is activated. The values/weight of neuron will depend on its correlation factor. If some factor is more dependent on the outcome, it may have higher weight. As input data is passed through these layers, the output is calculated (Fig. 7.3).

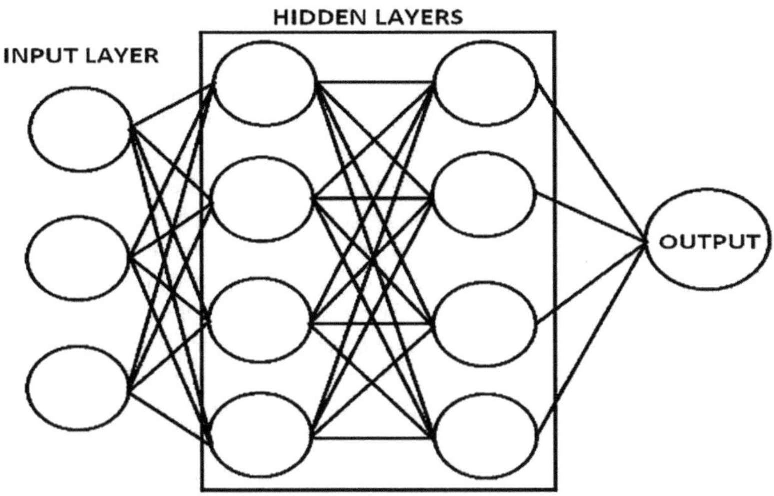

Fig. 7.3 Several layers of neurons [9]

7.2.3.2 Types of Neural Networks

1. Convolutional neural networks (CNNs): It can recognize patterns and attributes inside a picture, allowing it to perform tasks such as object detection and recognition. It is widely used in picture categorization and computer vision applications. In 2015, a CNN outperformed a human in an object recognition challenge for the first time [10]. This could be valuable for medical picture analysis in computer-aided diagnosis in healthcare informatics.
2. Recurrent neural networks (RNNs): RNNs are extensively used in natural language processing (NLP) and speech recognition applications because they use sequential or time series data. It uses the output from the previous step as input, and it contains a memory to keep track of prior results. The output and input of an RNN are normally independent, although it must remember the prior output in specific instances. When we're processing, for example, it needs to remember prior output in order to forecast the next word in a sentence. It is particularly beneficial in healthcare for making diagnosis based on the user's complaints [11–12].

7.3 Deep Learning Applications in Electronics Healthcare Report

For years, deep learning has been used in a wide range of industries, and it is always evolving. We have made a huge progress in deep learning. Deep learning is very useful in healthcare. Now you may wonder, how can deep learning be helpful in the field of healthcare. Here are some applications for it.

7.3.1 Deep Learning for COVID-19 Pandemic

During COVID-19 pandemic many people lost their lives. Deep learning can be helpful in checking if a person is infected by checking their CT scan. Let us say we have all data of patient in one centralized location. We can create a deep learning model from data of other patients who were infected earlier. So, by using deep learning we do not need to do RT-PCR (Reverse Transcription-Polymerase Chain Reaction) test which takes a long time to get result but using deep learning can be much faster and efficient than traditional RT-PCR test. It can also predict other aspects such as the chances of survival. We will need millions of data to make this model accurate. It can be used not only to predict infection but it can also be used for research purpose. It can be used to study how the virus is working. It has less chances of getting false results as CT scan is also taken into consideration. Yet, there are disadvantages to CT scan for COVID are there. CT scan can be harmful if it is done multiple times. The chances of spreading the disease are more. CT scan is costlier than RT-PCR. However, it is being used and is developing every day.

7.3.2 Deep Learning for Predicting Diagnosis in Patients

Data can predict what a disease or disorder of a patient based on the symptoms. It can be achieved by analyzing data of patients. This can create an AI doctor [13]. Natural language processing is used for this purpose (Fig. 7.4).

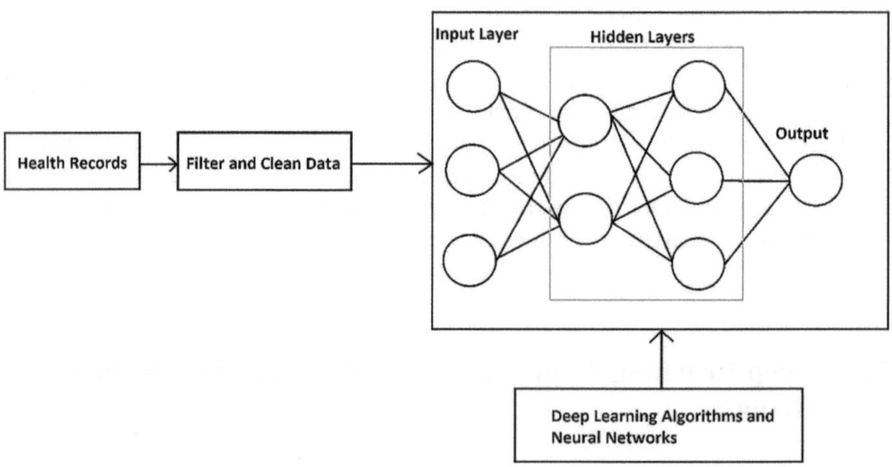

Fig. 7.4 Example of deep learning [11]

NLP is a program that can understand text or audio just as human beings do. A patient's symptoms are processed through NLP and by using data from patients, the disease can be analyzed. This is done by creating Recurrent Neural Network and feeding it into the healthcare records. Significant progress has been made in this field. There project is named Doctor AI which can be found on GitHub, and it has around 72% accuracy. This is being used on small scale as of now, but it can provide assistance to doctors. It can also analyze patient's data and store it in EHR directly; it can provide insights to doctor about what kind of treatment the patient needs. Now, you may wonder if these deep learning models can replace doctors? The answer to this question is no, because we cannot create super accurate doctor AI with 100% accuracy, and even if we could, it would require tremendous amount of computing power that we have now. Obviously, it cannot replace doctors, but will assist them.

7.3.3 Deep Learning for Predicting Chances of Heart Diseases

Heart diseases generally come at advanced age. If a patient's family has history of any heart-related disease, then there are chances that a person can also have it. For this purpose, data such as cholesterol level, cardiogram, blood pressure, age, and blood count are considered. We can create and train model with these features. This can be predicted by using deep learning model and health records of all members in the family. We can predict when a person is likely to be affected by heart disease in future so doctor can treat them accordingly. This is similar to Doctor AI (Fig. 7.5).

There are tons of applications of deep learning in EHR, and the basic aim is to predict something or analyze data. It can be also used to analyze data so is helpful for research purpose. Scientists have created a robot that can perform surgery using deep learning algorithms. Our aim is to make progress in healthcare by taking advantage of deep learning.

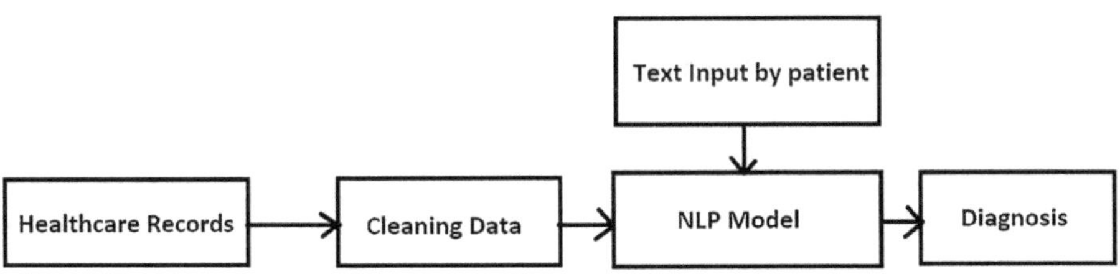

Fig. 7.5 Example of NLP [12]

7.4 Application of Deep Learning in Medical Tourism

7.4.1 Medical Tourism

The act of going outside one's own country to get medical treatment is called medical tourism. This involves person going from developing country to developed countries for medical treatment. There are several reasons why a person would travel to another country for medical treatment. For instance, it may be due to lack of skilled doctors, surgeons, etc., or it may cost more in their country of origin. Following are some applications of deep learning in medical tourism:

7.4.2 Electronic Health Records

It is the system of storing patients' data in digital format. Patients' medical histories, medications, and treatment plans are all included in this document. It can be accessed from anywhere. This will help increasing medical tourism. EHR will help doctors in other countries to know the patient's medical history. The adoption of IT and ICT in healthcare, particularly in medical tourism, is aided by the development of EHR platforms and applications, as well as Medical Registries at the patient level. We can feed this data to deep learning algorithms to predict diseases, proper medications, the population going to medical tourism in upcoming years, etc. We can feed data, such as age, country, diseases, medications, and prescription, to get the outcomes. It can also help classify data using DL algorithms. It can help in identifying hidden patterns in data which we cannot see. With computer-aided vision we can identify problems using medical images such as X-rays, MRI, and CT scans. The benefit of deep learning in EHR is that we can train model for many programs as all data is a click away. Deep learning can also be used for analyzing large datasets from EHR, so administrators can predict analytics such as the number of people who will get a certain disease in future. Some countries have different standards of health records; by using deep learning, we can make them work with other country's health record. We can use automatic feature extraction to accomplish this. These are some ways in which we can use deep learning in EHR system.

7.4.3 Electronic Health Card

It is a system in which information of patients is stored in a card such as your license which is valid document. It is of two types: administrative and medical. In the administrative category, it contains data such as prescriptions, insurance status, abroad treatment rights. In medical category, it contains data for which the patient has given permission to be shared, drug information, demographics, etc. All

European Union countries have implemented the Electronic Health Card, which is now operational in facilitating medical tourism and boosting patients' degree of decision. With the use of health card, we can predict many things, such as predicting the cost of treatment. Deep learning can predict chances of a person getting a certain disease by training the model with datasets from health cards of people. It uses methods like automatic feature extraction, regression methods, neural networks to predict outcomes. Now we feed the data from health card to model and make predictions from input. These techniques are also used in EHR for prediction as health card is also a part of the EHR system.

7.4.4 Telemedicine

It is the technology used to treat or monitor a patient from anywhere in the world. In locations where doctors are few, telemedicine is becoming more popular. For example, the usage of telemedicine in medical tourism, as well as the aspirations of healthcare executives regarding service model costs and the importance of health promotion and prevention. In the medical tourism industry, a patient from another nation might get valuable information about his health status through a tele-consultation with a physician and choose the best treatment alternatives for their travel itinerary. Deep learning can help by providing advice to patients over network. There are many websites featuring this. We can make bots on web with which we can talk with patients and provide them suitable advice. This can be done by making natural language processing (NLP) [12] using Recurrent Neural Network (RNN). We can use NLP to build a model that can decipher what a patient says.

7.4.5 Virtual Social Network

It is one of the oldest forms of tourism. It is designed to assist travelers for a better experience before, during, and after their trip. Virtual medical tourism will facilitate communication between visitors and healthcare providers. It includes social groups, web forums, channels, and Q/A system, which are examples of virtual communication systems. Today, there are many platforms for virtual social networks. You can consult a doctor overseas on many websites. Thus, making communication easier and efficient for medical tourism. There are many web forums available; we can use deep learning to check if the given information is correct or not. Thus, people can be saved from frauds and scams. We can integrate a deep learning model into a web forum so that it can moderate things. If a person posts wrong information or false claims, it will detect them and mark it as scam. This is very similar to scam email detector in email systems. We can also develop a chat bot in these forums using deep learning algorithms. These are some of the ways in which we can use deep learning in virtual social network [13].

7.4.6 Data Mining and Knowledge Discovery

The practice of processing massive datasets to scan and extract previously unknown patterns or correlations in order to develop knowledge for making decision. When an EHR system is combined with analytical tools, it gives useful insights to doctors to analyze a patient problem, and patients can know of cost-effective treatments without going anywhere. This is done by using deep learning algorithms. We will train the DL model using datasets of patients and their medical history. We can include data such as last visit, cost of treatment, medications, demographics, and country of residence to predict features like total cost of treatment, chances of successful treatment, and many more things.

7.4.7 Medical Tourism Recommender System (RS) and Decision Support System (DSS)

It is used to provide travel advice to tourists. It is implemented on various platforms such as the internet, mobile, ranking systems, and scheduling systems. This has reduced overload of information. It can give recommendation on which place is better for a certain treatment or recommends what kind of treatment one will need. These systems use deep learning modules such as recommendation systems and providing advice. In this, deep learning uses Convolutional Neural Network to generate advice and recommendations by training it with dataset of patients. These are some of the applications of deep learning in medical tourism.

7.5 Deep Learning Techniques Used in Health Informatics

It is possible for deep learning models to use medical images such as X-rays, MRI scans, and CT scans to provide accurate diagnoses. Algorithms may be able to detect any risk or anomalies in medical images. When it comes to cancer detection, deep learning is frequently used.

7.5.1 Real-Time Monitoring of Patient Health Information Simulation

Sensor-based cloud apps can capture real-time user data for monitoring and tracking purposes in a public space, such as a park, garden, or other public area. Our standard device for tracking users' whereabouts and health status is designed to help in times of crisis. A proper service cloud has been prepared and queries dispatched to deal with the nature of these emergencies. When a server-side system framework received an automated alarm for monitoring purposes, a rescue squad was dispatched to the scene. Latitude and longitude coordinates are used to track the user's location. There are multiple upper and lower threshold values that can be utilized to monitor the health of users with the new method. Inconsistencies in a user's data are automatically flagged by the system and sent to the user. To ensure the safety of our users as well as the efficiency of our system design, we have implemented a sensor device, a cloud-based data storage system (such as Google Big Query), and social media for monitoring purposes. The process of providing healthcare services is broken down into three distinct and sequential phases, as well as a number of methodological components. This is the first step in creating a decision matrix (DM) [14] that utilizes the crossover between "multi-healthcare services" and "hospital list" in an intelligent data and service management center [15] (Tier 4). The creation of a DM for hospital selection based on combined VIKOR-Analytic Hierarchy Process (AHP) approaches is discussed in the second part. Finally, the validation procedure for the proposed framework is examined. The figure given below explains the flow of how the Real-Time Monitoring is useful in the health informatics and how it works.

7.5.2 *Convolutional Neural Networks for Multimedia Medical Image Retrieval*

As the healthcare industry and hospitals expand, massive archiving databases are being used to save diagnostic test findings for treatment and future research. Data is becoming increasingly unmanageable for doctors to deal with on a daily basis due to the increasing number of patients. Medical picture annotation is a time-consuming process that might be affected by the diagnostician's language proficiency and therefore takes longer than expected. Faster diagnosis is achievable because of a powerful image retrieval system that can manage these big and complex picture sets. Content-based image retrieval (CBIR) analyses an image's content properties such as color and texture instead of utilizing textual descriptions. Machine learning techniques are becoming more prominent as a means of conducting complicated calculations in big databases. Convolutional neural networks (CNNs) and their mathematics are briefly discussed in this chapter, focusing on the state-of-the-art designs such as LeNet and AlexNet [16] (Fig. 7.6).

Medical image networks (MINs) and deep learning frameworks are used to assess and compare the performance of the content-based multimodality image retrieval system (CBMMIR) [17]. Data from seven different types of imaging are fed into the training model, and the derived features from the model are then used to get a multimodal dataset. Both the training and query images were sent into the CNN for feature extraction. It was determined by comparing the training and query characteristics using Euclidean distances. Iterational accuracy from the trained model,

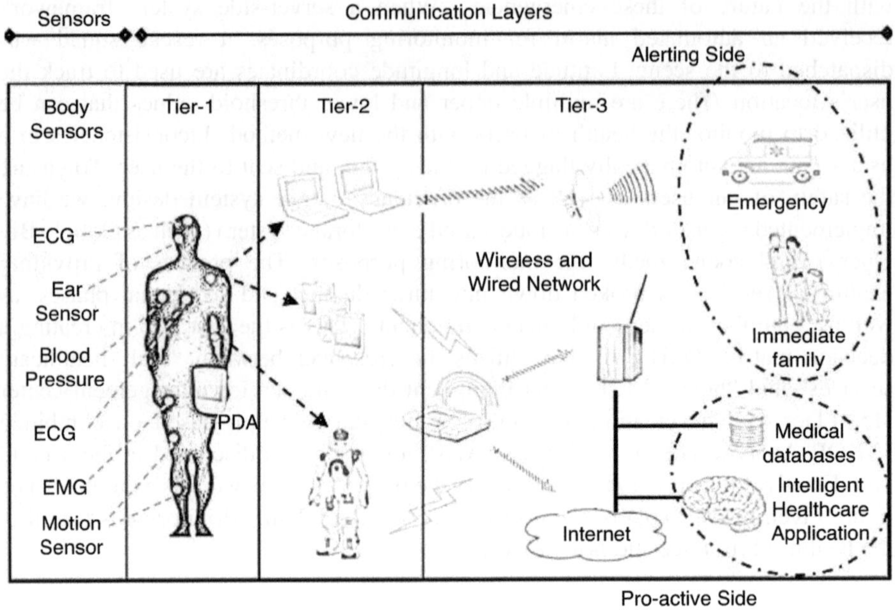

Fig. 7.6 Remote health monitoring system [16]

retrieval time, precision, recall, F score, and mean average precision are among the evaluation criteria determined by this experiment (MAP). The trained algorithm finds images that are similar to the query image in terms of modality and anatomy. In AlexNet and LeNet's MAPS, 83.9% and 86.9%, respectively, are their respective MAPS. Finally, the chapter will assess the pros and cons of the two design approaches. In the graphic shown below, deep learning in medical imaging is presented.

7.5.3 *Medical Big Data Optimization Through Deep Learning Techniques*

Over time, medical institutions are learning to navigate a dynamic and complicated environment in which scientific discoveries and new medical delivery model commercial models are the major variables. It is the primary goal of any medical professional to provide world-class care to each and every patient (Fig. 7.7).

Medical science is becoming more and more complicated and expensive and achieving its ultimate goal is a huge challenge. There are several applications of deep learning (DL) techniques in a wide range of scientific fields, from speech recognition to image processing to categorization. Additionally, when dealing with large amounts of data, standard data analysis and processing methods have a number of

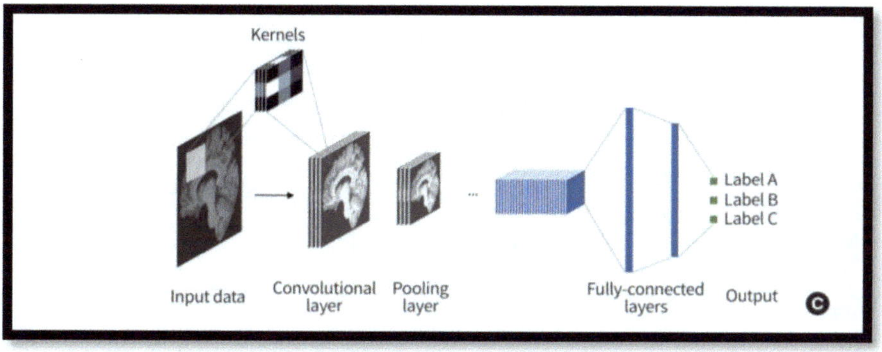

Fig. 7.7 Medical image analysis [17]

drawbacks. Deep learning and big data analytics are popular in the field of medical science right now. Big data is becoming increasingly relevant in the medical industry due to the large volumes of data that have been amassed. Innovative medical science delivery strategies and groundbreaking research are made possible by the ability to work with massive amounts of data. There is therefore a considerable presence in specialized contexts, such as medical and massive data machine learning landscapes, of existing deep learning algorithms used in generic settings. Human involvement in developing algorithms for big data and deep learning in medicine is also a contributing fact to bad results.

7.5.4 Melanoma Detection and Staging Can Be Automated Using Deep Learning in Histopathological Image Analysis

Pathology images can now be analyzed quantitatively for disease diagnosis and elucidation because of advancements in digital microscopy. In order to make digital whole slide images (WSI), a high-resolution slide scanner is used. Hematoxylin and eosin are commonly used to stain the slides (H&E). MART-1 (for melanoma) and PD-L1 (for lung cancer) are examples of immuno-specific stains that may be used to confirm a diagnosis. Lymph veins carry cancer cells to lymph nodes in advanced stages. A lymph node biopsy is therefore commonly performed to determine if the malignancy has progressed to the lymph nodes (Fig. 7.8).

WSIs with a high pixel count can contain billions of pixels. Preprocessing, segmentation, feature extraction, and classifications are some of the more traditional image analysis modules. Histopathology images have recently been successfully analyzed using deep learning algorithms such as SegNet and U-Net [18]. Melanoma detection and proliferation index computation using deep learning networks are described in detail and compared to traditional feature-based approaches. Testing shows that DNNs are superior to DNNs in terms of learning speed (Fig. 7.9).

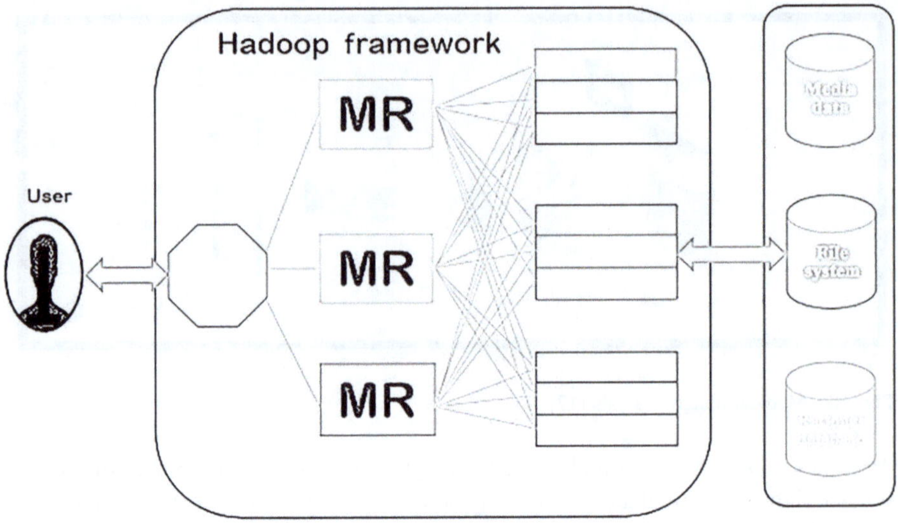

Fig. 7.8 Deep learning improves medical big data [18]

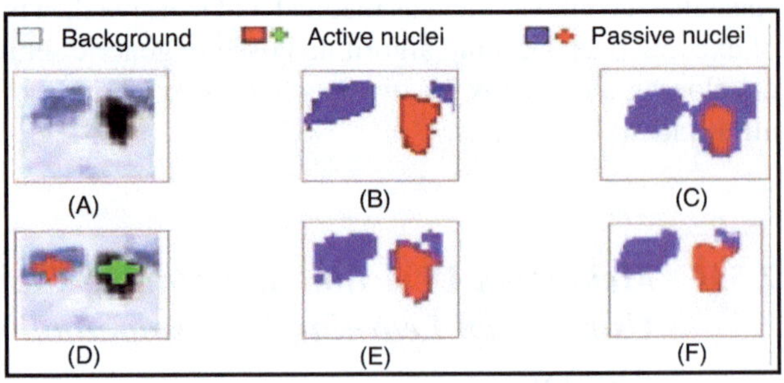

Fig. 7.9 (**a**) Original test image, (**b**) the ground truth image (**c**) FCM+KM [19], (**d**) Otsu+ SVM [20], (**e**) GMM+CNN [21], and (**f**) PI-SegNet [22]

7.5.5 Deep Learning-Based Approach in Identification of Cardiac Disease

Damage or obstruction to the heart muscle, valves, rhythm, and arteries can occur as a result of cardiovascular disease. As the leading cause of sudden mortality in humans, early detection is critical. The electrocardiogram (ECG) is the most frequent biological signal used by cardiologists to diagnose cardiovascular disease (ECG). Cardiac disease diagnosis can be improved with the help of ECG signal classification. Traditional machine learning and deep learning techniques have been used in the literature to automatically classify ECG readings. Traditional methods of machine learning necessitate the use of carefully designed attributes. Just some of the characteristics provided include morphological feature extraction, RR interval computation, QRS peak identification, ST segment, ST distance, and amplitude computation, among others. Deep - learning techniques extract features from training data, which exceed features created by typical machine - learning algorithms in terms of performance. Cutting-edge architectures include CNN, RNN, LSTM, and gated recurrent units (GRU). Existing architectures take a disease-by-disease approach. With the help of ECG and a transferable methodology, the goal of this chapter is to give a consistent framework for classifying cardiac illness. Using current deep - learning architectures such as CNN, LSTM, RNN, and GRU to classify heart disease in ECG signals is how we want to go about this. The proposed methodology was evaluated using precision, recall, and F1 score. In comparison to RNN and CNN, we discovered that LSTM and GRU performed well. For all three disorders, LSTM and GRU yield the highest precision and recall score, which ranges from 0.97 to 0.98. When compared to RNN, GRU has a lower computational cost. Deep learning architectures can be transferred, as our research shows. Contrary to deep learning, which is a process driven by data, machine- learning algorithms are neither configurable nor transferable. Different machine- learning techniques such as Naive Bayes, K-next neighbor, SVMs with RBF and linear kernels, random forest, decision tree, and logistic regression are compared for each of the three diseases studied in the article.

7.6 Security Issues and Challenges in Healthcare Informatics

Various approaches have been proposed for resolving confidentiality and security issues in the DL. To combat an adversarial attack on DL, a slew of defenses have been developed. These can be divided into three categories: input pre-processing, malware detection, and strengthening the model's robustness. Prior processing is designed to decrease the impact of immunity on a model by executing operations such as image transformation, randomization, and denoising that often do not require the model to be modified or retrained. For example, feature denoising, adversarial training, and regulation can be used to improve the model's robustness by requiring the model to be modified or retrained. Stateful detection, image transformation detection, and adaptive denoising detection are examples of third-category detection mechanisms that can be implemented before the first layer of the model (Fig. 7.10).

7.6.1 Control of Security Issues in Deep Learning

A number of defense techniques against deep learning security issues were identified and categorized.

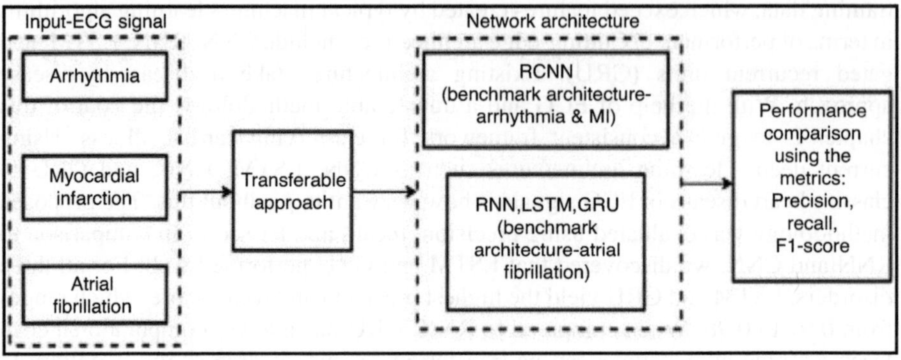

Fig. 7.10 Transferable approach for cardiac disease classification using deep learning [22]

7.6.1.1 Evasion Attacks Defense

Confrontation is the most effective defense against an evasive attack, but it is also the most time-consuming and difficult to implement.

7.6.1.1.1 Detecting Adversarial Examples

Various strategies were given by the researchers in order to recognize and create different benign and hostile samples in the input. The fundamental issue with detecting hostile examples is that the testing example used to forecast the adversarial example is imprecise and difficult to handle. In order to recognize an adversarial example, it is impossible for a human to manually mark the label. Using testing examples and the template for testing examples, Meng and Chen provided a method for verifying hostile examples. Once this operation is complete, the classifier will treat the testing sample as a Deep Neural Network.

7.6.1.1.2 Adversarial Training

The author suggested training benign instances against each training adversarial example in order to counter the evasion attempt. By comparing the initial benign and attack adversarial examples, the system learner will be able to build a deep understanding of the Deep Neural Network through backpropagation learning.

7.6.1.1.3 Defensive Distillation

According to their research, Deep Neural Network Training might be accomplished using a distillation-based technique developed by Sethi et al. A Deep Neural Network generates a set of confidence ratings for each training example. In addition, when hostile instances generated in purified Deep Neural Network are slightly greater than in non-Deep Neural Network, noise is added as a positive example.

7.6.2 *Poisoning Attack Defense*

Then, the authors remove any points that are not close enough to the main point of interest. A slab defense and defensive field that eliminates points outside the ball's radius are utilized to gather information. By modifying the attack label, an attacker/hacker can influence training point distribution. The author also describes reclassifying sites outside the resolution's scope. The exterior outcome can also be calculated in a variety of ways. The impact functions are said to be used to follow the model's predictions and locate the most convincing data points responsible for the supplied projection.

7.6.3 *Deep Learning Privacy Preserving Techniques*

Cryptographic primitives that are being used by organizations to protect the privacy of Deep Neural Networks (DNNs) will be explored in the following section.

7.6.3.1 Homomorphic Encryption (HE)

A party can encode data using Homomorphic Encryption (HE) before delivering it to another party. HE-256 uses basic HE encryption. Fully and partially homomorphic encryption exist. Homomorphic Encryption Scheme (Enc) [23] employs this equation. Over time, researchers developed a comprehensive Homomorphic Encryption method that could be applied on any data, allowing complicated computations.

7.6.3.2 Garbled Circuits (GCS)

Yao's [23] garbled circuit approach can be used to establish a secure two-party system and design an arbitrary Boolean function without revealing input information. One party encrypts the circuit while the other computes its output without knowing its value or information. Second party decrypts each first-party encrypted gate.

7.6.3.3 Goldreich Micali Wigderson (GMW)

It was designed in 1987 with the purpose of evaluating a circuit's wire values using a secure linear secret sharing method that is generic in nature. The linear complexity of the circuit is utilized since all AND gates are handled individually and in parallel.

7.6.3.4 Differential Privacy (DP)

An entry's "DP" is the amount of information that a database query discloses. It is important to keep the database's statistical properties intact when each data point is affected by the addition of more noise.

7.6.3.5 Share Secret (SS)

No information or data concerning the secret is published, but it may be put together from the posts. Choosing a random sample and creating a final message with the secret value communicates the secret.

7.6.4 Challenges and Opportunities

- The practical application of deep learning in healthcare faces a number of hurdles despite the encouraging findings gained utilizing deep architectures.
- *Datavolume:* A group of computationally demanding models is referred to as "deep learning." It follows that in order to train an effective and robust deep learning model, large amount of medical data would be required compared to other media.
- *Dataquality:* Data in the healthcare industry, in contrast to that found in other industries and fields, is often unstructured, unclear, and noisy. A good deep learning model is challenging to train with such big and diverse datasets because of factors such as sparsity, redundancy, and missing values.
- *Temporality:* It is impossible to predict how an illness will progress or change over time. For this reason, static vector-based inputs, such as those used by existing deep learning models in the medical field, are often used. An important component that necessitates the creation of new solutions is the design of deep learning algorithms that can handle time-varying healthcare data.
- *Domain complexity*: It is not feasible to request as many patients as we want in a healthcare setting because space is often at a premium.
- *Interpretability*: There has been a lot of success with deep learning models, but they are still viewed as black boxes by the general public. For healthcare, the

quantitative algorithmic performance as well as the rationale of the algorithmic work is important. This may not be an issue for more deterministic domains such as photo annotation.

- *Feature enrichment:* An essential and difficult research problem would be how to effectively integrate and utilize such diverse inputs in a deep learning model. In order to achieve a holistic abstraction of patient data, a solution in this area might take advantage of the hierarchical nature of deep learning and process each data source individually using the appropriate deep learning model (e.g., using layers of AEs or deep Bayesian networks).
- *Federated inference:* It is vital to note that this federated context necessitates the development of secure methods for learning deep models in a federated manner (e.g., homomorphic encryption and secure multiparty computation).
- *Model privacy*: Scaling deep learning creates privacy concerns. Current research has pushed the boundaries in this field to preserve the privacy of deep learning models. Given how much personal information deep models in clinical applications are projected to process, next-generation healthcare solutions must take these hazards into consideration and design a differential privacy policy.
- *Incorporating expert knowledge:* Semi-supervised learning, a method that uses only small number of labeled samples to learn from big unlabeled ones, has a lot of promise because it can use both labeled and unlabeled samples for the job.
- *Temporal modeling:* Deep learning models that are time-sensitive are critical to assess the patient's state and giving timely clinical decision support in many healthcare-related difficulties, particularly those incorporating electronic medical records and monitoring equipment.
- *Interpretable modeling:* For healthcare issues, model performance and interpretability are of equal importance. But how to communicate these results and make them more intelligible is critical in the development of trustworthy and dependable systems.

7.7 Future of Health Informatics

Between 2014 and 2024, the Bureau of Labor Statistics expects the employment of Health Informaticists to grow by 15%, which is much faster than the average growth of all occupations in the United States. The healthcare industry will make use of a variety of new technology. Patient consultation, physician training, pre-surgical planning, and surgical intervention will all be possible through the use of virtual reality in the future of health informatics, according to the industry. Efforts to improve interoperability in health informatics will have a significant impact on EHR data transfer efficiency in the future.

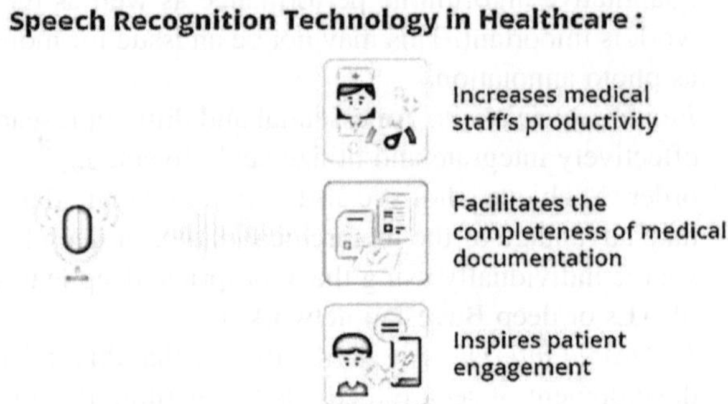

Fig. 7.11 Voice detection in health informative [23]

7.7.1 *Voice Dictation*

Health informaticists are studying AI speech recognition to transcribe healthcare practitioners' notes and directions in real time. This could save healthcare staff's time by minimizing data entry and allowing them to spend more time with patients. Voice transcription has a 7.4% error rate; hence, it faces opposition. Lack of proofreading by clinicians was associated to this error rate. In another study, proofreading reduced errors to 0.3%. Astute and creative health informaticists are needed to produce accurate and efficient voice recognition systems (Fig. 7.11).

7.7.2 *Predictive Analytics*

It is a sort of data analysis used in healthcare to discover indicators of frequent symptoms, diagnosis, processes, and other outcomes through the use of predictive analytics. It is possible to identify 80% of the time if an artificial intelligence software analyses children's speech patterns and compares them with past clinician interviews and parent questionnaires, for example. Predictive analysis can help us identify the disease in its earliest stages, allowing therapy to begin before the patient's health deteriorates (Fig. 7.12).

7.7.3 *EHR Alert Optimization*

One-way instantaneous alerts might benefit patient care is that they can provide healthcare professionals with a wealth of information regarding a wide range of topics such as screenings and drug interactions as well as information about managing long-term conditions such as chronic illness. All of a sudden, nothing seems essential because everything is raising an alert. Alert fatigue, when healthcare workers ignore alarms due to their frequency, is as risky as not having any.

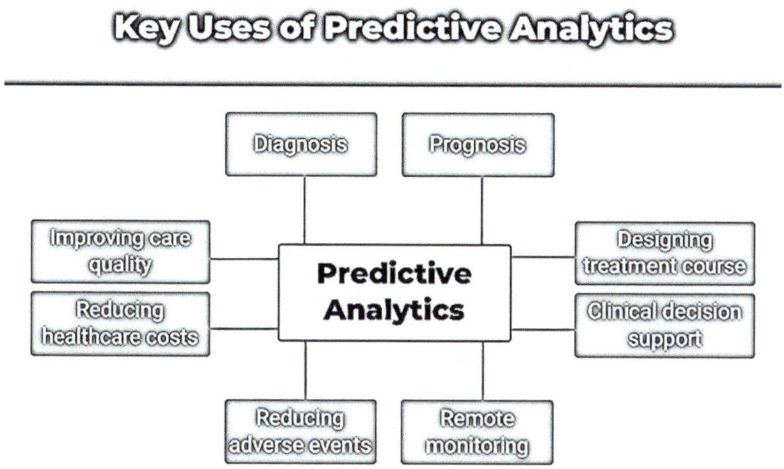

Fig. 7.12 Predictive analysis in health informatics [24]

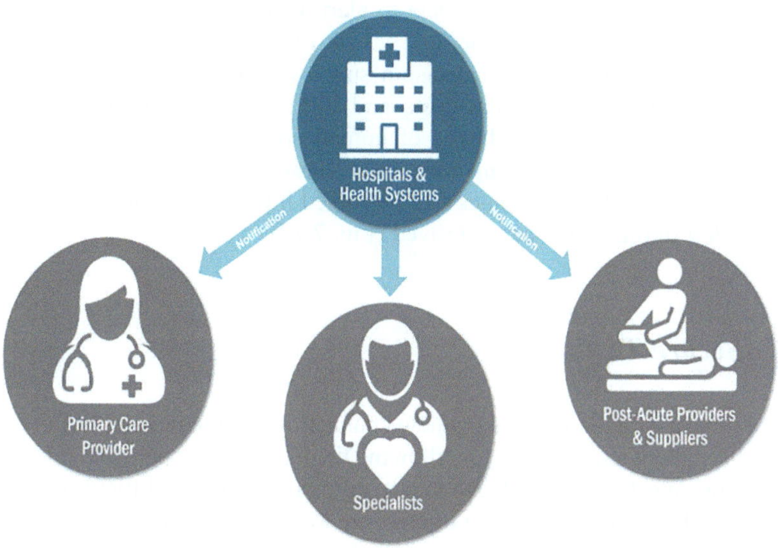

Fig. 7.13 EHR in health informatics [25]

Informaticists are reducing EHR warnings to improve their usefulness. Some of the suggested methods include tailoring warnings to the specific needs of each patient, classifying alerts based on severity, and altering the color or format of alerts to make them more or less apparent as required (Fig. 7.13).

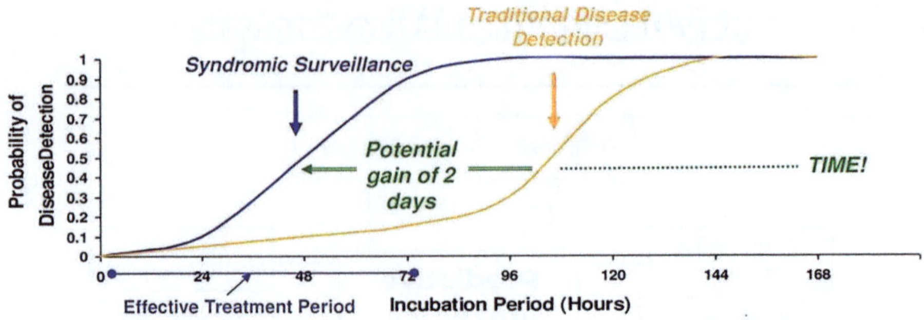

Fig. 7.14 Syndromic surveillance in health informatics [26]

7.7.4 Syndromic Surveillance

In real time, patients can be monitored for potential adverse events using predictive analytics and alarms from their electronic health records. Real-time clinical decision support tools can use the analyzed data to alert doctors to take urgent or cautious action. Poor usability, alert fatigue, and a lack of end-user knowledge hinder the introduction of real-time clinical decision support tools. Using these tools in the future could minimize healthcare costs and difficulties by offering faster, more tailored care, minimizing the chance of human errors, and even boosting public health by rapidly communicating infectious illness diagnoses, for instance. It is anticipated that the latter two issues will be solved if predictive analytics algorithms and EHR alert optimization are improved (Fig. 7.14).

7.7.5 Secure Texting

With the advent of patient portals, a new channel of communication has opened up between the patient and their doctor, allowing them to see their personal information, prescriptions, and lab results. However, many patients find it difficult to regularly access a portal. It has emerged that doctors are looking into ways to send encrypted SMS warnings to their patients, which can be automated and thus save both providers and patients' time. However, securing the safety of those texts is the most challenging part (Fig. 7.15).

7.7.6 Clinical Image Capture

As medical imaging has evolved, so have the data sizes. Imaging can be difficult to retain or access in the EHR after an MRI, CAT scan, X-ray, or other procedure.

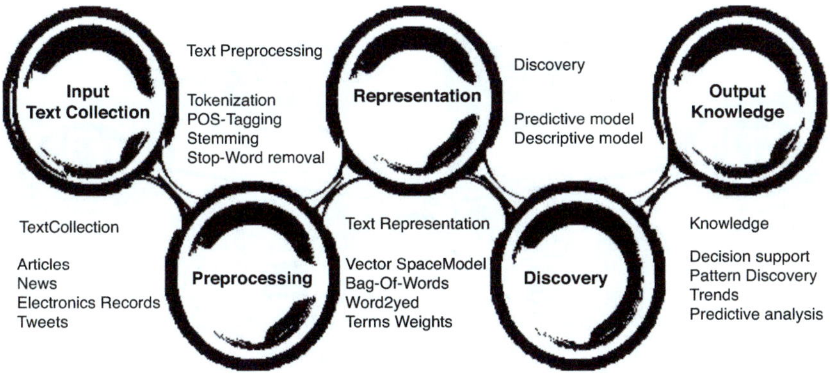

Fig. 7.15 Secure texting useful in health informatics with text mining [27]

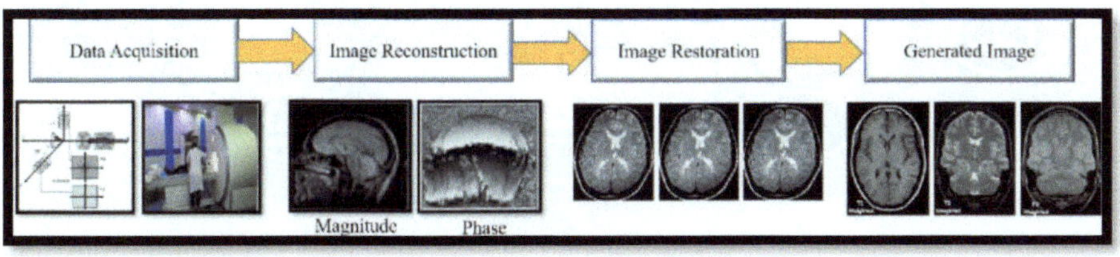

Fig. 7.16 Image capture process helped in health informatics [28]

Depending on its intended use and the technology used to create it, images can be kept in many formats and locations. Accessing and storing medical records requires a patient's name. Informaticists are working on a solution that considers all these considerations. In a perfect world, an imaging system could record any image and link it to the rest of the patient's data in a single, safe file. Future predictive analytics could be used on imaging data to assist doctors make more accurate diagnoses (Fig. 7.16).

7.7.7 *Shift to the Cloud*

Photos, music, films, and even medical records are being uploaded to the "cloud." No hardware or software installation is necessary, and users can access the system from anywhere with an internet connection. When combined, these benefits save money. Cloud-stored data is not error-free, so be careful. Health informatics experts maintain cloud-based systems (Fig. 7.17).

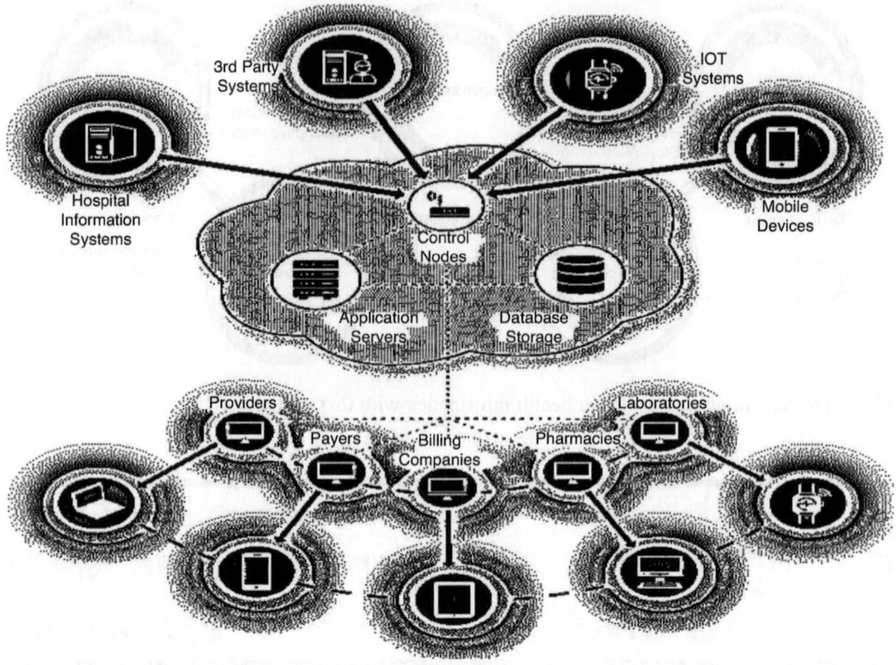

Fig. 7.17 Strategy of implementing cloud system in health informatics [28–29]

7.8 Conclusion

In light of the success of deep learning in other real-world applications, it is thought to offer innovative and precise solutions for medical imaging and is considered a significant technique for upcoming applications in the healthcare industry. Due to the fact that deep learning already has an advantage in many high-value applications, image analytics is expected to be the focus of attention on the clinical side for the foreseeable future. It is believed that an electronic health recorder, or EHR, plus predictive modeling, called Dara, will address the problem of individualized health quality in medicine. Therefore, we need a mechanism that removes the majority of the data from each patient's record while still extracting curated predictor variables from normalized EHE data. Without any site-specific data harmonization, deep learning can predict a variety of medical occurrences from different medical institutions using this representation. For a number of clinical resource scenarios, data learning algorithms can be employed to produce an accurate and scalable prediction. The identification of pertinent data from the patient's chart and records can be done using deep learning neural networks. In particular, because many academics in precision medicine are still unsure of exactly what they should be looking for, deep learning is an excellent method for researchers and pharmaceutical stakeholders hoping to highlight novel trends in these comparatively untapped datasets. Deep learning is the one that will help the health sector to analyze the process efficiently by shrinking the time for key components. Deep learning will soon be the tool for a handy diagnostic companion in the inpatient setting, which can remind healthcare professionals when high-risk situations such as sepsis and respiratory failure alter. On the basis of the research, we found that deep learning will be able to build the models like ASR that can handle multiple people's conversations from weather complexes to other serious medical diagnosis.

7.8.1 *Future Directions*

In light of the success of deep learning in other real-world applications, it is thought to offer innovative and precise solutions for medical imaging and is considered a significant technique for upcoming applications in the healthcare industry. Due to the fact that deep learning already has an advantage in many high-value applications, image analytics is expected to be the focus of attention on the clinical side for the foreseeable future. It is believed that an electronic health recorder, or EHR, plus predictive modeling, called Dara, will address the problem of individualized health quality in medicine. Therefore, we need a mechanism that removes the majority of the data from each patient's record while still extracting curated predictor variables from normalized EHE data. Without any site-specific data harmonization, deep learning can predict a variety of medical occurrences from different medical institutions using this representation. For a number of clinical resource scenario scenarios, data learning algorithms can be employed to produce an accurate and scalable prediction. The identification of pertinent data from the patient's chart and records can be done using deep learning neural networks. In particular, because many academics in precision medicine are still unsure of exactly what they should be looking for, deep learning is an excellent method for researchers and pharmaceutical stakeholders hoping to highlight novel trends in these comparatively untapped datasets. Deep learning will help the health sector to analyze the process efficiently by shrinking the time for key components. Deep learning will soon be the tool for a handy diagnostic companion in the inpatient setting, which can remind healthcare professionals when high-risk situations such as sepsis and respiratory failure alter. On the basis of the research, we found that deep learning will be able to build the models like ASR that can handle multiple people's conversations from weather complexes to various serious medical diagnoses.

References

1. Siau, K., & Shen, Z. (2006). Mobile healthcare informatics. *Medical Informatics and the Internet in Medicine, 31*(2), 89–99.
2. Beeler, P. E., Bates, D. W., & Hug, B. L. (2014). Clinical decision support systems. *Swiss Medical Weekly, 23*(144), w14073.

3. Haux, R. (2006). Individualization, globalization and health–about sustainable information technologies and the aim of medical informatics. *International Journal of Medical Informatics, 75*(12), 795–808.
4. Dick, S. (2019). Artificial intelligence. *Harvard Data Science Review, 1*, 1. https://doi.org/10.1162/99608f92.92fe150c
5. Mishra, M., & Srivastava, M. (2014). A view of artificial neural network. In *2014 international conference on advances in engineering & technology research (ICAETR-2014)* (pp. 1–3). IEEE.
6. Hsu, F. H. (1999). IBM's deep blue chess grandmaster chips. *IEEE Micro, 19*(2), 70–81.
7. Pueyo, S. (2018). Growth, degrowth, and the challenge of artificial superintelligence. *Journal of Cleaner Production, 1*(197), 1731–1736.
8. Samuel, A. L. (1959). Some studies in machine learning using the game of checkers. *IBM Journal of Research and Development, 3*(3), 210–229.
9. Burgess, J. (2020). Rtx on—the nvidia turing gpu. *IEEE Micro, 40*(2), 36–44.
10. Sarbadhikari, S. N. (2019). Digital health in India–As envisaged by the National Health Policy (2017). *BLDE University Journal of Health Sciences, 4*(1), 1.
11. Yang, L., Song, Q., Wang, Z., & Jiang, M. (2019). Parsing r-cnn for instance-level human analysis. In *Proceedings of the IEEE/CVF conference on computer vision and pattern recognition* (pp. 364–373).
12. Hirschberg, J., & Manning, C. D. (2015). Advances in natural language processing. *Science, 349*(6245), 261–266.
13. Ma, F., Ye, M., Luo, J., Xiao, C., & Sun, J. (2021, August 14). Advances in mining heterogeneous healthcare data. In *Proceedings of the 27th ACM SIGKDD conference on knowledge discovery & data mining* (pp. 4050–4051).
14. Sharma, M., & Sehrawat, R. (2020). A hybrid multi-criteria decision-making method for cloud adoption: Evidence from the healthcare sector. *Technology in Society, 61*, 101258.
15. Zhao, X., Liu, L., Qi, S., Teng, Y., Li, J., & Qian, W. (2018). Agile convolutional neural network for pulmonary nodule classification using CT images. *International Journal of Computer Assisted Radiology and Surgery, 13*(4), 585–595.
16. Liu, H., Li, B., Lv, X., & Huang, Y. (2017). Image retrieval using fused deep convolutional features. *Procedia Computer Science, 1*(107), 749–754.
17. Mahmood, T., Arsalan, M., Owais, M., Lee, M. B., & Park, K. R. (2020). Artificial intelligence-based mitosis detection in breast cancer histopathology images using faster R-CNN and deep CNNs. *Journal of Clinical Medicine, 9*(3), 749.
18. Abdollahi, A., Pradhan, B., & Alamri, A. M. (2020). An ensemble architecture of deep convolutional Segnet and Unet networks for building semantic segmentation from high-resolution aerial images. *Geocarto International, 30*, 1–6.
19. Mungle, T., Tewary, S., et al. (2017). Automated characterization and counting of Ki-67 protein for breast cancer prognosis: A quantitative immunohistochemistry approach. *Computer Methods and Programs in Biomedicine, 139*, 149–161.
20. Alheejawi, S., Xu, H., Berendt, R., Jha, N., & Mandal, M. (2019). Novel lymph node segmentation and proliferation index measurement for skin melanoma biopsy images. *Computerized Medical Imaging and Graphics, 73*, 19–29.
21. Saha, M., Chakraborty, C., Arun, I., Ahmed, R., & Chatterjee, S. (2017). An advanced deep learning approach for ki-67 stained hotspot detection and proliferation rate scoring for prognostic evaluation of breast cancer. *Scientific Reports, 7*, 3213.
22. Alheejawi, S., Mandal, M., Berendt, R., & Jha, N. (2019, May 6–8). Automated melanoma staging in lymph node biopsy image using deep learning. In *Proceedings of the IEEE Canadian conference on electrical and computer engineering (CCECE), Edmonton, Canada.*
23. Kim, H. J., Kim, H. I., & Chang, J. W. (2017, June 25). A privacy-preserving kNN classification algorithm using Yao's Garbled circuit on cloud computing. In *2017 IEEE 10th international conference on cloud computing (CLOUD)* (pp. 766–769). IEEE.

24. Lamba, D., Hsu, W. H., & Alsadhan, M. (2021). *Predictive analytics and machine learning for medical informatics: A survey of tasks and techniques*. https://doi.org/10.1016/B978-0-12-821777-1.00023-9
25. Miah, S., Shen, J., Lamp, J., Kerr, D., & Gammack, J. (2019). Emerging insights of health informatics research: A literature analysis for outlining new themes. *Australasian Journal of Information Systems, 23*. https://doi.org/10.3127/ajis.v23i0.2137
26. Northwest Center for Public Health Practice.
27. Luque, C., Luna, J. M., Luque, M., & Ventura, S. (2018, March 30). An advanced review on text mining in medicine. *WIREs Data Mining and Knowledge Discovery*. Submitted.
28. Kashyap, R., & Rahamatkar, S. (2019). Healthcare informatics using modern image processing approaches. In *Medical data security for bioengineers* (pp. 254–277). IGI Global. https://doi.org/10.4018/978-1-5225-7952-6.ch013
29. Shah, R., Shastri, J., Bohara, M. H., Panchal, B. Y. & Goel, P. (2022). Detection of different types of blood cells: A comparative analysis. In *2022 IEEE international conference on distributed computing and electrical circuits and electronics (ICDCECE)* (pp. 1–5). IEEE.

Chapter 8
Detection of Breast Cancer Diagnosis Algorithm Based on TWCNN Technique

Balbir Singh, Tousief Irshad Ahmed, P. Suganthi, S. Ananthi, Kumud Pant, and Maharaj Krishen Koul

8.1 Introduction

According to medical professionals and researchers in the medical field, breast cancer (BC) is one of the human body's most dangerous and life-threatening diseases. Later stage identification of BC will result in the patient going into comatose/coma, leading to death. This motivates researchers to identify and predict the BC in the suspected region with the early symptoms and identify the type of BC with the help of MRI lung images. With the help of an MRI lung image, the best method that predicts the accurate location of the region in the lung with the help of an IP and segmentation algorithms is identified. BC, generally recognised with the screening of sequential scan images, will be identified mainly by the symptoms of headache and other complications. Mammography, ultrasonography, MRI, and biopsies yielded categorizable images. Breast cancer mammography employs X-rays. If a mammogram reveals suspicious results, the doctor will test the tissues.

B. Singh (✉)
Administrative Staff College of India, Hyderabad, Telangana, India

T. I. Ahmed
Tutor Demonstrator Department of Biochemistry, Govt Medical College, Srinagar, J&K, India

P. Suganthi · S. Ananthi
Computer Science and Engineering, Sri Sairam Institute of Technology, Chennai, India
e-mail: suganthi.cse@sairamit.edu.in; ananthi.cse@sairamit.edu

K. Pant
Department of Biotechnology, Graphic Era Deemed to Be University, Dehradun, Uttarakhand, India

M. K. Koul
Galgotias University, Greater Noida, Uttar Pradesh, India
e-mail: krishen.koul@galgotiasuniversity.edu.in

F. J. J. Joseph et al. (eds.), *Computational Intelligence for Clinical Diagnosis*, EAI/Springer Innovations in Communication and Computing,
https://doi.org/10.1007/978-3-031-23683-9_8

Mammograms are followed with ultrasounds. If a breast area seems suspicious, your oncologist will order an ultrasound. If clinical testing is inconclusive, the doctor may recommend a breast MRI. It shows the exact position and perspective better. A biopsy is the primary technique for diagnosing cancer. Fortunately, 80% of women who had a cancerous tumour removed do not develop a breast cancer. Breast cancer detection requires machine learning. These photos (figs. 8.1 and 8.2) show various diagnosing processes, classifying diagnostic images with machine learning.

There seem to be numerous additional indicators of breast cancer, such as structural deformity, however these are inconsequential. Masses and micro-calcifications are two different forms of early illness indicators. Both benign and malignant tumours can be seen in the masses. The malignant tumour has a somewhat spherical shape, having whiter borders than the fibroid, whereas the benign tumour has an oval or curved shape [1]. The worst sort of BC that causes breast cancer cells to activate is cancer. The spread of these cells throughout the female organism and some other anthropomorphic body parts is erratic [2]. Women between the ages of 30 and 40 are brutalised by the BC. The scenario for women's survival is worrying as a result of this pitiful growth in breast cancer cases [3]. Approximately 50–60% of BC patients have survived during the last 5 years in the United States, compared to 70–80% in India and other nations. In India, the number of breast cancer patients arose by roughly two million in a given year [4].

Many developers retrain their models using machine learning. Linear data is machine-learned. When the knowledge is too extensive, machine learning does not work well. A learning algorithm is used to train the model. Supervisor-assisted machine learning leverages known data to execute tasks. Unsupervised machine learning is not monitored. Fewer patterns are reinforced. These algorithms use prior information to make accurate conclusions. Machine learning is a subfield of deep learning. Unsupervised data analysis, unstructured or unlabelled data may be present. Deep neural networks with several back propagation methods are called so. Input is on top and output is below. The intermediate layer has more layers than a neural network. Neurons house the layer. Deep learning is more successful than machine learning. Convolution neural network classifies breast cancer dataset.

Convolutional neural networks classify images. Breast cancer image inputs are used. CNN receives images and weights. Changing weights reduces errors and improves performance. CNN's layers include convolution, dumping, ReLU, and dense. Convolution layer feature map extract and compress picture features. Pooling reduces image pixels. ReLU is used as an activation function to determine if its value falls within a range. The last layer is entirely connected. It aggregates all layers' findings and assigns probabilities to each base classifier using softmax. Medical imaging applications are improving day by day with modern technology which improves the prediction, analysis, and prevention of diseases. Due to economic and environmental changes, new and innovative technology provides an opportunity for experts to contribute to and improve the identification of diseases. As a computer graduate, this motivates me to do this research work and resolve some issues that could help the medical society take preventive measures for various diseases. This work studies the identification of BB through image segmentation techniques, which is one of the most demanded medical fields. However, many people suffer from various types of BC without any age difference.

8.2 Literature Survey

A few intrusive estimation procedures are proposed to gauge breast cancer rates (BCR), such as electrical impedance tomography [5–7]. This algorithm covered the many various algorithms used to identify the region of an input frame that is affected by CRS. The two most important filters that should be used on magnetic pictures are smoothing and noise reduction. The filtering method developed by these two, and Malik is amongst the finest filters that produced the best findings for the database used in this investigation [8, 9]. Better outcomes in later phases, such as classification, categorization, and the extraction of the images, arise from using the right filter for the pre-processing procedure [1].

Based on how well it performs, this algorithm is contrasted with other ones that are already in use. FCM is important in this situation [10]. This technique uses non-local linear discriminant analysis in two stages to filter the noisy image. This sifted image is used as a guided image by the second channel using a non-local harsh filter [11]. This approach, which corrects the images with spatial parametric noise depending on local bias, automatically determines the total levels of noise represented [12].

In recent years, a number of industrial algorithms have been presented that are suitable for the identification and classification of many complicated breast cancer diseases. The ConvoNet approach has been developed to classify aggressive and non-invasive cancers. Additionally, it demonstrates how serious breast cancer is [8]. Furthermore, other researchers suggested the use of CNNS and their various variations, including deep learning and perceptron. Through the use of several cutting-edge machine learning algorithms, they also attempted to detect breast cancer [9]. Mammography is a type of X-ray technique used to detect breast cancer in its early stages and prevent premature mortality. It was once thought to be the best way to detect cancer. Only women over the age of 40 who have tiny tumours are diagnosed using this procedure. However, it has no effect on young females [13]. Classification of breast cancer density in a different method that produces superior results and the local quinary recognition system has been used [14]. A novel approach called near-infrared fluorescent has been proposed for the careful monitoring of early diagnosis in order to replace mammography technique. This method for detecting breast cancer in image processing uses continuous images of the disease that are very informative [8]. When breast cancer is discovered in its early stages, therapy can begin sooner.

Several researchers found it difficult to identify early breast cancer indicators such as breast body heat, depth, and diameter [15].Over the past 10 years, numerous studies have demonstrated the detrimental effects of using tomography to treat breast cancer. According to a study, the mammogram method for women who use it repeatedly has an impact ratio of about 50% [16]. This technique has also been used to diagnose breast cancer in other cases. The percentage of breast cancer spread is decreased in women using the sentinel lymph node approach [7]. Kennedy, Lee, and Seely [4] suggested a novel method for the detection of breast cancer that combines thermography and mammography. The results of this method showed that mammography-based detection had a sensitivity of 50%, combined thermogram and mammogram detection had a sensitivity of 82%, and thermogram-based recognition had a specificity of just 76%. This method depends upon the texturing in the nearby surroundings. Then, breast cancer thermogram detection was used. In the classification phase, they utilised a conjugate gradient training method and a tariff. They put their method to the test by using 100 images from the public DMR database. The recommended system is examined using an imbalance analysis method. The results showed that this approach has a high level of accuracy rate compared to earlier studies. To get this excellent result, a small dataset was used [17].

That said, support vector machines were really the best classifiers that had the most precision of all. SVM, KNN, ANN, and decision trees have all been compared. It was applied to the blood and picture datasets. As a result, Greneker [7] proposed a machine learning model using a different classifier. Accelerated Learning Algorithm, Svc, Artificial Neural Network. To get excellent performance, the classifier was slightly modified. That said, the Extreme Learning Machine produced the best outcomes. The machine learning-based model was proposed by Cao et al. [8]. It employed SVM, REPtree, Multilayer Perceptron, and Colonnaded Haas as four different classifiers. The author claims that KNN provided superior accuracy. SVM had its limitations. For binary variables, SVM produced better results. Multi-SVM was employed for this reason. Zhao et al. [9] completed the analysis of machine learning methodologies. The Milwaukee breast cancer dataset and entity framework were used in the comparison. The author claims that SVM produced superior performance matrix findings. Convolutional neural networks were created to address the issue with machine learning later.

The method of convolution neural network ensemble learning was proposed by Lee et al. [10]. There were other models utilised by CNN, but they primarily employed the Cellular Net and Inception templates. According to the author's evaluation of the two models, Inception V3 provides better accuracy. However, there was still a chance to treat breast cancer with machine learning. Ribeiro et al. [11] suggested a supervised machine learning model. This study used classifiers including KNN, SVM, and Bayesian Network. Results pertaining to efficiency were achieved once the sample was received from the extracted features. This indicates that SVM was an effective classifier with 83.6% technical accuracy. Haridy et al. [18] put forth a machine learning model using a different classifier. The Decision Tree model, VSI, Linear Regression, and Naive Bays were used by the author. Python's Anaconda Platform was used for the implantation. The author claims that Random Forest did well, with a prediction performance of 85.76%. When the classifier network was slightly altered, accuracy may have increased. Adrover-Jaume et al. [12] proposed an ANN-based model, and an SVM classifier assessed performance. According to the report, ANN offered 97% accuracy compared to SVM's 91%. Without SVM, the author added, it offered more accuracy. A search strategy and model-based SVM were recommended by Zhang et al. [1].

The author first applies the SVM research before using it with parameterization. The author conducted comparisons to determine which was best. The new model was created in comparison. A grid search was used to attain the higher accuracy. Jin et al. [19] suggested a model based on CNN and k-mean GMM. Prior to using the surface feature selection technique, the author determined the ROI. He finally used the classification algorithm to discover the best outcomes. The author achieved 75.6% accuracy. The author's choice of MIAS dataset [20] proposed a deep learning-based model. The author concentrated on CNN for classifications and Lloyd's technique for clustering. The suggested strategies were successful in achieving an accuracy of 86%. It employs histopathological pictures for the purpose of diagnosis.

Deep learning and sensor fusion were also explained in this paper. Jain et al. [21] suggested a model based on deep learning-enhanced histopathology image improvement. Many techniques, including PCA and LDA, were employed in this research for feature extraction. The author also discussed machine learning approaches, but since there was a vast dataset, these techniques did not yield any better results. Therefore, when CNN is used, it has an accuracy rate of 81%. However, when the photos were trained on a GPU, the accuracy increased to 79%. Kumar et al. [15] suggested a deep residual neural network-based technique for IDC prediction. Histopathology photos made up the author's dataset. The author's accuracy rate was 79.28% with a score of 0.7756. A neural network for the detection of breast cancer has numerous strategies for the survey and discovered that the learning algorithm raised the program's precision.

Based on the opinions, Neffati et al. [16] presented the model. The model was built using deep learning techniques with computer assistance. This article provided a concise overview of all current supervised learning trends [16]. Gopal et al. [22] conducted a survey on deep learning-based image recognition. It emphasised the deep learning application's key characteristics. It provided fundamental knowledge about every topic and demonstrated why deep learning algorithms produced better results employing a diagnosis method like mammography to classify the meningioma. For categorization, it made use of a CNNs. It ran on a modified Internet; according to his findings, simple changes may produce the best results. It made use of an activation function that produced superior outcomes to others. The author focused on data management and recommendation systems for breast cancer results from the past and current.

The author used the DSM dataset. The taxonomy of breast cancer was completed by Subramani et al. [23]. It provided the highest accuracy when compared to all CNN models. The Origami Recurrent Residual Convolutional Layer produced the best outcomes in this regard. The web was also utilised as an interface. Programming in R was used for the work. Anand, L., and S. P. Syed Ibrahim [17] suggested conducting research using a deep learning-based unsupervised feature extraction approach. This method was used solely for feature extraction. The author also employed stacked auto-encoders, which essentially decreased the dimensionality and produced more compact versions of the original data. The author employed an SVM classifier. The University of California acquired the analysed data. Anand, L., and V. Neelanarayanan [24] investigated using the genes. It employed gene signatures to foretell breast cancer relapse. The author utilised a Graph Convolution Neural Network as his model. In comparison to the previous algorithm, it provided the best result, therefore. Nandakumar et al. [25] proposed a system based on classification models. Numerous procedures were used in this work, including edge detection, picture improvement, separation, and the use of different classifiers. For that model, the MIAS database was utilised. Sound absorbing techniques such as median filtering and segmentation techniques such as thresholding were applied.

The approach based on k-nearest neighbours was proposed by Bagale et al. [26]. The author used the Breast Cancer dataset to analyse performance in relation to distance. The author employed two distance formulas and obtained accuracy using each code's distance. It achieved 87.37% distance accuracy and 98.70% Euclidian distance accuracy. The model based on the SVM classifier was proposed by Sharma et al. [27]. The Munich filter difference and stochastic filters were employed for detection in this model, which was based on mammography scans. From the micro dataset, only 55 histologic images were used. This method was 98.24% accurate. Using an SVM classifier, Omnia Saidani Neffati et al. [28] developed a mammogram-based model. This research was conducted in several stages. Pre-processing, ROI segmentation, feature extraction, and classification came first. The SVM provided the highest accuracy in the call-outs dataset used for this purpose. Accuracy of 83% was attained. The Classification Tree Classifier Model for Breast Cancer was put forth by Tina Catherine Mathew et al. [29]. Decision trees were used to implement the Badger breast cancer dataset. The naive Bayes tree and rotating forest for classification were also discussed in the paper.

Environmental research was conducted. Additionally, it examined batching, pushing, adaptable boosting, and REPtree and showed accuracy. The author employed a dataset related to breast cancer and applied classification methods to it. The scientist used the five classifiers both with and without the attribute selection procedure. These feature selection techniques mostly rely on correlation and data. Finally, it demonstrated how accurate these five classifiers were using feature selection methods and without them. The model was put forth and was based on classification techniques. Using data on Minnesota malignancy, it applied the random forest and SVM classifiers. The accuracy of the results, which took the carriage proportion into account, was 87.523%.

Both situations carry the risk of being fatal and disastrous. The techniques that successfully segregated worrisome areas in digital image data include CPS, MMSE, Electromagnetic Interference Optimization, and LPC [1]. Swarm-based notions are the basis for a lot of study, particularly in PSO. Segmenting MRI images presents a variety of difficult issues [18]. In addition to developing hybridised algorithms based on the idea of clustering algorithms in many disciplines, this academic's work included the implementation of PSO. Numerous applications have been developed for these algorithms [19].

The fuzzy logic approach is used to propose a novel method for modelling human vision based on colours. Because of fuzzy logic systems, the clusters are not limited to linear or rectangular lines. The most prominent cuckoo search algorithm outperformed the correlation and K-Means algorithms according to the testing results, and it also allowed for a wider variety of real-world applications [15, 20, 21, 30].

8.3 Proposed System

The optimal solution of the Median filter was modified to create the unique approach that has been presented, and voxel values are influenced by their immediate surroundings [31]. The principal application of this technology is the segmentation of MRI images tainted by salt and pepper sounds. Data from MRI lung scans was utilised to demonstrate the validity and effectiveness of the suggested technique [8]. The algorithm is evaluated for both synthetic and real data. Based on how well it performs, this algorithm is contrasted with other ones that are already in use. FCM is important in this situation [10]. This technique uses non-local Principal Component Analysis in two stages to filter the noisy image (PCA). This sifting image is used as a guided image with a non-local harsh filter in the second channel. This technique, which tries to correct the images with temporal Rican distortion based on regional bias, internally determines the total degree of noise represented [2, 4, 32–34].

8.3.1 Histogram Equalization (HE)

Histogram equalisation is used to adjust the images' intensity values, which enhances the contrast [3]. Then the histogram of the output region is matched with another specified histogram [35]. Histogram equalisation is used to improve the contrast of the fundus image [36–39]. This is carried out by modifying the histogram.

The histogram equalization is

$$r_k = \frac{n_k}{N} \tag{8.1}$$

Let the fundus image be represented by 'm', and pixel intensities of an integer may range from 0 to $L - 1$

$$\rho_n = \frac{\text{Number of pixels with intensity } n}{\text{Total number of pixels}} \quad n = 0, 1, \ldots\ldots\ldots, L-1 \tag{8.2}$$

Thus, the fundus image is enhanced and tends to achieve its brightness [13]. A uniform intensity distribution is created due to the reassigning of the intensity pixel value to the existing ones [14, 16, 17, 22, 23]. The contrast enhancement is performed on the filtered image by the histogram equalization. Due to economic and environmental changes [24–27], new and innovative technology provides an opportunity for experts to contribute to and improve the identification of diseases. As a computer graduate, this motivates me to do this research work and resolve some issues that could help the medical fraternity to take preventive measures for various diseases [28, 29]. This work studies the identification of BB through image segmentation techniques, which is one of the most demanded medical areas. However, many people suffer from various types of BC without any age difference.

Step 1: Load the MRI breast image from the MRI scanner in the DICOM format
Step 2: Using the available software convert it into standard image file format (.jpeg, .gif, .png, .bmp, etc.,)
Step 3: Store the image with the standard .jpeg extension
Step 4: Convert the image into a 3D matrix and read the image properties such as size, colour, and image type
Step 5: Apply HE to the MRI image using eq. (3.1)

$$f(x, y) = \text{HE} \in S_{xy}\{g(s, t)\} \ldots.$$

Step 6: Store the resultant images with their execution time, memory size, and pixel variation for further analysis.

8.3.2 *TWCNN*

A capable, measurable strategy is a central component of the investigation. This strategy can be utilised to recognise designs of tall measurements. FLA is utilised in design acknowledgement and to confront compression. The prepared pictures are put away in a vital component frame in design acknowledgement issues. After that, the information is utilised to discover the closeness or divergence between an obscure dataset and the stored information. FLA is viably utilised in optic plate discovery. In the proposed research, the localization phase includes the estimation of optical.

The following is the TWCNN Algorithm's systematic process

Step 1: Process FLA (Image set X, cluster K)
$X = (X_i)_{i=1}^{N}$ And K Return U and R.
Step 2: nU0 is casually originated
Step 3: Reiteration
Step 4: These parameters put away between 0 and 1, which speaks to the membership information focuses for each and each cluster, whereas the difficult c-means employments, as it were and 1 as the two values for the participation function

$$J^1(u,v) = \sum_{i=1}^{c} \sum_{j=1}^{n} u_{ij}^m \|X_j - V_i\|^2.$$

Step 5: Implement the equation

$$J^1(u,v) = \sum_{i=1}^{c} \sum_{j=1}^{n} u_{ij}^m \|X_j - V_i\|^2.$$

u is the membership value of j X to cluster i.

$$u_{ij} = \frac{1}{\sum_{k=1}^{n} \left(\|x_j - v_i\| / \|x_j - v_k\|\right)^{2/(m-1)}}$$

Step 6: End procedure

8.3.3 TWCNN Classifier

The following are some of the most critical layers used in the preparation and testing of TWCNN. The foremost aim of the TWCNN algorithm for this input MRI image is to detect the BB affected region from the images based on their intensity values. It randomly chooses the pixel values and iterates their values based on the TWCNN algorithm's functions and definitions. The TWCNN calculation is based on the objective and enrolment work spoken to by the U framework. The values are put away between 0 and 1, which speaks to the participation information focus for each cluster. In contrast, the two difficult c-means employments were 0 and 1, as the two values for the enrolment work.

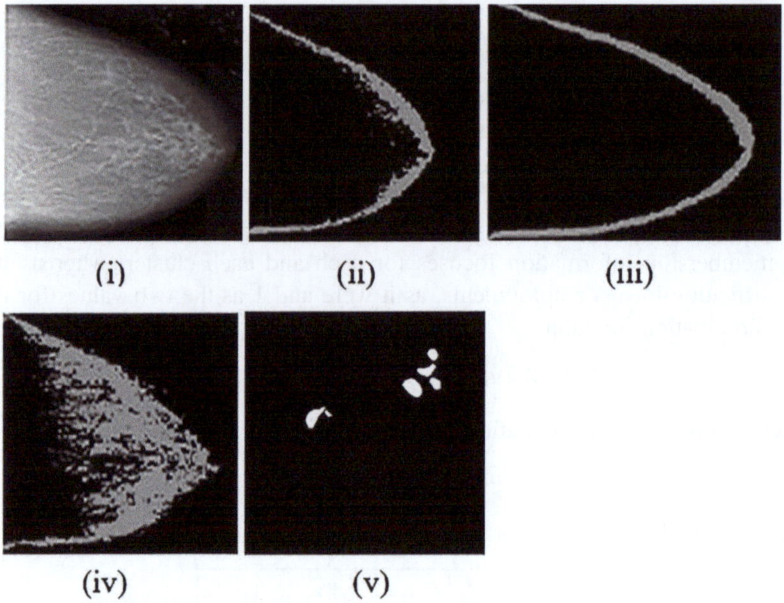

Fig. 8.1 Experimental result of sample image 1. (i) Affected system. (ii) Histogram Equalization image. (iii) Fuzzy C-Means threshed image. (iv) Ostu image. (v) Segmented region image

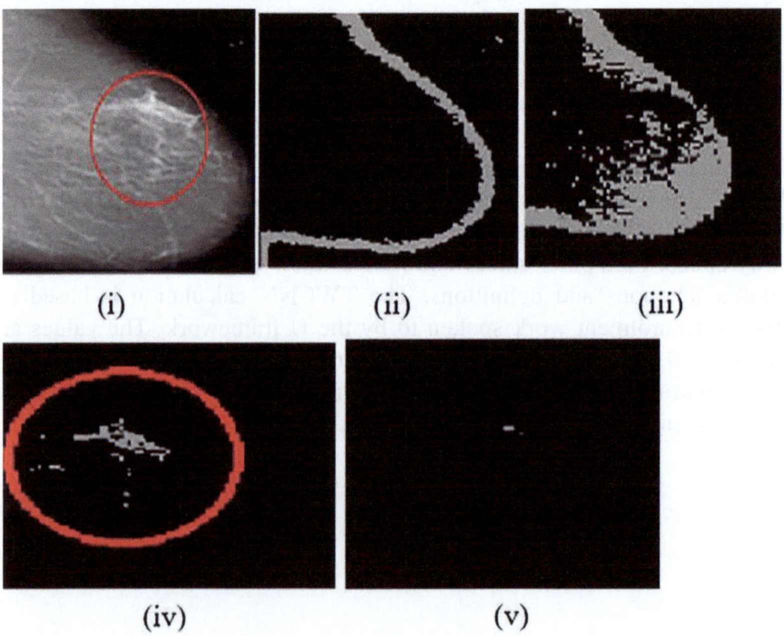

Fig. 8.2 Outcomes of experiments on the damaged system in sample picture 2 I. (ii) Gradient Comparative example. (iii) Hazy C-Means visual threshing. (iv) Image of Ostu. (v) Image with canny edge detection. (vi) Image of a segmented region. (vii) Labelled photo

Fig. 8.3 Neural network progress

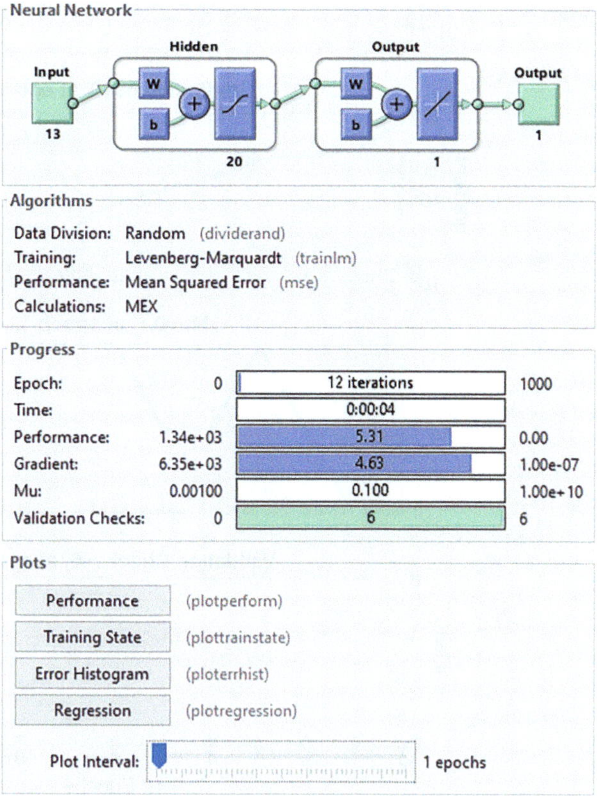

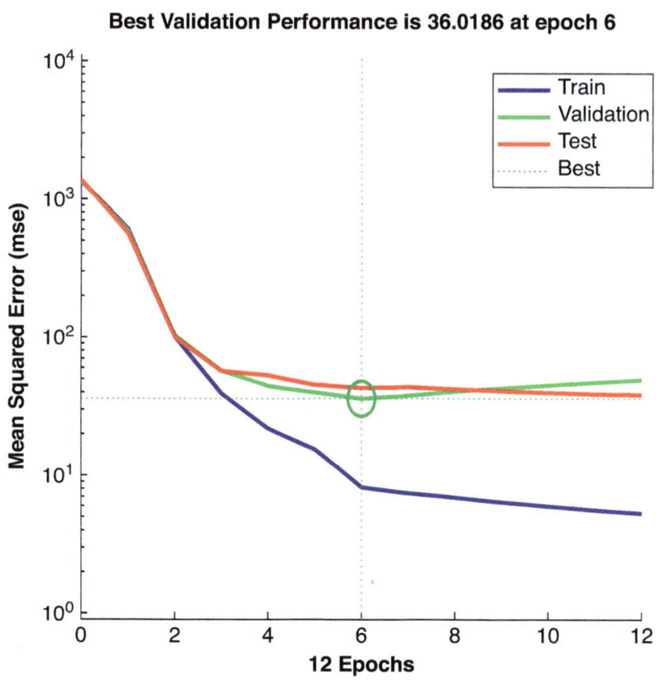

Fig. 8.4 Performance measures of validation
This figure does not show any major issues with the preparation. The approval and test bends are exceptionally comparative

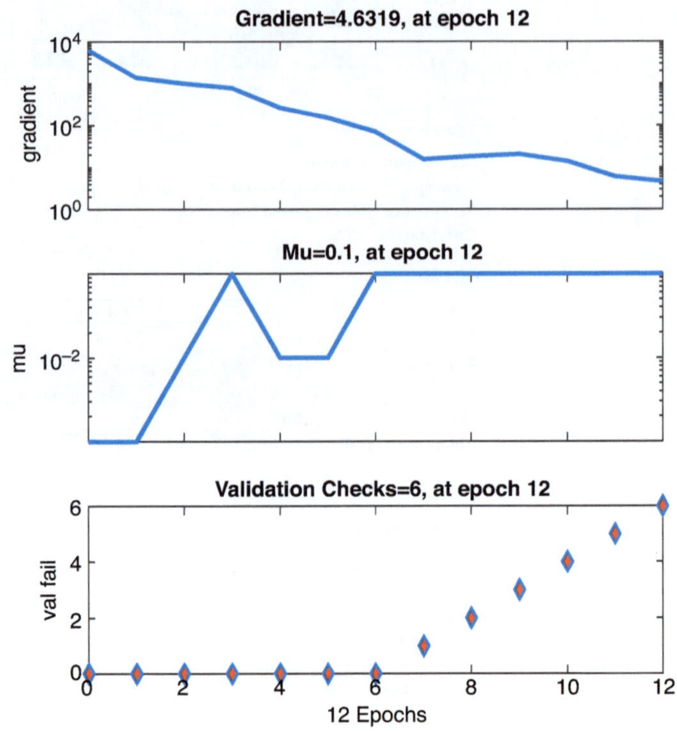

Fig. 8.5 Graph for neural network training

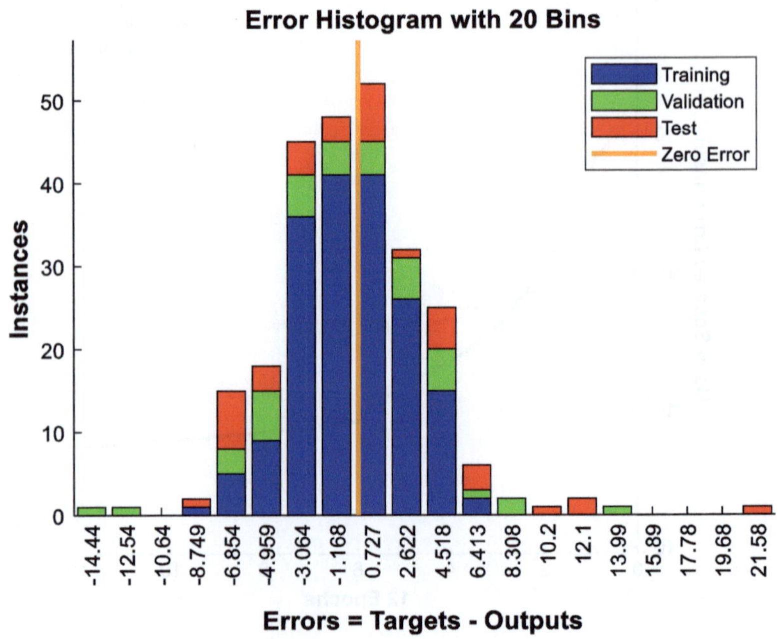

Fig. 8.6 Histogram error plot

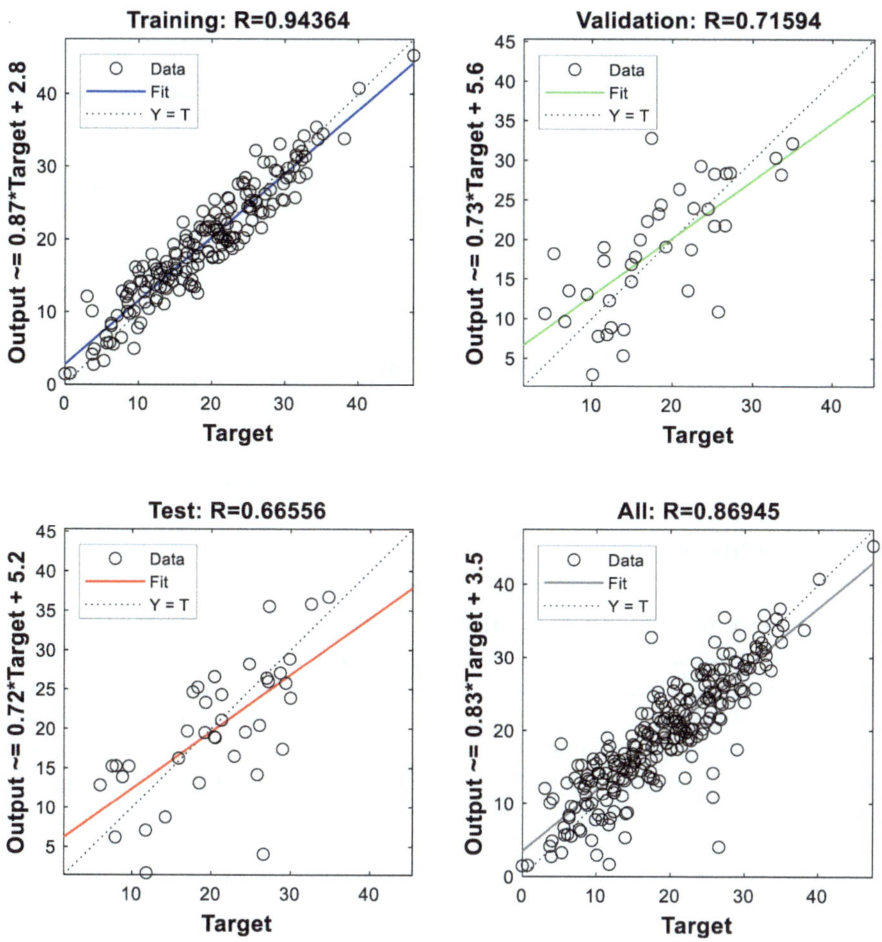

Fig. 8.7 Regression plot for TWCNN classifier

8.4 Result and Discussion

The experiments are carried out in the research work with MATLAB (R2019b) software. The hardware specification of the system used in this research work is with the Intel core2Duo processor and 16GB RAM, running on the Windows 10 operating system (Figs. 8.1, 8.2, 8.3, 8.4, 8.5, 8.6 and 8.7).

Figure 8.8 shows the output of CNN classifiers, which is the customary metric for numerous features. From the table, it is possible to recognise which feature amalgamations provide higher accuracy. Border error symbolises the rate of faultily breast images. This gives a more accurate 98.57%.

Fig. 8.8 Confusion matrix of CNN classifier

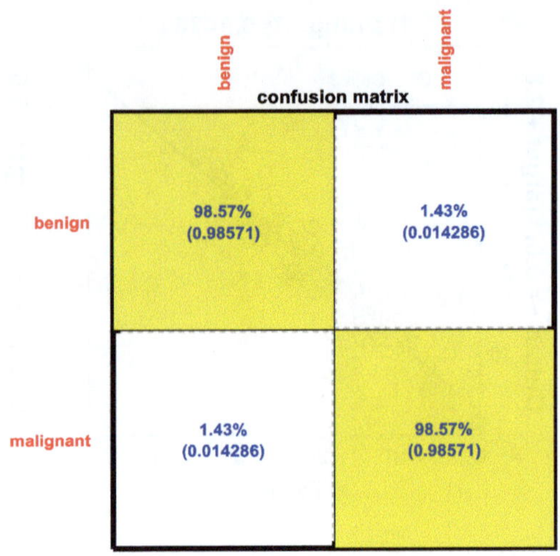

8.5 Conclusion

The purpose of this research is to offer a TWCNN classification approach for the detection of breast cancer systems. The method makes use of picture combining and a significant learning methodology. We have performed pre-processing on the input picture by applying a picture HE channels technique that is quadtree-based. In order to proceed with the dissolution of the RDS district, the HE procedure was carried out. After that, a modern TWCNN structure was presented to categorise tumour progression from MRI images into two categories (strong and unwanted pictures) and three categories (kind, hazardous, and conventional). Therefore, if it is utilised in supporting manner, it can be particularly dependable for the masters within the environment.

References

1. Zhang, J., Yang, Z., Liu, Q., & Liang, H. (2019). Electrochemical biotoxicity detection on a microfluidic paper-based analytical device via cellular respiratory inhibition. *Talanta, 202*, 384–391.
2. Misra, N. R., Kumar, S., & Jain, A. (2021). A review on e-waste: Fostering the need for green electronics. In *2021 international conference on computing, communication, and intelligent systems (ICCCIS)* (pp. 1032–1036). IEEE.
3. Agrawal, N., Jain, A., & Agarwal, A. (2019). Simulation of network on Chip for 3D router architecture. *International Journal of Recent Technology and Engineering, 8*, 58–62.
4. Kumar, S., Jain, A., Kumar Agarwal, A., Rani, S., & Ghimire, A. (2021). Object-based image retrieval using the U-net-based neural network. *Computational Intelligence and Neuroscience, 2021*, 4395646.

5. Chen, L., Menghan, H., Liu, N., Zhai, G., & Yang, S. X. (2020). Collaborative use of RGB and thermal imaging for remote breathing rate measurement under realistic conditions. *Infrared Physics & Technology, 111*, 103504.
6. Viola, P., Jones, M. (2001). Rapid object detection using a boosted cascade of simple features. In *Proceedings of the 2001 IEEE computer society conference on computer vision and pattern recognition. CVPR 2001* (Vol. 1, p. I–I). IEEE.
7. Greneker III, & Eugene F. (1997). Radar sensing of heartbeat and respiration at a distance with security applications." In *Radar sensor technology II* (vol. 3066, pp. 22–27). International Society for Optics and Photonics.
8. Cao, M., Qiuli Sun, X., Zhang, Y. M., & Wang, J. (2021). Detection and differentiation of respiratory syncytial virus subgroups A and B with colorimetric toehold switch sensors in a paper-based cell-free system. *Biosensors and Bioelectronics, 182*, 113173.
9. Zhao, Z., Huang, C., Huang, Z., Lin, F., He, Q., Tao, D., Jaffrezic-Renault, N., & Guo, Z. (2021). Advancements in electrochemical biosensing for respiratory virus detection: A review. *TrAC Trends in Analytical Chemistry, 139*, 116253.
10. Lee, H. G., Choi, W., Yang, S. Y., Kim, D.-H., Park, S.-G., Lee, M.-Y., & Jung, H. S. (2021). PCR-coupled paper-based surface-enhanced Raman scattering (SERS) sensor for rapid and sensitive detection of respiratory bacterial DNA. *Sensors and Actuators B: Chemical, 326*, 128802.
11. Ribeiro, B. V., Cordeiro, T. A. R., Oliveira e Freitas, G. R., Ferreira, L. F., & Franco, D. L. (2020). Biosensors for the detection of respiratory viruses: A review. *Talanta Open*, 100007.
12. Adrover-Jaume, C., Alba-Patiño, A., Clemente, A., Santopolo, G., Vaquer, A., Russell, S. M., Barón, E., et al. (2021). Paper biosensors for detecting elevated IL-6 levels in blood and respiratory samples from COVID-19 patients. *Sensors and Actuators B: Chemical, 330*, 129333.
13. Singhal, A., & Sharma, D. K. (2022). New generalized 'Useful' entropies using weighted quasi-linear mean for efficient networking. In *Mobile networks and applications* (pp. 1–11). Springer Nature
14. Kumar, R., Fadi Al-Turjman, L., Anand, A. K., Magesh, S., Vengatesan, K., Sitharthan, R., & Rajesh, M. (2021). Genomic sequence analysis of lung infections using artificial intelligence technique. *Interdisciplinary Sciences: Computational Life Sciences, 13*(2), 192–200.
15. Kumar, A., & Jain, A. (2021). Image smog restoration using oblique gradient profile prior and energy minimization. *Frontiers of Computer Science, 15*(6), 1–7.
16. Neffati, O. S., Sengan, S., Thangavelu, K. D., Kumar, S. D., Setiawan, R., Elangovan, M., Mani, D., & Velayutham, P. (2021). Migrating from traditional grid to smart grid in smart cities promoted in developing country. *Sustainable Energy Technologies and Assessments, 45*, 101125.
17. Anand, L., & Syed Ibrahim, S. P. (2018). HANN: A hybrid model for liver syndrome classification by feature assortment optimization. *Journal of Medical Systems, 42*(11), 1–11.
18. Haridy, S., Maged, A., Baker, A. W., Shamsuzzaman, M., Bashir, H., & Xie, M. (2021). Monitoring scheme for early detection of coronavirus and other respiratory virus outbreaks. *Computers & Industrial Engineering*, 107235.
19. Jin, B., Zhao, Y., & Liang, Y. (2021). Internet of things medical image detection and pediatric renal failure dialysis complicated with respiratory tract infection. *Microprocessors and Microsystems, 83*, 104016.
20. Bi, C., Ramos-Mandujano, G., Tian, Y., Hala, S., Xu, J., Mfarrej, S., Esteban, C. R., et al. (2021). Simultaneous detection and mutation surveillance of SARS-CoV-2 and co-infections of multiple respiratory viruses by rapid field-deployable sequencing. *Med 3*, 1–26
21. Jain, A., Dwivedi, R. K., Alshazly, H., Kumar, A., Bourouis, S., & Kaur, M. (2022). Design and simulation of ring network-on-chip for different configured nodes. *Computers, Materials and Continua*; Henderson, *71*(2), 4085–4100.

22. Gopal, V. N., Fadi Al-Turjman, R., Kumar, L. A., & Rajesh, M. (2021). Feature selection and classification in breast cancer prediction using IoT and machine learning. *Measurement, 178*, 109442.
23. Subramani, P., Al-Turjman, F., Kumar, R., Kannan, A., & Loganthan, A. (2021). Improving medical communication process using recurrent networks and wearable antenna s11 variation with harmonic suppressions. *Personal and Ubiquitous Computing*, 1–13.
24. Anand, L., & Neelanarayanan, V. (2020). Enchanced multiclass intrusion detection using supervised learning methods. In *AIP conference proceedings* (vol. 2282, no. 1, p. 020044). AIP Publishing LLC.
25. Nandakumar, K., Vinod, V., Akbar Batcha, S. M., Sharma, D. K., Elangovan, M., Poonia, A., Mudlappa Basavaraju, S., Dogiwal, S. R., Dadheech, P., & Sengan, S. (2021). Securing data in transit using data-in-transit defender architecture for cloud communication. *Soft Computing, 25*(18), 12343–12356.
26. Bagale, G. S., Vandadi, V. R., Singh, D., Sharma, D. K., Garlapati, D. V. K., Bommisetti, R. K., Gupta, R. K., Setsiawan, R., Subramaniyaswamy, V., & Sengan, S. (2021). Small and medium-sized enterprises' contribution in digital technology. *Annals of Operations Research*, 1–24.
27. Sharma, D. K., Singh, N. C., Noola, D. A., Doss, A. N., & Sivakumar, J. (2021). A review on various cryptographic techniques & algorithms. *Materials Today: Proceedings*. https://doi.org/10.1016/j.matpr.2021.04.583
28. Neffati, O. S., Setiawan, R., Jayanthi, P., Vanithamani, S., Sharma, D. K., Regin, R., Mani, D., & Sengan, S. (2021). An educational tool for enhanced mobile e-learning for technical higher education using mobile devices for augmented reality. *Microprocessors and Microsystems, 83*, 104030.
29. Narayanasami, S., et al. (2021). An enhanced trust-based Kalman filter route optimization technique for wireless sensor networks. *Wireless Personal Communications*, *127*, 1–19.
30. Gupta, N., Vaisla, K. S., Jain, A., Kumar, A., & Kumar, R. (2021). Performance analysis of AODV routing for wireless sensor network in FPGA hardware. *Computer Systems Science and Engineering, 39*(2), 1–12.
31. Gupta, N., Jain, A., Vaisla, K. S., Kumar, A., & Kumar, R. (2021). Performance analysis of DSDV and OLSR wireless sensor network routing protocols using FPGA hardware and machine learning. *Multimedia Tools and Applications, 80*(14), 22301–22319.
32. Kumar, S., Jain, A., Shukla, A. P., Singh, S., Raja, R., Rani, S., et al. (2021). A comparative analysis of machine learning algorithms for detection of organic and nonorganic cotton diseases. *Mathematical Problems in Engineering, 2021*, 1–18.
33. Jain, A., & Kumar, A. (2021). Desmogging of still smoggy images using a novel channel prior. *Journal of Ambient Intelligence and Humanized Computing, 12*(1), 1161–1177.
34. Ghai, D., Gianey, H. K., Jain, A., & Uppal, R. S. (2020). Quantum and dual-tree complex wavelet transform-based image watermarking. *International Journal of Modern Physics B, 34*(04), 2050009.
35. Sharma, S. K., Jain, A., Gupta, K., Prasad, D., & Singh, V. (2019). An internal schematic view and simulation of major diagonal mesh network-on-chip. *Journal of Computational and Theoretical Nanoscience, 16*(10), 4412–4417.
36. Agarwal, A. K., & Jain, A. (2019). Synthesis of 2D and 3D NoC mesh router architecture in HDL environment. *Journal of Advanced Research in Dynamical and Control Systems, 11*(4), 2573–2581.
37. Jain, A., Gahlot, A. K., Dwivedi, R., Kumar, A., & Sharma, S. K. (2018). Fat tree NoC design and synthesis. In *Intelligent communication, control and devices* (pp. 1749–1756). Springer.
38. Jain, A., Dwivedi, R., Kumar, A., & Sharma, S. (2017). Scalable design and synthesis of 3D mesh network on chip. In *Proceeding of international conference on intelligent communication, control and devices* (pp. 661–666). Springer.
39. Jain, A., Kumar, A., & Sharma, S. (2015). Comparative design and analysis of mesh, torus and ring NoC. *Procedia Computer Science, 48*, 330–337.

Chapter 9
Internet of Things (IoT) and Artificial Intelligence (AI) to Detect Urinary Tract Infections

Viswanatha Reddy Allugunti, Dhana Naga Kalyani Tummala, and Maitrali Marik

9.1 Introduction

Compared to upper respiratory contaminations, urinary plot diseases (UTIs) are the second in recurrence. Regardless of this, bacteriuria testing (a regular methodology for UTI conclusion) is the most often mentioned clinical technique, with enormous work stories checking 200–300 pee tests consistently. Unlike most upper respiratory contaminations, which are brought about by infections and consequently expect practically no clinical intervention, UTIs are generally brought about by gastrointestinal microorganisms. *Escherichia coli* (*E. coli*) is the most widely recognized bacterium among them, representing 80–85% of all cases. *Staphylococcus saprophyticus* is another microbe that causes 5–10% of UTI diseases [1]. UTIs can be brought about by viral or contagious contaminations in uncommon circumstances [2]. UTIs can also be induced by other organisms such as *Staphylococcus*, *Proteus*, *Salmonella*, and *Enterobacter*, yet they are usually connected with urinary framework abnormalities or urinary catheterization [3]. Figure 9.1a portrays the commonness of different urinary lot contaminations (uropathogens). Early discovery of the sickness can support the anticipation of additional serious intricacies [4, 5].

Be that as it may, the ongoing ways to deal with distinguishing UTIs are typically sluggish and require explicit gear. The customary reason for uropathogenic location depends on pee culture, which includes research facility testing. Before a clear

V. R. Allugunti (✉)
Solutions Architect, Arohak Inc, Monmouth, NJ, USA

D. N. K. Tummala
Mygo Consulting Inc, Naperville, IL, USA

M. Marik
Independent Researcher, New Brunswick, NJ, USA

F. J. J. Joseph et al. (eds.), *Computational Intelligence for Clinical Diagnosis*, EAI/Springer Innovations in Communication and Computing,
https://doi.org/10.1007/978-3-031-23683-9_9

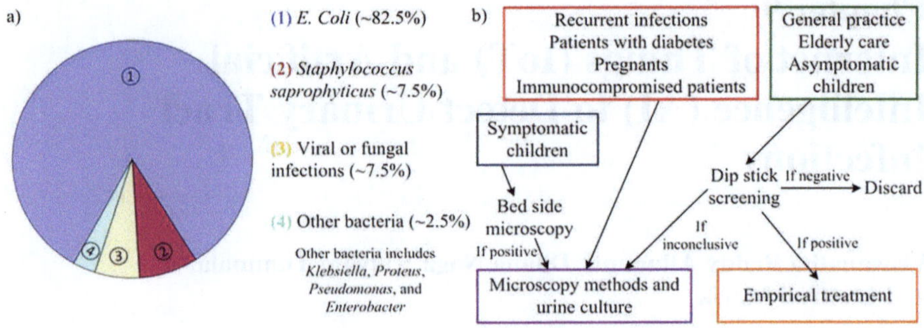

Fig. 9.1 (**a**) Incidence of the major infections caused; (**b**) standards for the commonly used dipstick vetting and contact microscopy urinary infection preliminary identification procedures. (Image modified from Graham and Galloway [4])

judgment is possible after the urine inspection, several days may have passed. The Malthus schema approach method and Gram's approach [12–14], Gram's approach [6], biocatalytic methods like the catalase test, glutathione peroxidase, or reagent strip checking (nosedive stick inspection) [7], colorimetric clarifier [8], luminescent replies [9], iodometric position of progress [6], electrochemical methods [10], microdilution vetting [11], Lysates amoebo-cyte lysate gyn. A pee culture from the patient's pee test is commonly expected by these ways to deal with recognizing and measuring bacterial development. Tiny strategies are the current "best quality level" among the previously mentioned innovations, by and large requiring an earlier cell culture [15]. There are as yet fast, starter approaches to evaluating new pee for UTI discovery prior to getting back to this methodology. Figure b portrays the rules for these strategies [16].

9.2 Symptoms

When you have a UTI, the coating of the bladder and urethra becomes red and bothered, similarly to when you have a virus [17]. The disturbance can cause torment in your lower mid-region, pelvic region, and even lower back and will normally cause you to want to pee on a more regular basis. Consuming or tormenting while peeing is the most well-known side effect [18]. You might try and feel a compelling impulse or have to pee, but just get a couple of drops. This is because the bladder is aggravated to such an extent that it causes you to feel like you need to pee, in any event, when you do not have a lot of pee in your bladder. You may occasionally let go completely and spill pee [19]. You may likewise find that your pee smells horrible and is shady. Kidney contaminations frequently cause fevers and upper back torment, normally on one side or the other. Kidney infections are also frequently associated with nausea and heaviness. These diseases should be treated immediately on the grounds that kidney contamination can spread into the circulatory system and cause hazardous medical problems (Table 9.1).

Table 9.1 Standards for urine tests

Assortment of parameters Hazard	Mysterious illness
Fructose >130.0 mg/dL	Hepatic illness, hyperglycemia, and brain tumor
Enzyme >20.0 md/dL	Infected kidneys and diabetic
Anaerobic metabolism >40.0 mg/dL	Mellitus
Hematoidin >1.0 md/dL	Liver failure and hepatitis
pH value <4.0 or >9	Obesity, hyperglycemia, rheumatism, and bacteremia
Relative density: >1.0	Pouchitis
Plasma >3.0	Erythrocytes inflammatory or a renal tumor
Erythrocyte >5.0	Infection, nephrolithiasis, and WBC/hpf
Bromate ≥ 0	Endometrial hyperplasia

The typical quality ranges between 1.005 and 1.025. Low unambiguous gravity might show a hindered capacity to focus pee because of medical issues such as diabetes insipidus, sickle cell nephropathy, or intense cylindrical rot. Alternately, high qualities might be demonstrative of high protein or ketoacid fixation in the pee.

9.2.1 Causes

Numerous germs reside in great numbers on your skin as well as in the vicinity of your urethra and vagina. Microorganisms could enter the bladder through the urethra and end up in the urine. They can attempt to stray up to the kidney. Whatever their extent, microbes in the urinary system can cause certain problems. Similar to how some people are more susceptible to colds, people are more susceptible to UTIs. Since women's urethras are smaller than men's, bacteria must travel a greater distance to reach the bladder in order for women to get a UTI.

9.3 CTSS Operating Precepts

A trackpad may be an effective tool for bio-sub-atomic ID, as demonstrated in [20], with the ability to carry out incredibly fine bioassays [21]. Contact screens are progressively being utilized in "cell phones," recognizing and restricting a touch occasion in a predefined show locale [22]. Infrared, subsurface acoustic energy, resistance recognition, and inductive location are just a few of the technological advancements utilized to identify impact occurrences. The latter is currently the standard in PDAs [23]. However, capacitive touch panels have two distinctly new standards and interactions here between touch board, the regulators, the contact occurrence [24, 25]. One approach makes use of the identity technique (or interface

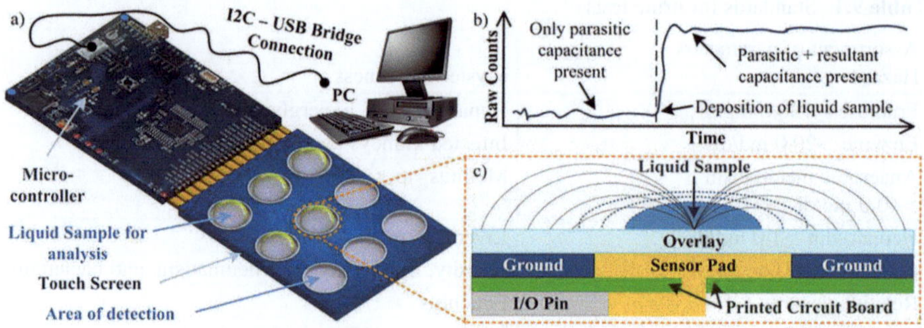

Fig. 9.2 Working principle of CTSS

capacitance reaction), in which a modest electrical flow (20–500 A) is generated by the interaction of the touch–occasion combination. The regulator distinguishes this created dog lease by working out the distance between the touch–occasion and the terminals situated in the touch board's corners. The touch screen can subsequently distinguish only each touch occasion in turn, confining its utilization. The shared capacitance approach (or projected capacitive reaction), then again, considers the synchronous identification of numerous contact occasions. This is performed by estimating capacitance alterations to the circuits imprinted on the touch board instigated by human finger commitment. Different touch occasions may consequently be limited and separated since each contact will have an interesting cathode blend and significant force.

Through the proposed study, a self-capacitance comparable model (displayed in Fig. 9.2c) is utilized to depict the carried-out touch screen [24, 25]. The touch sensor in this framework consistently screens a pattern capacitance esteem (CX) that shifts bearing upon the encompassing conditions. At the point when no material comes into multitouch interface, spurious inductance is estimated, i.e., CX = CP.

This capacitance considers each of the results of using a trackpad components, for example, the collaborations among the sensor cushion, substrate, neutral, or the lender's pin impedance. In this way, CP addresses the perplexing electric field created by the parts as a whole.

9.4 Modeling and Simulation of a CTSS

Preceding coordinating early preliminary testing, a couple of speculative preliminaries of the CTSS ideal model to be executed should be finished. A FEM re-enactment is suited for these tests because it gives students control over the model developed and prospective outcomes as figures of the certifiable model technique of performing. The ACDC element from the for-profit program COMSOL Multiphysics was used to run the 3D computations of the reactive touch screen. The model was built with no charges and charge insurance as assumptions. One key on

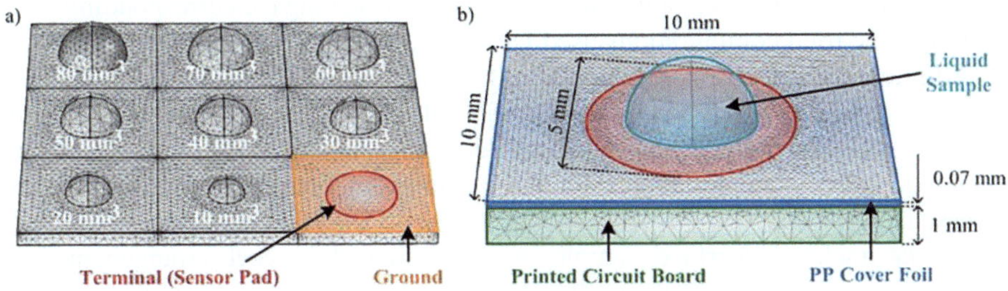

Fig. 9.3 Theoretical tests of the CTSS

the capacitive trackpad that was used for the assessments had a layout comparable to the model. The PCB substrate was displayed as a square surface having 10 mm edges and 1 mm width, with the recreation area visible on some of its top. The sensor pad was made by describing a round region (radium = 2.5 mm) in this layer as the terminal (1 V). A polypropylene (PP) cover foil with a thickness of 70 m was placed on top of the substrate as an overlay for insurance and security. Besides, an air zone was worked around the model to allow the conveyed electric field to multiply.

The reproductions analyzed the contact detectors response to distinct degrees of *E coli*, an absolute impedance (a) of 100 [26], pee, with $a = 76.1$ [27], and water, with $a = 80$, which are all notable in the writing. At the focal point of the model (lined up with the sensor cushion), a semi-circle addressing the fluid drop under test was characterized, and the amounts put to the test altered its volume. Several thoughts for *E. coli* considering the findings previously described in [28], bacterial testing was conducted. The basal concentration of UTI urine is 105 peace deal framing units/mL, and the largest volume of any solitary bacterium that will eventually form a colony is 1.1 m^3. All bacteria present (prior to submitting a request) would be set in the cushion area if a 1 mL test clings to the capacitive touch surfaces (via, for example, a bioassay), bringing about a complete volume of microorganisms of 1.1 105 m^3. For instance, a circle with a span of 30 m may be utilized to address this volume since the least complex shape can be rationally reenacted and best portrays the state of the microorganisms (Fig. 9.3).

9.4.1 Setting the Testing for the CTSS Test

The experiments were conducted using the capacitive touch CY3280-BSM Simple Contact Unit and the processor CY3280-20×66 Universal Cap Sensitive Processor. The two components might be altered and put to use after the accompanying programming was introduced. According to the manufacturer's procedures, the CY3280-20×66 Universal Cap Sense Operator was set up to provide an ongoing RC browse from a specific button. The perfect favorable griming of the touchpad in the CY3280-BSM Simple Contact Module was shown through simple testing, including as touching each button with a finger and watching the corresponding LED light up. The tried configurations used DI water as well as regular faucet water.

Additionally, 3.5 g of NaCl and 100 mL of tap water were combined to create a saltwater solution, which had a concentration of 35 g/L. The samples of post-night pee were collected halfway and stored in sealed tubes. In less than 2 hours after being gathered, these examples were stored in a climate-controlled environment and assessed.

On the trackpad interface, samples were terminated for each arrangement in a variety of buttons to conduct the tests. How many examples were increased by 10 L (10 mm^3) and moved from 10 to 100 L (100 mm^3). There were several tries at each arrange mental measure. A PP cover foil was attached to the surface of the touch screen to protect its electronic components, which was acquired from Biogenies in Mannheim, Germany.

This stratum was added to the device which had a considerable impact on the previous discoveries, according to preliminary analyses. The touch interface just observed the RCs for the single button on the off chance as each test was done autonomously. When a sample was being deposited, the fingertip sensor's RC value was recorded. For each test, a Raw Count Difference (RCD) was processed.

Nine tests were completed, and then the touching sensor was disinfected with an ethanol solution to keep away from the adherence of unwanted particles and extras from prior testing (particularly on account of pee tests).

9.4.2 Data Acquisition Layer

To beneficially expect and evaluate for pee tainting in the home environment, accurate information about various pee limits is required. As a result, the current proposal for data grouping introduces a layer that needs to be clearly characterized for the statistics layer. The info layer is the top layer in the educational activity that interacts with clients directly and is in charge of gathering client-related information about their urine, such as white blood cell count, pH concerned, bilirubin, ketones, and release cells. The sensors built inside the clever restroom holders are used to put this information together. There are several sensors for this in the floor near the quick bathrooms that are utilized to identify and calculate different pee restrictions such as tone, scent, etc., with essentially no person obstruction. For the distinctive confirmation of each and every client, different Radio Recurrence ID (RFID) names or special finger impression sensors are joined to the flush edge work.

9.4.3 Data Pre-processing

The most fundamental step before data test notion and route is probably data pretreatment. As a result, before doing any AI calculations, the PE data obtained by IoT sensors needs to be processed and transformed into a format appropriate for AI estimations. Our suggested structure makes use of a component depiction strategy for the equal encoding of various PE-related restrictions obtained through the data acquisition layer. Expecting the unique limit has a projected worth with the eventual goal of assigning a zero worth. However, if the value of the alternative limit crosses the protected edge, a value of 1 is assigned. For example, pH is assigned a value of 1 in the preprocessed dataset if it exists in the range of 4 or higher than 9, unambiguous gravity is assigned a value of 1, and similar encoding is carried out for other limitations existing in the dataset.

9.5 Categorization of Information

In order to examine the presence of pee sickness in individuals by evaluating various noteworthy limitations, the resampled data is then organized using various AI algorithms. Due to the cloud server's proximity to the home situation, the fog layer is useful in the comfortable evaluation of the validation set.

Additionally, the fog layer is in charge of calculating the overwhelming digital games in light of the data used to guide the course of action. IRF has been used to forecast the likelihood of a condition linked to urine pollution in each time interval. The IRF threshold is used to determine whether the patient is healthy or, alternatively, if there are any probable outcomes of any wager.

We model our structure so that pee data is assembled multiple times every day, integrating the morning, night, and night after each dining experience. This will look at the patient's prosperity incessantly and hence decrease any sort of danger by early acknowledgment of any peculiarities. In view of IRF's probability gauge, we can isolate the assembled information into two classifications: powerful and non-irresistible.

9.5.1 Antimicrobial Susceptibility Testing (AST)

Because of the range of likely microorganisms in the urinary plot, organism ID tests ought to be enhanced by AST to pick a fitting enemy of disease for ideal treatment. For the continuous standard, clinical lab examination organisms ought to initially be refined and isolated for AST. The microorganism is then filled in the nonappearance and presence of the counter-contamination specialists. Advancement inside an immunizing agent poison shows impediment. The phenotypic has been good in light of the fact that it remains constantly liberated from the genetic reason against disease resistance.

A genetic approach using massively parallel microarray of accordingly deterrent portions or PCR of established safe-giving qualities is an optional system. For differentiating between methicillin-weak S. aureus evidence and methicillin-safe

S. aureus, PCR-based AST has been clinically convincing. The population genetic system is not criticized for the fact that AST's genetic tools are always improving and could not always manifest as hereditary alterations.

9.5.2 Biosensor for Diagnosing UTIs

Safe microscopic organisms appear as a result of the lack of unquestionable UTI care end features and wide-ranging hostile current treatment trials. More than 30% of *E. coli* are resistant to sulphamethoxazole, while patient resistance to fluoroquinolones ranges from 11% to 50%. Broadened spectrum tech test *Escherichia coli* and oxacillin *S. aureus* are two bacteria that can cause contamination, and their prevalence is on the rise, creating a problematic clinical problem today.

Since its more sensitive and rapid sub-nuclear concept compared to other ways, factors have been implicated that UTI certification is growing in popularity in the puppy lease situation.

9.6 Conclusions

When contrasted with different diseases, the high pervasiveness of UTIs prompts a high demand for bacteriuria, and subsequently a rising prerequisite for substantial pee tests. Since recovering these examples is a tedious and bothering activity, dispensable diapers can be utilized to make the cycle more straightforward. Following that, a portable biomedical gadget in view of a CTSS may be utilized for face-to-face UTI detection. Primer examination on a CTSS-based UTI identifier was introduced. The FEM reproduction results uncovered that the touch sensor answered dramatically to expanding volumes of *E. coli* and fluid examples. The touch sensor showed variations in the request even after emergence of *E. coli* to the replica in the primary reproduction set, which can be reasonably noticed despite being small. In the second arrangement of reenactments, a tremendous contrast in the CTSS response to pee several water fragments were found. In exploratory testing, the CTSS's comment to assorted fluid arrangements with expanding measures of broken-up particles was assessed. The arrangements contemplated were DI water, fluid water, salt water, and new pee tests. The CTSS recognizes different volumes of fluid and shows an outstanding response as the sums rise. These outcomes are reliable with recreated results.

9.6.1 Future Work

Dementia is a neurological state of mind that influences immense number of people all around the world. At some random time in the United Kingdom, one out of four crisis facility beds is occupied by a person with dementia, while around 22% of these crisis center affirmations are result of preventable causes. In this chapter, we analyzed using Internet of Things (IoT) progress and at-home material contraption along with AI methodology to screen the concerning the behavior of the people with dementia. This will allow us to give seriously convincing and important thought and decrease preventable crisis center confirmations.

One of the unique pieces of this work is getting regular updates together with physiological test accumulated at negligible cost in at-home devices to eliminate critical information concerning the behavior of the people with dementia in their own home environment. The complexity of a UTI can involve recurring illnesses, particularly in women who have at least two UTIs in a 6-month period, or possibly four people experiencing kidney damage from severe or severe kidney disease (pyelonephritis) as a result of an untreated UTI. These sicknesses can be trailed by using test results. Bio-clinical sensors assume a significant part in empowering the IoT gadget to recognize the disease. Bio-clinical sensors will go probably as a data device and, with the help of pre-taken care of data, will recognize the urinary plot contaminations (UTIs) which are achieved by the pathogens.

References

1. Nicolle, L. E. (2008). Uncomplicated urinary tract infection in adults including uncomplicated pyelonephritis. *The Urologic Clinics of North America, 35*, 1–12.
2. Amdekar, S., Singh, V., & Singh, D. D. (2011). Probiotic therapy: Immunomodulating approach toward urinary tract infection. *Current Microbiology, 63*, 484–490.
3. Salvatore, S., Salvatore, S., Cattoni, E., Siesto, G., Serati, M., Sorice, P., & Torella, M. (2011). Urinary tract infections in women. *European Journal of Obstetrics, Gynecology, and Reproductive Biology, 156*, 131–136.
4. Graham, J. C., & Galloway, A. (2001). The laboratory diagnosis of urinary tract infection. *Journal of Clinical Pathology, 54*, 911–919.
5. Pezzlo, M. (1988). Detection of urinary tract infections by rapid methods. *Clinical Microbiology Reviews, 1*, 268–280.
6. Pezzlo, M. T., Tan, G. L., Peterson, E. M., & de la Maza, L. M. (1982). Screening of urine cultures by three automated systems. *Journal of Clinical Microbiology, 15*, 468–474.
7. Halloran, S., & Bennitt, W. (1999). Urine reagent strips: An MDA evaluation. *Professional Nurse, 14*, 791–796.
8. Longoria, C., & Gonzalez, G. (1987). FiltraCheck-UTI, a rapid, disposable system for detection of bacteriuria. *Journal of Clinical Microbiology, 25*, 926–928.
9. Males, B. M., Bartholomew, W. R., & Amsterdam, D. (1985). Leukocyte esterase-nitrite and bioluminescence assays as urine screens. *Journal of Clinical Microbiology, 22*, 531–534.
10. Lamb, V. A., Dalton, H. P., & Wilkins, J. R. (1976). Electrochemical method for the early detection of urinary-tract infections. *American Journal of Clinical Pathology, 66*, 91–95.

11. Livsey, S. A. (1995). Turbidimetric urine screening. *British Journal of Biomedical Science, 52*, 71–73.
12. Smith, T., Eggington, R., Pease, A., Harris, D., & Spencer, R. (1985). Evaluation of Malthus 128H microbiological growth analyser for detecting significant bacteriuria. *Journal of Clinical Pathology, 38*, 926–928.
13. Kunin, C. M. (1975). Detection, prevention, and management of urinary tract infections: A manual for the physician, nurse, and allied health worker. *Annals of Internal Medicine, 83*, 128–129.
14. Ouslander, J. G., Schapira, M., & Schnelle, J. F. (1995). Urine specimen collection from incontinent female nursing home residents. *Journal of the American Geriatrics Society, 43*, 279–281.
15. Gochman, R. F., Karasic, R. B., & Heller, M. B. (1991). Use of portable ultrasound to assist urine collection by suprapubic aspiration. *Annals of Emergency Medicine, 20*, 631–635.
16. Shvartzman, P., & Nasri, Y. (2004). Urine culture collected from gel-based diapers: Developing a novel experimental laboratory method. *The Journal of the American Board of Family Practice, 17*, 91–95.
17. Putnam, D. F. (1971). *Composition and concentrative properties of human urine*. National Aeronautics and Space Administration.
18. Sharief, N., Hameed, M., & Petts, D. (1998). Use of rapid dipstick tests to exclude urinary tract infection in children. *British Journal of Biomedical Science, 55*, 242–246.
19. Carlsson, S., Govoni, M., Wiklund, N. P., Weitzberg, E., & Lundberg, O. (2003). In vitro evaluation of a new treatment for urinary tract infections caused by nitrate-reducing bacteria. *Antimicrobial Agents and Chemotherapy, 47*, 3713–3718.
20. Won, B. Y., & Park, H. G. (2012). A touchscreen as a biomolecule detection platform. *Angewandte Chemie (International Ed. in English), 51*, 748–751.
21. Karlsen, H., & Dong, T. (2014). *Touch Sensor system for detection of urinary tract infection in disposable diapers*. Proceedings on the 36th Annual International Conference of the IEEE Engineering in Medicine and Biology Society (EMBC'14), Chicago, 26 August–30 August 2014.
22. Kim, H.-K., Lee, S., & Yun, K.-S. (2011). Capacitive tactile sensor array for touch screen application. *Sensors and Actuators A: Physical, 165*, 2–7.
23. Young, J. (2012). *A label-free DNA detection method utilizing capacitive touchscreen* [M.S.c Thesis]. Korean Advanced Institute of Science and Technology, Daedeok Innopolis, Daejeon, Korea, 27 November 2012.
24. Getting Started With CapSense®. Available online: www.cypress.com/?docID=50002. Accessed on 30 July 2014.
25. Kolokowsky, S., & Davis, T. *Touchscreens 101: Understanding touchscreen technology and design*. Available online: http://www.cypress.com/?docID=17212. Accessed on 28 July 2014.
26. Bai, W., Zhao, K. S., & Asami, K. (2006). Dielectric properties of E. coli cell as simulated by the three-shell spheroidal model. *Biophysical Chemistry, 122*, 136–142.
27. Yoon, G. (2011). Dielectric properties of body fluids with various hematocrit levels. *World Academy of Science, Engineering and Technology, 5*, 1646–1649.
28. Barbosa, C., & Dong, T. (2014). *Modelling and design of a capacitive touch sensor for urinary tract infection detection at the point-of-care*. Proceedings on the 36th Annual International Conference of the IEEE Engineering in Medicine and Biology Society (EMBC'14), Chicago, IL, USA, 26 August–30 August 2014.

Chapter 10
Early Detection and Analysis of Diabetics and Non-diabetics Using Machine Learning

Vikas Somani, Awanit Kumar, and Geetanjali Amarawat

10.1 Introduction

Multiple healthcare opportunities are generated because machine learning models have advanced predictive analytics potential. Machine learning models can also predict chronic diseases such as heart infections and intestinal disorders. There will also be several future machine learning models for predicting non-communicable conditions and increasing healthcare benefits. Researchers are working on machine learning models to predict particular diseases in patients at an early stage and to produce successful methods of disease prevention. This will also minimize patient hospitalization. This transition would be of great benefit to health organizations [1]. Healthcare systems that use advanced computing methods are the most studied field of healthcare research. The allied fields are moving toward more ready-to-to-assemble systems, as seen above. Patients with diabetes cannot generate insulin, resulting in hyperglycemia, a medical measure for increased sugar in the body. In other words, the body cannot repress the hormone insulin release. This leads to abnormal carbohydrate metabolism and high blood glucose levels. Because of the above causes, early detection of diabetes is very critical. Many people worldwide have diabetes, and this is increasing daily. This condition can involve multiple essential organs so that the medical equipment can heal it early in the diagnosis. The number of diabetic patients increasingly requires unnecessarily relevant medical information. Researchers need to create a system that stores,

V. Somani (✉) · A. Kumar
Sangam University, Bhilwara, Rajasthan, India
e-mail: vikas.somani@sangamuniversity.ac.in; awanit.kumar@sangamuniversity.ac.in

G. Amarawat
Swaminarayan University, Kalol, Gujarat, India
e-mail: deanengg@swaminarayanuniversity.ac.in

F. J. Joseph et al. (eds.), *Computational Intelligence for Clinical Diagnosis*,
EAI/Springer Innovations in Communication and Computing,
https://doi.org/10.1007/978-3-031-23683-9_10

updates, and analyses this diabetes knowledge and also recognizes threats using today's expanding technologies. [2] Diabetes is one of the diseases that spread over the world like epidemics. It was proved that every generation, including infants, teenagers, youth and the ages, suffers. Pro-long impacts on organs, such as hepatitis, kidneys, heart, stomach, and death, can be worse. Retinopathy and neuropathy conditions are also interlinked. Diabetes mostly forms type 1 and type 2 [3].

Type-1 Diabetes: In this case, the liver produces no insulin whatsoever. Insulin is a hormone necessary for the use of blood glucose in the body. Blood sugar will increase and lead to type 1 diabetes without insulin in the bloodstream. It is common for children and adolescents. It happens primarily due to genetic disorders. It is also referred to as a youth disease. Its frequent signs are frequent urination, loss of weight, increased hunger, blurred vision, and nerve problems. It can be treated with insulin.

Type-2 Diabetes: In people over 40 years, it is usually a long-term metabolic condition. High blood sugar, resistance to insulin and high insulin are apparent. Fatness and lack of exercise are the main factors. This bad lifestyle will lead to blood glucose storage and diabetes. Only 90% of people with type 2 diabetes are affected. Metformin is administered to treat insulin resistance.

Diabetic Neuropathy: These are the nerve abnormalities acquired over time in diabetic patients. They also happen in the hands and feet. The typical symptoms are pressure, numbness, pinching, and loss of a hand, foot, arms, etc.

Diabetic Retinopathy: It is a diabetic condition which leads to continuous blindness of the eye. At first, there is no noticeable symptom, and symptoms gradually occur. The second stage is the formation of blood vessels on the back of your eyes which can lead to agile bleeding.

10.2 Background and Key Issues

An analysis of computer and artificial intelligence (AI) techniques for the early detection of diabetes is given in Table 10.1.

The diabetes deduction literature survey reveals that a single approach to diabetes detection is not very sophisticated in early stages of diabetes. A hybrid solution with classificatory as primary elements, vector support machines analysis of genetic algorithms can improve the efficiency of artificial neural networks since this technique helps to minimize data noise by extracting features and then using learning methods to recognize hidden patterns, providing more accurate output.

Table 10.1 Survey for early diabetes detection using different machine learning and artificial intelligence techniques

Author	Central idea	Pros	Cons
Mohammed Imran et al.	Diabetic retinopathy (DR) detection using extended fuzzy logic 2. The OWE calculation is based on damage to the eyes Retina [4].	It enables the identification and calculation of retinal damage	Complex method and time taken
Mani Butwall Shraddha Kumar et al.	The approach to data mining for diabetes prevention is based on the random forest classification [5]	Classifiers are a good way of handling massive datasets	As compared to hybrid, a single classification the approach is not very successful
Kamadi V.S. R.P.Varma et al.	It uses the key component analysis and the modified Gini Index SLIQ Decision Tree Algorithm [6]	With fugitive SLIQ, sharp judgment limits can be overcome	Precision can be further improved by fluid membership
Kiarash Zahirnia Mehdi et al.	This document presents and compares various cost-sensitive methods of learning for type 2 diabetes diagnosis [7]	Cost-sensitive approach to resource use is successful	Assumptions in data sets, matrices are used to produce results
Kemal polat et al.	Combining c-means and SVM fuzzy is used for the dataset diabetes prediction [8]	Fuzzy C-means better classify data set with the membership feature	Real-time data is noisy, so that it can be used for processing
Nawaz Mohamudally et al.	Diabetes is shown in this study C4.5, neural network, K-means [9]	It is a successful approach because of the use of a hybrid system	Prediction, description, visualization demands enormous effort
Mostafa Fathi Ganji et al.	ACO is used to derive a set of FADD diagnostic rules [10]	FADD is an excellent solution to diabetes detection.	A single deduction method must be associated with others

10.2.1 Machine Learning Models for Diabetes Detection

The following techniques are used to detect diabetes in the early stages using machine learning techniques and discuss the advantages and disadvantages of the methods in this section.

10.2.2 SVM

SVM can be used for regression and classification applications but is better known for classification applications. This procedure, also known as the dimension plane, plots each point inside a data object into three-dimensional space, where n is the number of data attributes. Distinctions between classes serve as the basis for categorization; these classes can be thought of as tiers of information. Since this is a controlled learning method, data sets are prepared in advance for use [11]. It displays datasets in space as cloud points. The objective is to create a hyperplane that divides data into different categories. The hyperplane divides data collection into groups for data collection and classification. The overall margin of this hyperplane should be the other categories. However, advanced kernel configuration techniques are used if the data categories are wide-ranging.

10.2.2.1 Advantages

- SVM is used to efficiently identify diabetes data by assigning hyperplane information to various categories.
- It removes the fitness of the samples.

10.2.2.2 Disadvantages

- For massive datasets, SVM cannot be used.
- SVM is running slowly.

10.2.3 Fuzzy C-Means

It is an extension to a K-mean clustering algorithm that aims to form clusters and then discover the centers of the cluster, and that cluster with a minimum distance to its centroids is allocated the incoming dataset. However, often there is very little space for new data packages to fall for more than one cluster [12]. The fluid C-means that cluster algorithm prevented this because it uses a fluid partition that is the member variable. The findings are also more precise.

10.2.3.1 Advantages

- In this respect, participation in the fuzzy logic of the membership function helps produce better classification results.
- The learning method is unsupervised so that the effects are more real-time.

10.2.3.2 Disadvantages

- It takes time to calculate.
- It is more likely to be a misconception in the early stages.

10.2.4 PCA (Principal Component Analysis)

PCA is a statistical model for classifying datasets to have the highest correlation in data collection [13]. This aims to create an orthogonal plane to organize data along with this plane. Another plane, well known for its second relationship between the datasets, is perpendicular to that plane. It supports function extraction and measures the main component using Eigen values and Eigen vectors.

10.2.4.1 Advantages

- It helps to reduce the dimension and preserve the alteration between datasets.
- It helps to reduce noise by selecting the highest variance dataset.

10.2.4.2 Disadvantages

- Eigenvalues and covariance matrices are difficult to quantify.
- PCA alone does not provide excellent results when it comes to diabetes detection.

10.2.5 Naive Bayes Classifier

Bayes theorem is a controlled learning technique. It is the algorithm family, assuming that the value of one function is independent (native). It considers the conditional chance of determining the likelihood of an occurrence if any of the events have already occurred. It is used for diabetes diagnosis and diabetic retinopathy detection. The Generative Learning Model can also be referred to as his classificatory. The classification is based on Baye's theorem, which implies separate predictors. In short, this classifier assumes that certain features are not connected to any other function in a class. Success and failure are equally possible if there is a dependence on the characteristics of each other. This tool is handy and easy for databases with large volumes of data [14].

10.2.5.1 Advantages

- It helps reduce noise by averaging values.
- The higher likelihood value provides a better outcome.

10.2.5.2 Disadvantages

- The shape of the distribution is taken very strongly.
- Data is lost when the continuous functionality is discreet.

10.2.6 Decision Trees

Decision trees support very advanced techniques in support of decision making. A structure like a tree or a diagram is based on cost, classification, and effort. When all the requirements are in place, go from the root to the leaves (until the tasks are complete). Gini indexes are used to calculate the split node. The value of the Gini index aids in separating the nodes. Classification forests also have a random subset of decisions like these. This classification also helps us to diagnose diabetes. This algorithm constructs the regression models. These models are built in a tree-like system, which provides a tree-like structure. It also divides the set data into sub-sets and smaller subsets, creating a tree gradually. This tree includes the particulars of the decision to classify the leaf node, while the decision contains branches. The tree's top decision node will match the root node. This is the best forecast [15].

10.2.6.1 Advantages

- The best predictive model is a thorough analysis of the problem.
- Random forest classifications are ideally suited for vast amounts of data and incomplete data.

10.2.6.2 Disadvantages

- Random forests are quick to train but slow to predict once they are educated.
- Decision trees are unstable even if the input is minimal.

10.2.7 Random Forest

There are parallels between the classification system and this is the technique used for categorizing data. Different trees may use different methods for classifying data and making predictions about regression, but ultimately the goal is to construct a set of decision-making bodies at the data and class levels. This invariance in categorization is more important than gathering training data, especially for decision-making bodies [16].

10.2.8 Neural Network

This classifier's unit names reference vectors, referred to as "nodes," convert the inputs to the vectors known as "features" to their respective outputs. Each neuron enters an input, often a non-linear input, and an output function is given in the next step. The first level entry is the next level output, so the classification algorithm follows a feedback loop. This way, the previous level has no input so that signals passing through neurons and layers can be weighed, and these signals are then translated into a training process that eventually becomes a network to handle a given problem [17].

10.2.8.1 Advantages

- ANN is used for feature extraction with backpropagation for the detection of diabetes.
- When combined with fluid logic, uncertainty can be managed.

10.2.8.2 Disadvantages

- Training requires a great deal of work.
- It is hard to ensure that all inputs are prepared.

10.2.9 Nearest Neighbor

In reality, classification rules the nearest algorithm. The nearest algorithm for classification is a common term for this method. Labeled point clusters are used to shed light on how the other points were assigned their labels. When adding a new marker, it first looks for possible neighbors (those that are geographically close) to the spot being added. When a new item receives a neighbor's same rating, it becomes equivalent to the rating of other items in the vicinity, depending on the neighbor's vote. In the 'k' algorithm, this is the count of confirmed neighbors [18].

All of the necessary knowledge for implementing the categorization algorithms and procedures used to foresee the sickness has already been acquired. Following this poll, it was suggested that a combination of a hybrid classification algorithm and any kind of learning might increase the disease's predicted accuracy by more than 80%. When more than two classifiers are combined, accuracy improves. We build a model for assessing the quality of training data using a combination of the decision tree and other classifiers. In addition to the aforementioned techniques, we have also employed XGBoost for each classifier and analyzed its performance. With this combo, we can boost accuracy by over 80% [19].

10.3 Hybrid Classification Algorithm System

Specificity for the presence of diabetes in patients is maximized using the proposed strategy. In this discussion, we examine the many types of machine learning algorithms and how they can be used to produce predictions and inferences. More than one algorithm can be used to boost the reliability of predictions (Fig. 10.1).

After collecting information related to a disease, it is sent to a pre-processed device for analysis. Extractive functions will be used to glean information from unstructured, large, or otherwise uninteresting data sets. The necessary machine learning method is used for the data training and data gathering, and the results are then evaluated [20]. Then, to get the desired outcome, we employ a classifier

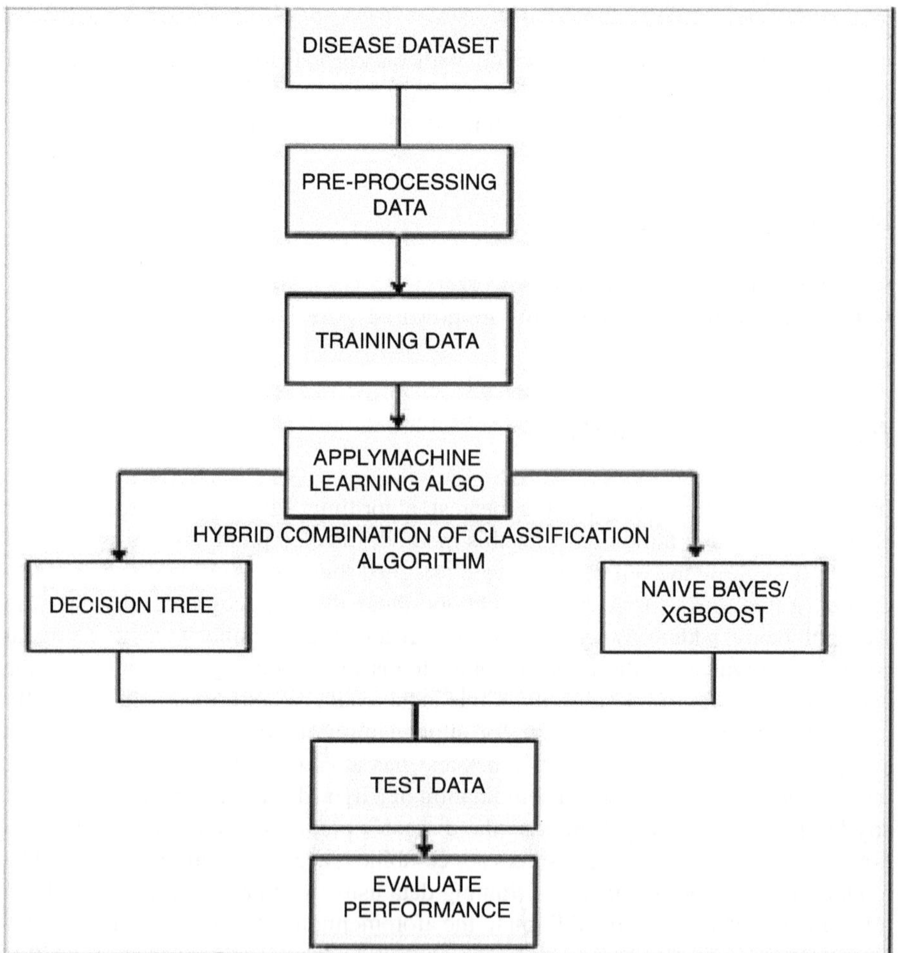

Fig. 10.1 Diagram of the proposed system architecture

combination. In this way, we recommend combining the Decision Tree with the Support Vector Machine, the Decision Tree with XGBoost and the Hybrid Results Test method. The information will then be monitored and the desired outcomes evaluated. We now study the various classifiers and explore the hybrid mix used in our scheme. There are multiple forms of classification; an algorithm is a classification system that maps data entered into a particular group.

10.3.1 System Flow

Figure 10.2 explains the device design flow map; we also made feature selection for pre-processing: advance feature selection and backward feature selection. This is to show how data can be provided using ADA Boost, XGboost, voting classifiers, and stacking classifiers to assist in the identification of people who are likely to develop diabetes. The proposed approach has two major phases in which the desired effects can be achieved together. Data are prepared in the first stage, and the second stage is classified. The machine input is then the PID dataset, and the output is a stable or diabetic class. Steps are taken to increase productivity. The data collection eliminates the noisy and inaccurate data, first of all.

The main goal is to identify whether or decrease the likelihood of diabetes. When the number of samples increases, so does the classification accuracy but with no real increase in statistical significance (Fig. 10.3).

In certain instances, but not all, the algorithm yields performance high in rhythm but low in classification. Our model's primary goal is to achieve high precision. Different methods for classifying diabetic and non-diabetic outcomes were

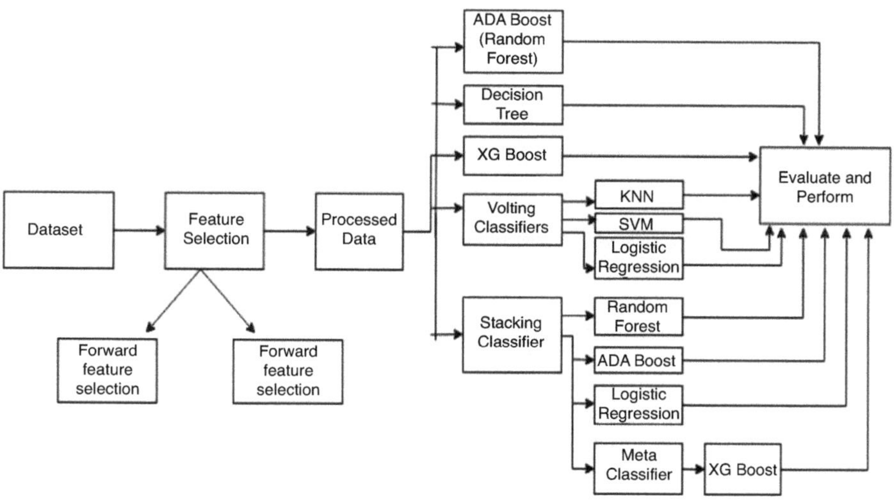

Fig. 10.2 Flow of proposed system

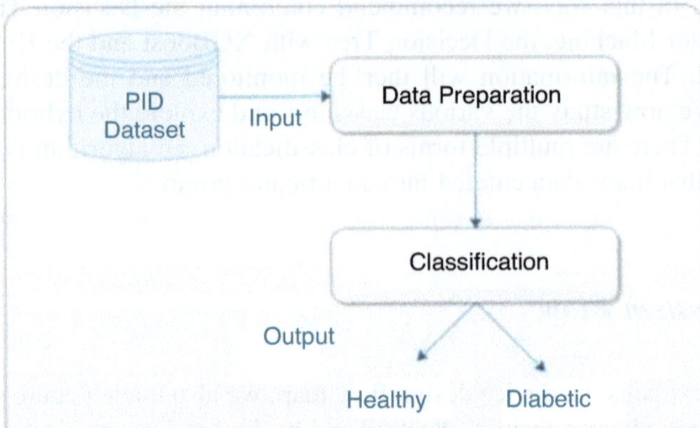

Fig. 10.3 Proposed system diagram

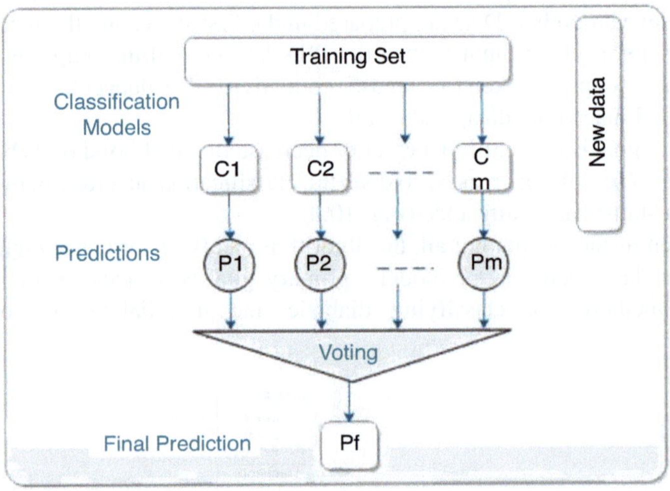

Fig. 10.4 Functional diagram for voting classifier

examined. This proposed approach uses techniques such as AdaBoost, Tree Classification Decision, XGBoost, voting classification, and Diabetes Prediction Stacking. We will go into classifiers now and then go through the classification of the stacking and voting in the following parts (Fig. 10.4).

- Stacking: Stacking is an ensemble learning strategy that integrates predictions from several simple models plus a new dataset. These new data are taken for another classifier as input data. The issue was resolved with the help of this rating. A synonym for stacking is mixing.
- Voting Classifier: "hard" and "soft" voting is carried out by the Vote Classifier Ensemble. When we vote strongly, the final class label in the classification

models is expected to be the most previewed class label. By averaging class probabilities in soft votes, we predict class labeling (advocated only if the classifiers are considered accurate).

10.3.2 Working Principle

Gives step-by-step instructions on how to use various classifiers to improve accuracy.

10.3.3 Hardware Requirements

For the device implementation, the following hardware was used:

- RAM SIZE: 4GB
- 10GB HDD
- Processor Type: Intel 1.66 GHz Pentium 4B.

10.3.4 Implementation Steps

PIMA Indian Diabetes Dataset has been selected as the diabetes data kit of choice. There are a total of 768 instances, both diabetic and non-diabetic, and four risk factors: the prevalence among pregnant women, the concentration of plasma glucose after 2 hours of oral glucose administration, diastolic blood pressure, and triceps skin thickness. Whether it is done automatically or manually, Feature Selection determines which features are most relevant to the desired prediction attribute or output. The quality of our models can suffer if our data contains extraneous information (Fig. 10.5).

- We use a PIMA Indian diabetic dataset.
- The system uses the function selection method: Advanced selection of features and backward feathering for pre-processing. We train five different graders and determine which graders are highly accurate. We used these AdaBoost, XGBoost, Voting Classifier, and Stacking Classifier classifiers.
- The Stacking Classifier is used as its basis by Random Forest, AdaBoost, Logistical Regression, and XGBoost for its Meta classifier.
- The Acoustic and Stacking Classifier is the most powerful because of its improved ability to classify power and class strength.
- In order to better comprehend the sequence of our measures and their intended results, we have included screenshots below. The ADA Boost classifier's output

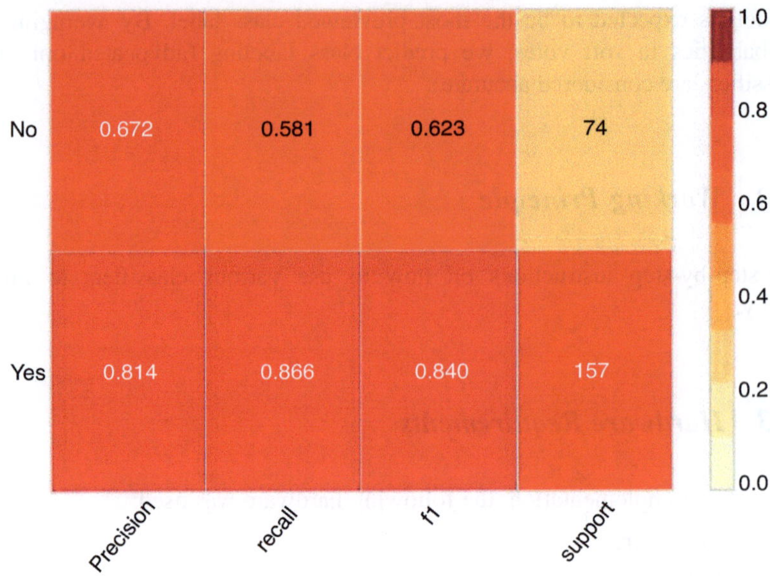

Fig. 10.5 AdaBoost classification report

will be displayed graphically. For Decision Tree, XG Boost, Vote, and Stacking, we have taken analogous measures.

We discuss the classification findings after first introducing the AdaBoost classification method. ROC curves were calculated using the same methodology applied to the decision tree, XGBoost, voting, and stacking classifiers. For more examples, check out the images below (Figs. 10.6, 10.7, 10.8, and 10.9).

We then determine the total number of diabetes sponsors. Next, a screen displays test results for a person with diabetes (Fig. 10.10).

10.4 Results

Achieving a success rate of 80% or above in predicting diabetes using five separate classification schemes is a major step forward. You may do some basic analysis using the graphs in Figs. 10.11 and 10.12. The AUC, accuracy, recall, and F1 results from various classifications are displayed in Fig. 10.11. Figure 10.12 depicts how histograms are appropriately displayed using different classifiers (Table 10.2).

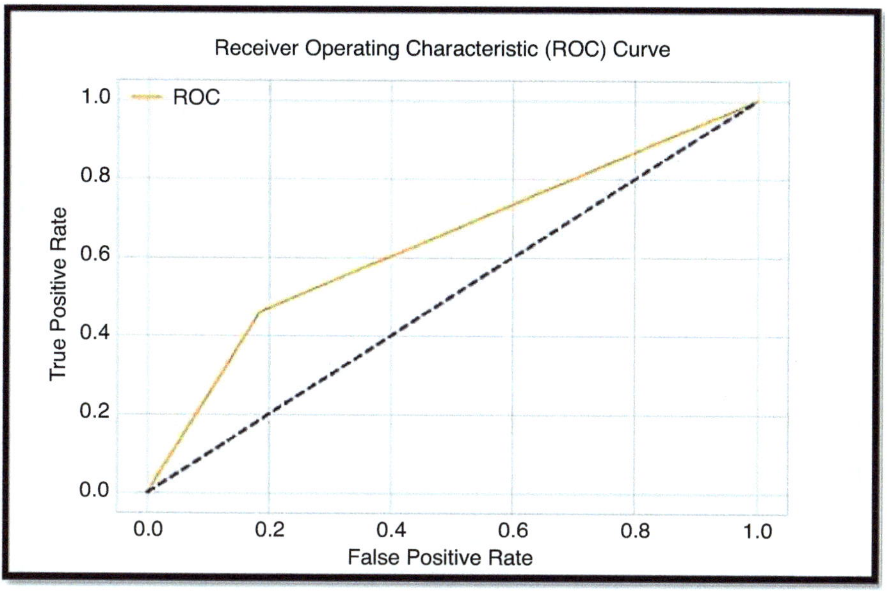

Fig. 10.6 ROC decision tree

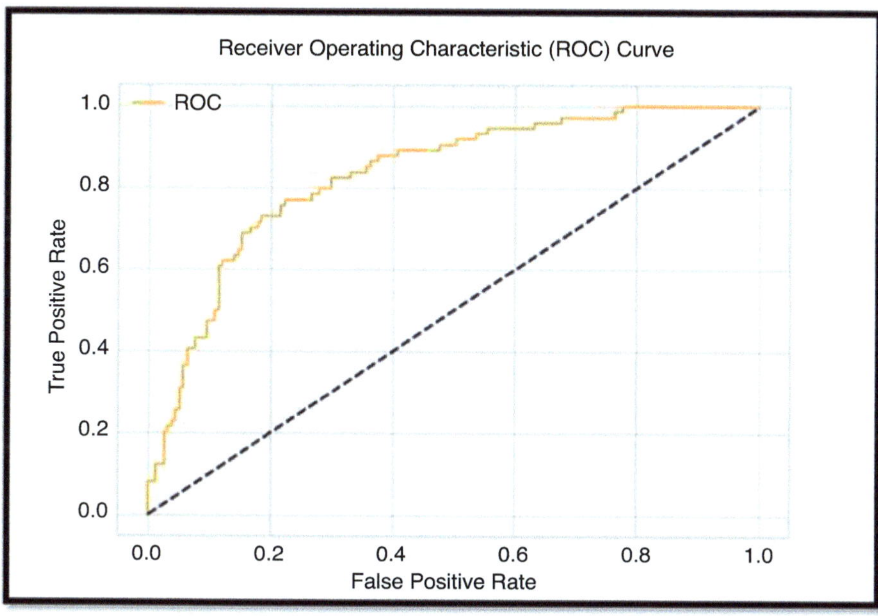

Fig. 10.7 ROC XGBoost

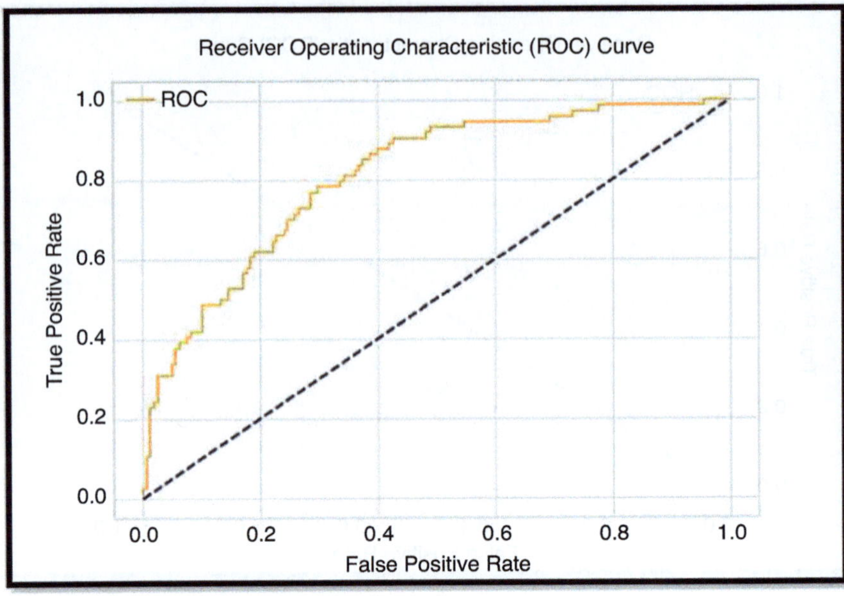

Fig. 10.8 Classifier ROC voting

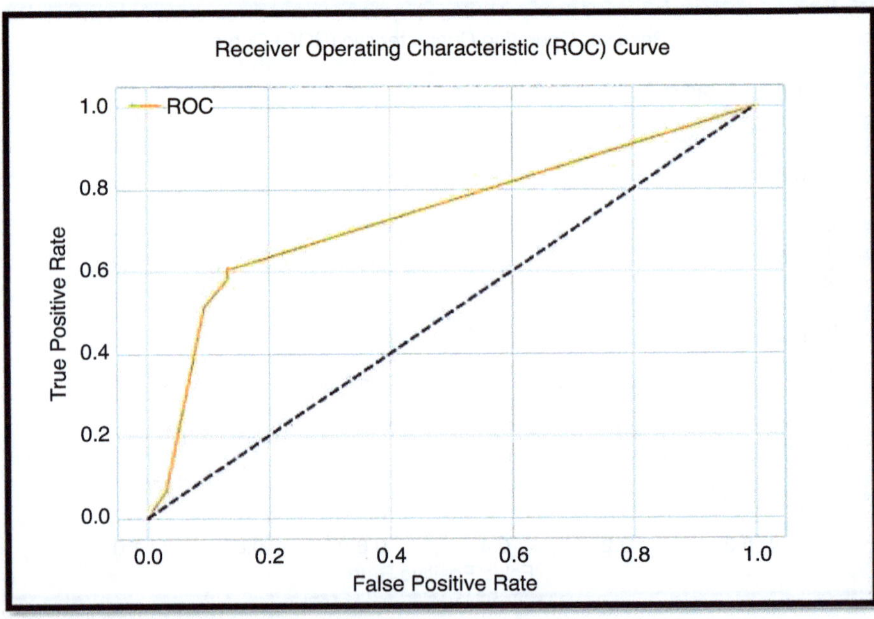

Fig. 10.9 Classifier ROC voting

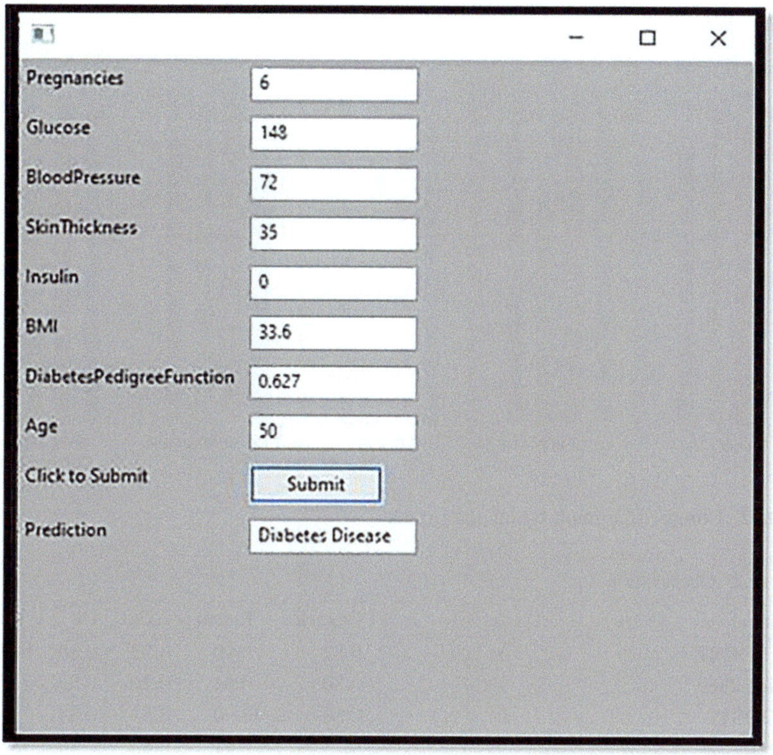

Fig. 10.10 Detected diabetes shown on the test screen

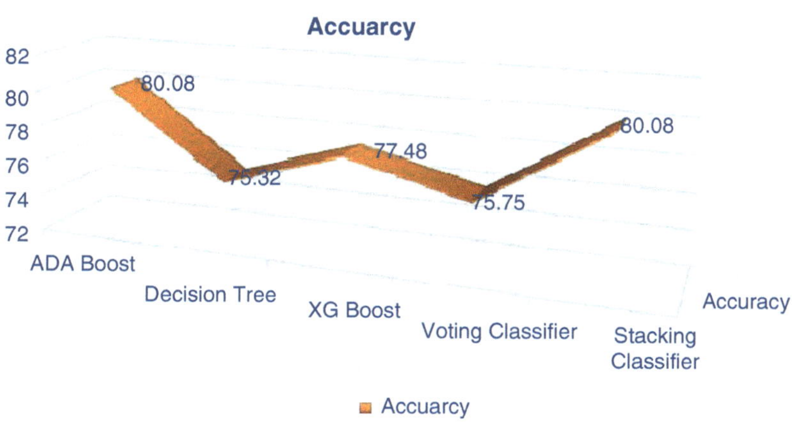

Fig. 10.11 Graph for precision, F1 score, AUC, and recall

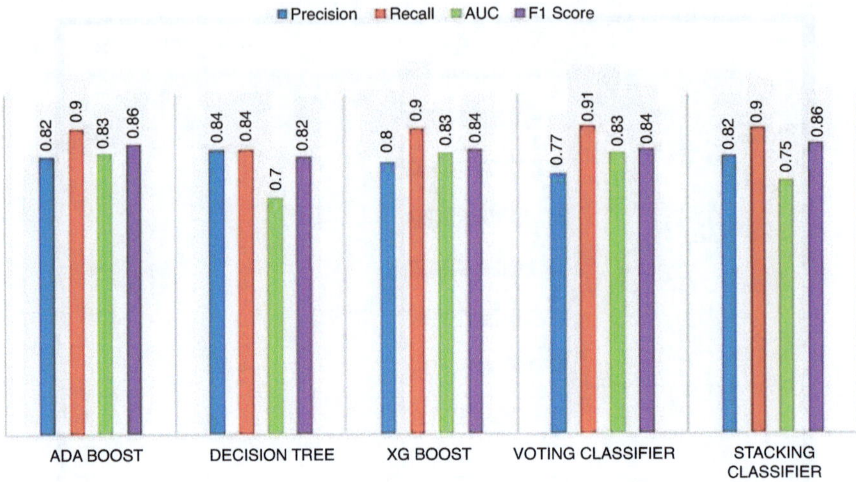

Fig. 10.12 Comparison graph for all algorithms

Table 10.2 Observations

Classifier	Precision	Recall	AUC	F1	Accuracy
ADA BOOST	0.82	0.90	0.83	0.86	80.08
Decision Tree	0.80	0.84	0.70	0.82	75.32
XGBOOST	0.80	0.90	0.83	0.84	77.48
Voting (KNN, SVM, Logistic regression)	0.77	0.91	0.83	0.84	75.75
Stacking (Random Forest, ADAboost, Logistic regression)	0.82	0.90	0.75	0.86	80.08

10.5 Conclusion

Medical professionals can benefit from the use of machine learning techniques for the diagnosis and treatment of diabetes. Finally, we will state that enhanced categorization accuracy paves the way for enhanced machine learning model outputs. The performance analysis focuses on the accuracy of all classification techniques and also found that the present method was less than 71% accurate, so we suggest using a mixture of classifications known as the hybrid approach. The hybrid solution is based on the advantages of two or more technologies. Our scheme provides 75.33% for decision-making tree classification, 77.47% for XGBoost, and 75.76% for voting classification. We have therefore found that Stacking Classifier and AdaBoost are the strongest of all the above classifiers.

References

1. Kaur, H., & Kumari, V. (2018). Predictive modelling and analytics for diabetes using a machine learning approach. *Applied Computing and Informatics.*
2. Carter, J. A., Long, C. S., Smith, B. P., Smith, T. L., & Donati, G. L. (2019). Combining elemental analysis of toenails and machine learning techniques as a non-invasive diagnostic tool for the robust classification of type-2 diabetes. *Expert Systems with Applications, 115*, 245–255.
3. Kavakiotis, I., Tsave, O., Salifoglou, A., Maglaveras, N., Vlahavas, I., & Chouvarda, I. (2017). Machine learning and data mining methods in diabetes research. *Computational and Structural Biotechnology Journal, 15*, 104–116.
4. Mahmud, S. M., Hossin, M. A., Ahmed, M. R., Noori, S. R. H., & Sarkar, M. N. I. (2018). Machine learning based unified framework for diabetes prediction. In *Proceedings of the 2018 international conference on big data engineering and technology* (pp. 46–50). ACM.
5. Patil, R., & Tamane, S. (2018). A comparative analysis on the evaluation of classification algorithms in the prediction of diabetes. *International Journal of Electrical and Computer Engineering, 8*(5), 3966.
6. Dagliati, A., Marini, S., Sacchi, L., Cogni, G., Teliti, M., Tibollo, V., et al. (2018). Machine learning methods to predict diabetes complications. *Journal of Diabetes Science and Technology, 12*(2), 295–302.
7. Barik, R. K., Priyadarshini, R., Dubey, H., Kumar, V., & Yadav, S. (2018). Leveraging machine learning in mist computing telemonitoring system for diabetes prediction. In *Advances in data and information sciences* (pp. 95–104). Springer.
8. Choudhury, A., & Gupta, D. (2019). A survey on medical diagnosis of diabetes using machine learning techniques. In *Recent developments in machine learning and data analytics* (pp. 67–78). Springer.
9. Samant, P., & Agarwal, R. (2017). Diagnosis of diabetes using computer methods: Soft computing methods for diabetes detection using iris. *Threshold, 8*, 9.
10. Dankwa-Mullan, I., Rivo, M., Sepulveda, M., Park, Y., Snowdon, J., & Rhee, K. (2019). Transforming diabetes care through artificial intelligence: The future is here. *Population Health Management, 22*(3), 229–242.
11. Joshi, T. N., & Chawan, P. M. (2018). Logistic regression and svm based diabetes prediction system. *International Journal For Technological Research In Engineering 5.*
12. Beam, A. L., & Kohane, I. S. (2018). Big data and machine learning in health care. *JAMA, 319*(13), 1317–1318.
13. Nnamoko, N., Hussain, A., & England, D. (2018). Predicting diabetes onset: An ensemble supervised learning approach. In *2018 IEEE congress on evolutionary computation (CEC)* (pp. 1–7). IEEE.
14. Yadav, B., Sharma, S., & Kalra, A. (2018). Supervised learning technique for prediction of diseases. In *Intelligent communication, control and devices* (pp. 357–369). Springer.
15. Joshi, R., & Alehegn, M. (2017). Analysis and prediction of diabetes diseases using machine learning algorithm: Ensemble approach. *International Research Journal of Engineering and Technology, 4*(10).
16. Singh, D. A. A. G., Leavline, E. J., & Baig, B. S. (2017). Diabetes prediction using medical data. *Journal of Computational Intelligence in Bioinformatics, 10*(1), 1–8.
17. Gujral, S. (2017). Early diabetes detection using machine learning: A review. *International Journal for Innovative Research in Science & Technology, 3*(10), 57–62.
18. Zia, U. A., & Khan, N. (2017). Predicting diabetes in medical datasets using machine learning techniques. *International Journal of Scientific & Engineering Research, 8.*
19. Naqvi, B., Ali, A., Hashmi, M. A., & Atif, M. (2018). Prediction techniques for diagnosis of diabetic disease: A comparative study. *International Journal of Computer Science and Network Security, 18*(8), 118–124.
20. Chen, J. C. H., Kang, H. Y., & Wang, M. C. (2018). Integrating feature ranking with ensemble learning and logistic model trees for the prediction of postprandial blood glucose elevation. *Journal of Universal Computer Science, 24*(6), 797–812.

Chapter 11
An Intelligent Air Quality Prediction System Using Neuro-Fuzzy Temporal Classifier with Spatial Constraints

S. Anu Priya and V. Khanaa

11.1 Introduction

The world is growing fast economically, especially since the majority of cities in fast-developing countries such as India and China are affected due to air pollution. Air pollution has affected all young and elderly people with lung and heart diseases. To protect the world from air pollution, researchers are developing warning systems for predicting air quality and also providing health alerts to people who are living in cities to protect themselves. The available techniques concentrate on the air quality prediction process only and do not reach the public. Air quality is useful for preparing the health index of a country. The health index is calculated by considering the air quality; then, it is called the air quality health index, which is useful for understanding the impact of air pollution on health. These systems are helpful for people to get awareness about air pollution and also try to reduce the air pollution level. Moreover, the way of improving the air quality is also considered to reduce the footprint of the surroundings, so this chapter proposed a new model for categorizing the quality of quality.

The PM 2.5 is being monitored since 2013 in India at New Delhi, and it has spread gradually to the important cities of India such as Chennai, Hyderabad, Mumbai, and Kolkata. This monitoring process is capable of predicting the day to day pollution in a city. Moreover, the archived and live PM2.5 data are to be

S. Anu Priya (✉)
Research Scholar, Department of Computer Science and Engineering, Bharath Institute of Higher Education and Research, Chennai, Tamil Nadu, India
e-mail: anupriya.mca@bharathuniv.ac.in

V. Khanaa
Department of Information Technology, Bharath Institute of Higher Education and Research, Chennai, Tamil Nadu, India

F. J. J. Joseph et al. (eds.), *Computational Intelligence for Clinical Diagnosis*, EAI/Springer Innovations in Communication and Computing,
https://doi.org/10.1007/978-3-031-23683-9_11

supplied for the researchers and public users for performing the analysis and also to enhance the understandability and the current trends of PM2.5 in various cities. Later on, the PM2.5 data are collected according to the variation of different places in a city. The seasonal trend is also captured for every city, and various trend analyses on PM2.5 were also conducted. Analyzing the trends of PM2.5 in various cities is done by applying machine learning algorithms that are capable of performing data preprocessing and classification.

Machine Learning (ML) techniques are utilized widely for categorizing the levels in different environments such as science field, industry, and business. The various ML algorithms, including Decision Tree (DT), Random Forest (RF), Naïve Bayes (NB), Support Vector Machine (SVM), and Neural Network (NN), are used as ensemble approaches for improving the performances in the process of classification. The majority of ensemble methods have used the baseline to combine the different classifiers. Here, stacking is a powerful method in the ensemble. Stacking is a learning method which combines the regression methods through a meta-regressor. These models are used to train the set according to the result column of the training data. The stacked model performed well than other models and is also capable of highlighting the poor performance [1]. It is widely applied to the method of winning the competition and is also used in various fields, including just-in-time and ski injury predictions [2, 3]. However, the available ML techniques have not achieved sufficient accuracy in prediction. To enhance prediction accuracy, Deep Learning (DL) algorithms are applied widely in this direction.

In this chapter, a new air quality prediction system is proposed for predicting air quality by applying a newly proposed neuro-fuzzy temporal classification algorithm with spatial constraints. Moreover, an existing Butterfly optimization algorithm is also applied for performing feature optimization. It helps in improving the neural classifier's prediction accuracy.

The contributions of this chapter are as follows:

1. To propose a new air quality prediction model for predicting the quality of the air using a neuro-fuzzy temporal classification algorithm (NFTCA).
2. To predict the air pollution level in different areas according to the air quality prediction result.
3. To incorporate the spatial constraints in the proposed neural classifier for making an effective decision on PM2.5 datasets.
4. To apply the existing Butterfly Optimization Algorithm (BOA) for performing an effective feature optimization process.
5. To achieve high prediction accuracy and low root mean square error rate.

The rest of the chapter is organized into four sections: Literature survey, System Architecture, Proposed Air Quality Prediction Model, Result and Discussion and Conclusion. The next section of this chapter is the Literature Survey which describes the relevant works available in the literature by highlighting the contributions, merits, and demerits of their work. The third section in this chapter is System Architecture, which demonstrates the workflow of the prediction model. In the fourth section, we provide context for the suggested approach for predicting air quality. The experimental findings and analysis are reported in Sect. 11.5. The final section wraps up the work by pointing out the various contributions and promising future efforts in this field.

11.2 Literature Survey

Bruno et al.'s [4–8] literature predicts that many air quality prediction models apply feature selection and classification algorithms to predict air quality in cities and countries. Bruno et al. [4] proposed a black box system for forecasting and mitigating air pollution. Their method forecasts weather and environment. Neagu, C.-D., Kalapanidas, et al. New neuro fuzzy air quality predictor. Fuzzy logic prediction uses back propagation neural networks. Ganapathy et al. [5] developed a temporal fuzzy min-max neural classifier to forecast diseases successfully. They used the Particle Swarm Optimization algorithm to optimize the features and achieved better prediction accuracy than existing neural classifiers due to fuzzy logic and temporal restrictions.

Gu et al. [1] developed a predictor that incorporates the heuristic recurrent for predicting air quality. The predictor uses machine learning algorithms for handling the pollution factors and estimating the air quality for more hours. Huang et al. [2] introduced an intelligent air index prediction method for past mining data and also realized the quality of brain health by using IoT technology. They performed data preprocessing to enable users to understand the air index from anywhere, anytime. Their method is helpful for managing cloud-based users by supplying relevant data. Soh et al. [9] aimed to predict the quality of the air up to 48 hours of time duration by using multi-neural classifiers including ANN, CNN, and LSTM for extracting the temporal features. In addition, their model extracts the air quality index from multiple places in a certain area. Gu et al. [1] developed a new air quality prediction system that incorporates the heuristic recurrent to predict air quality. To enhance the reliability in the prediction process, they have applied a 1-h prediction for estimating air quality after several hours successfully and proved it as better than the relevant models.

Zhao et al. [3] constructed a new model for mining new relationships in various regions. They considered the spatiotemporal features in their model for mining the local relationship and the regional relationships and to predict air quality. In the end, they evaluated their model and proved as scalable, reliable, and dynamic. Yatong et al. [10] proposed a new learning technique to predict air quality that applies gaseous pollutant concentration to enhance the prediction process. Zhang et al. [11] considered the issues of processing large-scale high-dimensional data by incorporating their new model to forecast the data for predicting the quality of air accurately. They applied a mechanism called sliding window that is useful for mining the temporal data to enhance the training process in various dimensions. They collected data from 35 stations that are available for monitoring air quality in China. Finally, they have proved that it was better than the other models. Jun Ma et al. [12] proposed a transferred learning-based LSTM to perform an air quality prediction process. Moreover, their approach considers temporal resolutions for predicting air quality.

Daniel et al. [13] built a new model to predict air quality using LSTM, and they have achieved better prediction accuracy. Quang et al. [14] developed a new method for enhancing the prediction accuracy that considers the indoor air pollutant profiles, stochastic nature, index, and humidity. They applied the Kalman filter with fractional order in their indoor air quality model that dealt with inaccurate and non-linear data from sensors. Finally, their model compared with the existing core relevant works and proved to be better. Wei Huang et al. [15] developed a new method to optimize the backpropagation neural classifier that incorporates the PSO for predicting the air quality index. In their work, an inertia weight is considered as a learning feature for searching the capability during the early and late stages with fast convergence. They also applied their own mutation method for performing an effective searching process and also omitted the particles that failed to meet the requirement of local optimality. Finally, they achieved better air quality index results than other works.

Hong Zheng et al. [16] proposed an air quality prediction model that is explored with a series of ML-based ensemble techniques. Zhang and Woo [17] identified the various air quality index patterns for particular regions by considering the IoT sensors that are placed in vehicles. They also demonstrated the feasibility of predicting air quality through ML techniques on live data. Finally, they achieved better performance in terms of prediction accuracy. Ying et al. [18] proposed a new method to predict air quality according to the multiple features through ML techniques and fusion. Their method considered 6 days of meteorological air quality data as input and applied a fusion technique for providing the prediction result in China. They used an extreme gradient boost decision tree for making final decision input data in the process of prediction. Yu-Chun et al. [19] developed a new neuro-fuzzy-aware air quality prediction system for forecasting air quality. In their system, they trained data by using clustering, fuzzy rules, genetic, particle swarm optimization, and neural classifier, and then suitable decision is made on input data.

Xu and Yoneda [20] devised an encoder that uses LSTM to forecast time-sensitive data models in various city areas. They used meteorological data for predicting. Edith Chen et al. [21] proposed using LSTM and S2S to forecast air quality. Extreme gradient boosting decision tree is used. Finally, they validated their method's accuracy and model expression power. Saravanan and Santhosh Kumar [22] suggested a bidirectional RNN approach for detecting air quality. Their technique used interconnected neurons to construct a cyclic network with current and historical inputs to monitor air pollution over time. Ritu et al. [8] discovered air quality patterns on a CNN to detect air pollution. Using scripting and Python, they preprocessed and analyzed data. Air quality data of 2015–2020 was utilized to determine the optimal CO, NO2, and SO2 levels. Finally, they forecasted the most contaminated location and calculated the highest prediction accuracy. Krishna et al. [23] built an air quality prediction framework that processes key dataset features to improve prediction accuracy. CNN, denoising encoder, and RNN handle the data. The suggested framework handles missing values and analyses data to estimate air quality. Lack of adequate training techniques prevents all present air quality prediction models from meeting the current needs. This work provides a novel model to better predict air quality in cities.

11.3 System Architecture

The working flow of the proposed air quality prediction system is explained diagrammatically in Fig. 11.1. The working flow of the prediction system has been explained with the help of various components, including the user interaction module, spatial agent, temporal agent, prediction manager, rule base, rule manager, feature optimization, and data classification.

The required PM2.5 data is extracted by the user interaction module from the PM2.5 dataset. The extracted required data are sent to the prediction manager to predict the quality of air. The prediction manager forwards the collected data into feature optimization to optimize the dataset by incorporating the butterfly optimization algorithm. After that, the data is sent to the classification phase, where a spatially constrained neuro-fuzzy temporal classifier is used to the data for efficient categorization. The prediction manager makes the ultimate call based on the rules contained in the rule base as well as spatial and temporal limitations. In this case, the rule base takes fuzzy logic into account and stores the available rules there. The fuzzy rules themselves were produced by the fuzzy rule manager and filed away in the rule base.

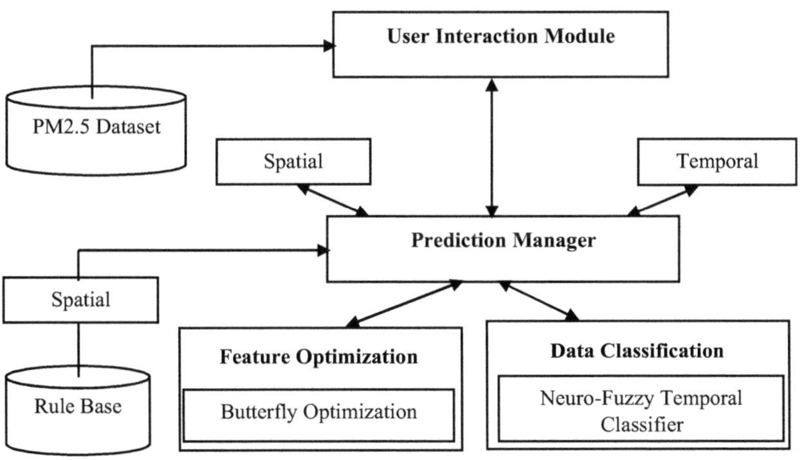

Fig. 11.1 System architecture

11.4 Proposed Work

Air quality in different cities and nations can be predicted with the use of a new system described in this section. In this chapter, we offer a new neuro-fuzzy temporal classification system for estimating air quality that takes geographical limitations into account. Arora and Singh's [24] Butterfly Optimization Approach (BOA) is another feature selection algorithm used in this work to boost prediction precision. There are two sections that detail the proposed air quality prediction system, one focusing on feature optimization and the other on data categorization. Initial context for the feature optimization procedure is also provided.

11.4.1 Feature Optimization

Feature optimization plays a vital role in the process of selecting the most contributed features. The prediction system applies the feature optimization process first to reduce the number of features for performing the classification and reduces the training and testing time. When it reduces the input data size, the classification time is also reduced. This work uses Butterfly Optimization Algorithm (BOA) by Arora and Singh [24] to optimize the dataset to improve classifier speed and accuracy. The user interaction module reads the PM2.5 dataset with the proper values for PM2.5, PM10, NO_2, CO, O_3, and SO_2 and delivers it to the feature optimization phase.

11.4.2 Data Classification

This subsection explains in detail the newly proposed Neuro-Fuzzy Temporal Classification Algorithm (NFTCA) with spatial constraints with necessary background information about the neural classifier and the working flow of the proposed classifier.

11.4.2.1 Neural Classifier

Neural networks (NNs) are the most useful technique to categorize the given input data effectively according to the fixed conditions that are set by the administrator. Recently, many research works have been done by using the NN aware classifiers in the direction of data classification. The NNs are applied in various emerging fields such as medical, military, and social service. First, the NNs are self-adaptive methods that equip the current information without any particular method. Second, the methods of NNs are considered a universal method that approximates any method along with sufficient prediction results. Third, the NNs are non-linear models that are capable of developing a flexible model to resolve complex live issues. In the end, the NNs are capable of estimating the probabilities of the posterior that supply the basic information to generate rules and also performing the statistical analysis. Generally, it consists of three layers: input layer, output layer, and processing layer. Among them, the input layer gets the necessary input from the user and forwards it to the processing layer. The processing layer processes the input data and produces the output. The output layer gets output from the processing layer and produces it for the users. The various NN algorithms, such as Artificial Neural Network (ANN), Back Propagation (BP), and Feed Forward Network (FN), are available in the literature.

11.4.2.2 Fuzzy Logic

Wei Zhang et al. [25] proposed Fuzzy sets that form a key technique to represent and process uncertain data. The uncertainty arises in various forms in the databases, such as imprecision, vagueness, non-specificity, inconsistency, etc. The fuzzy sets exploit the uncertainty for making a system complex. At the same time, fuzzy sets are created as a powerful method for considering incomplete data, noisy data, and imprecise data. These are useful in developing data uncertainty which provides better performance traditionally. Here, two important tasks, such as fuzzification and de-fuzzification processes, are performed in this fuzzy theory. The fuzzy intervals are also varying according to the fuzzy membership functions, including triangular, trapezoidal, Mamdani, and Gaussian fuzzy membership functions. The fuzzy rules are generated based on the intervals that are fixed by the specific fuzzy membership function and the expected outcome for the specific problem.

11.4.2.3 Temporal Constraints

Time (Temporal constraint) is playing a major role today in making effective decisions on day-to-day activities. Moreover, time is also important to collect the data from various resources. In addition, each system is considered as efficient when it takes less processing time to produce the output in all kinds of applications. Thus, this work also considers the temporal constraints to make a decision on the dataset and also gives importance to the data collection time duration in each location of the cities and countries. Generally, the temporal data is capable of producing good results than the normal data.

11.4.2.4 Spatial Constraints

The spatial data is also very important when collecting weather data, traffic data, medical data, etc. This work uses PM2.5 data for performing classification and also to predict air quality. The PM2.5 dataset is also containing date, time, and location (space) as well for mentioning the data collected location and time that are helpful for predicting the future air quality in the specific location by performing the training process on various data so that the spatial constraint is very important in the process of air quality prediction forever.

11.4.2.5 Proposed Neural Classifier

The proposed Neuro-Fuzzy Temporal Classification Algorithm (NFTCA) with spatial constraints is explained in detail in this section. The information about the neural networks, fuzzy logic, temporal constraints, and spatial 250 constraints. Moreover, the proposed NFTCA with spatial constraints is explained stepwise in this section. The spatial fuzzy temporal rules have been generated and incorporated into the neural network for making effective decisions on datasets. In this NN, a sigmoid function is applied as an activation method for performing the decision-making process. In addition, the trapezoidal fuzzy membership function is applied to create rules that are helpful for finalizing the decision-making process. The steps of the proposed NFTCA are as follows:

Algorithm NFTCA with Spatial Constraints (NFTCA-S)

Input: PM2.5 dataset, trapezoidal method, sigmoid method
Output: Prediction results

Step 1: Read the entire PM2.5 dataset.
Step 2: Choose 80% of the records from PM2.5 dataset randomly.
Step 3: Perform the training process and also assume that TR = {}
Step 4: Classify the records as "Good," "Moderate," and "Unhealthy".
For I =1 to NR // NR – No. of records
Begin
a. Substitute the primary class label with result column
b. Consider and include a new record into the training record set TR.
End
Step 5: Find the mean value for all the columns of the dataset.
Step 6: Rank the features according to the mean values and the threshold value by using the fuzzy temporal rules and spatial constraints.
Step 7: Apply the Butterfly Optimization Algorithm (Arora and Singh 2018)
Step 8: Generate the fuzzy temporal rules with spatial constraints for performing training process.
(a) Perform the fuzzification process using trapezoidal fuzzy membership function.
(b) Every record will be named and also stored in a file.
(c) Form rules for making decision using rules in testing process.
(d) Consider 20% of the data for performing the testing process from the total dataset.
(e) Apply spatio-fuzzy temporal rules to perform testing.
(f) Classified results will be returned.

Step 9: Display the prediction result according to the classification results and categorize as “Good,” “Moderate,” and “Not Good for Health.”
Step 10: Update the decision on records as results in the PM2.5 dataset.

The proposed NFTCA-S is working based on the above steps. The proposed algorithm is useful for predicting the environment in terms of air quality is “Good,” “Moderate,” and “Not Good for Health.” According to the prediction results, people can take remedy for managing the moderate and not good for health environment. This work applies neural networks, fuzzy logic, temporal logic, spatial constraints, and an optimization technique. The BOA is helpful for choosing the most useful features with valid input values to perform the decision-making process. Fuzzy temporal rules are generated with the consideration of spatial constraints for fine-tuning the decisions on records. The temporal and spatial constraints are very important in predicting air quality. The air quality may differ in different seasons and timing as well. So that this work applies all the necessary features for making better decisions on the PM2.5 dataset.

11.5 Results and Discussion

The evaluation measures, dataset description, and experimental outcomes are all broken off into subsections here. The indicators of quality are presented and discussed first.

11.5.1 Evaluation Metric

To measure how well the suggested system predicts, we employ the industry standard Root Mean Squared Error (RMSE) statistic. Using the following formula, we can determine the RMSE (11.1).

$$\mathrm{RMSE}=\sqrt{\frac{1}{N}\sum_{i=1}^{N}(y_i-\widehat{y}_i)^2} \tag{11.1}$$

where the variables y_i and $\widehat{y}_i$ are the real value and also perform the prediction process. The variable N indicates the length of the record. The RMSE reported the various horizons and the mean value of RMSE for all the horizons of the prediction process. Various experiments have been conducted in this work to prove the effectiveness of the proposed system.

11.5.2 Dataset Description

The PM2.5 dataset is accessible for no cost in the UCI Machine Learning Repository and was amassed from a number of sites in Beijing, China, that track air quality. Information on PM2.5, PM10, NO_2, CO, O_3, and SO_2 can be found in the dataset. In addition to the aforementioned information, the dataset also includes meteorological data for the specified time period, including details about the weather, pressure, temperature, humidity, wind speed, and wind direction. Also, the Meteorological Data Centre of Chennai provides the dataset that is used in the training and testing procedures.

11.5.3 Experimental Results

Various experiments have been conducted to evaluate the performance of the proposed air quality prediction system. In this work, 80% of the records are considered for performing the training process, and the remaining 20% of the total records in the PM2.5 dataset are considered for performing the testing process. The data is preprocessed by applying the existing BOA to achieve better prediction accuracy. In this data preprocessing stage, the irrelevant data is to be removed and the relevant data only is taken into considered for further process.

To illustrate how well the proposed air quality prediction system predicts both in and out of the lab, we present the results in Fig. 11.2. In this study, five separate experiments were performed, each one using a different database of records as input.

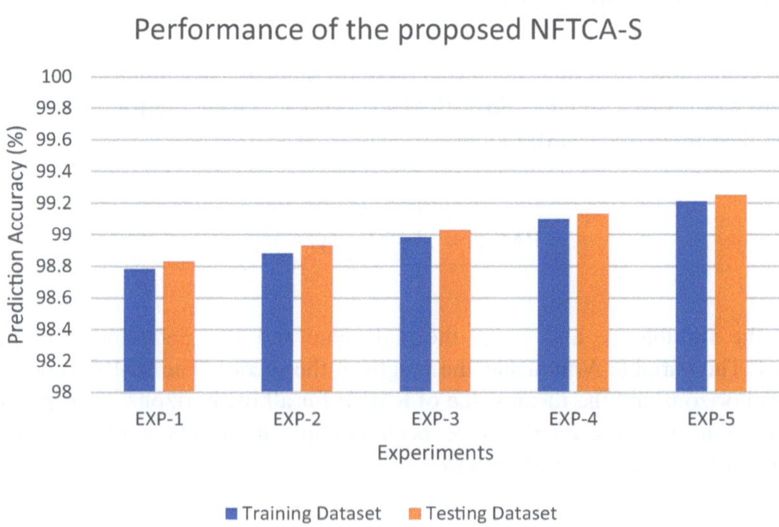

Fig. 11.2 Performance of the proposed NFTCA-S without feature selection

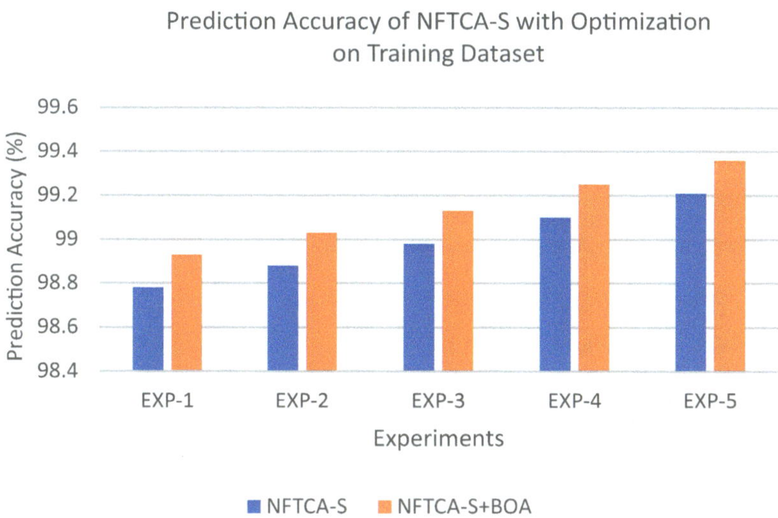

Fig. 11.3 Prediction accuracy of NFTCA-S with optimization on the training dataset

Figure 11.2 shows that the proposed air quality prediction system performs well across all five experiments, with forecast accuracy increasing steadily as the number of recordings grows. Incorporating the newly created spatio-fuzzy temporal rules that are helpful for making effective decisions on the datasets is the cause for the improved prediction result. To make a clear call on the dataset, fuzzy logic is applied, and the spatial and temporal restrictions are exploited to make forecasts about the area's weather and air quality in the past.

The accuracy of the proposed air quality prediction system on the training dataset and the testing dataset after including the current BOA is displayed in Figs. 11.3 and 11.4, respectively. Experiments can then be run with the optimized, featured dataset as input. In this study, five separate experiments were performed, each one using a different database of records as input.

In all five studies, NFTCA-S with feature optimization performs well, as shown in Figs. 11.3 and 11.4. Both graphs' prediction accuracy grows as the number of records increases. The upgrade is due to a new optimization method. The training and testing prediction accuracy was 99.36% and 99.56%, respectively.

Figure 11.5 compares the proposed NFTCA-S and BOA air quality prediction system to current classifiers such as SVM, RF, DT, and MLP (MLP).

Figure 11.5 shows that the suggested air quality prediction system (NFTCA-S +BOA) performs poorly compared to MLP, SVM, DT, and RF. Incorporating freshly produced spatio-fuzzy temporal rules improves prediction results for datasets. Fuzzy logic is employed to make sharp judgments on the dataset, and spatial and temporal limitations are applied to anticipate historical weather and air quality.

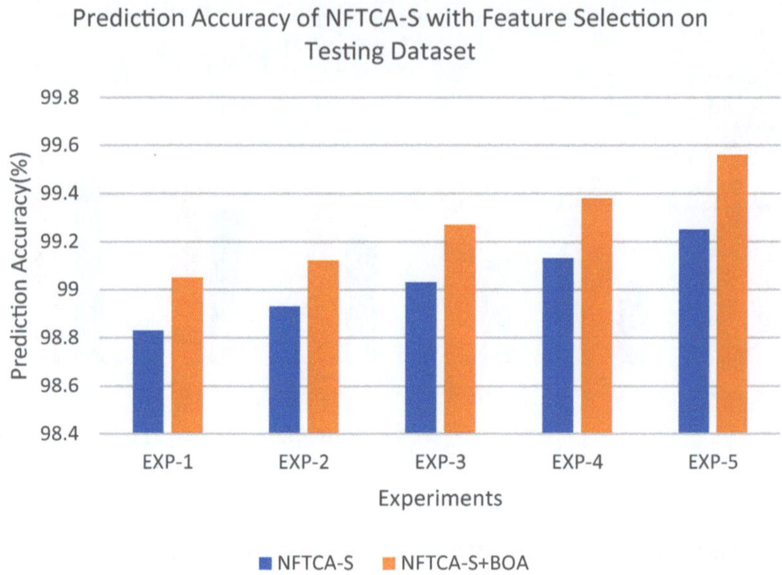

Fig. 11.4 Prediction accuracy of NFTCA-S with optimization on the testing dataset

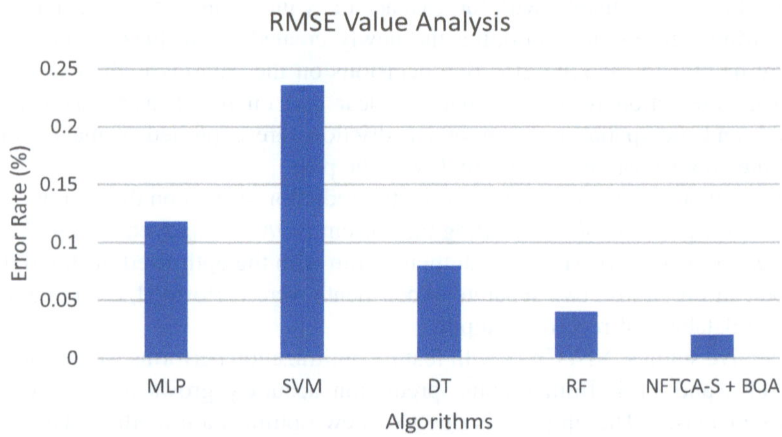

Fig. 11.5 RMSE value analysis between the proposed and existing algorithms

Figure 11.6 compares the proposed air quality prediction system to SVM, DT, RF, MLP, and prediction systems. The suggested prediction system combines NFTCA-S with BOA to achieve high accuracy and low error. This experiment tests the proposed air quality forecast system by comparing five sets of records.

Figure 11.5 shows that the proposed air quality prediction system (NFTCA-S +BOA) performs better than current classifiers (SVM, DT, RF, MLP) in all five experiments. Better performance is due to freshly produced spatio-fuzzy temporal

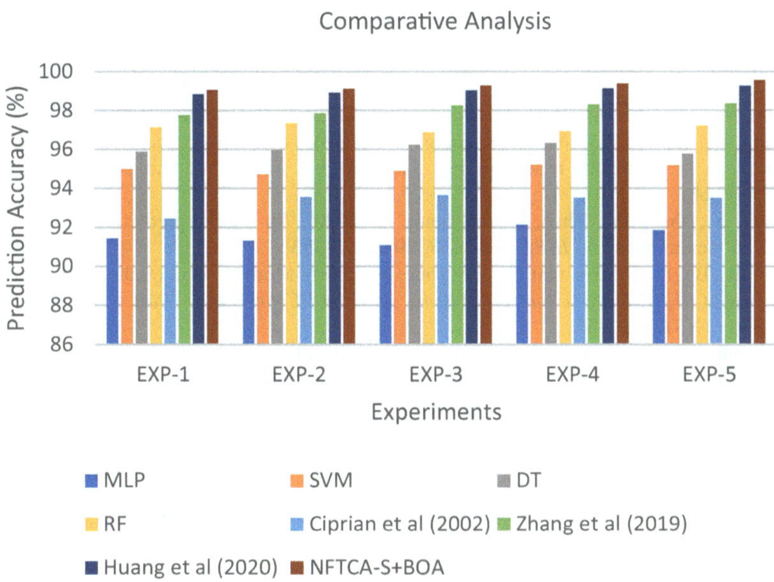

Fig. 11.6 Comparative analysis

rules that help make effective dataset selection. The trapezoidal fuzzy membership function is employed to fuzzify the dataset, and spatial and temporal restrictions are applied to estimate historical weather and air quality.

11.6 Conclusion and Future Works

This work proposes and implements an air quality forecast system. In this system, a newly proposed Neuro-Fuzzy Temporal Classification Algorithm with spatial constraints (NFTCA-S) is used for performing the prediction process. Moreover, an existing feature optimization technique called Butterfly Optimization Algorithm (BOA) is also used for performing the feature optimization process effectively, which is helpful for enhancing the prediction accuracy and also reduces the root mean square error. In this work, fuzzy logic, temporal logic, and spatial constraints are applied in a single neural network for making effective decision-making. The PM2.5 dataset is used as input for this prediction system and also proved the effectiveness of the proposed air quality prediction system by categorizing the day as "Good," "Moderate," and "Not Good for Health" according to the air pollution that considers the level of sulfur dioxide, carbon monoxide, and nitrogen oxides for decision making. This work can be enhanced further by applying a deep learning algorithm with innovation to improve the highest prediction accuracy.

References

1. Gu, K., Qiao, J., & Lin, W. (2018). Recurrent air quality predictor based on meteorology- and pollution-related factors. *IEEE Transactions on Industrial Informatics, 14*(9), 3946–3955.
2. Huang, Y., Zhao, Q., Zhou, Q., & Jiang, W. (2018). Air quality forecast monitoring and its impact on brain health based on big data and the internet of things. *IEEE Access, 6*, 78678–78688.
3. Huang, Y., Xiang, Y., Zhao, R., & Cheng, Z. (2020). Air quality prediction using improved PSO-BP neural network. *IEEE Access, 8*, 99346–99353.
4. Andò, B., Baglio, S., Graziani, S., & Pitrone, N. (2000). Models for air quality management and assessment. *IEEE Transactions on Systems, Man, and Cybernetics—Part C: Applications and Reviews, 30*(3), 358–363.
5. Ganapathy, S., Sethukkarasi, R., Yogesh, P., Vijayakumar, P., & Kannan, A. (2014). An intelligent temporal pattern classification system using fuzzy temporal rules and particle swarm optimization. *Sadhana, 39*(2), 283–302.
6. Kanimozhi, U., Ganapathy, S., Manjula, D., & Kannan, A. (2019). An intelligent risk prediction system for breast cancer using fuzzy temporal rules. *National Academy Science Letters, 42*(3), 227–232.
7. Huang, G., Zhao, G., He, G., & Wang, Q. (2019). Innovative spatial-temporal network modeling and analysis method of air quality. *IEEE Access, 7*, 26241–26254.
8. Chauhan, R., Kaur, H., & Alankar, B. (2021). Air quality forecast using convolutional neural network for sustainable development in urban environments. *Sustainable Cities and Society, 75*(103239), 103239.
9. Soh, P. -W., Chang, J. -W., & Huang, J. -W. (2018). Adaptive deep learning-based air quality prediction model using the most relevant spatial-temporal relations. *IEEE Access, 6*, 38186–38199.
10. Zhou, Y., Zhao, X., Lin, K.-P., Wang, C.-H., & Lie, L. (2019). A Gaussian process mixture model-based hard-cut iterative learning algorithm for air quality prediction. *Applied Soft Computing, 85*, 105789.
11. Zhang, Y., et al. (2019). A predictive data feature exploration-based air quality prediction approach. *IEEE Access, 7*, 30732–30743.
12. Ma, J., Cheng, J. C. P., Lin, C., Tan, Y., & Zhang, J. (2019). Improving air quality prediction accuracy at larger temporal resolutions using deep learning and transfer learning techniques. *Atmospheric Environment, 214*, 116885.
13. Schürholz, D., Kubler, S., & Zaslavsky, A. (2020). Artificial intelligence-enabled context-aware air quality prediction for smart cities. *Journal of Cleaner Production, 271*, 121941.
14. Ha, Q. P., Metia, S., & Phung, M. D. (2020). Sensing data fusion for enhanced indoor air quality monitoring. *IEEE Sensors Journal, 20*(8), 4430–4441.
15. Huang, W., Li, T., Liu, J., Xie, P., Du, S., & Teng, F. (2021). An overview of air quality analysis by big data techniques: Monitoring, forecasting, and traceability. *Information Fusion, 75*, 28–40.
16. Zheng, H., Cheng, Y., & Li, H. (2020). Investigation of model ensemble for fine-grained air quality prediction. *China Communications, 17*, 207–223.
17. Zhang, D., & Woo, S. S. (2020). Real time localized air quality monitoring and prediction through mobile and fixed IoT sensing network. *IEEE Access, 8*, 89584–89594.
18. Zhang, Y., Zhang, R., Ma, Q., Wang, Y., Wang, Q., Huang, Z., & Huang, L. (2020). A feature selection and multi-model fusion-based approach of predicting air quality. *ISA Transactions, 100*, 210–220.
19. Lin, Y.-C., Lee, S.-J., Ouyang, C.-S., & Wu, C.-H. (2020). Air quality prediction by neuro-fuzzy modeling approach. *Applied Soft Computing, 86*, 105898.
20. Xu, X., & Yoneda, M. (2021). Multi task air quality prediction based on LSTM autoencode model. *IEEE Transactions on Cybernetics, 51*(5), 2577–2586.

21. Chen, E., & Brauer, M. (2021). Traffic related air pollution and stress: Chen and Brauer respond. *Environmental Health Perspectives*, *116*, 9.
22. Saravanan, D., & Santhosh Kumar, K. (2021). Improving air pollution detection accuracy and quality monitoring based on bidirectional RNN and the Internet of Things. *Materials Today: Proceedings*. https://doi.org/10.1016/j.matpr.2021.04.239.
23. Krishna Rani Samala, K., Babu, K. S., & Das, S. K. (2021). Temporal convolutional denoising autoencoder network for air pollution prediction with missing values. *Urban Climate, 38*, 100872.
24. Arora, S., & Singh, S. (2019). Butterfly optimization algorithm: A novel approach for global optimization. *Soft Computing, 23*(3), 715–734.
25. Zhang, W., & Wang, T. (2010). Model integration anthropogenic heat for improving air quality forecasts over Beijing City. *IEEE Transactions in Pollution Environment, 25*(4), 815–824.
26. Neagu, C.-D., Kalapanidas, E., Avouris, N., & Bumbaru, S. (2001). Air quality prediction using neuro-fuzzy tools. *IFAC Proceedings, 34*(8), 229–235.

Chapter 12
An Analysis of the Use of Machine Learning in the Diagnosis of Autism Spectrum Disorder

M. Swedha and A. Devendran

12.1 Introduction

12.1.1 Diseases on the Autism Spectrum

Autism is a developmental disease characterized by impaired social interaction. While social interaction can now be used to diagnose ASD at 18 months, many children still go undetected until they are 3 or when they start school.

12.1.2 Autistic Disorder

Social engagement, stereotypical patterns or behaviors, interests, and unwavering repetition all work against those with autism. Lack of motor skills and the inability to make eye contact are symptoms of this disorder.

12.1.3 Asperger's Syndrome

Definition: Asperger's syndrome is a form of autism in which autistic persons show typical progress in communicating, even while they struggle to understand the social norms of traditional society or the etiquette of others.

M. Swedha (✉) · A. Devendran
Department of Computer Applications, Dr M.G.R. Educational and Research Institute, Chennai, Tamil Nadu, India

F. J. J. Joseph et al. (eds.), *Computational Intelligence for Clinical Diagnosis*, EAI/Springer Innovations in Communication and Computing,
https://doi.org/10.1007/978-3-031-23683-9_12

12.1.4 Childhood Disintegrative Disorder (CDD)

Those who suffer from CDD may also experience regressive autism. Up until the age of 2, children with this syndrome develop normally. Alterations in behavior typically take place between the ages of 3 and 4, but never later than 10 years of age. They can't even keep the skills they would have previously learned, such as motor abilities, social abilities, and play techniques.

12.1.5 Rett's Disorder

Female children are the ones who are affected by Rett's disorder, which is a disease that primarily impacts neurodevelopmental activities. Those affected by this disease typically show sluggish growth between the ages of 12 and 18 months, at which time their heads are typically abnormally small in proportion to their bodies. In medical terms, this impairment is known as "Microcephaly." Some children with this illness also have trouble walking because of muscle issues that make it hard for them to utilize their hands.

12.1.6 Pervasive Developmental Disorder-Not Otherwise Specified (PDD-NOS)

This sort of youngster may lack social skills, struggle with making and keeping friends, avoid eye contact, be unwilling to share tasks with others, prefer to work alone, and feel isolated.

12.1.7 Characteristic Features of ASD

Kids with ASD possess unique strengths; nonetheless, the most consistently seen characteristics of the disorder are difficulties with social interaction, repetitive behaviors, illogical thought processes, and sensory processing.

12.1.8 Machine Learning Techniques

Machine learning methods are based on a novel algorithm that allows for automated study, analysis, and comprehension. Methods from the field of machine learning are applied to the problem of identifying individuals with autism spectrum disorders in this investigation.

12.2 Related Work

Cheol-Hong Min [1] uses two different sensors: wearable and static. It is completely based on self-stimulatory patterns. For wearable sensors, they used an accelerometer to detect the behavioral patterns of a subject. For static sensors, they use a microphone and webcam to capture sound, photographs, and motion pictures, i.e., videos of subjects within a particular area/room. For feature extraction, they have used time frequency methods. For analyzing the Accelerometer signal Hidden Markov Model (HMM). Accuracy in classification is 91.5%. Wearable sensors are fixed and managed in various parts of the body like the wrist, stomach, legs, and ankles to provide the motion of sensors (3-axis accelerometer). The readings from the microphone and webcam sensor are sent from the sensor system to the computer directly. To analyze the behavioral patterns of children with autism, the sensor, which is wearable only, is not sufficient. Therefore, an audio sensor like a microphone detects the sound of the subject needed. Video records at 15 fps. Audio records at 22 kHz. To reduce the burden of video analysis, video labelling capability is used. The disadvantage is that it requires sensors that are patched on the skin of the body to measure the signals. This will cause some discomfort to the children, and it is difficult for us to track their true affective states.

The dataset used by Ayse Demirhan et al. [11] is available from the UC Irvine Machine Learning Repository, catalogued as adolescent scan data for autism spectrum disorders. Ten of the features have been taken (behavioral). KNN, SVM, and RF are the algorithms employed. Here, MATLAB is employed as a preprocessing method. Furthermore, the teenage group had 20 features taken. In order to accomplish this classification task, SVM employs a supervised learning algorithm and an non-linear strategy. SVM is trained using a combination of the Gaussian RBF Kernel Function and Sequential Minimal Optimization (SMO) methods. In order to prevent parameter-dependent bias, ten-fold CV (Cross-validation) is used. The output model is used for estimating the model's effectiveness. The accuracy of the categorization is measured using a ten-fold cross-validation procedure. Accuracy, sensitivity, and specificity performance measures are employed in the categorization process. The results of applying the algorithms, specifically the SVM, kNN, and RF techniques, for binary classification achieved accuracy percentages of 95%, 89%, and 100%, respectively. The kNN method is the least effective in classifying ASD occurrences, the results showing.

Sumi Simon et al. [9] related their work to empirical evaluation. They have used six features in total, which are behavioral features. The commonly used feature selection algorithms are fish filtering, relief and run filtering, and step disc. Among all those feature selection algorithms, the filters used for the feature selection of behavioral data are relief and runs filtering, which is best suited. The dataset is taken from National Institute for the Mentally Handicapped. The algorithms they have used are SVM, J48, Multilayer Perceptron, and IBI Classification Algorithm.

Aishwarya et al. [2] employ an autistic patient examining model with the utilization of machine-learning techniques and implement it as a web application to detect ASD in toddlers. To identify autism by means of precision, specificity, sensitivity, precision and f1 score, several algorithms are used, namely, Support Vector Machines (SVM), Random Forest (RF), Ada Booster Algorithms, and Decision Tree (DT). The dataset is taken from the UCI repository. The dataset is further divided into training and testing phases, i.e., 80% and 20%. It involves five processing phases, namely, data collection, data syncretization, developing a model for predicting the autism spectrum disorder, and comparing the model, which was developed for the purpose of prediction and implementation as a web application. The dataset contains 15 features which is a combination of both numerical and categorical data. It contains 10 behavioral characteristics and a few individual characteristics: 10 binary fields, one continuous field, four categorical fields, and one binary class variable. It is then tested with the AQ-10 dataset to identify autism, and it achieves an accuracy of 92.89%, 96.20%, 100.00%, 79.14% for the respective algorithms. The results show that AdaBoost and Random tree algorithms are successful algorithms in the examination of autism.

Erinas. Dewi et al. [3] use two datasets for the work: one is child and the other is adolescent. The dataset is taken from the UCI repository. It contains 21 attributes. For the purpose of ASD classification, the author used KNN, SVM, Random Forest, Deep Learning, and Back Propagation. Each algorithm is used with different parameters. The algorithms KNN, SVM, Random Forest, Deep Learning, and Back Propagation achieve the accuracy of 89.7, 99.65, 100, 95.89, and 99.65 for the classification process in children and achieve the accuracy of 93.08, 89.42, 100, 88.46, and 89.42 for the classification process in adolescents. This paper concludes that the Random Tree algorithm achieves the greatest accuracy than the other algorithms. This proves that Deep Learning is no better than the Random Forest algorithm.

Since Ramya et al. [4] Get the VAERS Dataset in a Common Separated Values (CSV) format [24]. There are eight different features to it. In order to provide accurate ASD predictions, this study integrates three separate algorithms: Deep Learning, Random Forest, and Naive Bayes. A DRN model combines the strengths of Deep Learning, Random Forest, and Nave Bayes into one cohesive framework. It is a part of the rapid miner tool that measures things such as accuracy, precision, recall, error during categorization, and execution time. Results from this study demonstrate that the DRN model outperforms other popular methods such as Stacking, Bagging, Ada Boost, Vote, and Bayesian Boosting. Classification error is reduced and accuracy is increased with the DRN model.

The dataset used by Kaushik Vakadkar et al. is derived from the Q-CHAT (Quantitative Check List for Autism in Toddlers) and contains 1054 cases with 18 attributes. The models used include the Support Vector Machine, Random Forest classifier, Nave Bayes, Logistic Regression, and kNN. When compared to training with a non-linear kernel, SVM‘s accuracy improves significantly when using a linear RBF kernel. When compared to other methods, logistic regression has the highest accuracy (97.15%). This algorithm’s strength lies in its simplicity, but its weakness is that it is only effective with tiny datasets.

Geetha Ramani and Sivaselvi [5] have come up with a supervised learning methodology for examining autism. This work uses a new measure for weighting

Table 12.1 Performance of random forest technique

Author	Dataset	Algorithm	Metrics used	Findings
Ramya et al. [4]	VAERS	DRN (deep learning, Random forest, Naïve Bayes)	Kappa statistic, classification error, mean absolute, and root mean squared error	DRN model provides higher accuracy and lower classification error than the already available models, namely vote stacking Ada boost, bagging, and Bayesian boosting models
Aishwarya et al. [2]	UCI repository (2020)	Support Vector Machines (SVM), Decision Tree (DT), Random forest and Ada Booster Algorithms	Classification error	AdaBoost and Random Forest algorithm works well for good prediction of ASD than Decision Tree and Support Vector Machine (SVM)
Erina and Elly [3]	UCI repository (2020)	KNN, SVM, Random forest, deep learning and back propagation	Kappa statistic, K-folds cross-validation	The Random Forest algorithm achieves the highest accuracy of the other algorithms
Geetha Ramaniand and Sivaselvi [5]	UCLA's CART	Random Forest (RF)	Fisher, runs, help with feature selection, new centrality norm in neuroimaging, RS-functional MRI	The random tree technique is established along with Fisher for feature selection Feature selection that acquires a greater precision of 88.46%
Kaushik Vakadkar et al. [17]	Q-CHAT	SVM, Random Forest, Naïve Bayes, kNN, logistic regression	F1 score, Precision recall	Logistic Regression achieves a greater accuracy of 97.15% than all the other algorithms, but it is possible only when the dataset is small

the leverage variants, and this measure is called the centrality measure. Random Forest algorithm with Fisher feature selection and also Sparsity Thresholding achieved higher reliability of 88.46% in examining autism. Table 12.1 tabulates the performance of the RF algorithm in the autism dataset.

Vaishali et al. [19] extracted data from the UCI Machine Learning repository. Optimal feature selection is done using binary firefly algorithm and takes 10 features automatically out of 12 so that the ASD and non-ASD patients are separated automatically. Accuracy was attained at an average of 92.12–97.97%. There is no misbalancing class issue because out of 292 subjects in the dataset, 151 subjects with class “yes” and 141 subjects with class “No”. The algorithms utilized are Naïve Bayes, J48, Support Vector Machines, and k-Nearest Neighbor. The disadvantage with this work is that due to the fewer instances, there arises an issue called “overfitting” in the dataset.

Sumi et al. [6] utilize the dataset from the National Institute for Mentally Handicapped for the detection of autism. Six attribute groups are taken into consideration. Support Vector Machine (SVM), J48 for examining the data both categorically and continuously, Multilayer Perceptron and Instance-Based learning classification algorithm are employed side by side to check the precision of the behavioral model. Support Vector Machine (SVM) achieves the greatest classification reliability, i.e., 95–97%. For learning skills analysis, SVM and decision tree J48 are used. Filters, namely, relief and runs, are well matched for the feature selection of behavioral data. Bag Valve Mask, Classification and Regression Trees, Decision Tree namely C4.5, CS-CRT, C-SVC, Iterator Dichotomize 3, and k Nearest Neighbor, Linear discriminant, Multilayer perceptron (MLP), Naïve Bayes, Multinomial Logistic Regression, PLS-DA, PLS-LDA, and Random Tree are the classification methods that are compared on M-Chat R dataset. BVM, CVM, and MLR obtain accurate results in classifying the autistic data. SVM, J48, BVM, and decision tree provide high accuracy and low error rate in classifying the autistic data.

Suman and Sarfaraz [7] use the dataset from the UCI repository. Three types of data are taken into consideration, namely, ASD screening data for adults, children, and adolescents. Totally, 21 attributes are taken for each set of age groups. SVM, LR, NB, CNN, K-Nearest Neighbor, and ANN are compared. The problem of missing values is handled by imputation methods. The result shows that CNN acquires a higher accuracy than all the other models. The accuracy level of CNN for adults is 99.53%, for children 98.30% and for adolescents, 96.88%. Results of this classification model show that the model that is grounded on CNN can be implemented for the detection of autism.

Bi et al. [9] established a random Support Vector Machine cluster because the classification precision of a single SVM is usually very less, so the author combines several support vectors machines to identify autistic children and typical developing (TP). This work focuses on classifying between two, namely, ASD and TD. For the purpose of classifying the above-mentioned types, this work uses four graph metrics such as degree, shortest path, local efficiency, and clustering coefficient of brain activity association. The superior results achieved and the identified dependability are backed by the ideal attribute set, which includes the inferior frontal gyrus (IFG), the hippocampal formation, and the praecuneus. A 96.15% degree of accuracy is attained with this procedure. Using scan data from adolescents with ASD, this study employs SVM, kNN, and RF learning approaches to correctly diagnose the illness.

Bone et al. [11] implemented a classifier with the help of a Support Vector Machine to improve the commonly used screening and examining methods for autism.

The dataset contains the data of children of age 10 of 1264 subjects having autism habits as well as 462 children who have no autism habits, and they have made

Table 12.2 Comparative study of SVM in autism dataset

Author	Dataset	Algorithm	Metrics used	Findings
Sumi et al. [6]	National Institute for the Mentally Handicapped	SVM, J48, BVM	Relief, runs filtering	SVM, J48, BVM and decision tree provide high accuracy and low error rate in classifying the autistic data
Bi et al. [9]	The ASD Brain Imaging Data Exchange – 2014	Random SVM cluster	Local efficiency, shortest path	SVM cluster gives high performance than a single SVM
Demirhan [10]	UCI Machine Learning Repository – 2017	kNN, SVM, Random Forest	Sigmoid, polynomial, RBF kernel function, tenfold cross validation	SVM, kNN, and RF achieve very good performance, and therefore lowest performance is obtained from the kNN algorithm
Bone et al. [11]	Data consists of ADI-R, SRS, and Developmental Disorder (DD)	SVM classifier	Nested cross validation	Due to the limited number of datasets, the work is focused only on verbal experiments

clinical diagnoses among the children who are having mild symptoms of autism and children without symptoms in various phases of cross-validation. This work provides a method that uses five behavioral attributes for diagnosing children lower and higher than 10 years and establishes that children who are less than 10 years attain the sensitivity and specificity of 89.2% and 86.7%, respectively, and children above 10 years were 59.0% and 53.4% respectively. Table 12.2 tabulates the comparative study of SVM in the dataset for autism.

Duda M et al. [17] used forward feature selection and undersampling. The dataset is taken from the Q-CHAT method by [17]. Project Description: Six Machine Learning models were trained and evaluated, including SVM (linear kernel), which reaches 96.5% accuracy using just two attributes from a possible 65, and on a set of 65 attributes, the Random Forest Classifier gets 95% accuracy using just nine of them, the Logistic Regression model gets 96% using just five of them, the Decision Tree model gets 93% accuracy using just two of them, and the Categorical Lasso model and the Linear Discriminant Analysis model get 96% and 96.4% accuracy using just two of them, respectively. Among the 65 behaviors measured by the Social Responsiveness Scale in a sample of 2925 people with ASD or ADHD, just five were sufficient to differentiate the two conditions with a 96.4% level of certainty. Due to the skewed composition of the dataset, which was predominantly comprised of autism-related datasets, we conclude that the ASD group is significantly overrepresented.

Al Banna et al. [19] developed an Artificial Intelligence system with an attached sensor with the help of a dataset taken from Kaggle containing 35,887 images of autism patients. The images used for the detection are of grayscale type. The sensor is used to analyze the data about the patient with autism with the help of expressions and emotions delivered from the patient's face. During the Co-vid pandemic times, this work sends proper alerts to the caretakers of the patient. This system works by attaching a smart band fixed on the hands of the patients with a screen to monitor them and a camera which is connected to the mobile device. The highest accuracy attained by the Inception-ResNetv2 architecture is of 78.56%. The major drawback of this work is it produces the lowest accuracy compared to other research work in the early stages of detection.

Cheol-Hong Min [7] uses two different sensors: wearable and static. Self-stimulatory means repetitive actions. For wearable sensors, they used the accelerometer to detect the behavioral patterns of the children. For static sensors, they used a microphone and webcam to capture the sound, image, and motion videos of the person within a particular area. For feature selection, time-frequency methods are implemented. For analyzing the accelerometer signal, Hidden Markov Model (HMM) is utilized. Accuracy in Classifying Autistic children is 91.5%. Here the wearable sensors are deployed in multiple parts of the body like the wrist, waist, torso, legs, and ankles to give motions of the sensor (3-axis accelerometer). Microphones, webcams, and readings from sensors are exported from the sensor system to non-public computers instantaneously. Wearable sensor only is not enough to interpret the behavioral models of autistic children. Therefore, sensors used for audio, such as microphone, detect the sound of the children's needs. Video records at 15 fps. Audio records at 22 kHz. Video labelling capability is enabled here, and the advantage of this video labelling capability is to show the decreasing load of the study video. Hidden Markov models are employed to analyze the wearable accelerometer data. The disadvantage of this work is it requires sensors to be attached to the subject's body to examine the signals concurrently. This will give rise to few discomforts to the subject and to track their real affective states. Table 12.3 shows the performance of sensor-based models.

Gong et al. [12] used the dataset collected from 35 children in the United States that can simply be implemented as an application on mobile devices. Support Vector Machine. It uses Correlation Based Feature Selection Algorithm (CBF). It aims to develop a hands-on and completely automated autism detecting solution which can be developed as a mobile application on modern child-specific devices and used at home without any official or professional assistance. A 17-month research on 35 children confirms the capability of the proposed method for Typically Developing and Autism children classification. Therefore, the inexpensive accessibility and

Table 12.3 Performance of sensor-based models

Author	Algorithm	Sensors used	Findings
Cheol-Hong Min [7]	Hidden Markov Model (HMM)	Accelerometer, microphone, and web camera	Sensors need to be patched on the children's bodies that may cause discomfort
Al Banna et al. [19]	Inception-ResNetv2	Web camera	Produces lower accuracy of only 78.56%

capability of the proposed model tend to be potentially very beneficial to autism children, specifically those in regions where there are inadequate mental health resources. Moreover, the utilization of such a model may not be just restricted to autism screening, it could also help measure the capability of involvement and mask the growth of a toddler. Hence, we require our outcome will deliver purposeful understanding for future expeditions and growth models concentrating on ASD populations.

Salwa o slim et al. [13] emphasized a system to examine the activities of children who have autism with the use of accelerometer data provided by a mobile device that can be wearable. The movements of autistic children are recognized by using the DTWDir algorithm, i.e., Dynamic Time Wrapping. The dataset is gathered by a Lenovo smartphone sensor. It works on four behaviors. One is communication, and the other three deal with the interaction behaviors, namely, goodbye, drinking, and clapping. This algorithm is grounded on formulating displacement and both the signals of the direction. In contrast to the kNN algorithm, classical Dynamic Time Warping (DTW) and One Dollar Recognition ($1) algorithms DTWDir are calculated. To compare these algorithms, a C++ application was developed. The outcome of this work proves that Dynamic Time Wrapping Dir accuracy is better than the other algorithms in both the acceleration and orientation data. The disadvantage here is that it consumes higher execution time. Table 12.4 tabulates the comparative study of wearable devices used for the prediction of autism.

Work by Thabtah et al. [20] is grounded in rule induction, more specifically Rules-Machine Learning (RML). It makes use of covering learning, which produces non-repetitive rules in an easy-to-understand format. Specifically, it uses a cross-validation technique called ten-fold to partition the datasets into 10 equal parts. When compared to other methods like Boosting, Bagging, and Decision trees, the RML approach delivers better accuracy. According to this work, the RML method is not very effective when dealing with an uneven dataset that has been well labelled.

Ganesh et al. [14]'s work compares autistic and non-autistic children by differentiating between various emotions, namely, happiness, sadness, and anger. It performs the segmentation using the K-means algorithm; GLCM is used to characterize the features of the image and develops a CAD tool. The classification

Table 12.4 Comparative study of wearable gadgets used in autism dataset

Author	Dataset	Tool	Algorithm	Metrics used
Gong et al. [11]	35 kids in the US between April 2016 and September 2017 using an app on modern child-specific gadgets	Correlation coefficient	SVM, CFS	The covered toolkit, statistic functions, confusion matrix
Salwa O Slim et al. [14]	Through Lenovo's 98-sample-per-second smartphone sensor. Every action attempt took 6 seconds	C++	DTWDir	K-fold cross-validation

algorithm used to classify an autistic and non-autistic child is by Support Vector Machine (SVM). The regions taken to attain the temperature are the eyes, cheek, forehead, and nose. The accuracy obtained using the SVM classifier is 88%, Random Forest obtains 73%, Naïve Bayes 66%, and Dense-net 121 obtains 89.47%.

Kavya Ganesh et al. [15]s work uses the thermal imaging technique, and this work also compares 50 autistic and 50 non-autistic children with the help of customized CNN and ResNet. The regions taken into consideration are the eyes, cheek, nose, and forehead. Three kinds of emotions are taken into consideration, namely, happiness, sadness, and anger, from which anger shows the highest temperature. The accuracy obtained from customized CNN and ResNet is 96% and 90%, respectively. The sensitivity obtained from both is 100% and 87%.

The thermal imaging modality is used by Rusli et al. [16] as a tool for studying biosignals. According to this study, alterations in core body temperature are a direct result of arterial blood flow. In order to identify shifts in the face, we use a wavelet-based method for pattern technique in time series. A success rate of 88% is attained. Children between the ages of 5 and 9 are studied, with the goal of hiding their "real" effective ages, and the authors restrict themselves to studying only the three basic emotions of happiness, sadness, and anger.

In order to illustrate the anatomical and functional features of the brain's functional mapping [16], devised a novel algorithm. The outcomes demonstrate that by combining the multimodal information for classification, a higher level of accuracy is achieved. When the machine learning model is used, the accuracy of the model improves by 4.2%. As a downside, this approach is plagued by substantial variances in the datasets used and a machine learning method directly into the diagnostic tool for ASD, and it has an accuracy of 97.6%. This technique has limitations, in that it only applies to smaller datasets (612 autism studies and 11 non-autism datasets).

Deshpande et al. [21]'s study is based on the metrics of brain activity used for the prediction of ASD. This uses SVM to achieve accuracy of 95.9% with two clusters and features of 19 in total. The drawback is a constrained sample size or data.

12.3 Result and Discussion

Several methods are compared and contrasted in this survey using a variety of criteria. The accuracy gained by these methods on the autism dataset is summarized in Table 12.5 [22]. As shown in Fig. 12.1, the Random Forest (RF) method outperforms competing algorithms when it comes to achieving a satisfactory result in the context of classification approaches.

Table 12.5 Comparison of classification algorithms

Technique	Precision	Tool	Metrics
DRN	98.6%	Rapid Miner	Classification, kappa, mean absolute, and root mean squared error
Random Forest	88.46%	DISCO AI	Fisher-
J48	90.2%	Java	k-fold CV, one-away
SVM	88.9%	Correlation Coefficient	TOOLKIT, statistics functions, confusion matrix
DTWDir	93%	C++	K-fold cross-validation
CBA	85.27%	DSM-IV	K-fold, DSM-IV, ADOS
RF	100%	MATLAB	Sigmoid, RBF, polynomial, ten-fold CV

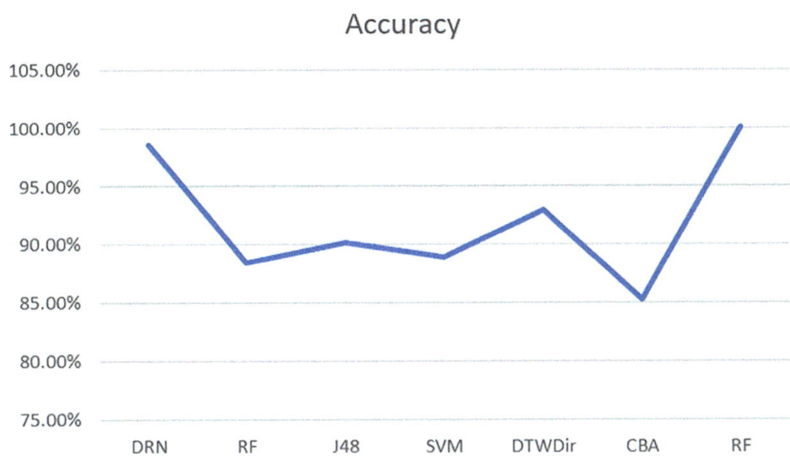

Fig. 12.1 Accuracy chart of various classification techniques

12.4 Conclusion

Based on the findings of this research, Machine Learning algorithms are being implemented into the assessment of people with autism who have difficulties with social participation, behavior models, difficulties in understanding (also known as "Cognoscible issues"), and audio-visual components, as well as with increased developmental disorderliness. Until certain symptoms of the illness become apparent, it is difficult to understand how to identify autism spectrum disorder in its early stages because so many questions emerge for parents, caregivers, clinicians, therapists, etc. This usually happens between 16 and 18 months of age, when kids have not yet developed any significant communication difficulties, have engaged in relatively few routine behaviors, have not yet developed significant social deficits, etc. This work offers a systematic approach to evaluating autism severity and treatment options, which therapists and doctors can use to inform their daily assessments of patients.

12.4.1 Future Scope

Clinicians and therapists can benefit from a more nuanced understanding of ASD through future work that focuses on establishing a system for an excellent comprehension of the children with ASD and predicting the autism condition in the embryonic period by using an improved Machine Learning algorithm.

References

1. Min, C. -H. (2017). *Automatic detection and labeling of self-stimulatory behavioral patterns in children with autism spectrum disorder.*
2. Aishwarya, J., Akshatha, N., Anusha, H., Shishira, J., & Mahadev, D. (2020). Engagement detection with autism spectrum disorder using machine learning. *International Journal of Engineering and Technology.* e-ISSN: 2395-0056 p-ISSN: 2395-0072.
3. Dewi, E. S., & Imah, E. M. (2020). *Comparison of machine learning algorithms for autism spectrum disorder classification.* In International Joint Conference on Science and Engineering (IJCSE 2020).
4. Dewi, E. S., Imah, E. M. (2020). *Comparison of machine learning algorithms for autism spectrum disorder classification.* In International Joint Conference on Science and Engineering (IJCSE 2020).
5. Ramya, R., & Zoraida, B. S. E. (2017). DRN hybrid model for predicting autism using rapid miner tool. *International Journal of Advanced Research in Computer Science, 8.*
6. Ramaniand, G., & Sivaselvi, K. (2017). Autism spectrum disorder identification using data mining techniques. *International Journal of Pure and Applied Mathematics, 117*(16), 427–436.
7. Min, C.-H., & Member of IEEE. (2018). Automatic detection and labelling of self-stimulatory behavioural patterns in children with autism spectrum disorder. *Mugla Journal of Science and Technology. Annu Int Conf IEEE Eng Med Biol Soc, 279–282.* https://doi.org/10.1109/EMBC.2017.8036816. PMID: 29059864.
8. Raj, S., & Masood, S. (2019). *Analysis and detection of autism spectrum disorder using machine learning techniques.* In International conference on computational intelligence and data science.
9. Simon, S., Chandra, J., & Saravanan, N. (2016). Empirical evaluation of data mining classification methods for autistic children. *International Journal of Trend in Research and* Development (IJTRD), ISSN: 2394-9333, Special Issue | EIT-16, March 2016, URL: http://www.ijtrd.com/papers/IJTRD3531.pdf.
10. Bi, X. A., Wang, Y., Shu, Q., Sun, Q., & Xu, Q. (2018). Classification of autism spectrum disorder using random support vector machine cluster. *Frontiers in Genetics, 9*, 18.
11. Demirhan, A. (2018). Performance of machine learning methods in determining the autism spectrum disorder cases. *Mugla Journal of Science and Technology, 4*(1), 79–84.
12. Bone, D., Bishop, S., Black, M. P., Goodwin, M. S., Lord, C., & Narayanan, S. S. (2016). Use of machine learning to improve autism screeningand diagnostic instruments: Effectiveness, efficiency, and multi-instrument fusion. *Journal of Child Psychology and Psychiatry, 57*, 927. https://doi.org/10.1111/jcpp.12559
13. Gong, Y., Yatawatte, H., Poellabauer, C., Schneider, S., & Latham, S. (2018). Automatic autism spectrum disorder detection using everyday vocalizations captured by smart devices. In *Proceedings of the 2018 ACM international conference on bioinformatics, computational biology, and health informatics* (pp. 465–473). ACM.
14. Slim, S. O., Atia, A., & Mostafa, M.-S. M. (2016). DTWDIR: An enhanced Dtw algorithm for autistic child behaviour monitoring. *International Journal of UbiComp, 7*(2), 1–8.

15. Ganesh, K., Umapathy, S., & Thanaraj Krishnan, P. Computer aided diagnosis of autism spectrum disorder based on thermal imaging. *Proceedings of Communications in Computer and Information Science*.
16. Ganesh, K., Umapathy, S., & Thanaraj, K. P. (2021). Deep learning techniques for automated detection of autism spectrum disorder based on thermal imaging. *Proceedings of the Institution of Mechanical Engineers, Part H: Journal of Engineering in Medicine, 235*(10), 1113–1127.
17. Vakadkar, K., Purkayastha, D., & Krishnan, D. (2021). Detection of autism spectrum disorder in children using machine learning techniques. *Proceedings of Springer Nature Journal, 2*, 386.
18. Duda, M., Ma, R., Haber, N., & Wall, D. P. (2016). Use of machine learning for behavioral distinction of autism and ADHD. *Translational Psychiatry, 6*(2), e732. https://doi.org/10.1038/tp.2015.221. PMID: 26859815; PMCID: PMC4872425.
19. Vaishali, R., & Sasikala, R. (2017). A machine learning based approach to classify autism with optimum behaviour sets. *International Journal of Engineering & Technology, 7*, 18.
20. Al Banna, M. H., Ghosh, T., Taher, K. A., Kaiser, M. S., Mahmud, M.. (2020). A monitoring system for patients of autism spectrum disorder using artificial intelligence. In *International conference on brain informatics* (pp. 251–262). Springer.
21. Thabtah, F., & Peebles, D. (2020). A new machine learning model based on induction of rules for autism detection. *Health Informatics Journal, 26*(1), 264–286.
22. Deshpande, G., Libero, L. E., Sreenivasan, K. R., Deshpande, H. D., & Kana, R. K. (2013). Identification of neural connectivity signatures of autism using machine learning. *Frontiers in Human Neuroscience, 7*, 670.
23. https://vaers.hhs.gov/data/data. Accessed 21 May 2022.

Chapter 13
A Cost-Effective, Agar-based Phantom for Thermogram- Guided Malignancy Analysis

R. Ramyadevi

13.1 Introduction

Light is still a significant source for the establishment of images. However, visible light does not allow us to perceive inside the body. The earliest medical images used light to create pictures, either of natural anatomic structures or using a microscope to visualize specimens [1]. As a result, a variety of imaging techniques are used to detect infections and abnormalities in human tissue.

13.1.1 Imaging Modalities for Malignancy Screening

Imaging modalities are being established to diagnose cancer as promptly as possible to recover survival rates and reduce the need for medications and therapies, resulting in fewer side effects. Some of these imaging modalities are used for screening, while others are used for diagnosis, and a few are used for additional examination. Cost-effective and efficient screening techniques should be cast off to range the infection [2]. When breast cancer is identified during screening exams, more in-depth examinations are typically accomplished using analytic modalities that can also be used for early identification. Imaging modality reports are used by doctors and physicians to boost their confidence in their initial diagnosis [3, 4]. Presently reprocessed methods include breast ultrasonography, electrical impedance-based imaging, mam-

R. Ramyadevi (✉)
Department of Computer Science, SRM Institute of Science and Technology, Ramapuram, Chennai, Tamil Nadu, India

F. J. Joseph et al. (eds.), *Computational Intelligence for Clinical Diagnosis*, EAI/Springer Innovations in Communication and Computing,
https://doi.org/10.1007/978-3-031-23683-9_13

mography, thermography, positron emission tomography (PET), optical imaging, magnetic resonance imaging (MRI), and computed tomography (CT). The procedures of each imaging technology are defined in this study, and their clinical performance is assessed independently.

13.1.1.1 Mammography

Using low-dose x-rays, mammography examines the breast's structure and detects a variety of abnormalities. Mammography has been the standard of care for detecting breast cancer since its introduction in 1960 [5]. However, sensitivity and specificity are affected by factors like age, breast density, family history, and infection phase. Increased worry, tension, and anxiety are brought on by the high incidence of false-positive mammography results.

Women under the age of 50 with thick or fibrocystic breasts are not typically advised to get a mammogram [6]. When viewed through mammography, thick breast tissue and cancer might look quite similar, making it difficult to tell; apart from increasing breast thickness, mammography's ability to detect abnormalities declines. Breast tissue density was categorized by the American Cancer Society [7] into four categories.

The breast muscles are crushed to compression of around 40 pounds throughout the screening process [4]. This results in the release of malignant tumor cells into the bloodstream by causing the rupture of the tumor's encapsulation. Radiation exposure is another potential danger with mammography [8]. Mammograms expose women to low doses of radiation, which has been linked to an increased risk of breast cancer. Younger women are more susceptible to the side effects of ionizing radiation than older women because their cells are more homogeneous [9]. BRCA1/2 mutations may be caused by radiation, according to this theory. Women who have the BRCA1/2 gene or a strong family history of breast cancer should not get regular mammograms.

13.1.1.2 PET/CT Imaging

PET/CT views for positron emission tomography in addition to computed tomography, which combines traditional radiology (CT) with nuclear medicine (PET) imaging towards the blend of structural and functional data [10]. By incorporating anatomic image registration and localization, this combination improves imaging accuracy. It provides an accurate diagnosis by using a radiotracer to measure metabolism and find alterations by the side of the cellular stage.

13.1.1.3 Ultrasound

Ultrasound stands for a diagnostic technology that uses wide-ranging high-frequency waves to distinguish dense from liquid-rich masses [11, 12]. Breast ultrasonography is a helpful technique for describing abnormalities found in mammograms, particularly in thick breasts. Asymmetrical masses, abnormally distended ducts, or concentrated foci of prolonged echogenicity with augmented Doppler vascularity are all signs of lesions. Although ultrasound has been shown to aid in the valuation of irregularities discovered by mammography, it should not be utilized as the sole method of cancer screening. However, ultrasound's sensitivity drops when it comes to detecting non-palpable cancers such as microcalcifications.

13.1.1.4 Magnetic Resonance Imaging (MRI)

This results in the rupture of the tumor's encapsulation, releasing malignant cells into the body's circulatory system. There is also the possibility of radiation poisoning from a mammogram. Mammography increases the risk of breast cancer since it uses low-dose radiation [8]. Since younger women have more homogeneous cells, they are more susceptible to the effects of ionizing energy than older women [9]. This hypothesis proposes that radiation is a potential trigger for BRCA1/2 mutations. Women who can verify a family history of breast cancer or who carry the BRCA1/2 gene should not get regular mammograms.

13.1.1.5 Phantom Development

Agar is a gelatinous polysaccharide made from the cell walls of certain seaweed and red algae species. Agar and agarose (the pure form) are commonly employed for the production of thermal phantoms due to their favorable physical and thermal properties.

Materials that look like breast tissue such as tissue-mimicking materials must be tested and verified in a variety of new biomedical applications. The following qualities should be present in an ideal phantom [13, 14]:

- The phantom structure should be anatomically similar to human tissue and have dimensions that can be measured.
- The ultrasonic and microwave properties of the phantom are similar to those of the target human tissue and can be maintained throughout time.
- The phantom can withstand mild pressure and distortion while being measured, but it will not shatter or leak.
- The ingredients should ideally be low-cost resources that do not necessitate the use of expensive equipment. In addition, the manufacturing process is simple.

13.2 Proposed System

13.2.1 Experimental Procedure

Thermal images at a resolution of 640 × 480 pixels were captured in this study using a CAT S60 smartphone with inbuilt thermal imaging. The CAT S60 has an inbuilt thermal camera; in addition to this, it is the first waterproof smartphone capable of diving to depths of up to 5 m for 1 hour. This camera includes an implanted thermal camera manufactured by FLIR, the world frontrunner in thermal imaging technology. CAT phone allows users to use their phones for a diversity of applications, as well as predicting heat radiation around doors and windows, detecting dampness and lining gaps, recognizing overheating e-machines and circuits, and viewing in complete darkness [15]. The thermal camera detects heat that is not apparent to the naked eye, showing temperature contrast. The background of the phantom is constructed to look like healthy tissue. Table 13.1 shows Agar phantom compositions. The resistor, which is put at various depths into the phantom, resembles cancerous tissue. The purpose of putting a resistor inside the phantom is to provide a regulated heat source. As the current passes through the resistor, it absorbs some of the electrical energy and releases it as heat, raising the resistor's temperature above the ambient temperature.

Before taking the measurement, a voltage of 5 volts is placed between the resistors, and the phantom is allowed to stabilize and reach a steady state [16]. The phantom is thermally stimulated for roughly 60 seconds by connecting a resistor to the DC source. Thermal photos were captured using a CAT S60 smartphone thermal camera during the rise in surface temperature and subsequent cooling [17]. For both the heating and the integrated resistor, a 1 s time step was used.

13.2.2 Datasets Used

The background of the phantom is constructed to look like healthy tissue. And the resistor, which is put at various depths into the phantom, resembles cancerous tissue. One hundred and twenty-five phantoms were created in total [18]. The experiment was carried out on five different resistor values: 22 Ω, 50 Ω, 100 Ω, 1kΩ, and 100kΩ. Under each resistor value, 25 sets of phantoms were created [19]. The resistors were embedded under the depth for each resistor value as follows:

Table 13.1 Agar phantom compositions

Material	Measure	Method
Distilled water	500 mL	Solvent
Agar	20 g	Mechanical strength
NaCl	2.3 g	Modifying thermal properties
Egg white	2 g	Modifying thermal properties
Formalin	3 mL	Preservative

- Heat Source embedded at depth 1 mm = 5
- Heat Source embedded at depth 2 mm = 5
- Heat Source embedded at depth 3 mm = 5
- Heat Source embedded at depth 4 mm = 3
- Heat Source embedded at depth 5 mm = 3
- Heat Source embedded at depth 7 mm = 2
- Heat Source embedded at depth 9 mm = 2

13.2.3 Image Acquisition of Phantoms

Meanwhile, the goal of the study was to assess the visualization of the phantoms with each imaging modality and determine their spatial accuracies; the phantoms were imaged with standard clinical imaging systems, using basic imaging protocols rather than specific clinical protocols or heat transfer measurements [20]. Thermal images at a resolution of 640 × 480 pixels were captured in this study using a CAT S60 smartphone with inbuilt thermal imaging. Figure 13.1 shows the schematic diagram and photo of the experimental setup with an embedded resistor.

13.3 Result and Discussion

Breast phantoms, as stated in [15], are a standard consistent patient with the proven clinical reality that can be used for a variety of purposes. Operator training for image-guided or imaging interventional processes is problematic with phantoms. They also recommend a quality assessment tool for initial imaging protocol implementation and quality control of image modality routines to ensure that the scanning system is working properly over time.

Phantoms can be used to help optimize scanning parameters. Imaging phantoms are created in accordance with the guidelines for active dynamic image examination [21]. Thermal cameras are used to examine, analyze, and modify the performance of thermography on phantoms. The phantom, which is utilized for active thermographic research, mimics the physical properties of biological tissues. To prevent water degradation during phantom manufacturing, agar powder is used as an essential component (Fig. 13.2).

Phantoms can be used to help optimize scanning parameters. Imaging phantoms are created in accordance with the guidelines for active dynamic image examination [22]. Thermal cameras are used to examine, analyze, and modify the performance of thermography on phantoms. The phantom, which is utilized for active thermographic research, mimics the physical properties of biological tissues [23]. To prevent water degradation during phantom manufacturing, agar powder is used as an essential component. Thermal excitation is used to simulate cancerous tissue on the phantom. An agar phantom is created with the components specified in Table 13.1 to simulate the women's breast tissue.

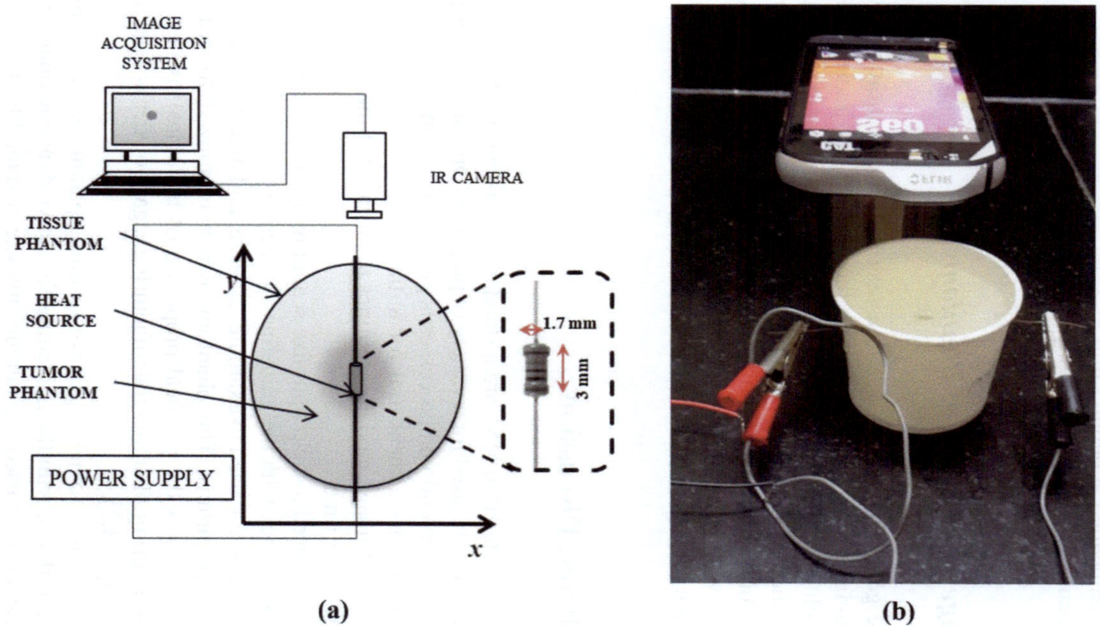

Fig. 13.1 (**a**) Schematic; (**b**) photograph of the experimental setup with an embedded resistor

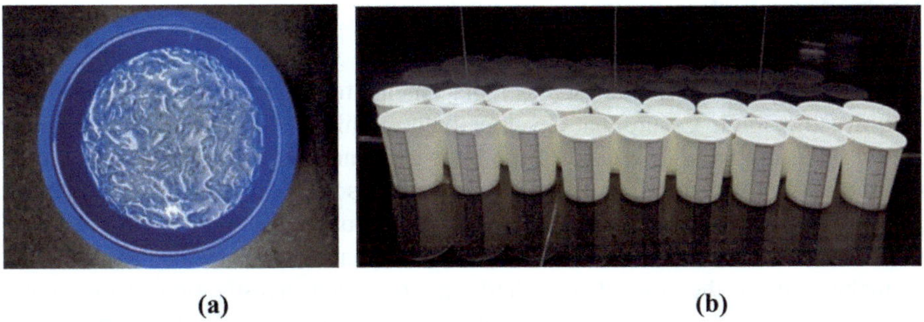

Fig. 13.2 (**a**) Agar socked in distilled water; (**b**) Agar gel in the mold

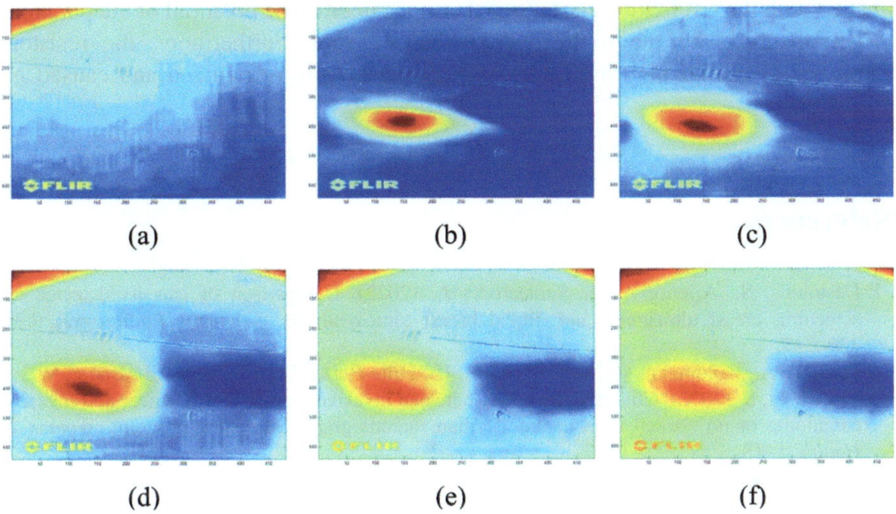

Fig. 13.3 Raw thermal images collected at heat source 1 mm depth at (**a**) 5 s, (**b**) 25 s, (**c**) 50s, (**d**) 75 s, (**e**) 100 s, and (**f**) 130 s

After soaking agar in distilled water for half an hour, healthy tissue is prepared. Sodium chloride (NaCl) and formalin solution are added after the solution has been dissolved [24]. The solution is now heated to 80 °C until bubbles begin to form and the mixture becomes clear. After the heat has been turned off, the combined solution is poured into molds to imitate the anatomical structure [25]. To prevent the agar mixture from sticking to the molds, they should have a flat surface. After that, the molds are kept in the refrigerator to shape and preserve them [26]. When pouring into the molds, keep in mind the depth at which the resistors will be embedded. The thickness of the phantom is 50 mm, and the radius is 20 mm [27]. The phantom has a radius of 20 mm and a thickness of 50 mm. Figure 13.3 shows a 100-ohm resistor implanted at a distance of 1 mm from the surface.

13.4 Conclusion

Medical imaging phantom is used as replacements for living tissues in the biomedical investigation to ensure that developed algorithms for imaging the human body are working properly. The need of the hour is for an imaging technique that lacks radioactivity risk, distress, anxiety, and false alarms and is non-invasive. Phantoms are used to calibrate or compare imaging systems utilized in real-world scenarios, such as significant clinical trials. The agar-based phantom was created for the study of malignancy in the context of a thermogram-guided investigation of the breast. Agar phantoms are simple to manufacture, don't require refrigeration, and have a number of advantages over other tissue-mimicking materials. They are also an excellent substrate for thermography tests. The breast phantoms were effectively imaged with the CAT S60 smartphone thermal camera. The potential of the phantom is demonstrated by the multi-modality testing tool. Furthermore, the resistors employed as malignancy indicators, which were easily recognized and caused no distortions.

References

1. Destounis, S., Arieno, A., & Santacroce, A. (2022). Comparison of cancers detected by screening breast ultrasound and digital breast tomosynthesis. *Academic Radiology, 29*(3), 339–347.
2. Farrokh, A., Goldmann, G., Meyer-Johann, U., Hille-Betz, U., Hillemanns, P., Bader, W., & Wojcinski, S. (2022). Clinical differences between invasive lobular breast cancer and invasive carcinoma of no special type in the German mammography-screening-program. *Women & Health*, 1–13.
3. Terao, T., & Matsue, K. (2022). Progress of modern imaging modalities in multiple myeloma. *International Journal of Hematology*, 1–12.
4. Mann, R. M., Athanasiou, A., Baltzer, P. A. T., Camps-Herrero, J., Clauser, P., Fallenberg, E. M., Forrai, G., et al. (2022). Breast cancer screening in women with extremely dense breasts recommendations of the European Society of Breast Imaging (EUSOBI). *European Radiology*, 1–10.
5. Clift, A. K., Dodwell, D., Lord, S., Petrou, S., Brady, S. M., Collins, G. S., & Hippisley-Cox, J. (2022). The current status of risk-stratified breast screening. *British Journal of Cancer, 126*(4), 533–550.
6. Martins, A. R. C., Di Maria, S., Afonso, J., Pereira, M., Pereira, J., & Vaz, P. (2022). Assessment of the uterine dose in digital mammography and digital breast tomosynthesis. *Radiography, 28*(2), 333–339.
7. Calisto, F. M., Santiago, C., Nunes, N., & Nascimento, J. C. (2022). BreastScreening-AI: Evaluating medical intelligent agents for human-AI interactions. *Artificial Intelligence in Medicine, 127*, 102285.
8. Fathi, I., Mkimel, M., & Mesradi, M. R. (2022). GATE/GEANT4 simulation of radiation risk induced cancer from mammographic screening. *Radiation Physics and Chemistry, 193*, 109929.
9. Mehedi, I. M., Rao, K. P., Al-Saggaf, U. M., Alkanfery, H. M., Bettayeb, M., & Jannat, R. (2022). Intelligent tomographic microwave imaging for breast tumor localization. *Mathematical Problems in Engineering, 2022*, 1.

10. Tiberi, G., Ghavami, N., Sánchez-Bayuela, D. Á., Sani, L., Vispa, A., Bigotti, A., Badia, M., et al. (2022). Mammo wave breast imaging device: Path to clinical validation, results and implications in future population-based breast screening programs. In *2022 16th European Conference on Antennas and Propagation (EuCAP)* (pp. 1–4). IEEE.
11. Venmathi, A. R., & Vanitha, L. (2022). Data visualization on breast phantom mammogram images using kernel performance of SVM. In *Advances in Data Science and Management* (pp. 385–395). Springer.
12. Matsumoto, Y., Katsumura, A., & Miki, N. (2022). Pressure-controlled ultrasound probe for reliable imaging in breast cancer diagnosis. *Japanese Journal of Applied Physics, 61*(SD), SD1035.
13. Prasad, A., Pant, S., Srivatzen, S., & Asokan, S. (2021). A non-invasive breast cancer detection system using FBG thermal sensor array: A feasibility study. *IEEE Sensors Journal, 21*(21), 24106–24113.
14. Jacob, G., Jose, I., & Sujatha, S. (2021). Computational and experimental investigation on the breast tumor depth characteristics performed using infrared Thermography. In *Proceedings of the 26th National and 4th International ISHMT-ASTFE Heat and Mass Transfer Conference December 17–20, 2021, IIT Madras, Chennai-600036, Tamil Nadu, India*. Begel House Inc.
15. Nguyen, D. H., Stindl, J., Slanina, T., Moll, J., Krozer, V., & Zimmer, G. (2021). High frequency breast imaging: Experimental analysis of tissue phantoms. *IEEE Open Journal of Antennas and Propagation, 2*, 1098–1107.
16. Schmidt, G., Gerlinger, C., Endrikat, J., Gabriel, L., Müller, C., Baus, S., Volk, T., et al. (2021). Teaching breast ultrasound skills including core-needle biopsies on a phantom enhances undergraduate student's knowledge and learning satisfaction. *Archives of Gynecology and Obstetrics, 304*(1), 197–202.
17. RamyaDevi, R., & Anandhamala, G. S. (2018). Recent trends in medical imaging modalities and challenges for diagnosing breast cancer. *Biomedical and Pharmacology Journal, 11*(3), 1649–1658.
18. Ramya Devi, R., & Anandhamala, G. S. (2019). Analysis of breast thermograms using asymmetry in infra-mammary curves. *Journal of Medical Systems, 43*(6), 1–9.
19. Amiri, S. A., Van Berckel, P., Lai, M., Dankelman, J., & Hendriks, B. H. W. (2022). Tissue-mimicking phantom materials with tunable optical properties suitable for assessment of diffuse reflectance spectroscopy during electrosurgery. *Biomedical Optics Express, 13*(5), 2616–2643.
20. AlFares, B., AlJabr, A. J., Zainalabedin, M., AlMuzain, M., Saleh, G., & AlHashim, M. (2021). Heterogenous breast phantom with carcinoma for ionizing machines. In *2021 IEEE International IOT, Electronics and Mechatronics Conference (IEMTRONICS)* (pp. 1–6). IEEE.
21. Teixeira, A. M., André, A., & Martins, P. (2021). 3D bioprinting: Parameters optimization for agarose. In *Advances and Current Trends in Biomechanics: Proceedings of the 9th Portuguese Congress on Biomechanics, CNB2021, 19–20 February 2021, Porto, Portugal* (p. 39). CRC Press.
22. Becker, A. E. (2021). *Multisource x-ray systems for digital breast tomosynthesis and breast CT imaging*. PhD diss., University of California, Davis.
23. Antoniou, A., & Damianou, C. (2022). MR relaxation properties of tissue-mimicking phantoms. *Ultrasonics, 119*, 106600.
24. Song, C., Yang, Z., Jiang, S., Zhou, Z., & Zhang, D. (2022). An integrated navigation system based on a dedicated breast support device for MRI-guided breast biopsy. *International Journal of Computer Assisted Radiology and Surgery, 17*(6), 993–1005.
25. Lennie, E., Tsoumpas, C., & Sourbron, S. (2021). Multimodal phantoms for clinical PET/MRI. *EJNMMI Physics, 8*(1), 1–24.
26. Er, W. X., Lim, W. J., Dwihapsari, Y., Awang, M. N. A., & Yusoff, A. N. (2021). Signal-to-noise ratio uniformity and stability of agar gel phantom with iron (III) oxide as relaxation modifier. *Beni-Suef University Journal of Basic and Applied Sciences, 10*(1), 1–13.
27. Eve, L., Charalampos, T., & Steven, S. (2021). Multimodal phantoms for clinical PET/MRI. *EJNMMI Physics, 8*(1).

Chapter 14
Multimodality Brain Tumor Image Fusion Using Wavelet and Contourlet Transformation

S. Anu Priya and V. Khanaa

14.1 Introduction

In recent years, imaging and its modalities have grown widely due to advancement in technology as well as human requirement, which led to research and development in the field. Image acquisition can be broadly classified into digital imaging and medical imaging with processing and analysis.

The study of image analysis is to read data logically for searching, finding, organizing, and computing, as well as evaluating the consequences based on physical and cultural objects and related patterns with the spatial relationship. To enhance the performance in analysis, more than one modality, dimension, and phase are required in the medical domain for efficient prediction and diagnosis.

Medical imaging is evolution of new modalities of the image with methods like cone beam/multislice computed tomography (CT), positron emission tomography (PET), magnetic resonance imaging (MRI), electrical impedance tomography which furthermore diffuses optical tomography. Recent applications are notified in the field of medical images. The applications of medical imaging/images include the following list, however unrestricted [1]:

- Computer-relevant discovery/diagnosis like breast cancer, liver cancer, lung cancer.

S. Anu Priya (✉)
Department of Computer Science and Engineering, Bharath Institute of Higher Education and Research, Chennai, Tamil Nadu, India
e-mail: anupriya.mca@bharathuniv.ac.in

V. Khanaa
Department of Information Technology, Bharath Institute of Higher Education and Research, Chennai, Tamil Nadu, India

F. J. J. Joseph et al. (eds.), *Computational Intelligence for Clinical Diagnosis*, EAI/Springer Innovations in Communication and Computing,
https://doi.org/10.1007/978-3-031-23683-9_14

- AI and expert systems (e.g., SVM, Statistical Method, Manifold-Space-based Method, and ANN) utilize machine learning in 2D, 3D, and 4D.
- Multimode fusion techniques like CT or PET, estimation of X-ray or CT, X-ray or Ultrasound (CT/MRI,CT/SPECT).
- Preventive medical image investigation such as classification, segmentation, pattern identification of injury, stage, organs, anatomy, context disease, along with medical facts.
- The medical image redesign for EM design, statistical procedure for CT, PET, MRI, and X-ray images.
- Image fusion is applied for multiple modalities of images.
- Zhaodong Liu A et al. [2] proposed a fusion process that can be applied for multiple phases and angles.
- Retrieval of images based on similarity, context, and medical image processing tasks as well as application visualization analysis.
- It enables quantitative method along with perception of medical images using different techniques via CT, MRI, PET.

MIPAV satisfies the following objectives:

- The quantification and medical data analysis can be archived by means of computational procedure and innovation.
- The professorate at the National Institutes of Health employs information analysis and visualization to address issues in medical research.
- Different levels of the fusion process can occur, such as pixel, signal, feature extraction, and symbolic level.

14.1.1 Pixel-Level Method for Image Fusion

Om Prakash et al. [3] proposed that the pixel-level method can be applied for image fusion to yield results. The composite image pattern conservation can be realized by means of sustaining an exactly similar type of knowledge from input imagery. Pixel-level image fusion might be categorized into two:

- Spatial domain fusion.
- Transformation domain fusion.

Every geographical domain union is the simplest way to perform directly on the source image, i.e., it will not need any transformation or decomposition with the original image. The transformation is utilized on the registered images to describe the key information of the image. Every image decomposes towards transform coefficients. Also, the fusion rule is applied to check the fusion decision plan and transformation coefficients.

Every integrated model image is attained in each process of inverse transformation. In this chapter, the following algorithms are chosen for fusion since each one contributes more toward its unique identity.

Numerous situations in imaging concurrently need huge spatial and large spectral information on every image.

Instruments are not capable of providing information on design because of observational conditions.

In infusion, more than one modality image is combined as per the requirement. The term image fusion has recently been used commonly, surrounded by medical complaints along with analysis. The patient images in distinct patterns are fused by the image fusion method. Various kinds of data evolution are as follows:

- SPECT – Single photon emission tomography.
- CT – Computed tomography.
- MRI – Magnetic resonance imaging.
- PET – Positron emission tomography.

In the area of radiology and radiation oncology, the images are different, such as CT images to ascertain the difference in density of the tissue. MRIs are mainly used to examine the spinal cord and brain on different conditions. The efficient way for disease diagnosis is carried out by radiologists by combining knowledge from multiple images using fusion procedure.

14.2 Review of Literature

Gaurav Bhatnagar et al. [4] proposed that image fusion (IF) is a key area in medical imaging, and it is applied widely level. Several techniques are available for fusion which include average method, Laplacian pyramid, ratio pyramid, morphological pyramid, contrast pyramid, discrete wavelet transform, shift invariant discrete wavelet transform, principal component analysis, redundancy discrete wavelet transform, contourlet transform, non-subsampled contourlet transform. In this section, we elaborate on these techniques based on the proposed method and also the way of measuring the information of fused images is discussed.

A.P. James et al. [5] proposed that the quality of images can be improved by way of registering and combining multiple images. The image might be a single image or multiple modalities of images. It results from improvement in the quality of the image and moreover reduces randomness with redundancy. This process yields increased scientific suitability of medical images for diagnosis and assessment of medical issues, known as medical image fusion. The survey summarizes the scientific challenges identified in the field of image fusion.

Hong Zhang et al. [6] proposed that contourlet transform is redefined for pixel-level fusion for multimodality medical images. The fusion integrates region-based contourlet contrast, local energy, and weighted averaging. This fusion method provides a systematic way to extract learning of multimodality images.

The contourlet transform is refined for pixel-level multimodality medical image fusion. The fusion constraints are activated which depends on region, bounded energy, as well as integration of weighting averaging.

L. Yang et al. [7] proposed contourlet transform the issue of wavelet transform since this in attempt to improve anisotropy, multiresolution, directivity as well as locating effects considering 2D signals. So, higher quality image fusion improvement can be expected. The method for contourlet transform fusion is as follows: transformation based on region position is enforced with two steps. In step one, double filter bank method holds as long as it is registered for transformation. Along with the second step, decomposition is carried out among fusion rules. At last, the fused image is reclaimed, adopting a reconstruction strategy.

Melkamu H et al. [8] proposed a global energy fusion procedure along with region-based image fusion techniques. They examined the match computed as a whole to select the wavelet coefficients coming from distinct sub-images of the identical scale. More generous facts about the boundary could be attained along with higher appropriate image obtained from the perspective of human vision. The actual meaning of wavelet coefficients known as discrete wavelet transform, including a novel coefficients selection procedure, holds the primary goal of multi-focus image fusion.

DWT procedure can be applied for source image decomposition with a low-frequency domain, including maximum sharpness. The dimensions were chosen for the fused image and utmost coefficients adjoining activity technique is recommended for high-frequency sub-bands coefficients. The authentication method can be substituted for the combined coefficients correlation with a resultant fused image. Every suggested procedure was applied two times in sync with real multi-focus images. Empirical impact explains the suggested way to improve visual quality.

14.3 Proposed Work

The proposed system aims to implement three types of fusion techniques for multimodality brain tumor images with quantitative analysis.

Images from two different modalities of the same patient are considered as input. The images are needed via the organ (brain) with respect to various modalities, namely CT, MRI (T1, T2, C+, with FLAIR), PET, and SPECT. Each set of the image is a combination of any two modalities (Fig. 14.1).

In medical imaging, more than one type of information (anatomical and pathological) is required for efficient diagnosis, but it is not possible to have both the information from a single modality. For that reason, a fusion technique can be used to combine two or more images taken from different modalities for the same patient with a specific organ.

The system aims to facilitate different fusion techniques as long as medical images are taken from multiple modalities. In this system, three different fusion techniques are proposed, namely, DWT and contourlet transform. The above-mentioned techniques were chosen because, according to the literature, it is declared that wavelet decomposition particularly occurs superior with isolated discontinuities, never adequate at edges along with textured region. In addition, it records finite

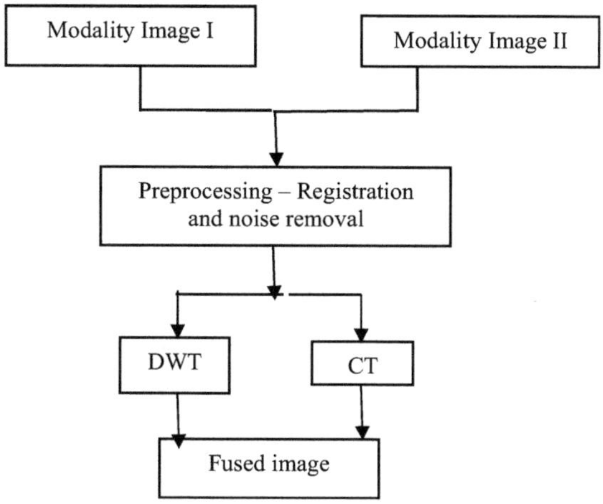

Fig. 14.1 System design

directional messages with vertical, horizontal, as well as diagonal directions. The particular case is corrected in the latest multiscale decomposition contourlet for images taken from two different modalities such as MRI, CT, and SPECT.

The whole dataset file (images) is composed [9]. These images were obtained through the organ (brain) toward distinct modalities such as CT, MRI, PET, and SPECT. A particular agreed image is appropriated and taken away from the same patient with a contrasting process of modality [10]. The system deals with three different fusion techniques, except multimodality image fusion along with quantitative analysis. A technique like this is determined in detail in the following sections:

- Preprocessing – Image registration and noise removal.
- Fusion techniques – DWT and CT.

14.3.1 Pre-processing

V.P.S. Naidu and J.R. Rao [11] proposed that source images are registered and pre-processed for noise/artifact removal before the fusion process. In registration, the source images of different modalities with different sizes are aligned to a similar size. Then the noise/artifact of the images is removed using the median filtering process. Digital image processing mostly applies to median filtering with certain conditions to preserve edges and at the same time remove the noise.

14.3.2 Fusion Technique

Fusion techniques are of two types:

- Discrete wavelet transform (DWT).
- Contourlet transform (CT).

14.3.3 Discrete Wavelet Transform (DWT)

The concept of image fusion methodology is applied efficiently for various modalities of registered images. It can be carried out in two-stage processes of decomposition and fusion.

Yong Yang et al. [12] considered A_1 and B_1 to be the types of registered images in various kinds of modalities such as CT and PET. Decomposition can be achieved through three levels by applying Daubechies filters for the pair of images via acquiring an appropriate wavelet band represented in Figs. 14.2 and 14.3.

In the primitive phase, the I_1 image fused with I_1^{a}, I_1^{v}, I_1^{d}, and I_1^{h} are the DWT sub-bands; furthermore, I_2^{a}, I_2^{v}, I_2^{d}, and I_2^{h} are the corresponding DWT sub-bands of image I_2. The pair of image coefficients taken away from the specific band of I_1 and I_2 was averaged to show the image features.

$$I_F^{a} = \text{mean}\ (I_1^{a,}\ I_2^{a}) \tag{14.1}$$

Position I_F^{a} is known as fused image estimation.

Fig. 14.2 Decomposition levels

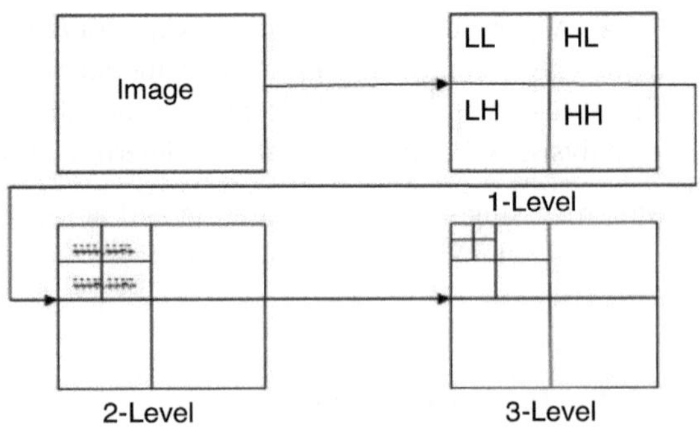

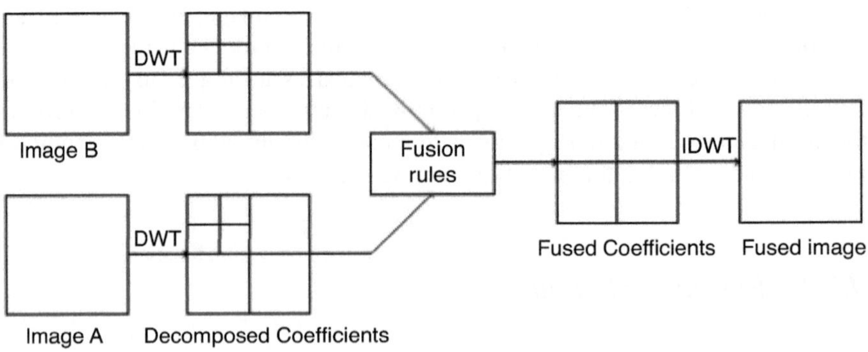

Fig. 14.3 Decomposition and fusion procedure of DWT

In that respect, the succeeding step and every sub-band such as LH, HL, HH are partitioned into blocks of size 3 × 3 with entropy for every block is estimated using the following equation.

$$e_i^{jk} = \ln \sqrt{\mu_i^{jk}} - \sum_{x,y=1}^{3,3} I_i^{jk} \frac{x, y}{\sigma_i^{jk}} / m^2 \tag{14.2}$$

K. Rajakumari et al. [13] proposed the position called $j = (v,d,h)$ and identifies its sub-bands where the value of m can be 3 and identifies the size of all blocks. Block number represented as K along with $i = 1, 2$ passed down to modify with two types of multidimensional images like I_1 with $I_{2.}$ The mean and the standard deviation for DWT coefficients are $\mu_{\rm i}^{\rm j,k}$ and $\sigma_{\rm i}^{\rm jk}$. Employ the entropy values for sub-bands of fused images $I_{\rm F}^{\rm v,}$ $I_{\rm F}^{\rm d}$, and $I_{\rm F}^{\rm h}$ are formed in Eq. 14.3. Fused image block extracted by $I_{\rm F}^{\rm jk,}$ DWT coefficients across $I_{\rm I\ is\ to}$ be chosen. The entropy value of the specified block of I_1 is greater than $I_{2,}$, but also $I_2^{\rm jk}$ is chosen.

$$I_{\rm F}^{\rm jk} = I_1^{\rm jk}, \text{if } \left(e_1^{\rm jk}\right) > \left(e_2^{\rm jk}\right) I_2^{\rm jk}, \text{otherwise} \tag{14.3}$$

Throughout, IDWT is correlated for all four fused sub-bands to bring out a final medical image fusion called $I_{\rm F}$.

$$I_{\rm F} = \text{IRDWT}\left(I_{\rm F}^{\rm a}, I_{\rm F}^{\rm V}, I_{\rm F}^{\rm d}, I_{\rm F}^{\rm h}\right) \tag{14.4}$$

14.3.4 Contourlet Transform

L. Yang et al. [14] proposed that smoothness in a fused image together with any two various modalities of the image can be achieved by contourlet transform. The transformation process depends on the region and is categorized into two different phases. The first phase carried out by double filter bank is implied for the benefit of transformation and decomposition is carried out with specific fusion rules in phase 2. Finally, fused images were retrieved by reconstruction method. Here, the proposed image fusion flow graph is represented in Fig. 14.4. The input source images are A, B, and F called the end result of the fused image after contourlet transformation.

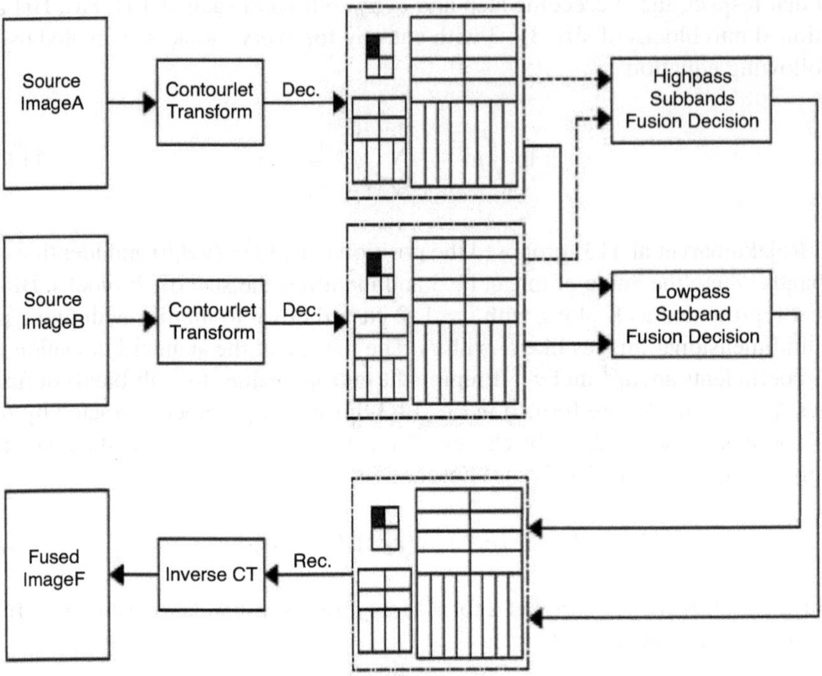

Fig. 14.4 Block diagram of the contourlet-based image fusion algorithm

14.3.5 Transformation Stage

Transformation phase Laplacian pyramid and directional filter bank method is correlated effectively for sub-band decomposition. Laplacian Pyramid Filter captures edge points. Discontinuities point in linear structure identified by applying directional filter bank.

14.3.6 Laplacian Pyramid Algorithm

The implementation of algorithm steps is as follows:

- Every input source image decomposes into low-frequency and high-frequency bandpass sub-bands.
- Input photos were downsampled with LP filter H to estimate (lowpass sub-band).
- The upsampled image is run via filter G.
- By subtracting the synthesis filter output from the input image, every high pass sub-band is imitated.

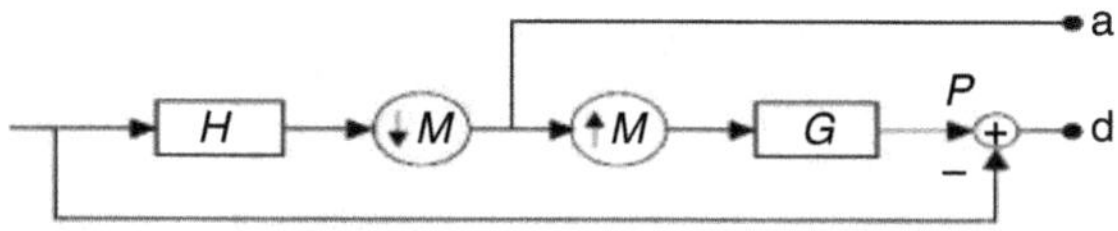

Fig. 14.5 Construction of LP

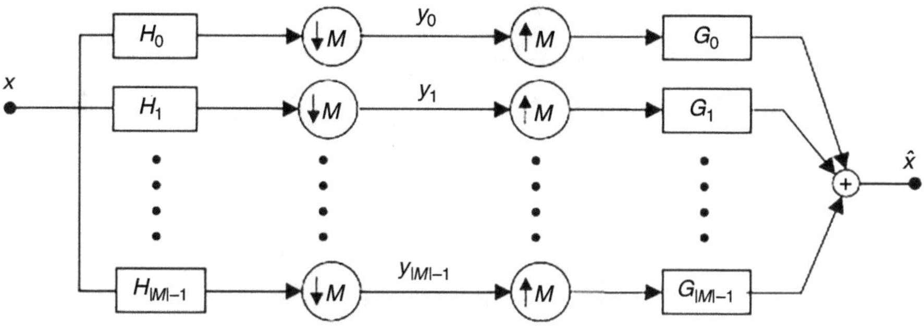

Fig. 14.6 Construction of DFB

- Low-frequency sub-bands in contourlet decomposition levels are treated similarly. Figure 14.5 depicts Laplacian pyramid decomposition.

14.3.7 Directional Filter Bank Algorithm

The steps are as follows:

- The high pass sub-band employs Quincunx Filter for deriving a tree-like image. Figure 14.6 shows directional filter bank.
- Since individual of each highpass sub-band down as well as upsampling is achieved, the resultant image is sent through synthesis filter G.
- Finally, the result of the synthesis filter is merged.

14.3.8 Decomposition Stage

Contourlet decomposition provides an improved anisotropy directionality multiresolution along with localization prospects for 2D signals than the actual image representation procedure. The withered sub-bands of transformation stages are combined as follows (Figs. 14.7, 14.8, 14.9, 14.10, and 14.11).

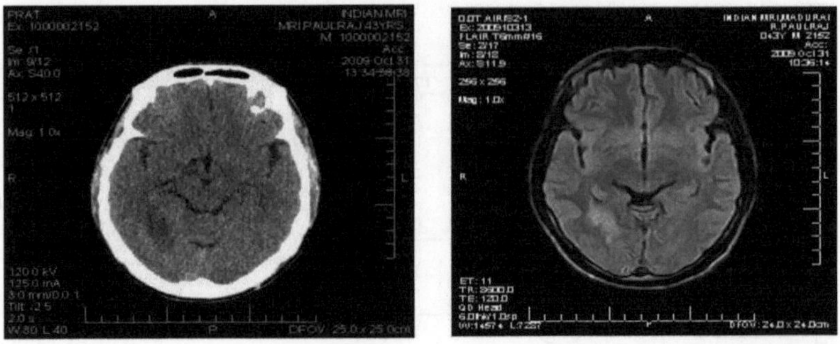

Fig. 14.7 Input images CT and MR images

Fig. 14.8 Decomposed images of DWT

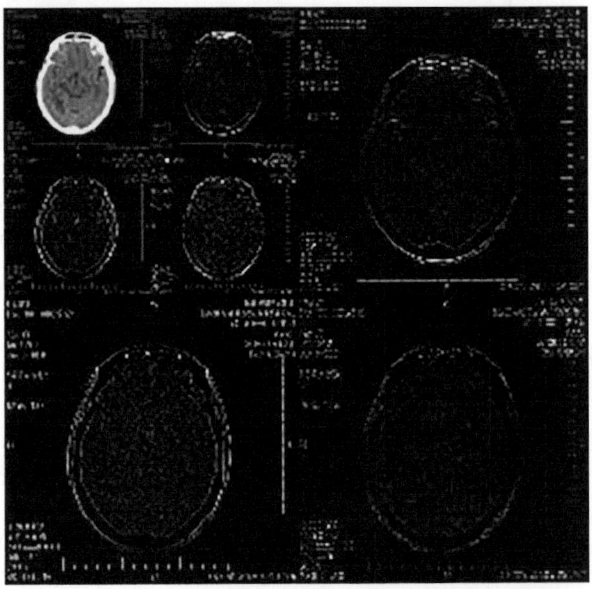

Fig. 14.9 Fused image of DWT

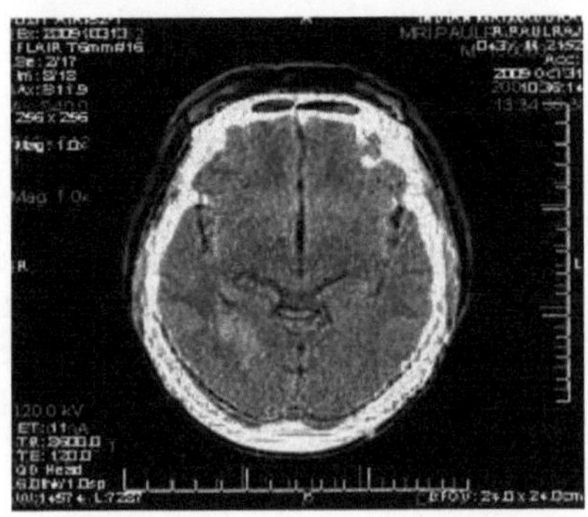

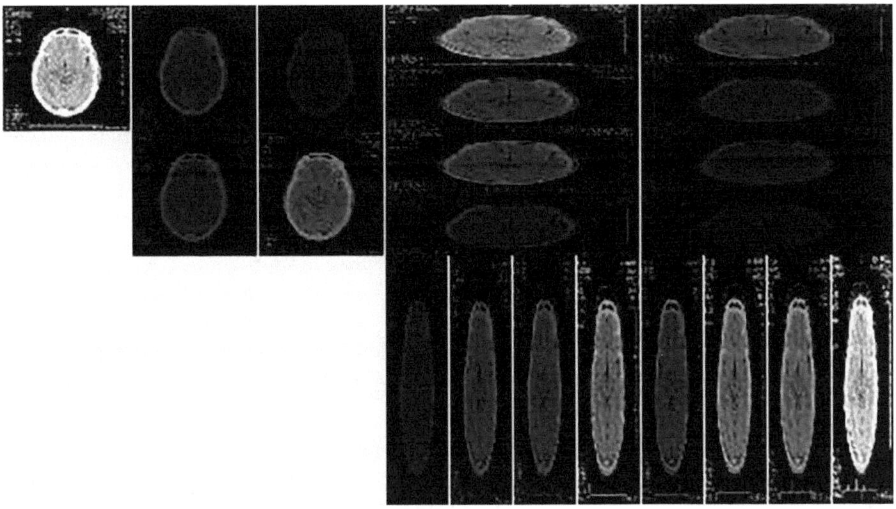

Fig. 14.10 Decomposed image of CT

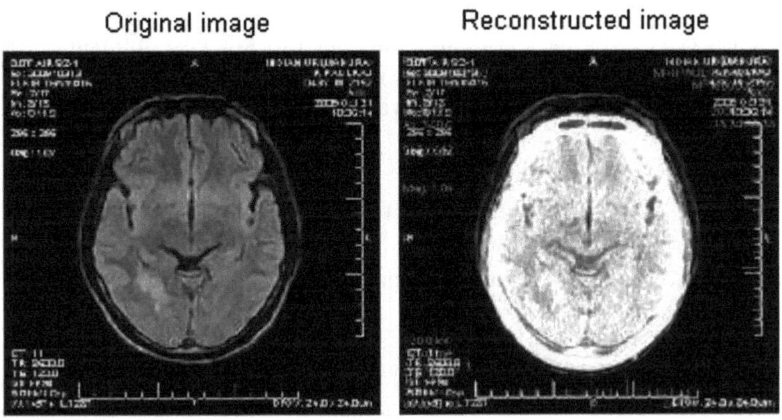

Fig. 14.11 Reconstructed image of CT

14.3.9 Low Pass Sub-band Fusion

The coefficients present along with the coarsest scale sub-band show an approximate composition of the source image. In the guidance of local energy, the contourlet domain is put together like a measurement. Later processes of selection, as well as averaging concepts are utilized to compute end coefficients.

$$E(x,y) = \sum_m \sum_n a_j \ (x+m, y+n)^2 \ W_L(m,n) \tag{14.5}$$

Within reach (x, y) estimates present contourlet coefficients $W_L(x, y)$ in figure size like 3 × 3

$$W_L = \frac{1}{9} * \begin{matrix} 1 & 1 & 1 \\ 1 & 1 & 1 \\ 1 & 1 & 1 \end{matrix} \tag{14.6}$$

Later prominence aspect was computed to identify the types of modes applied in fusion processes such as selection and averaging mode.

$$M_j^{AB}(x,y) = \frac{2\sum_m \sum_n a_j^A \ (x+m, y+n) a_j^B \ (x+m, y+n)}{E^A(x,y)} + E^{B(x,y)} \tag{14.7}$$

Here, $a_j^x(x,y); x = A, B$ stand for low pass contourlet coefficients of source image A/B and contourlet coefficients of the source image *A* or *B and M_j^AB (x,y).*

This aspect is given back with similarity such as low pass sub-bands with two types of source images. Furthermore, it is correlated to predefined threshold $T_L(T_L = 1)$. $M_j^{AB}(x,y) > T_L$ Since the averaging mode is identified for fusion with Eq. 14.8

$$a_j^F(x,y) = a_A a_j^A(x,y) + a_B a_j^B \ (x,y) \tag{14.8}$$

At this point, $a_j^F(x,y)$ are fused to a position(x). α_A, as well as α_B, depends on constraints given in Eq. 14.9

$$\alpha_A = \alpha_{min} \text{ for } E^A \ (x,y) < E^B(x,y)\alpha_{max} \text{ for } E^A \ (x,y) \geq E^B(x,y) \tag{14.9}$$

Here, $\alpha_B = 1 - \alpha_A \alpha_{min} \in (0,1)\alpha_{min} + \alpha_{max} = 1$.

The option mode is chosen for the constraints $M_j^{AB}(x,y) \leq T_L$, as well as the fusion condition represented in Eq. 14.10.

$$\begin{aligned} a_j^F(x,y) = a_j^A(x,y) \text{ for } E^A(x,y) \geq E^B(x,y) \\ a_j^B(x,y) \text{ for } E^A(x,y) < E^B(x,y) \end{aligned} \tag{14.10}$$

High pass sub-band fusion

The average approach says that after contourlet transform, high-frequency sub-bands $d_{j,k}$ are fused as follows

$$E_{j,k}^{F}(x,y) = d_{j,k}^{A}(x,y) + d_{j,k}^{B}(x,y) \tag{14.11}$$

Here, the local energy and high-frequency coefficients are $E_{j,k}^{F}(x,y)$, $d_{j,k}^{X}(x,y)$

Reconstruction of final fused image

The final result of the fused image is from $a_j^F(x,y)$ and $E_{j,k}^{F}(x,y)$ adopting inverse contourlet transform.

14.4 Implementation

14.5 Conclusion

This chapter compared two different types of image modalities as single imaging is not sufficient for better diagnosis. Discrete wavelet transform method was chosen since it produces better results for isolated discontinuities; however, it is less efficient for identifying edges as well as the textured region. Moreover, it grasps confined directional info in addition to vertical, horizontal, as well as directional knowledge. Here, fusion procedure may be efficiently applied for registered images with different types of modality into two-step processes such as decomposition and fusion. Daubechies filters are used to decompose image pairings in three steps. Non-subsampled contourlet transformation based on region was implemented twice. First, double filter banks were used. The second method decomposes using fusion rules. Next to the contourlet transform, higher absolute value coefficients in $d_{j,k}$ are averaged. Before fusing, the source photos were registered and noise/artifact-were removed. Wavelet and contourlet techniques were compared with the support of multimodality brain tumor images. From the snapshots, it has been observed that the DWT performs level-by-level decomposition, whereas the contourlet performs horizontal and vertical decomposition at various angles. Hence, the reconstructed fused image of the contourlet is better than the wavelet method (DWT). So the work can be enhanced further by applying deep-learning methodology with the guidance of innovation which may improve better prediction accuracy.

References

1. Median Filtering. (2014). http://homepages.inf.ed.ac.uk/rbf/HIPR2/median.htm
2. Liu, Z., Yin, H., Chai, Y., & Yan, S. X. (2014). A novel approach for multimodal medical image fusion. *Expert Systems with Applications, 41*, 7425–7435.
3. Prakash, O., Kumar, A., & Khare, A. (2014). Pixel-level image fusion scheme based on steerable pyramid wavelet transform using absolute maximum selection fusion rule. In *IEEE*

international conference on issues and challenges in intelligent computing techniques (ICICT) (pp. 765–770).
4. Gaurav Bhatnagar, Q. M., Wu, J., & Li, Z. (2013). Directive contrast based multimodal medical image fusion in NSCT domain. *IEEE Transactions on Multimedia, 15*(5), 1014–1024.
5. James, A. P., & Dasarathy, B. V. (2014). Medical image fusion: A survey of the state of the art. *Information Fusion, 19*, 4–19.
6. Zhang, H., Liu, L., & Lin, N. (2007). A novel wavelet medical image fusion method'. In *International conference on multimedia and ubiquitous engineering* (pp. 548–553).
7. Yang, L., Guo, B. L., & Ni, W. (2008). Multimodality medical image fusion based on multiscale geometric analysis of Contourlet transform. *Neurocomputing, 72*, 203–211.
8. Asmare, M. H., Asirvadam, V. S., Iznita, L., & Hani, A. F. M. (2010). Image enhancement by fusion in Contourlet transform. *International Journal on Electrical Engineering and Informatics, 2*(1), 29–42.
9. Types of brain images. (2014). http://www.abta.org/
10. Brain tumor images. (2014). http://www.braintumor.org/
11. Naidu, V. P. S., & Rao, J. R. (2008). Pixel-level image fusion using wavelets and principal component analysis. *Defence Science Journal, 58*(3), 338–352.
12. Yang, Y., Huang, S., Gao, J., & Qian, Z. (2014). Multi-focus image fusion using an effective discrete wavelet transform based algorithm. *Measurement Science Review, 14*(2), 102–108.
13. Rajakumari, K., & Nalini, C. (2014). Improvement of image quality based on fractal image Compressio. *Middle-East Journal of Scientific Research, 20*(10), 1213–1217, ISSN 1990-9233, © IDOSI Publications, 2014.
14. Yang, L., Guo, B. L., & Ni, W. (2007). Multifocus image fusion algorithm based on contourlet decomposition and region statistics. In *Fourth international conference on image and graphics* (pp. 707–712).

Chapter 15
Performance-Based Analysis of K-Medoids and K-Means Algorithms for the Diagnosis and Prediction of Oral Cancer

S. Sivakumar and T. Kamalakannan

15.1 Introduction

Oral cancer is one of the major causes of death in India [1]. According to the World Health Organization [2], one-third of people suffer from oral cancer due to the frequent usage of tobacco and liquor, including pipes, biting tobacco, cigarettes, cigars, betel nut, and snuffs. Radiotherapy and chemotherapy are applied to eliminate cancerous growth. Data mining [3] is the procedure of evaluating huge volumes of datasets to discover the intelligence of businesses that help companies solve problems and find new opportunities. Data mining is largely used in many real-time applications like health care systems, insurance systems, educational institutions, product development and marketing, finding the prediction of various diseases, discovering the customer characteristics for their product purchases, developing suitable marketing strategies for improving business, increasing revenue for their product, reducing costs of the works, and many more. Data mining techniques [4] like clustering and classification are used to find diagnosis and prediction of oral cancer [5].

Clustering [6] is an unsupervised learning method and an effective technique for data analysis. Clustering can be categorized into three types: partitioning, hierarchical, and grid-based and model-based models. Partition-based clustering divides the data into two groups of objects. Each cluster is more identical to objects in another

S. Sivakumar
Department of Computer Science, School of Computing Sciences, Vels Institute of Science, Technology and Advanced Studies, Chennai, Tamil Nadu, India

T. Kamalakannan (✉)
Department of Information Technology, Vels Institute of Science, Technology and Advanced Studies, Chennai, Tamil Nadu, India
e-mail: kkannan.scs@velsuniv.ac.in

F. J. Joseph et al. (eds.), *Computational Intelligence for Clinical Diagnosis*, EAI/Springer Innovations in Communication and Computing,
https://doi.org/10.1007/978-3-031-23683-9_15

cluster. K-Means, Clarans, and K-Medoids are the best illustrations of partition-based clustering algorithms. In this research, we have studied and applied different clustering techniques called K-Means and K-Medoids algorithms, along with their limitations and strength. We identified the best algorithm from the above-mentioned algorithm with the intention of predicting oral cancer. The oral cancer dataset is used for the purpose of the prediction of oral cancer using partition-based clustering algorithms.

The remaining part of the chapter is covered as follows. Section 15.2 provides data mining techniques for oral cancer analyses that are utilized for diagnosis and prediction of oral cancer examination. Section 15.3 highlights the application of oral cancer examination. Clustering calculations for oral cancer examination are examined in Sect. 15.4. The final section closes with an overview of the work done on oral cancer.

15.2 Related Works

Data mining (DM) is used to analyze large datasets and produce useful information. The main objective of DM is to change over the huge volume of data into helpful information for investigating different fields in the clinical field [7]. Many researchers have proposed distinctive volumes of clustering algorithms and utilizing diverse valuable areas in healthcare applications for survivability examination. The main idea behind their research papers is to attain high clustering accuracies in their applications. We have projected some of the clustering algorithm-based research papers that predict healthcare applications like breast cancer, lung cancer, oral cancer, and others.

Ahmed et al. [8] have submitted a research paper on the K-means clustering algorithm survey and the performance evaluation of the same. This paper provided an organized and comprehensive overview of the K-means algorithm and its flaws. The phases of K-means are outlined, and datasets were used to test them. They highlighted the work from other previous papers and included their detailed experimental analysis and the comparison of K-means clustering. This analysis disclosed that there is no global solution for the drawbacks of the K-means algorithm. They suggested that this work will assist the DM research community in designing novel methods of clustering algorithms.

Alsayat et al. [9] have proposed on K-means clustering algorithm using Kohonen Map [SOM]. The main purpose of this research paper is to reduce the number of centroids in K-means clustering. K-means algorithm works in two phases and uses SOM. In the first phase, they make the prototypes, and in the second, they use the prototypes to build clusters. The performance of the K-means clustering algorithm is found using SOM with two healthcare datasets. In the end, they came to the conclusion that the suggested outcome is accurate and exhibits improved clustering performance in addition to significant insights for each cluster.

Ogbuabor et al. [10] have proposed DBSCAN and K-means algorithms using Silhouette Score Value [SSV]. In this research, they analyzed various clustering techniques with the use of a healthcare dataset to find the best algorithm to bring the optimized group clusters. The DBSCAN and K-means algorithms are analyzed using SSV in two steps. They examined the K-means algorithm utilizing various cluster sizes and different distance parameters. Next, they examined the DBSCAN algorithm applying various distance metrics to form a cluster which needs very less number of points. According to the experimental findings, both DBSCAN and K-means clustering are quite strong in inter-cluster separation and intra-cluster cohesion. The K-means clustering algorithm outperformed the DBSCAN algorithm in terms of execution speed and accuracy.

Arora et al. [11] discussed K-means and K-medoids algorithms and tested both the algorithms with a dataset of KEEL. In their paper, they used randomly distributed data points to gather their input data, and then clusters were formed based on similarities. The datasets were examined and compared using K-means and K-medoids. This work proves that K-medoids clustering outperforms K-means clustering in terms of the cluster head selection time and space complexity of coverage. Furthermore, K-medoids outperform K-means in terms of noise reduction, evaluation time, and non-sensitivity to outliers.

Sya'iyah et al. [12] have proposed the K-means clustering algorithm using student data. This research is comprised of various steps such as data cleaning, data selection, data transformation, clustering, and knowledge performance. They divided three categories of student data based on the characteristics of student performance such as poor, average, and excellent. K-means clustering algorithm is then experimented using 724 student data and taking four variables such as study period, grade point average, thesis length, and score of English proficiency. The three student characteristics that emerged from this research are as follows: students in cluster 1 have a scaled GPA of 3.28, an LS age of 4.52, an EP score of 404, and an LT age of 7.46. Students in cluster 2 have a GPA of 3.29 on a scale of 4, an LS age of 4.48, an EP score of 481, and an LT age of 7.26. Students in cluster 3 have a GPA of 3.31 on a scale of 4, an LS age of 4.50, an EP score of 437, and an LT age of 7.14.

Shah et al. [13] have presented on K-medoids and K-means algorithms with modified K-means algorithm and their comparative study. This paper offers a novel modified K-means clustering algorithm and evaluates numerous strategies for selecting the initial cluster. When compared to K-medoids and K-means algorithms, the modified K-mean algorithm produces more clusters and takes less time to execute. The proposed approach is tested in health care, and the output is compared with K-medoids and K-means algorithms. The output provides less time to compute and performs better than K-medoids and K-means algorithms.

Najdi and Er-Raha [14] published their research paper with the intention of finding the educational outcomes based on the characteristics of student profile using unsupervised clustering. In this paper, they have discussed the K-means clustering algorithm and used R programming for their implementation with the intention of grouping graduate students. From this paper, they formed three student groups based on similar learning habits and their academic performance in the study period. They used student datasets, including six-semester marks and their final grades for their performance evaluation. Based on their experiments, they conclude that K-means clustering produced better results in identifying students learning characteristics with their performance each semester. Finally, they proposed that Moroccan universities adopt these innovative ideas and strategies to improve performance and educational outcomes.

Surya et al. [15] have analyzed unsupervised clustering algorithms of K-medoids and Kmeans and their performance. In this research, they used the agriculture dataset for the analysis of the above algorithms. They also compared the different characteristics of K-medoids and K-means algorithms such as precision, accuracy, MAE, and RMSR for their evaluation. Finally, they concluded that the K-medoids algorithm provided the best performance compared with the K-means algorithm.

Saravananathan et al. [16] proposed the prediction of disease using diabetes data with their analysis of clustering algorithms. In this paper, they surveyed different unsupervised learning algorithms with the intention of predicting diabetic diseases by using the diabetic dataset. For their research, they analyzed prescriptions of more than 15,000 diabetic patients. The algorithms were compared with different clusters and execution times. In each, the best algorithm was discovered based on their performance. Finally, they came to a conclusion that the K-means algorithm is suitable for diabetic disease prediction.

Velmurugan et al. [17] analyzed the performance of fuzzy C-means algorithm and K-means algorithm. They used arbitrary data points for their research and tested both algorithms with different input values. The cluster value rises when there is an increase in the number of input values. Finally, he claimed that k-means clustering is superior to the fuzzy C-means clustering algorithm.

Biradar et al. [18] suggested three algorithms – hierarchical, expectation maximization, and K-means clustering – for their research using the diabetes dataset. They experimented with both algorithms by using Weka and Tanagra tools. Finally, they compared all algorithms and suggested that the K-means algorithm is the best based on the outcome.

15.3 Materials and Methods

We analyzed K-medoids and K-means algorithms for the purpose of diagnosis and detection of oral cancer. Numerous inputs and different cluster ranges were considered for further analysis. Cluster formations are calculated based on the distance between data points and their midpoints. All clusters are identified using different symbols.

Table 15.1 Dataset for oral cancer

Sl. No	Attribute
1	Case
2	Gender
3	Age
4	Site
5	TNM
6	Stage
7	Histopathology
8	Smoking
9	Alcohol
10	Alive/Dead
11	Cause of Death
12	Survival time
13	Recurrence
14	Disease-free survival
15	The number of loci Ai
16	Number of loci informative
17	FAL Score
18	p53 IHC
19	Rb IHC

15.3.1 Dataset

We collected 2000 reports of patients from various hospitals, laboratories, and other sources. We used 19 different attributes from oral cancer datasets as inputs. The attribute of the oral cancer dataset is given in Table 15.1.

In this chapter, we discuss both K-means and K-medoids algorithms separately from the four steps defined. By comparing these two algorithms, we were able to find their accuracies and identify the best algorithm.

15.3.2 Methods

Two different algorithms, namely K-medoids and K-means, are examined for our research purpose, and a detailed explanation of these algorithms is described below.

15.3.3 K-Means Clustering Algorithm

K-means clustering algorithm is a partition-based and stepwise algorithm that splits the dataset into k-predefined recognizable non-overlapping subgroups, and all data points correspond to one group identically. It determines the data points to a cluster and defines the centroid for each cluster that is at a minimum. These centroids are created in dissimilar ways at different locations based on their results. The following steps give the representation of the K-means clustering algorithm.

- Place P points into the space represented by the objects that are being clustered. These points represent the initial group of centroids.
- Assign each object to the group that has the closest centroid.
- When all objects have been assigned, recalculate the positions of k-centroids
- Repeat steps 2 and 3 until the centroids no longer move.

The algorithm is designed to locate the medoids, which are objects that are centrally positioned in clusters. Objects that are provisionally classified as medoids are grouped together in a set K of selected objects. The K-means clustering algorithm can be executed several times to decrease the effect and is a good candidate to work for the randomly generated data points. This algorithm is mainly applied for finding a simple initiative scheme.

15.3.4 K-Medoids Clustering Algorithm

The K-medoids clustering is a partition around medoids (PAM). PAM splits the dataset into observations and searches through them for K representative objects among them. By associating each observation with the closest medoid based on the results, a set of K-medoids is created, and then K numbers of clusters are created. The key concept is to find the k-representative objects that minimize the sum of the observation differences from their nearest representative object. The detailed step-by-step algorithm is given below.

- Take K first points.
- Assume the outcome of displacing the individual of the chosen objects through one of the unselected objects.
- Choose the pattern among the lowest cost.
- Otherwise, correlate each unselected point with its nearby chosen point and stop.

Medoids are typical objects of a cluster within a dataset, and they have the minimum amount of differences between them and the other objects in the cluster. The main purpose of this algorithm is to calculate a K-representative object which minimizes dissimilarities of the observations with their nearest representative objects. With each iteration, the location of the medoid may be changed.

15.4 Experimental Results

We have used the tool R-programming for the purpose of diagnosis and prediction of oral cancer. The R-programming language is applied in many data mining and machine-learning algorithms, including classification, clustering, regression, and association rule extraction. Two unsupervised learning algorithms called K-medoids and K-means are tested and observed in the oral cancer dataset. The oral cancer dataset is divided into three, five, and seven sets of cluster centres. The dataset is initially partitioned into three sets of cluster centres using the K-medoids algorithm and K-means algorithm. We determine the outcome value for three clusters of the K-means algorithm and K-medoids algorithm based on the execution. Three clusters of partition-based clustering algorithms are presented in Table 15.2.

We used an oral cancer dataset for the purpose of analyzing and diagnosing oral cancer with ranges of 20–70 and smoking levels of 1–30. Figure 15.1 depicts the visualizations of three clustering for the K-means clustering algorithm.

Figure 15.2 depicts the visualizations of three clustering for the K-medoids clustering algorithm.

For five clusters, we used both K-means and K-medoids algorithms on a continuous basis. The time complexity and five clustering point of both algorithms are shown in Table 15.3.

Table 15.2 Three clustering

Algorithms	Execution time (in milliseconds)	Number of clusters 1	2	3
K-Means	4672	731	391	877
K-Medoids	5690	618	393	989

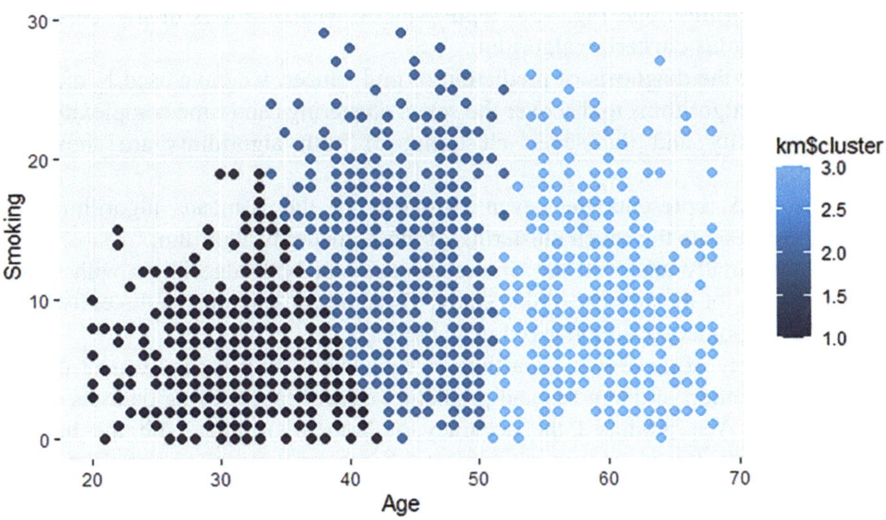

Fig. 15.1 Visualizations of three clusters (K-means)

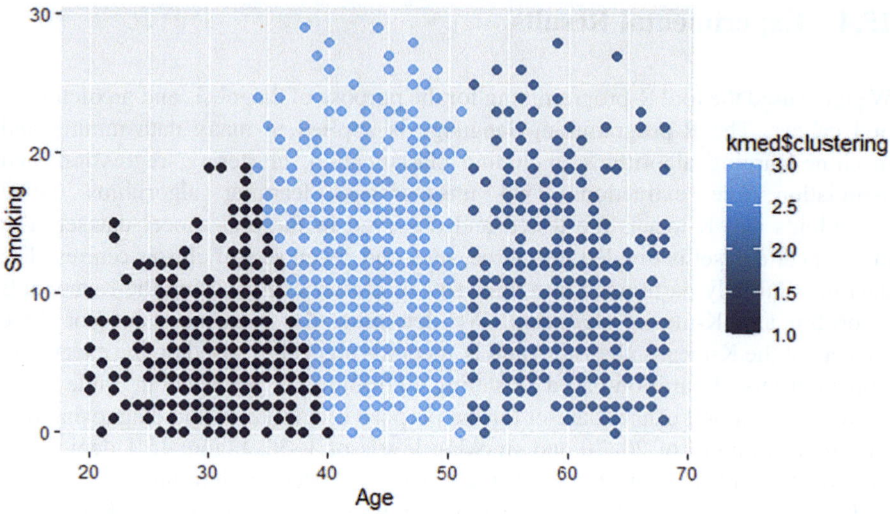

Fig. 15.2 Visualizations of three clusters (K-medoids)

Table 15.3 Five clustering points

Algorithms	Execution time (in milliseconds)	Number of clusters				
		1	2	3	4	5
K-Means	5037	397	353	358	485	407
K-Medoids	6347	411	361	425	457	346

Figure 15.3 represents the visualizations of five clustering for the K-means clustering algorithm, and Fig. 15.4 represents the visualizations of five clustering for the K-medoids clustering algorithm.

Finally, for the diagnosis of prediction of oral cancer, we have used K-medoids and K-means algorithms to discover the seven clusterings and time complexity. The time complexity and the seven clustering of both algorithms are shown in Table 15.4.

Figure 15.5 represents the seven clustering of the K-means algorithm, and Fig. 15.6 represents the seven clustering of the K-medoids algorithm.

We have finally analyzed the time complexity of both algorithms with varied clustered sizes for the purpose of this study. The time complexities of three, five, and seven cluster points are summarized in Table 15.5.

The accuracy of these two algorithms is calculated using an oral cancer dataset with a the intention of diagnosis and prediction of oral cancer using datasets of age and smoking. We produced the accuracy of both algorithms with the help of R-programming. Based on our experiments, K-means have an accuracy of 85.18 and K-medoids have an accuracy of 80.71. As a result, when compared to the K-medoids algorithm, the K-means algorithm is efficient.

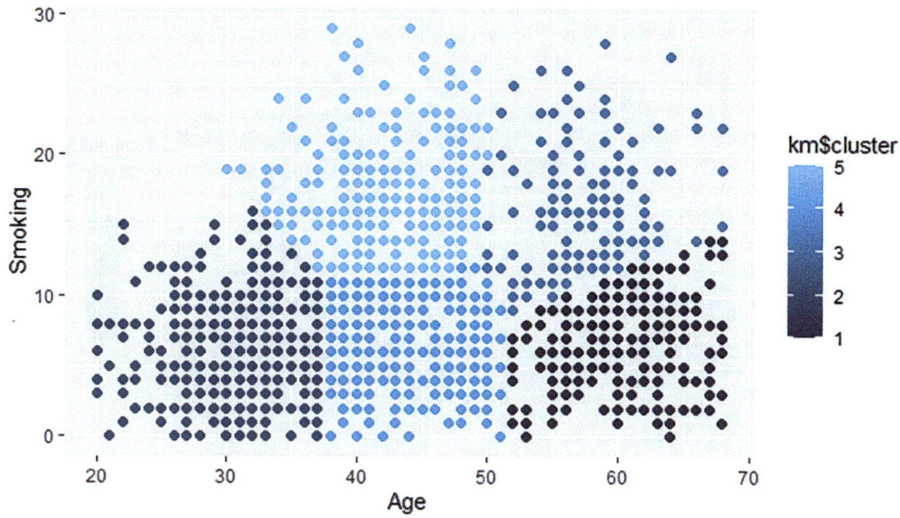

Fig. 15.3 Visualizations of five clusters (K-means)

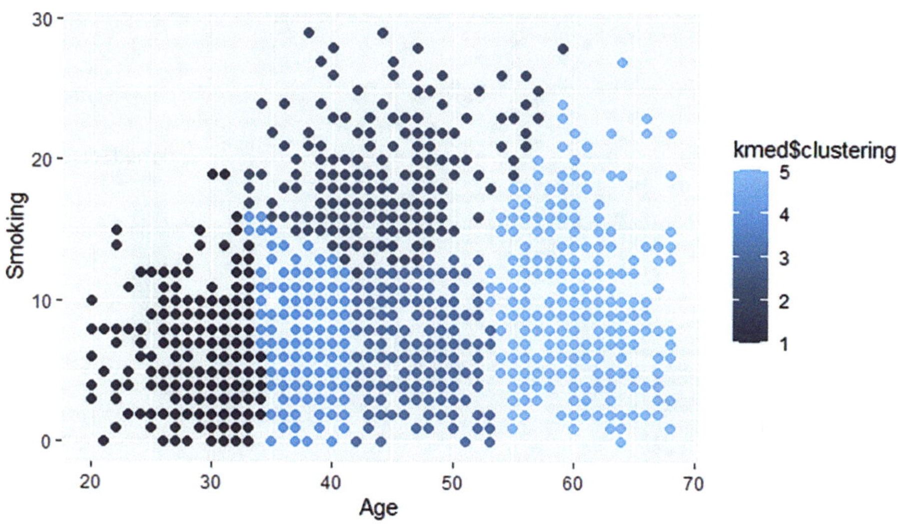

Fig. 15.4 Visualizations of five clusters (K-medoids)

Table 15.4 Seven clustering

Algorithms	Execution time (in milliseconds)	Number of clusters						
		1	2	3	4	5	6	7
K-Means	6934	169	260	334	332	262	393	250
K-Medoids	8034	402	253	291	331	283	216	224

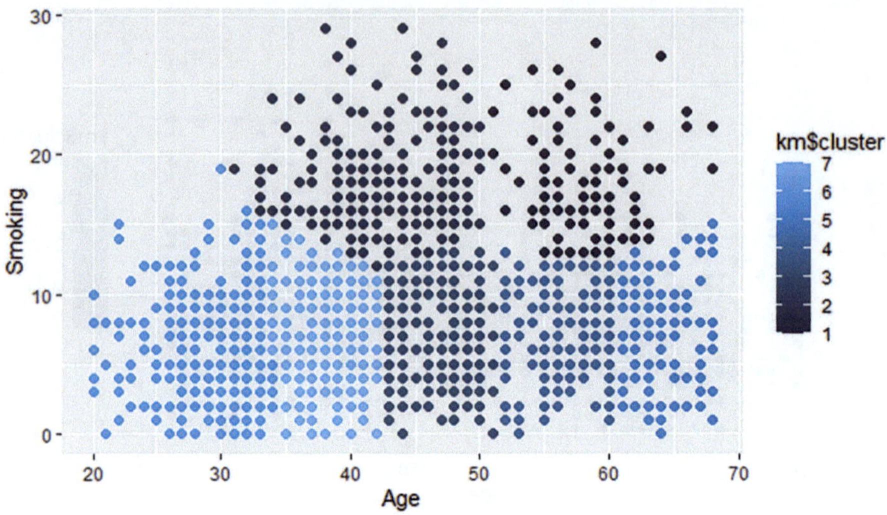

Fig. 15.5 Visualizations of seven clusters (K-means)

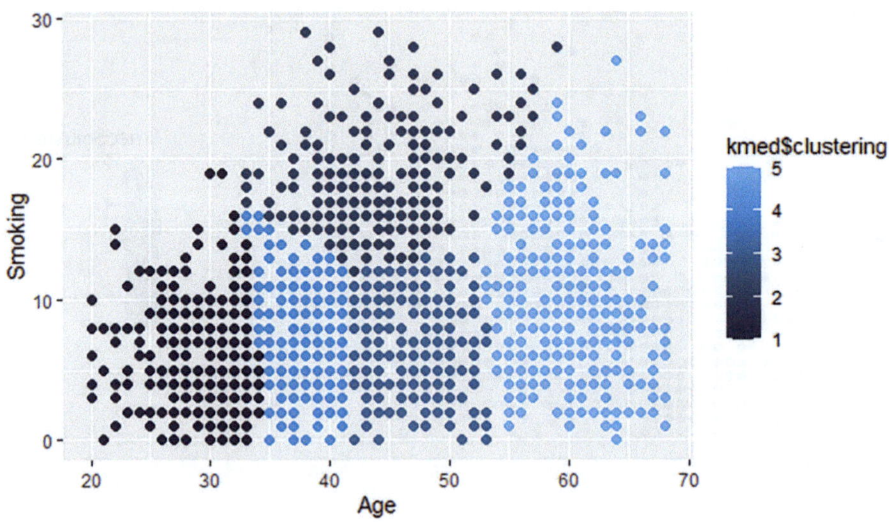

Fig. 15.6 Visualizations of seven clusters (K-medoids)

Table 15.5 Summarization of cluster points

	Number of clusters		
Algorithms	3	5	7
K Means	4672	5037	6934
K Medoids	5690	6347	8034

15.5 Conclusion

The proposed work points to the significance of various clustering algorithms for the diagnosis and prediction of oral cancer. The analysis of these algorithms is calculated based on accuracy and execution time to provide a comparison between them. For the purpose of our study, we have utilized a dataset on oral cancer for the diagnosis and prediction of oral cancer. In this study, we came to the conclusion that the K-Means algorithm is superior to the K-Medoids algorithm in terms of both the amount of time it takes to execute the algorithms as well as the level of accuracy they produce. Clustering algorithms are, according to the findings of studies conducted by researchers and conclusions drawn from those studies, the most effective method for diagnosing and forecasting oral cancer due to their necessity and excellent performance. Clustering strategies will be investigated with the purpose of advancing and bettering the methods for studying data in order to suggest a new facet of oral cancer. Several different partitioning approaches, such as Fuzzy C-means, K-medoids, and K-means, have highlighted the necessity of conducting investigations and determining the extent of oral cancer based on the results of laboratory tests.

References

1. ICMR- National Institute of Cancer Prevention and Research: http://nicpr.icmr.org.in/
2. World Health Organization: https://www.who.int/health-topics/oral-health
3. Witten, I. H., & Frank, E. (2016). *Data mining: Practical machine learning tools and techniques* (4th ed.). Morgan Kaufmann. ISBN: 9780128042915.
4. Consoli, S., Recupero, D. R., & Petkovic, M. (2019). *Data science for healthcare*. Springer. ISBN: 9783030052492.
5. Sivakumar, S., & Kamalakannan, T. (2021). A survey on oral cancer using data mining techniques. *Strad Research, 8*(2).
6. Han, J., Kamber, M., & Pei, J. (2011). *Data mining: Concepts and techniques*. Morgan Kaufmann Publishers. ISBN 978–0123814791.
7. Reddy, C. K., & Agarwal, C. C. (2020). *Healthcare data analytics*. CRC Press, Taylor & Francis Group. ISBN 9780367575687.
8. Ahmed, M., Seraj, R., & Islam, S. M. S. (2020). The K-means algorithm: A comprehensive survey and performance evaluation. *Electronics, 9*, 1295.
9. Alsayat, A., & El-Sayed, H. (2016). *Efficient genetic K-means clustering for health care knowledge discovery*, SERA 2016, June 8–10.
10. Ogbuabor, G., & Ugwoke, F. N. (2018, April). Clustering algorithm for a healthcare dataset using silhouette score value. *International Journal of Computer Science & Information Technology, 10*(2).
11. Arora, P., Dr, D., Varshney, S., Ogbuabor, G., & Ugwoke, F. N. (2016). Analysis of K-means and K-medoids algorithm for big data, Elsevier. *Procedia Computer Science, 78*, 507–512.
12. Sya'iyah, K., Yuliansyah, H., & Arfiani, I. (2019, August). Clustering student data based on K-means algorithms. *International Journal of Scientific & Technology Research, 8*(08).
13. Shah, S., & Singh, M. (2012, May). Comparison of a time efficient modified K-mean algorithm with k-means and K-medoids algorithm. *IEEE Xplore*. https://doi.org/10.1109/CSNT.2012.100

14. Najdi, L., & Er-Raha, B. (2016). Use of unsupervised clustering to characterize graduate students profiles based on educational outcomes. *International Journal of Computer Techniques, 3*(2).
15. Surya, P., & LaurenceAroquiaraj, I. (2019, January). Performance analysis of K-means and K-medoids clustering algorithms using agriculture dataset. *Journal of Emerging Technologies and Innovative Research, 6*(1).
16. Saravananathan, K., & Velmurugan, T. (2019, September). Quality based analysis of clustering algorithms using diabetes data for the prediction of disease. *International Journal of Innovative Technology and Exploring Engineering, 8*(11S2).
17. Velmurugan, T. (2012). Performance comparison between K means and fuzzy c-means algorithms using arbitrary data points. *Wulfenia Journal, 19*(8), 234–241.
18. Biradar, U. G., & Mugali, D. S. (2017). Clustering algorithms on diabetes data: Comparative case study. *International Journal of Applied Science and Engineering Technology, 5*(4), 1575–1581.

Chapter 16
Comparative Correlation of Markers of Inflammatory Metamorphism in the Peripheral Blood of Patients with Dorsopathies of Different Genesis

Khakimova Sohiba Ziyadulloevna

16.1 Introduction

A blood test for acute phase proteins and inflammation markers is a comprehensive study of various proteins, the level of which in the blood increases during various inflammatory processes in the organism [1]. Dorsopathy is a common pathology accompanied by aseptic inflammation in the spine but has not been studied for markers of inflammation [2–4].

An increase in fibrinogen is not only a component of the blood coagulation system but also an indicator of acute and chronic inflammatory, immune, and tumor phenomena [5, 6]. The current views of inflammation on the development of radiculopathies are based on the fact that the process was limited to one or several segments of the spinal column, having a local character [7, 8]. An increase in the concentration of fibrinogen above the physiological norm in these diseases is moderately pronounced and is well-stopped by NSAIDs [9, 10].

16.1.1 Purpose of the Study

Study of indicators and comparative correlation of markers of inflammatory metamorphism in the peripheral blood of patients with chronic pain syndrome in dorsopathies of various origins.

K. S. Ziyadulloevna (✉)
Department of Neurology and Neurosurgery, Faculty of Postgraduate Education, Samarkand State Medical University, Samarkand, Uzbekistan
e-mail: hakimovasohoba@lisr.ru

F. J. Joseph et al. (eds.), *Computational Intelligence for Clinical Diagnosis*,
EAI/Springer Innovations in Communication and Computing,
https://doi.org/10.1007/978-3-031-23683-9_16

The task of the work was to study the concentration of fibrinogen, C-reactive protein, and interleukin-1β in blood plasma in patients with chronic pain syndrome in dorsopathies of compression-ischemic genesis, brucellosis, rheumatic, and herpetic genesis.

16.2 Materials and Research Methods

320 patients with chronic pain syndrome with dorsopathies of various origins, who are being treated in the department of neurology of the city medical association of the city of Samarkand in the period from 2018 to 2021, were selected.

For further scientific research, the patients were divided into the following groups:

- First group: Chronic dorsopathy of compression-ischemic genesis (DCIG) – 82 patients
- Second group: Dorsopathy in chronic brucellosis (CBR) – 84 patients
- Tthird group: Dorsopathy of rheumatic genesis (DRheuG) – 76 patients
- Fourth group: Dorsopathy in chronic herpes (DHerH) – 78 patients
- The control group consisted of 40 conditionally healthy people with signs of dorsopathies, commensurate in sex and age with the above groups (employees of the city medical association were selected).

The studies were carried out within the framework of the Declaration of Helsinki of the World Association, "Ethical principles for scientific and medical research involving humans," as amended in 2000. All information about patients was collected, analyzed, and recorded in writing with the consent of the patients themselves. The scientific work was approved by the local ethics committee of the institute in accordance with the agreements on joint scientific work.

All patients with CPS were in the age range of persons from 16 to 75 years, with predominantly 30–39 years old – 96 (30%), and also 50–59 years old – 67 (20.9%).

Gender gradation of 320 patients: women – 205 (64.1%), men – 113 (35.4%) (Table 16.1).

Dorsopathies of various origins aroused the greatest interest: dorsopathy of compression-ischemic origin, dorsopathy in chronic brucellosis, dorsopathy of rheumatic origin, and dorsopathy in TORCH infection, namely herpes.

In this chapter, our goal was to highlight the obtained laboratory studies. We have analyzed the clinical and biochemical blood tests and urinalysis.

1. Rheumatic tests: (a) rheumatic factor (RF) – venous blood was examined by immunoturbidimetry, and a result of more than 8 IU ml was considered positive; (b) C-reactive protein (CRP) – venous blood was examined, where the patient was asked not to eat for 12 hours before the study, to exclude physical and emotional overstrain 30 minutes before the study, not to smoke for 30 minutes before the study. Readings greater than 10 mg/l indicate acute inflammation and

Table 16.1 Gradation by sex and age

Age (years)	Women (abs/%)	Men (abs/%)	Total (abs/%)
Under 19	13 (4,1%)	11 (3,4%)	24 (7,5%)
20-29	44 (13,7%)	13 (4,1%)	57 (17,8%)
30-39	59 (18,4%)	37 (11,6%)	96 (30%)
40-49	30 (9,4%)	23 (7,2%)	53 (16,6%)
50-59	44 (13,7%)	23 (7,2%)	67 (20,9%)
60 and older	17 (5,3%)	6 (1,9%)	23 (7,2%)
Total	207 (64,7%)	113 (35,3%)	320 (100%)

chronic disease; (c) antistreptolysin (ASLO) – venous blood was examined, where the patient was asked to donate on an empty stomach on the eve of the study to exclude alcohol, intense physical activity, and medication. Readings above 200 IU/mL are considered positive [11].

2. Tests for the detection of brucellosis: (a) Heddelson's reaction – they took blood on an empty stomach from a finger on a glass slide, and brucellosis diagnostic was dripped into it. The appearance of an agglutination reaction was considered positive; (b) Wright's reaction – venous blood was examined for the presence of antibodies to the brucellosis antigen. Titer values of 100–200 indicated a positive result, in which an acute process may become chronic.
3. Blood test for TORCH infection, which included tests for antibodies to four infections: herpes, toxoplasmosis, cytomegalovirus, and rubella virus. We selected patients with antibodies to herpes since, according to many authors, in this pathology, sensory ganglia and peripheral nerves are most often affected. AB to herpes 1 and 2 types IgG and IgM were checked. A positive IgG response meant chronic carriage [12].

To study endothelin-1, blood taken on an empty stomach from the cubital vein (14 hours after eating) was used. The blood was examined twice, at admission and at the end of the treatment. Not later than 2 hours after blood sampling, the serum was separated by centrifugation (3000 revolutions per minute), and then the study was immediately carried out.

16.2.1 Determination of Fibrinogen Concentration

Fibrinogen in blood plasma was determined in a standard, modified laboratory-clinical method according to Glauss [12], using a new test system, "Multi Tech-Fibrinogen." This method made it possible to determine the concentration of fibrinogen in a wide range, in which there is no dilution step that could affect the accuracy, correctness, and dilution. The essence of the method was to determine the clotting time of citrate platelet-poor plasma with excess thrombin. To conduct the study, venous blood was added to a plastic tube with sodium citrate, then it was incubated for 2 minutes at 37 °C, and only then 50 ml of thrombin solution was added. The clotting time of the studied plasma ranged from 5 to 100 seconds. The calibration of the test system was performed on coagulograms with different principles of recording the time obtained during clot formation. The calibration curve was linear in the range of 0.5–6 g/l [4].

C-Reactive Protein (CRP) is a glycoprotein belonging to the proteins of the inflammatory process, the synthesis of which increases after 6 hours under the influence of anti-inflammatory cytokines: interleukin-1, interleukin-6, and tumor necrosis factor-alpha, the concentration in the blood increases in almost 2 days 100 times. CRP is listed as a marker of the inflammatory response, taking part in the reactions of humoral and cellular immunity. Significant increases are observed with a viral or bacterial infection, as well as with tissue necrosis. The reasons for the increase in CRP can also be autoimmune processes (rheumatoid arthritis, vasculitis, spondyloarthritis, and so on), exacerbations of chronic diseases, and others. The material for the study is blood from a vein, which is taken after a 4-hour fast. On the eve of blood donation, intense physical activity, smoking, and drinking alcohol are excluded. When the reaction reached the endpoint, the increase in absorption as a result of precipitation was measured. The calibration curve had a linear character and was derived within the range of given values according to the standards in antiserum to CRP [13].

Interleukin-1β is a broad-spectrum pro-inflammatory cytokine that plays an important role in the development and regulation of nonspecific defense and specific immunity. Being synthesized and released by monocytes and macrophages, it is quickly included in the body's defensive response to pathogenic agents. In our study, interleukin-1β was determined by ELISA.

16.3 Discussion

The concentration of fibrinogen in blood plasma in patients with dorsopathies of compression-ischemic genesis (group I) did not exceed 4.3 g/l, corresponding to the physiological norm.

Fig. 16.1 Fibrinogen concentration in patients with radiculopathies of various origins

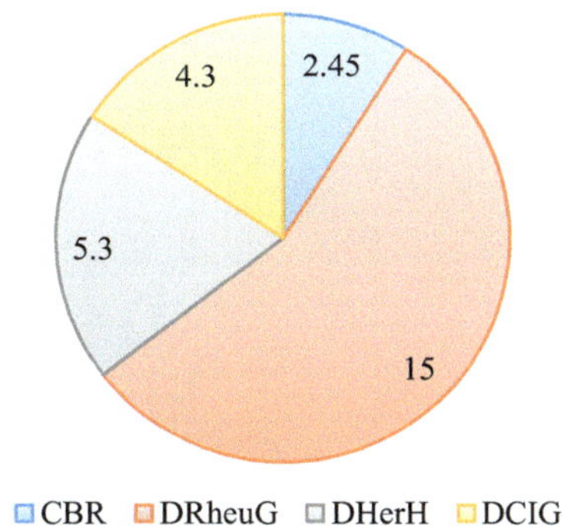

In patients with chronic pain in dorsopathies of brucellosis origin (group II), fibrinogen levels varied from 1.7 to 3.2 g/l, averaging 2.45 g/l, which also corresponded to the norm.

However, in the third group of patients with radiculopathies of rheumatic origin, fibrinogen increased from 12 to 18 g/l, which averaged 15 g/l.

Fibrinogen levels in blood plasma in patients with herpetic radiculopathies were slightly increased and amounted to 4.8–5.8 g/l, which averaged an average of 5.3 g/l.

Thus (Fig. 16.1), based on the data obtained, the presence of native fibrinogen in the blood plasma can be chosen as an additional biochemical criterion for the differential diagnosis of patients with chronic pain syndrome in dorsopathies of various origins.

CRP is one of the proteins of the acute phase of inflammation with a wide range of biochemical and immunochemical markers of inflammation. The development of chronic pain syndrome in radiculopathy of compression-ischemic genesis is facilitated by degenerative-dystrophic processes in the spine and intervertebral discs. For the development of pain, mechanical, biochemical, and immunological factors act on the spinal roots. As a result, aseptic autoimmune inflammation develops.

In our work, C-reactive protein was studied to assess the activity of the inflammatory process. In the blood serum of healthy people, CRP is detected in the form of traces and is below 3 mg/l. With inflammation of low intensity, CRP in the blood serum is up to 7 mg/l. 7.1–50 mg/l is an indicator of the average intensity of the inflammatory process. In severe inflammatory and autoimmune diseases, CRP levels exceed 50 mg/l.

The day before blood donation, patients were asked to exclude intense physical activity and refrain from smoking and drinking alcohol. Blood was taken from a vein in the morning on an empty stomach. The study was conducted on all 82 patients. The CRP concentration was determined by a highly sensitive quantitative method using a set of reagents from "Thermo Scientific."

In the first group of patients, the results showed that in 12 (14.6%) patients, the CRP values were 3–6 mg/l; in 61 (74.4%) patients, the CRP values were 7–12 mg/l; in 9 (11%) patients, the CRP values were 13–16 mg/l. According to modern concepts, this increase in the concentration of CRP in the blood plasma in the

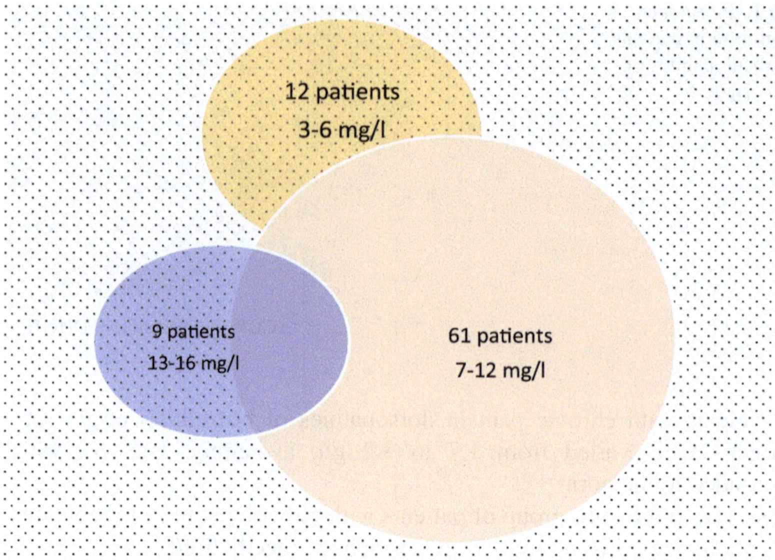

Fig. 16.2 Indicators of C-reactive protein in group I

studied patients indicated a subclinical inflammatory process. It displayed the activity of systemic inflammation and immunopathological processes in the body of patients with chronic pain syndrome with radiculopathy of compression-ischemic genesis.

In the second group of patients, the study of C-reactive protein had its own characteristics. We know that the causative agent of brucellosis is located inside the cell, resulting in recognition of loose connective tissue cells and their binding to receptors, the signals of which contribute to the launch of the innate immune system. Exogenous pathogens in the cell contribute to the synthesis and secretion into the blood of pro-inflammatory cytokines in loose connective tissue [14]. In response to cytokine synthesis, hepatocytes induce C-reactive protein. All 84 patients of group II underwent a study of C-reactive protein, the values of which were as follows: in 28 (33.3%) patients – 3–6 mg/l; in 39 (46.4%) – 7–12 mg/l; in 17 (20.3%) – 13–19 mg/l (Fig. 16.2).

The parameters of C-reactive protein in patients of group III were specific and indicative since, in diseases of rheumatic origin, this study is usually carried out for all patients. In the rheumatic process, in response to the entry of toxins into the blood, C-reactive protein is produced, which, by binding to them, renders them harmless. In some cases, C-reactive protein rises more actively than symptoms, and it is an indicator of both the development of the disease and the regression of the disease. In all 76 patients of group III, a study was conducted on the parameters of C-reactive protein. The results were as follows: in 8 (10.5%) patients – 3–6 mg/l; in 12 (15.8%) – 7–12 mg/l; in 56 (73.7%) – 13–19 mg/l (Fig. 16.3).

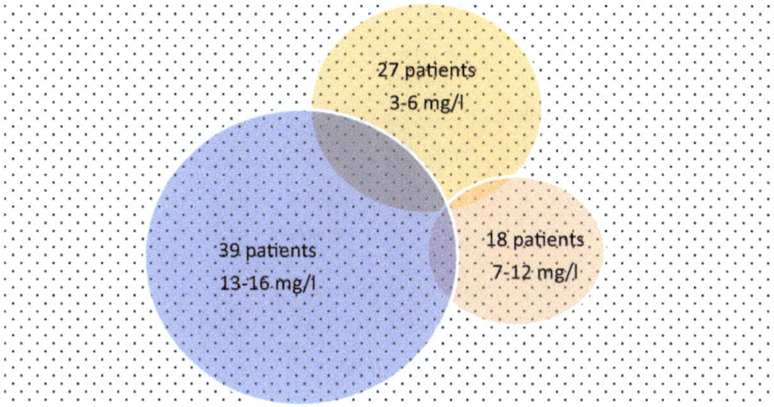

Fig. 16.3 Indicators of C-reactive protein in group II

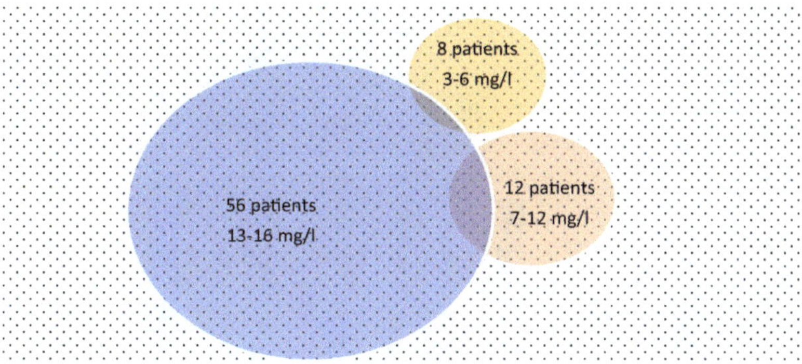

Fig. 16.4 Indicators of C-reactive protein in group III

All patients of group IV also had blood taken for the analysis of C-reactive protein, which, according to the literature, was not specific since it is an acute phase protein of inflammation and helps in the diagnosis of a bacterial infection. In all 78 patients of group IV, a study was conducted on the parameters of C-reactive protein. The results were as follows: in 27 (34.6%) patients – 3–6 mg/l; in 50 (64.1%) – 7–12 mg/l; in 1 (1.3%) – 13–19 mg/l (Fig. 16.4).

Summing up the results of the study of C-reactive protein in patients with chronic pain syndrome, we obtained the following results (Fig. 16.5).

Thus, the study of the concentration of CRP in the blood serum of patients with chronic pain syndrome in dorsopathies of various origins is a highly sensitive quantitative method that can be considered an additional diagnostic sign in the development of chronic pain syndrome. CRP can be considered a pathogenic factor in inflammation leading to pain, as well as a factor stimulating the production of pro-inflammatory cytokines (Fig. 16.6).

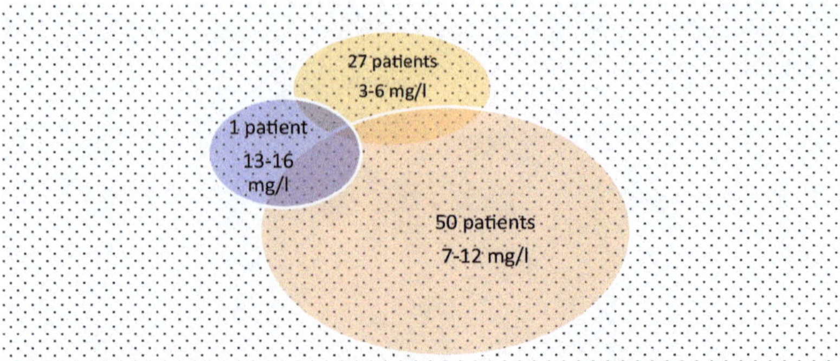

Fig. 16.5 Indicators of C-reactive protein in group IV

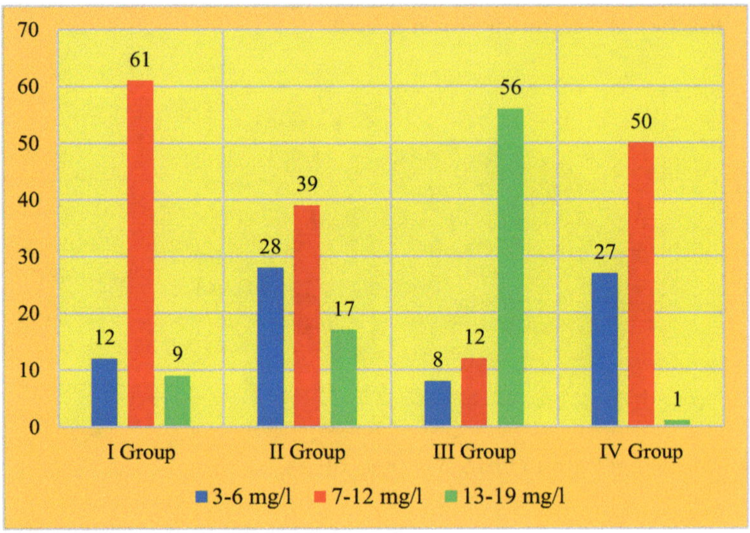

Fig. 16.6 Parameters of C-reactive protein in the blood plasma of patients with chronic pain syndrome in dorsopathies of various origins

Interleukin-1β, a secreted serum cytokine, is secreted by phagocytic mononuclear cells, participates in the development of both specific and nonspecific protective reactions of the body, and is active against a variety of target cells, including those in dorsopathy.

To conduct this study, we decided to select 25 patients from each group and, for comparison, take 10 people in the control group.

We selected 25 patients from group I for the determination of interleukin-1β by ELISA using standard reagent kits (Bender MedSystem 224/2, Austria) according to the instructions.

In patients with chronic pain due to radiculopathy of compression-ischemic genesis, the following results were obtained: in 11 (44%) patients, a pronounced

Table 16.2 The content of interleukin-1β in blood serum in patients of group I

Examined patients	11 (44%)	5 (20%)	9 (36%)	10 people in the control group
Interleukin-1β pg/ml	4.51 (4.47–4.55)	1.35 (1.29–1.41)	0.56 (0.54–0.58)	0.58 (0.55–0.61)

Table 16.3 The content of interleukin-1β in blood serum in patients of group II

Examined patients	2 (8%)	15 (60%)	9 (36%)	10 people in the control group
Interleukin-1β pg/ml	5.61 (5.60–5.62)	2.35 (2.29–2.41)	1.56 (1.54–1.58)	0.58 (0.55–0.61)

Table 16.4 The content of interleukin-1β in blood serum in patients of group III

Examined patients	17 (68%)	5 (20%)	3(12%)	10 people in the control group
Interleukin-1β pg/ml	7.65 (7.59–7.71)	5.32 (5.26–5.38)	3.75 (3.72–3.78)	0.58 (0.55–0.61)

Table 16.5 The content of interleukin-1β in blood serum in patients of group IV

Examined patients	17 (68%)	4 (16%)	4 (16%)	10 people in the control group
Interleukin-1β pg/ml	1.55 (1.49–1.61)	0.75 (0.69–0.81)	0.58 (0.56–0.60)	0.58 (0.55–0.61)

expression of interleukin-1β was detected, which amounted to 4.51 (4.47–4.55) pg/ml; in 5 (20%) patients – 1.35 (1.29–1.41) pg/ml, which indicated a mild degree of inflammatory reaction; and in 9 (36%) patients – 0.56 (0.54–0.58) pg/ml; the results indicated the absence of inflammatory processes (Table 16.2).

For the convenience of correlation of the obtained data on the concentration of interleukin-1β (IL-1β) in the blood serum of patients of group II, 25 patients were also selected. The results were as follows: in 2 (8%) patients – 5.61 (5.60–5.62) pg/ml; in 15 (60%) – 2.35 (2.29–2.41) pg/ml, which indicated a mild degree of inflammatory reaction, and in 8 (32%) patients – 1.56 (1.54–1.58) pg/ml, which indicated a weak degree of inflammatory processes (Table 16.3).

The content of IL-1β in the blood serum of patients of group III was as follows: in 17 (68%) patients – 7.65 (7.59–7.71) pg/ml; in 5 (20%) patients – 5.32 (5. 26–5.38) pg/ml, which indicated a pronounced degree of inflammatory reaction, and in 3 (12%) patients – 3.75 (3.72–3.78) pg/ml, which indicated a moderate degree of inflammatory processes (Table 16.4).

The concentration of IL-1β in blood serum of 25 patients of group IV was checked by the same methods, and the following results were obtained: in 17 (68%) patients, an unexpressed expression of interleukin-1β was detected, which was 1.55 (1.49–1.61) pg/ml; in 4 (16%) patients – 0.75 (0.69–0.81) pg/ml, which indicated a low degree of inflammatory reaction, and in 4 (16%) patients – 0.58 (0.56–0.60) pg/ml, which indicated the absence of inflammatory processes (Table 16.5).

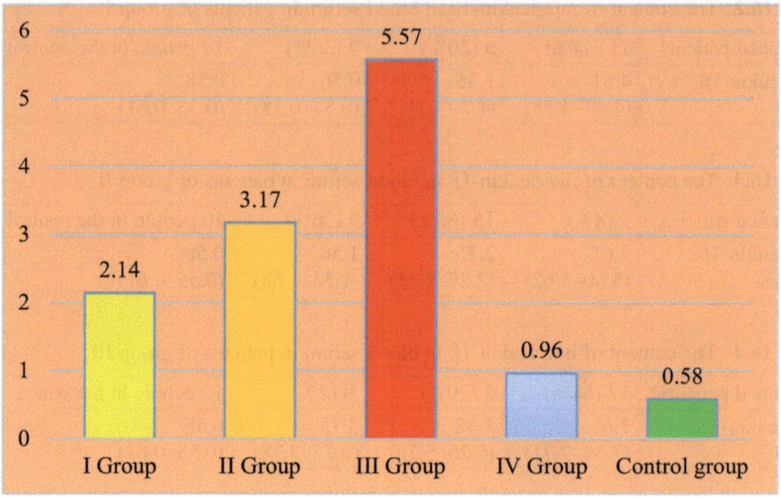

Fig. 16.7 The content of interleukin-1β in blood serum in patients with chronic pain syndrome in dorsopathies

The established level of IL-1β in patients with chronic pain syndrome (CPS) with radiculopathy of rheumatic origin (RRO) was comparable with the values characteristic of non-specific and specific infectious and non-infectious inflammatory processes [5].

As shown in the tables above, the content of IL-1β in the control group corresponds to the reference normal values for healthy examined individuals and is consistent with the data of other authors who used similar methods [7, 9].

According (Fig. 16.7) to the results obtained in our studies, a pronounced expression of IL-1β was detected in the third group of patients (Table 16.3) with CPS with RRO and averaged 5.57 pg/ml, which was 10 times more than normal. In patients of the second group with CPS with radiculopathy in chronic brucellosis (RCBr), the indicators were 5.5 times higher than the norm and showed an average of 3.17 pg/ml. Next, in terms of the significance of the obtained indicators, was the first group of patients with CPS in RCIG, the values of which were the following 2.14 pg/ml and were increased by almost 4 times. The value of the content of IL-1β in the blood serum of group IV with CPS in RG showed an average value of 0.96 pg/ml, which was increased by 2 times, but nevertheless indicated a decrease in the production of this cytokine in herpes infection, compared with other groups.

16.4 Conclusion

The study of inflammation markers in the blood serum of patients with chronic pain syndrome in dorsopathies of various origins makes it possible to identify signs of the inflammatory process. The study of native fibrinogen in blood plasma can be chosen as an additional biochemical criterion for the differential diagnosis of patients with chronic pain in dorsopathies of various origins. In the study of the concentration of CRP in the blood serum of patients with chronic pain syndrome with dorsopathies of various origins, it is a highly sensitive quantitative method that can be considered as an additional diagnostic sign in the development of chronic pain syndrome. Also, CRP can be considered as a pathogenetic factor of inflammation leading to pain, as well as a factor stimulating the production of pro-inflammatory cytokines. The detected concentrations of interleukin-1β in the blood serum indicated various indicators of the presence of an inflammatory process that provoked chronic pain. An increase in the concentration of endothelin-1 in the blood serum of the studied patients can be considered as evidence of damage to the peripheral vascular endothelium in dorsopathy, depending on the etiology and pathogenesis, which also determine the nature of chronic pain.

References

1. Khakimova, S., Gapparova, N., Samiev, A., Hamdamova, B., Kodirov, U., & Karabaev, S. (2021). Peculiarities of ENMG examinations in patients with chronic pain syndrome dorsopathies of compression-ischemic genesis. *Journal of Biomedicine and Practice, 6*(6), 80–87.
2. Aminov, Z. Z., Khakimova, S. Z., & Davlatov, S. S. (2020). Improvement of treatment protocols of pain syndrome in patients with chronic brucellosis. *European Journal of Molecular & Clinical Medicine, 7*(3), 2540–2545.
3. Lebedyuk, M. N., Zapolsky, M. E., & Goransky, Y. I. (2011). Herpetic lesions of the nervous system. *Ukrainian Journal of Dermatology, Venereology and Cosmetology, 2*(41), 92–97.
4. Khakimova, S. Z., & Dzhurabekova, A. T. (2016). Clinical diagnosis and treatment of chronic brucellosis in the real practice of a neurologist. *Medicine (Almaty), 7*(169), 68–72.
5. Ziyadullayevna, S. K., & Alisherovna, D. A. (2020). Results of examination of patients with radiculopathies in chronic brucellosis. *The American Journal of Medical Sciences and Pharmaceutical Research, 2*(10), 37–43.
6. Dadasheva, M. N., & Agafonov, B. V. (2016). Dorsopathies: Modern tactics of patient management. *Breast Cancer, 3*, 163–165.
7. Khakimova, S., Hamdamova, B., & Kodirov, U. (2022). Features of clinical and neurological results of examination of patients with dorsopathy of rheumatic genesis. *Journal of Biomedicine and Practice, 7*(1), 145–153.
8. Samiyev, A., Xakimova, S., & Soibnazarov, O. (2022). Rehabilitation of patients under spine surger. *Journal of Biomedicine and Practice, 7*(1), 139–144.
9. Khakimova, S. Z., Khamdamova, B. K., & Kodirov, U. A. (2022). Features of clinical and neurological results of examination of patients with dorsopathies of rheumatic origin. *Journal of Biomedicine and Practice, 7*(1), 145–154.

10. Akhmedova, D. A., Khakimova, S. Z., & Jurabekova, A. T. (2015). Features of post-stroke depression in the early and late recovery periods. *Innovative Science, 6*(2), 224–227.
11. Khakimova, S. Z., & Khakimova, G. K. (2021). Features of psychopathological and vegetative disorders in patients with chronic pain syndrome with radiculopathies of compression-ischemic origin. *Dr. Ahborotnomashi., 1*(98), 100–102.
12. Samiev, A. S., Khakimova, S. Z., & Soibnazarov, O. E. (2022). Rehabilitation of patients undergoing spinal surgery. *Journal of Biomedicine and Practice, 7*(1), 139–145.
13. Khakimova, S. Z., Mamurova, I. N., & Samiev, A. S. (2019). Clinical role of neurobrucellosis among patients with chronic dorsopathy. *Academy, 10*(49), 66–69.
14. Simbirtsev, A. S. (2019) Immunopharmacological aspects of the cytokine system, *Bull. Sib. Med., 18*(1), 84–95.

Chapter 17
AIOps Observability and Performance Impact of AI and ML Applications for Central Nervous System Drug Discoveries

Ajay Reddy Yeruva and Vivek Basavegowda Ramu

Abbreviations

AD	Alzheimer's Disease
ASD	Autism Spectrum Disorder
PD	Parkinson's Disease
SCH	Schizophrenia

17.1 Introduction

Probably, integrating several processes efficiently will determine the ultimate success of new drug discoveries for central nervous system (CNS). In order to maintain a network running smoothly and reliably, administrators must perform tasks such as problem detection, isolation, and restoration, all of which fall under the umbrella term "operations, administration, and maintenance" (OAM) [1]. Automated OAM that uses artificial intelligence for IT Operations (AIOps) is necessary because of the growing complexity of networks and ICT. By utilizing the principles of big data analytics and machine learning, AIOps optimizes data analysis and detection with fully automated IT processes. The discovery of new drugs has historically been an expensive proposition, with the research failure rate increasing by almost 90% in some cases. This results in a loss of almost 70% of the funds allocated for the research if the clinical trials are unsatisfactory or show a lack of efficacy or the

A. R. Yeruva (✉)
Independent Researcher, Pleasanton, CA, USA
e-mail: ajayr.yeruva@gmail.com

V. B. Ramu
Independent Researcher, Hartford, CT, USA
e-mail: vivekgowda.br@gmail.com

F. J. J. Joseph et al. (eds.), *Computational Intelligence for Clinical Diagnosis*,
EAI/Springer Innovations in Communication and Computing,
https://doi.org/10.1007/978-3-031-23683-9_17

possibility of adverse drug reactions. Consequently, introducing a new drug to the market can take more than 10 years at times. This is highlighted further in drugs related to the Central Nervous System, where appropriate research is lacking on account of insufficient evidence obtained from trials. Thankfully with the intervention of AIOps and with advancements in AI, ML, and Deep Learning (DL), there are a significant number of new research work being undertaken worldwide. Gradually, the dark-gray unknown world of neurological disorders is unfolding.

AIOps, MLOps, and Deep Learning have all contributed to the development of AIOps, which in turn has influenced the field of computer-assisted drug discovery [2]. The complexity of finding effective uses for drugs has been transformed by the broad adoption of machine learning, especially Deep Learning, and the advancements in computing power and software. Statistically, the human Central Nervous System (CNS) remains the most afflicted and responsible for a host of neurological disorders. Historically, this system had posed the toughest challenges as there was no consistency in diagnosing the disease; besides, the degree or intensity of the neurological illness varies considerably. Today, AIOps tools can automate closed-loop remediation of known issues by highlighting the variations concerning the historical data; consequently, the quantity and strength of the drug dosage to be administered to a patient is no longer an unknown quantity and can be better defined.

Computer-assisted drug discovery is a more effective process thanks to AI. This progress is being driven by a number of causes, including, but not limited to, advancements in computing hardware and software. Recently, the pharmaceutical business has emerged as one of the most promising early adopters of AI's many potential uses in other words, [3].

Over the course of the past 5 years, artificial intelligence (AI) and machine learning algorithms have been gradually but surely starting to disrupt the pharmaceutical sector and medication development, with new drug developments and drug repurposing, improved manufacturing standards in the pharma sector with dynamic clinical trials, and resulting acceleration of all manufacturing processes [4].

There has consistently been an issue with drug repositioning/repurposing in patients with CNS. Thankfully, with the augmented analytics of AIOps, systems like AI, ML, and Deep Learning can now assume a pole position, several success stories have been revealed, and the future shows immense positivity [5]. The evidence collected thus far demonstrates the potential for accelerating new drug discoveries and expediting their applications and manufacture despite their being in their infancy stages.

Collaboration between pharmacists, computer scientists, statisticians, physicians, and others in the drug development processes, as well as the adoption of AI-based technologies for the speedy discovery of medications, enhance the answers acquired by AI/ML. Drug repurposing and the discovery of new medications for a wide range of complicated human ailments are both viewed as being greatly aided by the use of AI techniques, in conjunction with large amounts of data. This is what the research shows [6].

Various drug prediction strategies have evolved alongside AI and ML techniques, as AIOps can administer timely resources at the appropriate time to optimize discovery efficiency. Primarily, datasets are selected and preprogrammed by accounting for the quality of data that can be obtained after due filtration. These datasets can be used as training datasets and input in machine learning techniques. Essentially, the data are derived from human cells and can offer valuable responses to drug treatment therapies. The resulting prediction algorithm can be labelled as a classification or regression model. It follows that this predictive model can be further validated in other similar datasets. Several other machine learning techniques can be employed to suit other models. Consequently, it will be possible to acquire several accurate cell lines or clinical samples for better drug discoveries [7].

The benefits of AIOps in drug discoveries have been enhanced with recent sophisticated digitalization. They have today become an essential part of the procedures, and the pharma industry will be lost without their presence [8]. Observability has improved and powered IT teams to act spontaneously to address issues that are of prime importance. Researchers confront significant obstacles when attempting to forecast a patient's reaction to medicine using machine learning algorithms and pipelines. The two main types of machine learning are supervised methods, which use labelled data to make predictions, and unsupervised methods, which instead use the data themselves to generate clusters [9].

Artificial intelligence is at the forefront of many fields, including structural design and clinical studies. Given the novel and complex ways in which information is interpreted to uncover patterns for the study's scope, it is crucial to have access to huge data sets for drug candidates [2]. The purpose of this study is essentially targeted at understanding the shortcomings in dealing with CNS diseases. There is insufficient research in this domain, and lower success rates have been observed in comparison with other medical studies, mainly due to the lack of knowledge of CNS conditions and more so in the physio-pathological context. Due to the existence of the blood-brain barrier (BBB), there has been a lack of efficiency in the diagnosis of many illnesses, especially in the early stages. The average time it takes for a medicine to get from discovery to regulatory approval for use in the central nervous system is now 15–19 years, due in large part to the difficulties inherent to developing drugs for this area [10].

17.1.1 Research Studies Review: Specific Procedures Employing AI and ML in Drug Discovery

17.1.1.1 Target Identification

For target identification, AI applications combine heterogeneous data into similar sets according to their patterns (molecular mechanisms associated with a disease). Predictive models are generated by AI/ML programs by analyzing massive amounts

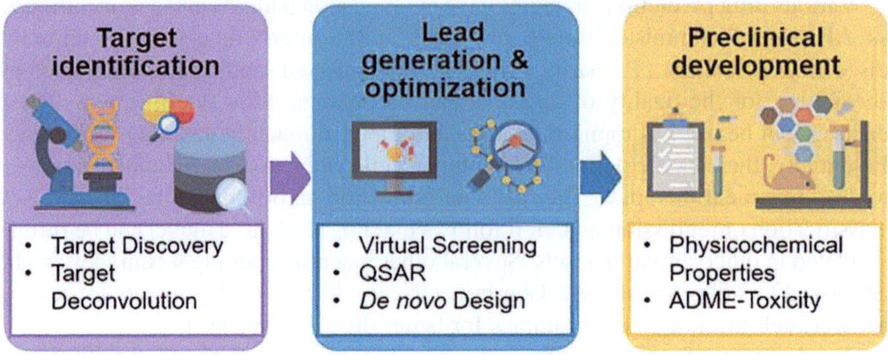

Fig. 17.1 The three stages of the AI/ML application processes involved in drug discovery and enhancing decision-making [11]

of data about a drug's physicochemical qualities in accordance with their ADME-T profiles; this is done to improve the lead generation and optimizations stage and to facilitate virtual screening of pipelines and the initial development stage (Fig. 17.1).

17.2 Background

AIOps (or "AI for IT operations") uses artificial intelligence so that big data can help IT teams work faster and more effectively. ML is "an artificial intelligence technique that may be used to create and train software algorithms to learn from and act on data."

17.2.1 Essentially, There Are Two Principal Types of AIOps

Adopting a traditional approach wherein Machine Learning models develop a correlation with IT events to assess the system failure that has occurred previously due to a common cause and at similar times. This helps in troubleshooting discovery operations/experiments in progress and eliminates errors from occurring. Besides, this approach can pinpoint the root cause of the problem and eliminate it forever.

A modern approach to AIOps in drug discoveries is to extend critical capabilities beyond a mere correlation and goes deeper into the underlying root cause that triggered the failure. Consequently, Health AIOps has evolved to be a core technology and unfolds the mysteries of the complexities in the new cloud activity to drive faster innovation, more efficiency, and better patient care outcomes.

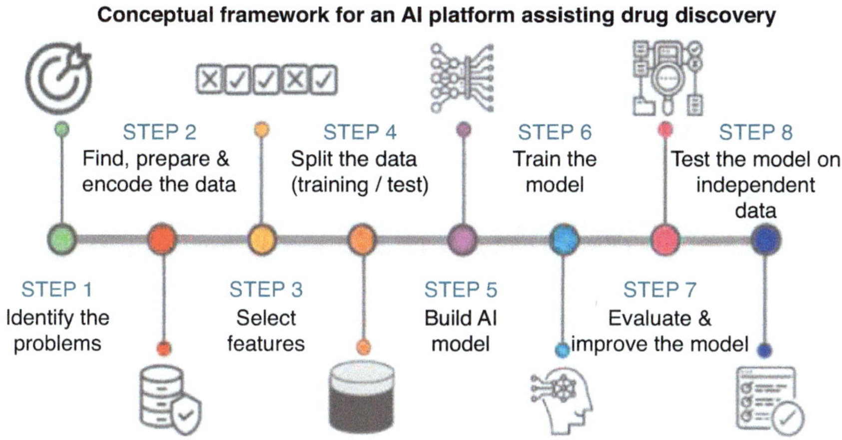

Fig. 17.2 The steps involved in establishing an AI platform for drug discovery [11]

Encoding: Specifically, in new drug discoveries, creating codes for clinical trials, and the results obtained, AI is empowered with definite algorithms that can be integrated into an information technology system directly to support programmers when it comes to finding and solving software glitches, as well as when it comes to creating a code [12]. Some AI technologies have been used to provide feedback when it comes to coding, and this has helped to enhance the performance of the developer, which has resulted in cleaner code, in turn improving productivity and offering a bug-free coding setting. After analyzing the structure of the code, the AI system provides valuable feedback. It not only improves overall productivity but also significantly reduces downtime during the development process [13].

Robotics: A robot is efficient in doing routine tasks with minimal (or no) human intervention. While using artificial intelligence in IT applications, IT departments will take big steps in automating backend processes that can allow various efficiency gains and reduce the requirement of human hours that are needed for these tasks. AI-powered methods will improve with time as the algorithms of the methods learn from their mistakes [13].

Beyond this broad definition, the actual approaches included in Artificial Intelligence will involve additional processes that will rely on adaptive techniques such as supervised, unsupervised, semi-supervised, active, reinforcement, transfer, and multi-dimensional learning methods (Fig. 17.2). Multiple algorithms are developed for each activity to get optimal outcomes and performance.

(i) Identifying a problem
(ii) Data preparation
(iii) Feature extraction
(iv) Datasets for both training and testing
(v) Constructing, training, and evaluating a model and then using it to tackle real-world problems

17.2.2 Target Identification with AI/ML

Finding chemicals that can both counteract a disease's effects and keep the body from reacting negatively is crucial to the success of medication research. One typical approach in drug discovery is to alter the function of a target to stop the development of a disease.

Successful learning strategies are crucial to the overall process of drug identification. Figures 17.1, 17.2, 17.3, and 17.4 expound on the fundamental approaches regarding the efficiency of the learning model to use and, afterward, describe the algorithms that are used for each individual task [14].

17.2.3 Drug Targets

Target discovery and target deconvolution are two of the most common examples of the uses of the phrase "target identification" that can be found in published works (Fig. 17.3).

17.2.4 Targeting

Targeting a particular physicochemical structure, and the nature of a disease can be a complicated process due to the molecular mechanics of the disease and the successful adjustments it has made to a patient [15]. Here is where AI and ML applications, when used properly, really shine. In addition, they have the ability to combine multi-scale data in order to better comprehend the various disease subtypes under consideration.

17.2.5 Analysis of Disease Genes

Researchers have been able to collect enormous volumes of genomic data with the assistance of ML classifiers, which has sped up the process of predicting genes that

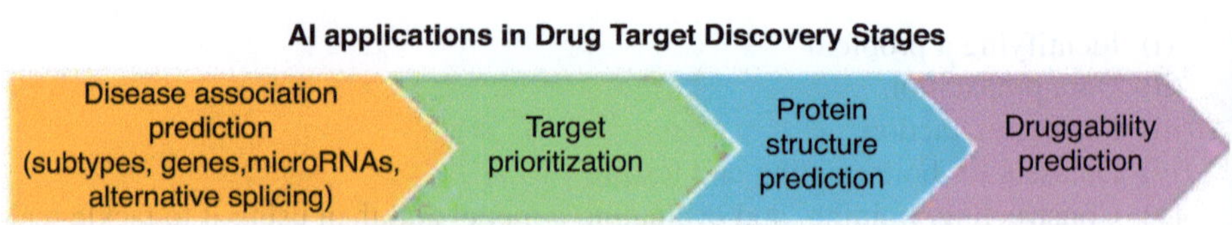

Fig. 17.3 AI-optimized target discovery [11]

are responsible for the disease. For an in-depth understanding of mutation data and driver genes, Dl-based methods (deep driver) and convolutional neural networks (CNN) have been fruitfully applied in understanding breast and colorectal cancers, respectively. Similarly, when dealing with Parkinson's disease, SVM's with DNN (deep neural networks) and protein-protein interaction (PPI) with suitable autoencoders have been effective in their gene analysis. Once the genes have been thoroughly analyzed, the drug detection process can be pursued as the target is identified. Other related gene discovery processes where AI, ML, and Deep Learning can play pivotal roles include the following procedures:

(i) An analysis of the micro-RNA that regulates gene behavior
(ii) Prediction of alternate splicing for understanding protein diversity

17.2.6 Druggability

Before concluding that the identified target can be treated with a specified drug, it is critical to understand the effect of the proposed drug by administering a small molecule into the disease area and analyzing the obtained results. Models based on machine learning can use a variety of inputs to make educated guesses about a target's druggability. Surface Cavity Recognition and Evaluation (SCREEN) webserver was one of the first programs of its kind and was developed using a radio frequency (RF) classifier.

17.2.7 Target Fishing

The current methods of identifying experimental approaches to establishing the efficacy of particular medications against possible targets have been time-consuming and costly. Several research has integrated AI/ML algorithms into computational target deconvolution instruments to improve their forecasting ability. For predicting drugs' macromolecular targets, for instance, self-organizing maps (SOMs) have been widely used, thanks to the work of Schneider and colleagues [16]. Several research has integrated AI/ML algorithms into computational target deconvolution instruments to enhance their forecasting ability. For predicting drugs' macromolecular targets, for instance, self-organizing maps (SOMs) have been widely used, thanks to the work of Schneider and colleagues. In most cases, they used unsupervised SOM algorithms to create "fuzzy" chemical representations that encircled the molecule of interest. Consequently, the trained SOM algorithm could share its expertise with nearby molecules, making their identification much less of a challenge.

17.2.8 AI/ML Applications for Lead Discovery

One of the best strategies that have evolved from AL and ML applications is the implementation of virtual screening (VS). The previously used technology was very expensive and had a poor performance ratio. VS has now made it possible to identify compounds that are most likely to combine with a useful protein. Besides, VS helps to build better pharmacore models that can be invaluable in lead discovery.

17.2.9 QSAR Prediction

This method, which is more mathematical in nature, can be used to determine whether or not a given chemical has a biological effect. As this method of prediction can selectively specify the amount of activity and the toxicity of the substances involved, it is widely utilized for medication optimization. According to a study [17], using the QSAR technology, a huge number of potential resources can be ruled out and exploited more efficiently [18]; notably, the RF method is the de facto standard in QSAR research due to its efficacy as a regression and classification tool. As a result, it is common practice to evaluate the efficacy of new QSAR prediction techniques by contrasting them to RF. There is a plethora of RF-based QSAR models available.

17.2.10 Extended Multi-dimensional Uses of AI and ML Applications

Security is at the forefront of minimizing risks associated with malicious attacks or data breaches, but the applications of AI and ML extend to numerous other predictions. Whenever a "new drug" is discovered in the pharmaceutical business, the government and private companies must take extra precautions to safeguard the associated sensitive data lest it falls into the wrong hands. A high-security layer can be built into all of these applications and IT systems with the help of advanced algorithms and the use of AIOps applications. The healthcare industry can benefit from the use of artificial intelligence as a framework for detecting and preventing future data breach assaults and receiving the necessary recommendations to avoid any other potential weaknesses in the present IT system.

Other areas of importance include the following:

- For accurately predicting physicochemical properties
- Enabling ADME-T predictions in de novo drug design
- Providing a deeper understanding of drug sensitivity
- Effects of drug-drug interactions
- Appropriately positioning drug repurposing

17.3 Methodology

17.3.1 *Drug Discoveries for Central Nervous System (CNS) Employing AIOps Software and Advanced AI/ML Applications*

CNS diseases are complex neurological disorders that can vary in intensity from patient to patient. Besides, there are no clear detectable patterns and tests that can help in evaluation. It follows that the process of treatment suffers as a consequence and suitable drug discovery is less obvious. Comparatively, other diseases are easier to diagnose and treat accordingly. Diseases of the central nervous system (CNS) are directly linked to difficulties in crossing the blood-brain barrier (BBB). Recent uses of AI and ML have offered insights that had previously been lacking.

17.3.2 *Predicting BBB Permeability*

The essential purpose of BBB is to shield the brain from blood composition variations, which include hormones, amino acids, and potassium. The primary step involved before attempting to build drugs for neurologic disorders is to devise strategies to increase the permeability of the brain membrane to allow concentrated amounts of CNS drugs. Formerly, time-consuming and expensive experiments were conducted to understand BBB permeability. With the introduction of AI, most of these elaborate steps have been eliminated with simultaneous accuracy being observed (Fig. 17.4).

17.3.3 *Neurological Disorders: Schizophrenia*

It has been established that schizophrenia is probably the most baffling neurodevelopmental disorder of all, and consequently, there is no appropriate treatment established to date. Thankfully, AI and ML applications are the only alternative treatments that have demonstrated immense promise.

When compared to other mental illnesses, schizophrenia is among the most mysterious. Since it is a problem of brain development [19], between 0.30% and 0.66% of the population will develop schizophrenia at some point in their lives. According to a 2015 study [20], complex pathophysiology is still a mystery after more than a century of study. An SVM classifier was used to identify the most effective indicators of presynaptic dopamine overactivity, which has been linked to schizophrenia [21]. QSAR models for the medications that inhibit the reuptake of gamma-aminobutyric acid (GABA), which can be useful in the treatment of Schizophrenia, were also predicted using a set of SVM classifiers. QSAR models of the

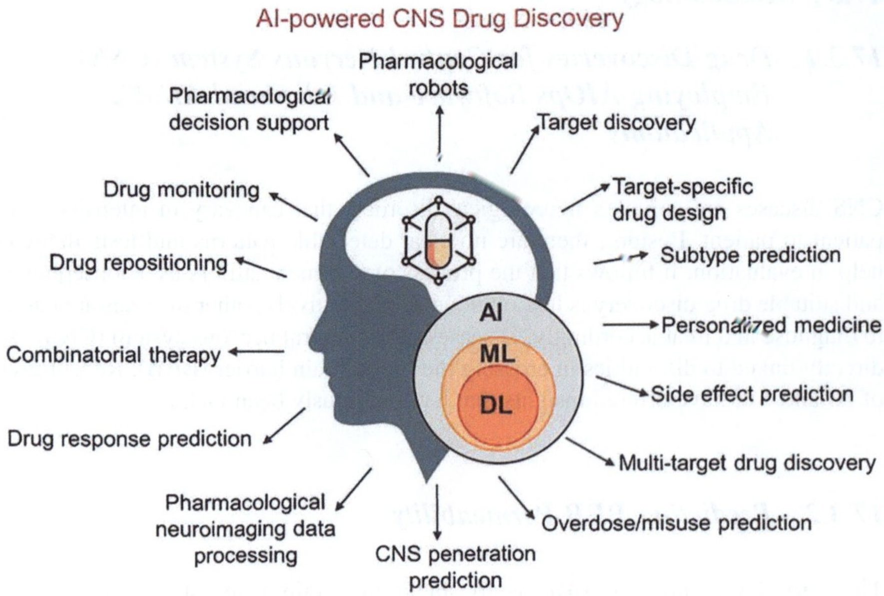

Fig. 17.4 The various components of AI for neurological disorder drug discovery. (Color image courtesy [11])

medications that block the reuptake of the neurotransmitter gamma-aminobutyric acid (GABA) were also predicted using VM classifiers, and these compounds have shown promise in the treatment of schizophrenia [21].

When SVM was trained on drug expression patterns, it was able to predict the repositioning of medications for schizophrenia better than any of the other ML approaches. All of these approaches rely heavily on a small number of molecular descriptors, and their predictive power is thus constrained to the case of passive diffusional uptake. By comparing their model's performance to that of existing SVM-based BBB permeability predictors, they found that incorporating physico-chemical features and fingerprints led to more accurate predictions. So far, we have only discussed AI/ML-based models, and all of them have been trained solely on molecular attributes, leaving out information about central nervous system (CNS) therapeutic efficacy.

17.3.4 *AI/ML for Depression-Related Drugs*

The development of psychiatric medications has recently benefited from the application of AI- and ML-based approaches; specifically, an elastic net has been used to identify predictors, and then a gradient boosting machine has been used to investigate their potential role in determining whether or not antidepressants are effective in alleviating current symptoms. This artificial intelligence-based service is being put to the test in real-world clinical settings, making it a strong candidate for direct research translation.

17.3.5 The Role of AI/ML in Treating Parkinson's Disease

More than 1% of adults over 60 are diagnosed with Parkinson's disease (PD), and that number rises to 5% in those over 85. Neurological disorders make them the second most common, however, whereas AI/ML applications have recently centred on discovering diagnostic biomarkers in CSF and have received minimal attention in PD medication discovery despite the fact that there is currently no known effective treatment in PD research [22].

17.3.6 AI/ML Applications for Anesthesia and Pain Treatment

During procedures like general anesthesia and sedation, pharmacological robots are increasingly useful because they provide patients with individualized dosing of anesthetic drugs, helping to keep their bodies in a stable state [23].

17.3.7 Performance Testing of AI and ML Models

With the advancement of AI and ML models, it is very important to ensure one can execute these models individually and also in parallel without any performance degradation. Any system where AI and ML models will be executed should be performance tested before officially rolling out.

17.3.8 Non-functional Requirements

Non-functional requirements related to AI and ML models should be clearly identified; this will be the target against which model performance will be measured. Below are some high-level non-functional requirements which should be captured:

- Concurrent users
- Total time for the model to execute and generate output
- Total transactions/hour
- Maximum or peak users expected to execute the model in parallel

17.3.9 Performance Testing and Tuning

Performance testing of the model will reveal if the infrastructure against which these models are executed is capable of handling the load, server utilization with respect to CPU, memory, etc., to be closely monitored and to make sure it stays within an acceptable threshold of 80%. If server computing power is not sufficient, then hardware capacity is to be increased; the cloud is another option to deploy the AI and ML models because of the flexibility with scaling. If the model takes more than the expected time to complete, memory distribution, process consumption, query execution times, data processing, etc., are to be analyzed, an appropriate fix is to be implemented, and performance testing is to be re-executed.

17.3.10 Bid Data Processing

It is important to use the right kind of data when training AI and ML models, and in some circumstances, you will need a lot of data to get a good result. Data storage, data sanitation, data transformation, and data processing are all processes involved in data management and should be efficiently managed. If the quality of data or computing power is not optimal, it will directly impact the model accuracy and outcome; in a performance test, if any data limitations are identified, then additional storage or computing power is to be leveraged, or cloud deployment is adopted for scaling flexibility.

17.4 Conclusion and Results

With AIOps assisting health care, it is gaining significant importance over most other segments. There is a strong push to find and create novel medications, especially for underserved areas like the treatment of CNS illnesses. Advanced digitization techniques have been necessitated to handle the huge volume of data and the millions of clinical trials being carried out worldwide. Importantly, with AIOps, tools like virtual healthcare and telehealth have become an integral part of patient care. Also, with the ease of converting large volumes of paper records into optimized digital data, very large amounts of clinical trials and relevant research papers can be assessed swiftly and accurately. Performance testing is another area of focus before officially allowing multiple users to run the model, and it will ensure the model is performance-optimized and desired results are provided in the expected time. Diseases of the central nervous system remain largely untreated due to their complexity and variable nature. While there can be broad signs, most symptoms differ from individual to individual. These can be a result of the dissimilarity of the mental state of human beings. Nevertheless, there is significant positive hope for the future with the application of AI and ML tools. The differences in the efficacy of treatment with AI/ML applications are promising and well accepted by academia and the pharmaceutical industries.

One of the main obstacles to using AI/ML in CNS drug discovery is the lack of high-quality, well-labelled datasets for training the necessary algorithms. It is difficult to make direct comparisons across the various extant generic databases due to the inconsistency of the methods used to gather them. Some datasets may even be at odds with one another, highlighting the need to screen and assess raw input data before proceeding. Therefore, this will be a crucial step in applications, including AI and ML, to verify the accuracy of the outcomes. Importantly, as the quantity and quality of input data improve, the corresponding result will look far more convincing than presently. In due course, there will be specific successful training of algorithms that will be more suited for CNS drug discovery and precise and permanent treatments. With the intervention of AI and ML techniques, much more accuracy in firstly detecting the nature of CNS and the affected cells and secondly offering suitable drug formulations to achieve better success rates than what has been achieved this far, there is finally a visible light at the end of the tunnel.

References

1. Qin, |. K. S., Ichibha, T., Hongo, K., & Maezono, R. (2020, January). Inconsistencies in ab initio evaluations of non-additive contributions of DNA stacking energies. *Chemical Physics, 529*, 110554. https://doi.org/10.1016/j.chemphys.2019.110554
2. Musella, S., Verna, G., Fasano, A., & Di-Micco, S. (2021, October). New perspectives on machine learning in drug discovery. *Current Medicinal Chemistry, 28*(32), 6704–6728. https://doi.org/10.2174/0929867327666201111144048
3. Paul, D., Sanap, G., Shenoy, S., Kalyane, D., Kalia, K., & Tekade, R. K. (Eds.). (2020, October). Artificial intelligence in drug discovery and development. *Drug Discovery Today, 26*(1), 80. https://doi.org/10.1016/j.drudis.2020.10.010
4. Koromina, M., Pandi, M.-T., & Patrinos, G. P. (2019, November). Rethinking drug repositioning and development with artificial intelligence, machine learningo and Omics. *OMICS: A Journal of Integrative Biology, 23*(11), 539–548. https://doi.org/10.1089/omi.2019.0151
5. Yang, X., Wang, Y., Byrne, R., Schneider, G., & Yang, S. (2019, July). Concepts of artificial intelligence for computer-assisted drug discovery. *Chemical Reviews, 119*(18), 10520–10594. https://doi.org/10.1021/acs.chemrev.8b00728
6. Farghali, H., Kutinová Canová, N., & Arora, M. (2021, December). The potential applications of artificial intelligence in drug discovery and development. *Physiological Research, 70*, S715–S722. https://doi.org/10.33549/physiolres.934765
7. Azuaje, F. (2016, July). Computational models for predicting drug responses in cancer research. *Briefings in Bioinformatics, 18*, bbw065. https://doi.org/10.1093/bib/bbw065
8. Moriwaki, H., Tian, Y.-S., Kawashita, N., & Takagi, T. (2018, February). Mordred: A molecular descriptor calculator. *Journal of Cheminformatics, 10*(1). https://doi.org/10.1186/s13321-018-0258-y
9. Yap, C. W. (2010, December). PaDEL-descriptor: An open source software to calculate molecular descriptors and fingerprints. *Journal of Computational Chemistry, 32*(7), 1466–1474. https://doi.org/10.1002/jcc.21707

10. Mohs, R. C., & Greig, N. H. (2017, November). Drug discovery and development: Role of basic biological research. *Alzheimer's & Dementia: Translational Research & Clinical Interventions, 3*(4), 651–657. https://doi.org/10.1016/j.trci.2017.10.005
11. Vatansever, S., Schlessinger, A., Wacker, D., et al. (2021). Artificial intelligence and machinelearning-aided drug discovery in central nervous system diseases: State-of-the-arts and future directions. *Medicinal Research Reviews, 41*, 1427–1473. https://doi.org/10.1002/med.21764
12. Isaias, P., Issa, T., Chang, V., & Issa, T. (2015, October). Outlining the issues of cloud computing and sustainability opportunities and risks in European organizations. *Journal of Electronic Commerce in Organizations, 13*(4), 1–25. https://doi.org/10.4018/jeco.2015100101
13. Sugumaran, V., & New, H. *Distributed artificial intelligence, agent technology, and collaborative applications*. Accessed August 26, 2022. [Online]. Available: https://ndl.ethernet.edu.et/bitstream/123456789/35112/1/Distributed%20artificial%20intelligence%20%20agent%20technology%20and%20collaborative%20applications.pdf
14. Center for Devices and Radiological Health. (2019). *Artificial intelligence and machine learning in software*. US Food and Drug Administration. https://www.fda.gov/medical-devices/software-medical-device-samd/artificial-intelligence-and-machine-learning-software-medical-device
15. Moffat, J. G., Vincent, F., Lee, J. A., Eder, J., & Prunotto, M. (2017, August). Opportunities and challenges in phenotypic drug discovery: An industry perspective. *Nature Reviews Drug Discovery, 16*(8), 531–543. https://doi.org/10.1038/nrd.2017.111
16. Shen, R., Olshen, A. B., & Ladanyi, M. (2010, January). Integrative clustering of multiple genomic data types using a joint latent variable model with application to breast and lung cancer subtype analysis. *Bioinformatics, 26*(2), 292–293. https://doi.org/10.1093/bioinformatics/btp659
17. Kumar, R., et al. (2015, July). An in silico platform for predicting, screening and designing of antihypertensive peptides. *Scientific Reports, 5*(1). https://doi.org/10.1038/srep12512
18. Briard, J. G., Fernandez, M., De Luna, P., Woo, T. K., & Ben, R. N. (2016, May). QSAR accelerated discovery of potent ice recrystallization inhibitors. *Scientific Reports, 6*(1). https://doi.org/10.1038/srep26403
19. Sullivan, P. F. (2012, February). Puzzling over schizophrenia: Schizophrenia as a pathway disease. *Nature Medicine, 18*(2), 210–211. https://doi.org/10.1038/nm.2670
20. Kambeitz, J., et al. (2015, January). Detecting neuroimaging biomarkers for schizophrenia: A meta-analysis of multivariate pattern recognition studies. *Neuropsychopharmacology, 40*(7), 1742–1751. https://doi.org/10.1038/npp.2015.22
21. Hsu, K.-C., & Wang, F.-S. (2017, June). Model-based optimization approaches for precision medicine: A case study in presynaptic dopamine overactivity. *PLoS One, 12*(6), e0179575. https://doi.org/10.1371/journal.pone.0179575
22. Shao, Y.-M., et al. (2018, January). Discovery of indolylpiperazinylpyrimidines with dual-target profiles at adenosine A2A and dopamine D2 receptors for Parkinson's disease treatment. *PLoS One, 13*(1), e0188212. https://doi.org/10.1371/journal.pone.0188212
23. Hemmerling, T. M., Taddei, R., Wehbe, M., Cyr, S., Zaouter, C., & Morse, J. (2013, February). First robotic ultrasound-guided nerve blocks in humans using the Magellan system. *Anesthesia & Analgesia, 116*(2), 491–494. https://doi.org/10.1213/ane.0b013e3182713b49

Chapter 18
Prediction and Classification of Aerosol Deposition in Lung Using CT Scan Images

K. Karthika and G. R. Jothi Lakshmi

18.1 Introduction

A wide variety of imaging technologies are employed in medical imaging to get diagnostic images that provide an accurate portrayal of the human body for the goals of disease diagnosis, monitoring, and therapy. In the absence of surgery or other invasive treatments, it is considered one of the most potent tools available for gaining a direct understanding of the human body. The problematic area being researched or treated can be studied using a variety of medical imaging technologies, each of which offers a unique perspective [1].

Infection and fibrosis of the lungs' tissue cause respiratory arrest in people with interstitial lung disease (ILD), one of more than 200 chronic lung diseases. In many circumstances, the disease is referred to as idiopathic because the evidence is inconclusive. For the most part, ILD is diagnosed by radiologists using magnetic resonance scans, which are used to identify various ILDs [2]. Because it provides such a precise picture of the tiniest structures as in lung tissue, computed tomography (CT) is the method of choice for diagnosing ILD. An automated diagnosis system (computer-aided diagnosis, CAD) has been widely utilized to overcome the flaws created by the quantitative method of the characteristics of emphysema and improve automatic detection [3]. To measure deposited aerosol particles in the respiratory system, there are numerous limitations to the methods used. Models for predicting the deposition of aerosol have now been developed to tackle these difficulties. Inside the lungs, there are nanoparticles [4]. To begin the process of finding lung nodules, the image's lung region must first be segmented. Step one is to divide the lung into sections where the tumors are expected to be. After that, a nodule

K. Karthika (✉) · G. R. J. Lakshmi
Department of ECE, VISTAS, Pallavaram, Chennai, Tamil Nadu, India
e-mail: jothi.se@velsuniv.ac.in

F. J. Joseph et al. (eds.), *Computational Intelligence for Clinical Diagnosis*,
EAI/Springer Innovations in Communication and Computing,
https://doi.org/10.1007/978-3-031-23683-9_18

augmentation procedure is performed on the segmented area. Input images are used to classify the strength of lung nodules based on their location in relation to the nodule center [5]. The offered approach makes use of a new idea to calculate the physical attributes of the designs in order to determine the value of the accruals concept zone.

The digital mammogram's input image is first binned to acquire the lesion's physical characteristics. Binning is a separation technique of the pictures into sub-regions, and it is especially successful for moving closer to the lesion area and performing additional analysis solely with the stratified sampling. Binning is a powerful tool for analyzing photos taken underwater [6]. An image processing technology will be used to calculate the reflection co-efficient and mass density concentration of a CT scan picture to aid in the prediction and classification of lung disorders. It is possible to identify photos based on similarities in specific attributes using a pattern recognition algorithm [7]. Pattern recognition [8] in photo editing is becoming increasingly important, and it must be presented in a user-friendly manner to assist practitioners in providing patients with the immediate advice they need to address specific areas of concern. Using a current image processing technique and pattern identification linked with micro-calcification, this research proposes an easy way for a doctor.

To determine the magnitude of the segments and sub-region, the proposed technique uses a new method of calculating the physical properties of the detected micro-calcification in images. Determine the connected properties of a lesion in order to find a pattern. Typically, a variety of segmentation methods are employed to determine the ROI. Enhancement [9], segmentation [10], feature extraction [11], and classification [12] are all conventional methods for detecting and classifying micro-calcifications. Tweaking and region-based approaches are used to segment data [13].

18.1.1 Proposed Work

The biopsy technique would be the most powerful method to evaluate and detect the health of the lung. This invasive method involved the extraction of tissue samples straight from the lung CT scan image. Segmentation of the lung CT scan image is the very first step for the analysis of the lung image, which is an essential way to prepare an accurate image of lung CT image analysis, for example, lung cancer detection. This process is fully based on computer-aided diagnosis (CAD). Using the U-net architecture, the work proposes a lung CT scan image segmentation. The architecture extracts the required information and also creates an asymmetrical way to recover the needed information. Micro-calcifications and macro-calcification are the two types of calcifications that are widely used. Huge calcium depositions in the lung tissue are known as macro-calcification. Smaller calcium depositions are known as micro-calcification if there is a high susceptibility to cancer developing in the lung tissue.

18.2 Work Principle

In current medical imaging, computer-aided diagnosis (CAD) is a very important diagnostic tool. It is also a prerequisite for the present medical field. This is an additional option for diagnosis accurately. This is widely used by physicians to get effective treatment. A particular way of segmentation method for a particular organ is needed for many CAD systems. To get an efficient quantitative lung CT scan image analysis, CAD is the initial step. However, for abnormal lung parenchyma, designing a lung segmentation process is a very challenging process. That time with the lung parenchyma, the blood vessels and nodules need to be segmented. However, for abnormal lung parenchyma, designing a lung segmentation process is a very challenging process, where the blood vessels and nodules need to be segmented separately. Automatic separation of the lung parenchyma region in CT scan has been proposed by a huge number of medical image analysis techniques. Most of the techniques are based on the contrasted information which is mentioned in the reviews. Deep learning is the appropriate kind of machine learning, which is the composition of multiple processing layers to get a standard abstraction when it tries to learn data.

The reflection coefficient and mass density are the considered physical characteristics for the lesion of CT scan images.

18.3 Methodology

In order to identify the patterns associated with a laceration, the related features of methods are obtained, which reflect co-efficiency, independent tissues, and mass identity in the CT scan image. The ways of recognizing the patterns help to classify the features of the image, which depend on the commonalities in a few aspects. To emphasize particular characteristics, present in the image, image enhancement is very important. Then, the physical parameters, textures, and features are extracted and measurements were taken. Then classifiers help to identify different classes and which decision needs to be taken. In ROI detection, segmentation takes the instrumental part.

18.4 Related Work

18.4.1 Pattern Recognition

A freely accessible medical image search tool called (OPEN I) provides the CT lung images. Normal and aberrant photos were included in the collection. This group of anomaly photos included lesions of benign or malignant origin, as depicted in Fig. 18.1.

Fig. 18.1 Flow chart. (Self-created)

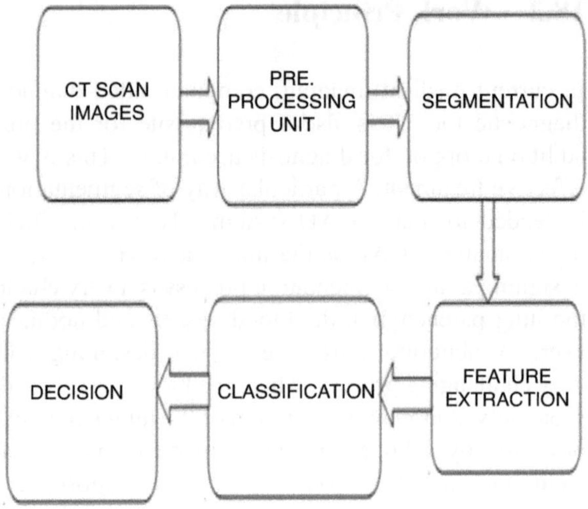

Image enhancement is essential to emphasize particular characteristics present in images. Thresholding and region detection are the common techniques applied while segmenting the images. Then features are extracted, and measurements are done.

18.4.2 Image Extraction

When the whole CT image is binned with less number of rows and columns, the binned image will be of larger size. Then the undesired irrelevant components may present together with deposition. The multiple binned images need to be studied at the second level of binning in order to extract the shape and size of the deposition. From detected ROI, features are obtained by applying fuzzy c-means clustering and SVM clustering to classify based on the recognized pattern.

18.4.3 Image Acquisition

The result of segmentation is for the particular case in the public data set where, with the help of U-net (R-231), the mask generates a low device is more coefficient than the ground truth. High-density areas in the segmentations are not included in the public dataset. For example, the segmentation includes tumors in the lung area but does not include the liver area. This overview is based on the testing and training program. Here we collected a database from the public, and two of them are the result of the routine checkup. This database is used in the training program of four generic semantic segmentation models. This model is also used for training purposes and also to make routine data.

18.5 Experimental Setup and Results

18.5.1 Image Binning

Binning is a technique that divides a single image into multiple smaller ones, allowing you to get close to the injured section and focus your area observed solely on that considered low. Equal-sized photos must be grouped together. The size of each first-level binned photo will be reduced when the CT image is junked with a certain number of rows. One or more binned photos may be created from it. As a result, the size and morphology of the aerosol deposition must be extracted from several binned photos by studying them at the second level of binarization. As shown in Fig. 18.2, the input picture size is 512 × 512, and it was reduced to 128 × 128 and represented in the first level of binning.

Second-level binning is performed on the bin containing ROI, which has been spotted. Second-level binning, as represented in Fig. 18.3, results in each binned image having a 75 × 75 resolution.

This is where researchers can get their hands-on off-the-wall photos and use them in their work. One hundred images from the lung CT diagnosis are selected, each with 512 rows and 512 columns of dimensions, i.e., each image. As a result, the ROI is designated with a blue color, whereas the intensity level in normal areas is lower or non-existent.

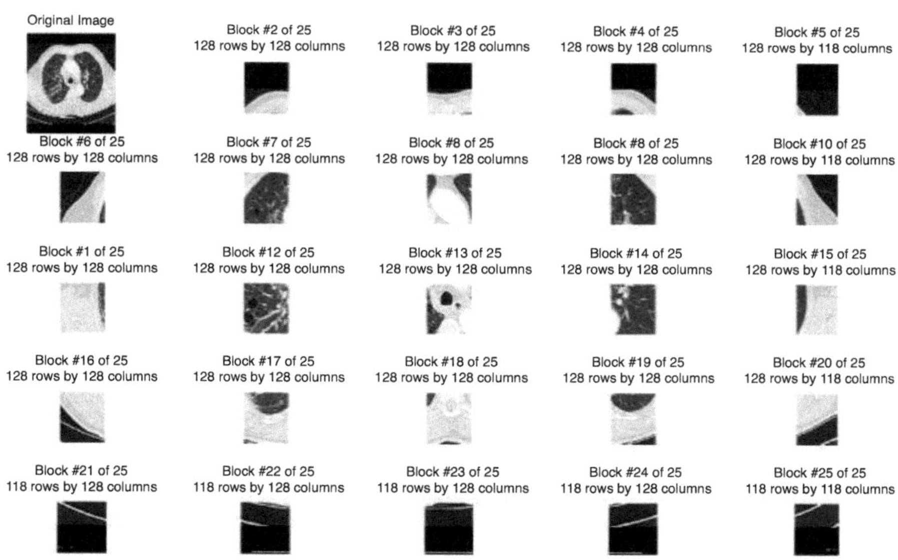

Fig. 18.2 First-level binning

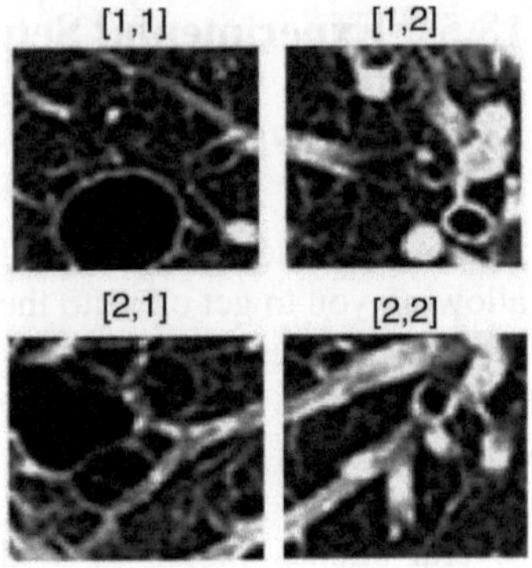

Fig. 18.3 Second-level binning

18.5.2 *Measurement and Plot of Reflection Coefficient*

The soft tissues of the lung make up the organ. Calcium and aerosol deposits form a solid coating in these tissues. The reflection coefficient can be calculated for the entire image, including the lesion area. Reflected energy and reflection ratio are also both high in the lesion region. A two-dimensional function $f(x,y)$ can be used to model an image.

$$f(x, y) = r\,(x, y)\; i(x, y)$$

where $i(x,y)$ is the illumination component and $r(x,y)$ is the reflectance component.

$$0 < i(x, y) < \infty \text{and } 0 < r(x, y) < 1$$

where $r = 0$ represents total absorption and $r = 1$ represents total reflectance.

Reflection values are shown as shown in Fig. 18.4 for each row, with the x-axis showing the respective column of the bin and the y-axis showing the reflection coefficient value. The reflecting coefficients must be evaluated for the minimum to identify ROI.

18.5.3 *Measurement of Mass Density*

Mass is calculated as the ratio of mass to volume. The damaged area's mass density can be determined thanks to the presence of aerosols and calcareous deposits in the lesion. Calcium oxalate is found in benign abnormal cells, while it is mainly seen in malignant, benign tumors. MATLAB's volume viewer function can be used to determine the micro-calcification mass density. The volume of the second-level bin is used to measure the weight of the split ROI. Table 18.1 shows the precise set of reflection coefficients that is used as a limit in ROI identification by fitting a curve with least squares.

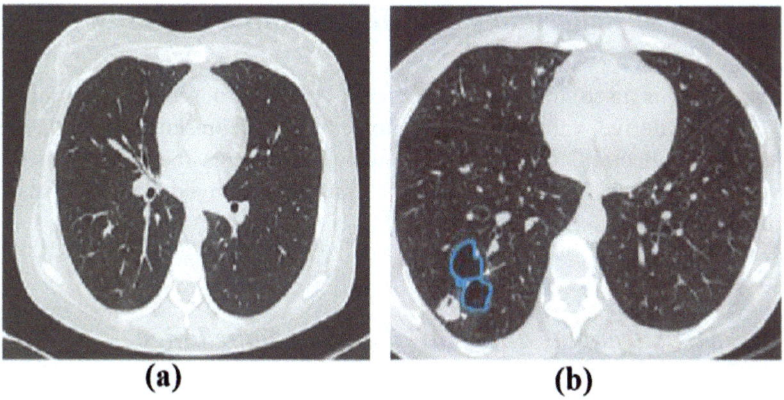

Fig. 18.4 (**a**) Normal lung. (**b**) Abnormal lung

Table 18.1 Reflection coefficient and mass density value

	Reflection coefficients				Mass density			
Sl. No	Bin [1,1]	Bin [1,2]	Bin [2,1]	Bin [2,2]	Bin [1,1]	Bin [1,2]	Bin [2,1]	Bin [2,2]
Abnormal images								
1	0.7929	0.3867	0.1757	0.8164	1.64	0.43	0.59	1.28
2	0.7070	0.0429	0.7890	0.1210	0.74	0.18	0.75	0.25
3	0.7226	0.6718	0.8242	0.1640	1.02	0.61	1.63	0.37
4	0.6835	0.6210	0.8359	0.3906	0.61	0.54	1.19	0.45
5	0.0703	0.7929	0.8303	0.6601	0.15	1.34	1.07	0.80
6	0.3007	0.4921	0.5273	0.8281	0.71	0.80	0.81	1.05
7	0.6093	0.7460	0.7929	0.4335	0.84	1.22	1.58	0.79
8	0.8164	0.0156	0.75	0.7226	1.29	0.78	1.60	0.41
9	0.7539	0.7851	0.0976	0.6601	1.40	0.39	0.70	0.92
10	0.7656	0.2695	0.2773	0.0312	0.93	0.44	0.59	0.66
11	0.7148	0.3984	0.8164	0.1054	0.95	0.58	1.32	0.62
12	0.7890	0.0390	0.5117	0.0156	1.03	0.64	0.70	0.48
Normal images								
13	0.7304	0.6171	0.5937	0.6757	0.94	0.35	0.53	0.97
14	0.6875	0.6914	0.6679	0.6796	0.65	1.04	0.86	0.81
15	0.6406	0.1484	0.6757	0.0390	0.89	0.81	0.61	0.49
16	0.6523	0.2617	0.0976	0.6953	0.81	0.74	0.21	0.62
17	0.0703	0.1054	0.1054	0.6132	0.34	0.33	0.17	0.75
18	0.1757	0.6835	0.0390	0.4687	0.38	0.84	0.39	0.53

18.5.4 Plot of Reflection Coefficient and Mass Density

A linear scale is used to compare different photos to second-level bins from Table 18.1 to derive values for the *x*-axis, which represents the value of the coefficient of reflection, and the *y*-axis, which represents the mass density. This achievement is shown in Fig. 18.5, and the morals are derived from comparisons of various pictures with second-level bins.

18.5.5 Measurement and Plot of Tissue Impedance

Each row is represented as a combination of the *x* and *y* values of a block's tissue impedance matching, which is derived using the given formula based on dispersion relation from the associated bin column value and the tissue resistance.

$$\Gamma = \frac{z_L - z_O}{z_L + z_O} \tag{18.1}$$

ZL is the tissue impedance and ZO is the air impedance, all of which is 376 ohms (Fig. 18.6)

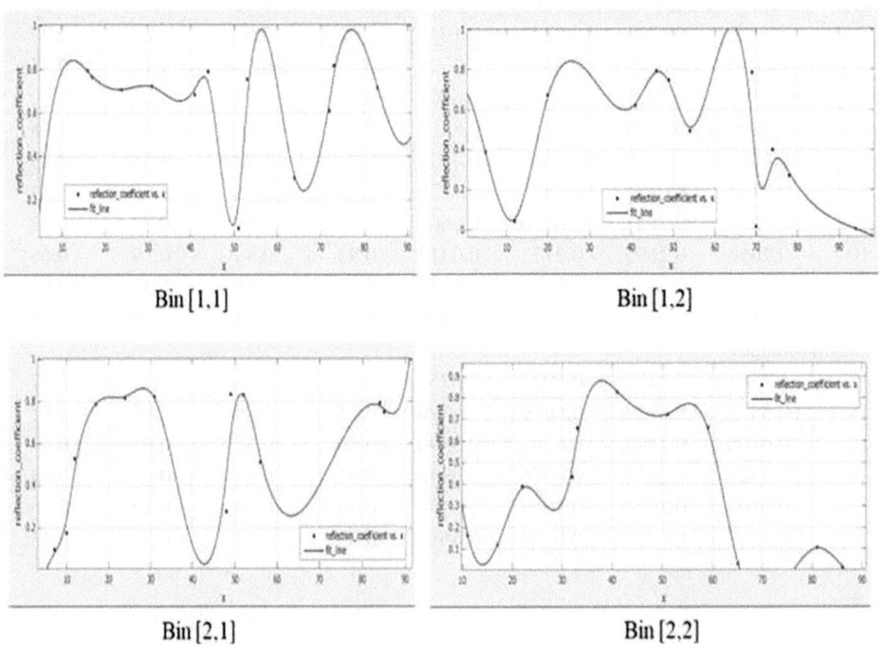

Fig. 18.5 Reflection coefficient plot

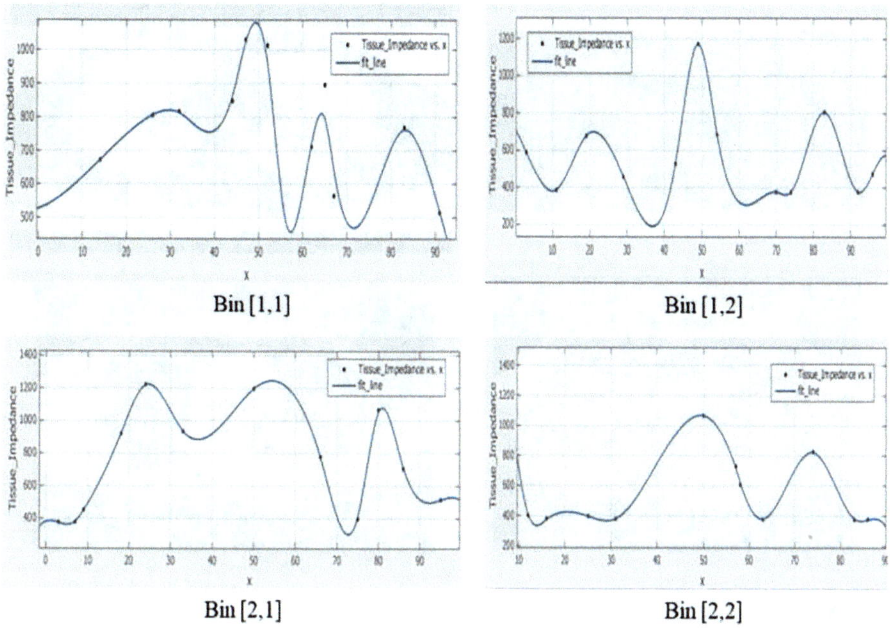

Fig. 18.6 Light transmission impedance plot

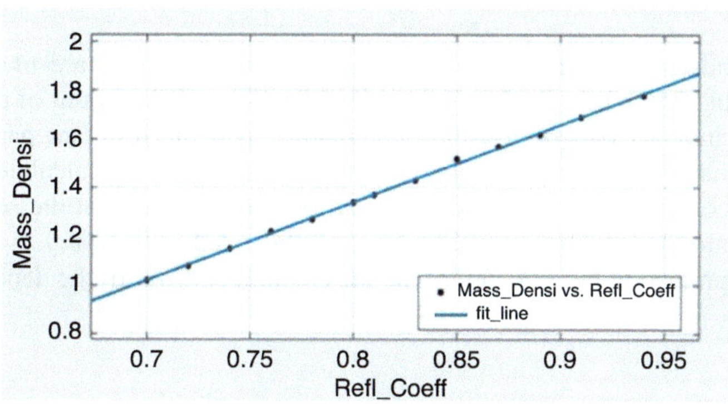

Fig. 18.7 Reflection coefficient versus mass density plot

18.5.6 Fuzzy C-Means Thresholding

There is an improvement in computational efficiency when the statistic gray-level photos are used as input. With this model, noise is accepted more readily (Figs. 18.7 and 18.8).

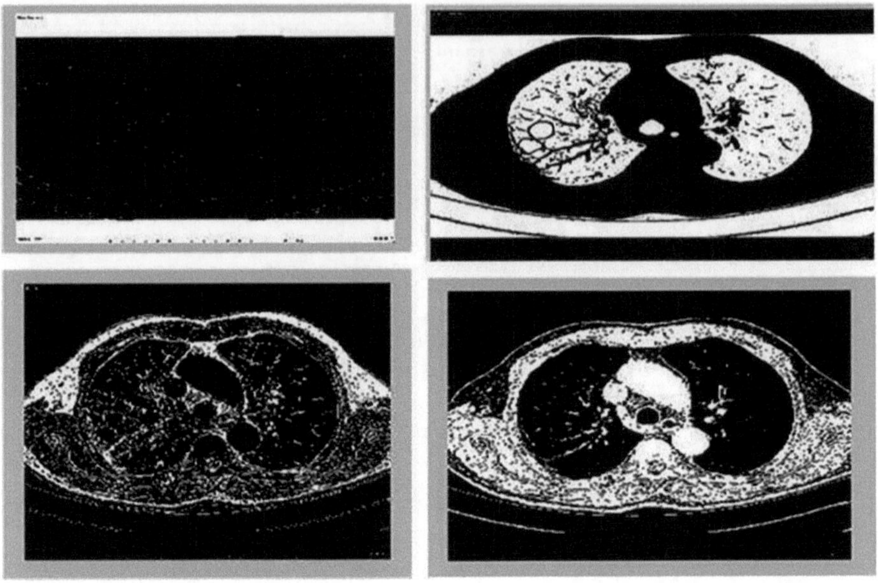

Fig. 18.8 Fuzzy c-means thresholding

18.5.7 3D Projection

On the foundation of the produced CT picture, the intensities are likely to vary between 0 and 255 when converted to gray scale. The small amount of precipitated air and calcium, its patterns on the bin imaging, and the resultant pattern in 3D projections have been computed and recognized. For the micro-calculated ROI, we project the columns and rows of pixels from our binned image at the second-level scrapping onto the two-dimensional z-axis, as illustrated in Fig. 18.9.

This 3D projection helps to determine the position and size of the deposition area ROI.

18.5.8 SVM Classification

A supervised ML model known as the SVM employs classified methods to solve classification issues involving two groups. To evaluate the classification performance of the models on a ("set of tests"), set values are computed. A pseudo code is employed as illustrated in Fig. 18.10 of anticipated and cheaper. There are a number of metrics that can be assessed with this tool.

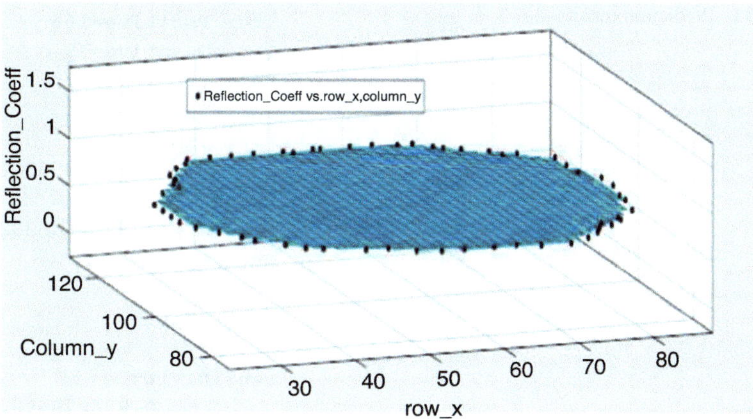

Fig. 18.9 3D projection plot

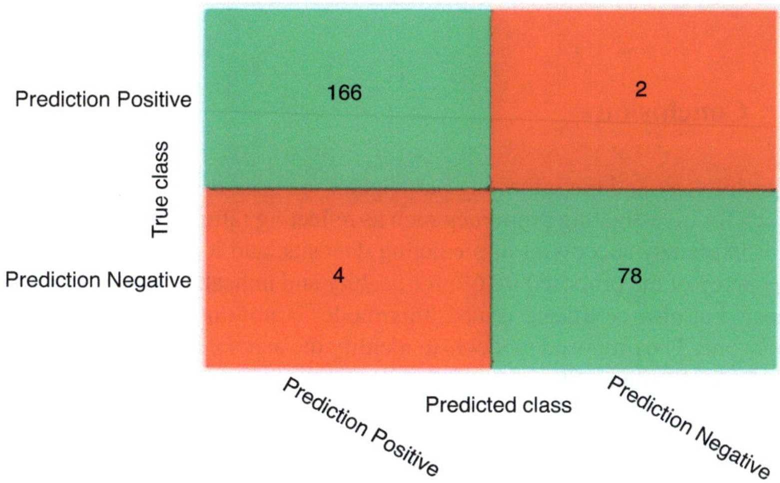

Fig. 18.10 Confusion matrix

The pictures that have been taught are divided into four categories: "True positive," "True negative," "False positive," and "False negative," respectively (FN). In Fig. 18.11, you can see the expected precision and error rate, determined using the method below.

From the above formula, the classifier predicts the result with an accuracy of 97.6% and also with an error rate of 2.4%.

Fig. 18.11 Prediction result

```
True_Positive=166
True_Negative=78
False_Positive=2
False_Negative=4
Precision =
        0.988095238095238
Recall =
        0.976470588235294
Accuracy =
                    0.976
Error_Rate =
                    0.024
Sensitivity =
        0.976470588235294
Specificity =
                    0.975
F_Measure =
        0.982248520710059
```

18.6 Conclusion

CAD technology and the informing participants are used to develop an autonomous approach for investigating properties such as reflecting ratio and mass densities. The SVM is extremely successful in predicting deposits, and it achieves a classification and accuracy of the proposed 97.6% for healthy and unhealthy lung CT images. For diagnosis but also certificate issued, this model is now more productive than the previous one. The proposed model is to identify the aerosol deposition in CT images using physical features like binning, reflection coefficient, mass density, and tissue impedance, and 3D projection is made for abnormal lung images. An accuracy of 96.78% is achieved in classifying and predicting the normal and abnormal lung CT images. The computation of deposition was carried out using interpolation over image intensity and the reflection coefficient. There, the deposition was precisely identified using a 3D projection of it, and thereby its size was accurately detected. The prediction of deposition is very accurate with the help of the SVM classifier. So this model is more efficient for the diagnosis and classification of lung disorders.

References

1. Hasan, A. M., Jalab, H. A., Meziane, F., Kahtan, H., & Al-Ahmad, A. S. (2019). Combining deep and handcrafted image features for MRI brain scan classification. *IEEE, 7*.
2. Anthimopoulos, M., Christodoulidis, S., Ebner, L., Geiser, T., Christe, A., & Mougiakakou, S. (2018). Semantic segmentation of pathological lung tissue with dilated fully convolutional networks. *IEEE, Journal of Biomedical and Health Informatics*.

3. Pang, T., Guo, S., Zhang, X., & Zhao, L. (2019). Automatic lung segmentation based on texture and deep features of HRCT images with interstitial lung disease. *Hindawi, BioMed Research International, 2019*, 1.
4. Bui, V. K. H., Moon, J.-y., Chae, M., Park, D., & Lee, Y.-C. *Prediction of aerosol deposition in the human respiratory tract via computational models.* Multidisciplinary Digital PublishingInstitute.
5. Veerakumar, & Ravichandran, C. G. (2013). *Intensity, shape and size based detection of lung nodules from CT images.* Springer.
6. Roman, C., Inglis, G., & Rutter, J. (2010). *Application of structured light imaging for high resolution mapping of underwater archaeological.* University of Rhode Island.
7. Junior, J. R. F., Koenigkam-Santos, M., Cipriano, F. E. G., Fabro, A. T., & de Azevedo-Marques, P. M. (2018). Radiomics-based features for pattern recognition of lung cancer histopathology and metastases. *Elsevier.*
8. Satoto, K. I., Nurhayati, O. D., & Isnanto, R. R. (2011). Pattern recognition to detect breast cancer thermogram images based on fuzzy inference system method. *IJCST, 2.*
9. Wang, W., & Shuguang, W. (2016). A study on lung cancer detection by image processing. *IEEE.*
10. Song, Q. Z., Zhao, L., Luo, X. K., & Dou, X. C. (2017). Using deep learning for classification of lung nodules on computed tomography images. *Journal of Healthcare Engineering, Hindawi, 2017*, 1.
11. Al-Bayati, M., & El-Zaart, A. (2013). Mammogram images thresholding for breast cancer detection using different thresholding methods. *SciRes.*
12. Jothilakshmi, R., Raaza, A., Rajendran, V., Sreenivasa Varma, Y., & Raj, R. G. N. (2018). Pattern recognition and size prediction of micro calcification based on physical characteristics by using digital mammogram images. *Springer, Journal of Digital Imaging*. https://doi.org/10.1007/s10278-018-0075-x
13. Karthika, K., & Jothilakshmi, G. R. (2021). Prediction and classification of liquid deposition in lung through physical characteristics using CT scan images. *Design Engineering*, ISSN:0011-9342 (Issue 8).

Chapter 19
3D Cyst Sonomammogram Projection Using Reflection Coefficient and Mass Density in Python

G. R. Jothi Lakshmi, V. Adarsh, Shalini Kumari, D. Ravi, A. Santhiya, and E. Ram Natesh

19.1 Introduction

Image processing is a technique for manipulating images using mathematical procedures. When a photo or video frame is used as the input, the result is either an image or a collection of characteristics or other factors related to the image. Another way to say it is processing the input image to meet the needs of the application. Images make up a crucial portion of all assessments made in the modern environment. Examples include 3D appealing resonance or marked scanning imaging, RNA genotyping, microscope slides, galactic sensations, global maps, artificial eyesight catch, and made opening Radar images. Investigating these extensive data sources calls for contemporary programming tools that should be simple to use, free of cost and restrictions, and prepared to handle all the challenges presented by such a diverse field of study. This paper presents scikit-image, a collection of Python-based image processing algorithms created by a vibrant volunteer community and distributed under the permissive Open Source license. It is the ideal time to introduce an image handling toolbox because of the growing popularity of Python as a conceptual computer language and the improved access to a wide range of related

G. R. Jothi Lakshmi (✉) · V. Adarsh · S. Kumari · A. Santhiya · E. Ram Natesh
Department of ECE, Vels Institute of Science, Technology and Advanced Studies, Chennai, Tamil Nadu, India
e-mail: jothi.se@velsuniv.ac.in

D. Ravi
Department of Mechanical Engineering, Bharath Institute of Higher Education and Research, Chennai, Tamil Nadu, India
e-mail: ravi.mech@bharathuniv.ac.in

F. J. J. Joseph et al. (eds.), *Computational Intelligence for Clinical Diagnosis*, EAI/Springer Innovations in Communication and Computing,
https://doi.org/10.1007/978-3-031-23683-9_19

devices. The majority of image processing algorithms treat the image as a two-dimensional signal and employ standard signal processing techniques.

A two-dimensional representation of a three-dimensional scene in terms of $f(x,y)$ is referred to as an image. The spatial coordinates are represented by (x,y). The amplitude of f at any point (x,y) is used to define the gray or intensity levels of the image at a point. The image is referred to as a digital image when the intensity values of f and the x and y are both discrete and uniform as well. Pixels are the finite number of elements present in the digital image. A particular location and value are provided by each pixel. When a digital image is manipulated by means of a processor, it is defined as digital image processing. The $f(x,y)$ value of the pixel is changed through a digital computer through some function. Based on the required application, this operation can be segregated into three groups. Finding proper ways to mathematically describe and analyze images is the primary goal of this image modeling or representation. We must understand that this may not be the best representation as there are various representations and thus different results as well. Image acquisition, image enhancement, segmentation, color image processing, image restoration, and classification are the fundamental steps in image processing.

Breast cysts are noncancerous fluid-filled sacs inside the breast. In one or more breasts, there is a possibility of one or more breast cysts. When a cyst becomes large and some anxiety is seen, then treatment is required; otherwise, this can be ignored. Breast cysts develop as a result of fluid accumulation in the glands of the breasts.

19.2 Related Work

The evaluation of mammographic images is very useful for detecting the abnormal nature of the tissues through a system that has been developed called mammographic computer-aided diagnosis [1], as studies show that increases and decreases in breast sensitivity, the density of the region in computer-aided design (CAD) [2] are used to detect the region of the interest. The accuracy of the lesion is deflected through the calculation of specificity [3]. The problem of adding normal tissues along with abnormal lesion region could be overcome by using the powerful direct correlation of the breast 51 parenchyma time–intensity curves (TICs) and density in the mammograms and carcinoma in the development of the CAD [4]. Local statistical and textural parameters were used to segregate fatty and dense mammograms [5]. The correlation between four mammographic risk assessment metrics was carried out using intra- and inter-observer variation [6].

The images are converted to the 2D view because it plays a major role in carcinoma, in diagnosing the region for treating cancer, and the cancer tissue is superimposed by its artificial creation showing its density [7]. Often they report false-positives and false-negatives, which affect the patient's risk of painful, undesirable procedures. To overcome the problem, magnetic resonance imaging (MRI) can be a procedure, that provide high resolution 3D images of the breasts. MRI is more advance than the mammography projection and the implication the tissue on the parochial it interest structures [7, 8]. The increase in the visibility margin of the dense breast region boosts the lesion part the projection of the X-ray is moved inner arc where the breast is fixed, and detection in the digital image [9] probability of detection of cancer in the woman can be estimated of the breast cancer indication with frequent screening, so that the cancer can be identified as early as possible [10].

The first process of spotting the affected region is to remove background properties such as the pectoral muscles; labels have been used previously in the developing process [11]. But the pixels have an identical gray scale combined with dense clustering, and fat is collected with the properties. The region of Interest is identified with many featured vector to indicate its particularity during the test of LBP operator [12]. The detection of clusters is difficult by using microcalcifications, and its use factors are shape, size, and the region of the cancer cells with a low-contrast background. Other features are gray-level, texture, and intensity of the image [13]. Images are segmented using boundary detection and seed-based region-growing techniques to segment microcalcifications in the given input images [14]. Jothilakshmi et al. [15] proposed a novel method of measuring the size of microcalcifications on the mammogram images through the 3D projection of the region of interest (RoI) by using only two physical characteristics, the reflection coefficient and mass density. Feature extraction and SVM classification [16] and the back propagation neural network [17] was used to identify microcalcification. A survey on cancer detection on ultrasound images was carried out [18], and a morphological edge detection algorithm [19] was proposed for detecting RoI edges using lung CT images.

19.3 Proposed System

For detecting abnormalities developed in the breast, various image processing techniques are being used. In addition to microcalcification-based analysis, abnormal masses can also be found using image-processing techniques. To detect and classify the exceptional growth, it has been observed that the analysis went the usual way. Image enhancement, image restoration, segmentation, and classification are the regular methods in use. Support vector machines (SVMs), Bayes, KNN, etc., have been used to achieve results. Over the past 10 years, the stabilizing time for photon tomography images has drastically decreased, going from minutes to seconds [1]. For radiography, new techniques such as single-pack imaging provide times down to the millisecond [3].

The time necessary to process the images, nevertheless, has not decreased to the point where the results of a successful beam imaging run are frequently transformed into logical results over the course of weeks or months. Changing billions of pixels and voxels to a few large numbers indicates a considerable loss of information. The grouping of operations that are often anticipated to generate this knowledge is frequently unknown beforehand or may change owing to antiquated rarities [5] or an unexpected change in the example. In order to choose the handling work approach, trial stages are fundamentally involved in picture preparation.

Therefore, image processing and analysis devices need to provide significant usage flexibility, a variety of computation options, and skillful operations to accommodate quick changes in focus while adjusting the workflow. A few programming and libraries are accessible to many customers. Owing to its intuitive menus, graphical tools, and the wealth of modules provided by a distinct group [17], ImageJ [4–6, 9], is widely used and is a universally helpful tool for 2D and 3D images. Programming used to interpret synchrotron data is also available, for instance [13], for diffraction images obtained from powder diffraction research. For 3D images, business tools such as Avizo 3D programming [15] are well-known for their intuitive graphical workflow and advanced 3D perception. Some synchrotrons have even developed their own volume preparation equipment, such as Pore3D [9] at Elettra.

However, if classically handled methods can be called to form frameworks, using a programming language offers more management, better consistency, and more difficult analysis contemplations, hence limiting the complexity of the programming task and the risk of mistakes. The academic field of computer vision and image handling is dominated by Open Object Recognition [15] and its image preparation tool segment. Scikit-image [3] is a Python library for image processing that is beneficial for everyone. It is also a part of the biological group of logical Python modules referred to as Sci Python [5]. Scikit-Picture is released under an open-source license and is freely available, just like the rest of the biological process. As the majority of scikit-picture work well with both 3D images, it can be applied to a wide range of modalities, including microscopes, radiographs, and scanning.

The interpretation of images is not perfect for doctors to analyze as the outputs through the existing algorithm may lead to false-positive and false-negative results. A different algorithm is proposed in this paper to detect the early occurrence of cysts by analyzing sonomammogram images through the calculation of the physical characteristics of the corresponding input images. The algorithm is also very useful in finding the size of the RoI. The size of the abnormalities can be easily measured through the 3D projection. The reflection coefficient for the lesion part of the image can be calculated in an easy method. Both reflection energy, as well as the reflection coefficient are high in the lesion part, and thus the ratio of the amplitude of the reflected wave to the incident wave gives the reflection coefficient. The reflection coefficient always lies between 0 and 1. 0. A flow diagram of the proposed methodology is shown in Fig. 19.1

As per the flow diagram, the images were acquired from a doctor with reports (Fig. 19.2). The size of the images is 768 × 1024 with respect to pixel count and 4.5 cm × 7 cm in height and width. The measurement of the lesion part is mentioned in the bottommost part of the image. There are two levels of binning involved as well. The whole image is binned with four columns and three rows at the first level of binning. The matrix size of the bins and the corresponding width and height of the image are calculated simultaneously. To find the exact RoI by omitting the unwanted region, the corresponding bin is divided further, two by two in second-level binning. There are four bins at the second level of binning, each measuring 256 × 256.

The reflection coefficient of all second-level bins is calculated. When the image pixel values are divided by the incident energy value, that gives a reflection coefficient in each coordinate of the image. As the lesion part is darker, the range

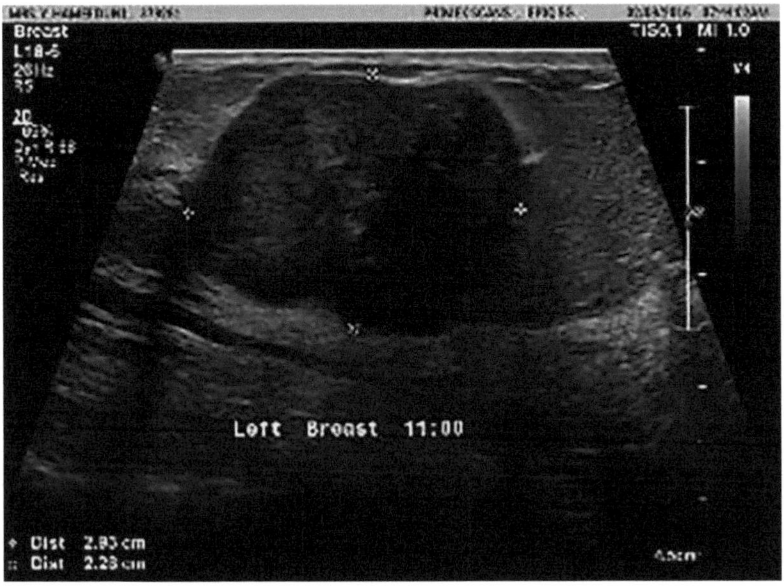

Fig. 19.1 Breast cyst: sonomammogram image

of the reflection coefficient lies between 0.02 and 0.225. Based on this range as a threshold, the RoI is segmented out. For the segmented region, the mass density is calculated. The mass density of all four second-level bins is calculated and has a maximum value of 0.9–1.01 g/cm^3. Then, the mapping between the range of the reflection coefficient and the range of mass density is performed. The mapping between reflection coefficient to mass density exhibits linear mapping between these two variables. Then, the second level bin with RoI is projected in 3D with the corresponding height and width values on the X and Y axis and the range of reflection coefficient on the Z axis.

19.4 Results and Discussion

As mentioned in the proposed method, the outputs are shown step by step as follows. Figure 19.3 shows the considered input image. Figure 19.4 exhibits the first level of binning, which consists of 12 bins. Bins 6 and 7 contain the RoI. Bin 6 is further subdivided into four bins, as shown in Fig. 19.5.

In Bin 2 of Fig. 19.5, the variation of the reflection coefficient in each row was shown in Figs. 19.6, 19.7, 19.8, and 19.9. The RoI is obtained by the thresholding of the reflection coefficient range as shown in Fig. 19.10, and the exact RoI is projected in Fig. 19.11. The calculated mass density of four second-level bins is shown in Fig. 19.10. The linear mapping between a measured range of reflection coefficient and mass density is shown in Fig. 19.11, as well as the projected 3D RoI.

Fig. 19.2 Flow diagram of the proposed methodology

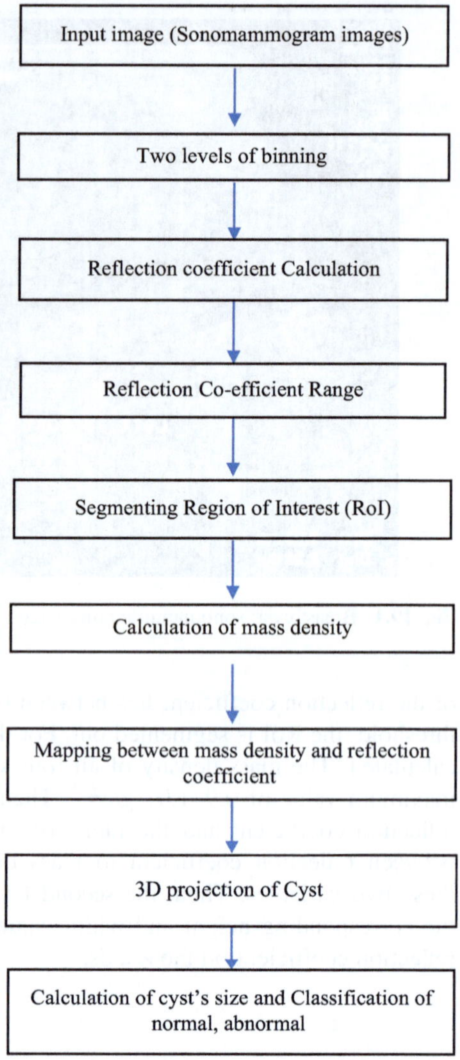

A desktop computer is created by each process, which can then be operated on individually. The usual order in which these actions are carried out results in a segmented image from which data can easily be extracted. For instance, from Figs. 19.4 and 19.5, it is clear that the image only requires a few seconds to apply, a chronological filter, a threshold to produce a color mask, and to simultaneously visualize each middle step to make sure that the specifications are optimized for the signal being studied. This is useful when trying a strategy that exists in a specific spatial–temporal frequency spectrum.

In Figs. 19.6 and 19.7, we will go through image, a program that combines Python's numerous and potent image analysis packages with a simple-to-use

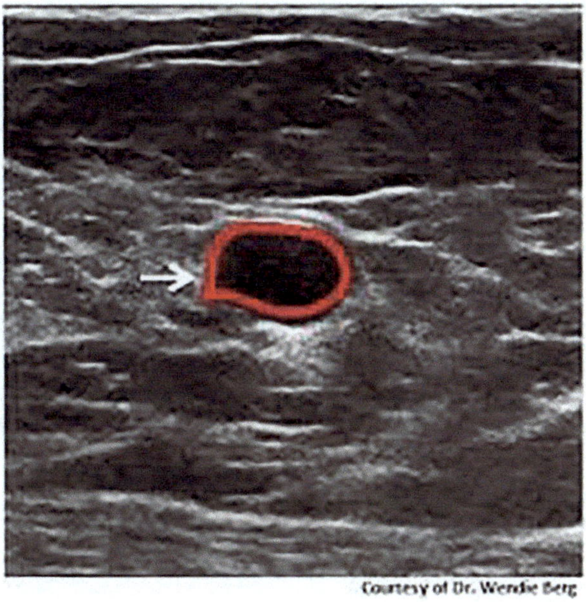

Fig. 19.3 Input image

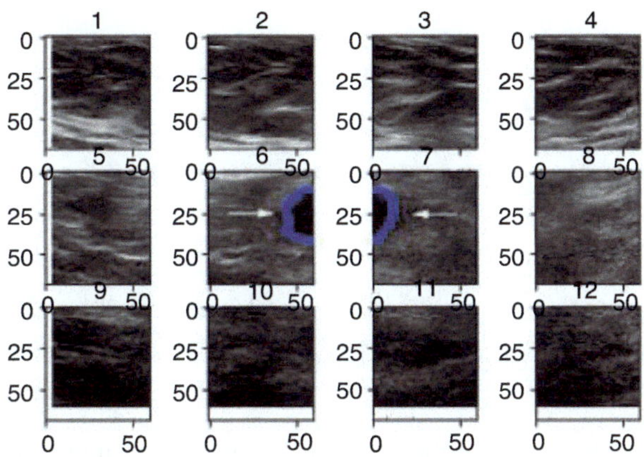

Fig. 19.4 First level binning

graphical user interface. Image also includes a number of integrated image recognition tools that make it simple and quick to visualize image information in order to accelerate imaging techniques.

As a result, activities that produce modest, non-integer outcomes, such as creating ratio imaging compared with ambient light, can be easily carried out without the requirement to build up the numbers, as is necessary for software programs that exclusively work with integer image data. Also, Figs. 19.8 and 19.9 indicate that there are options to convert the pixel to unregistered and verified integers with lengths ranging from 8 to 64 bits, which can help with interfaces with other software applications or cut down on computational load.

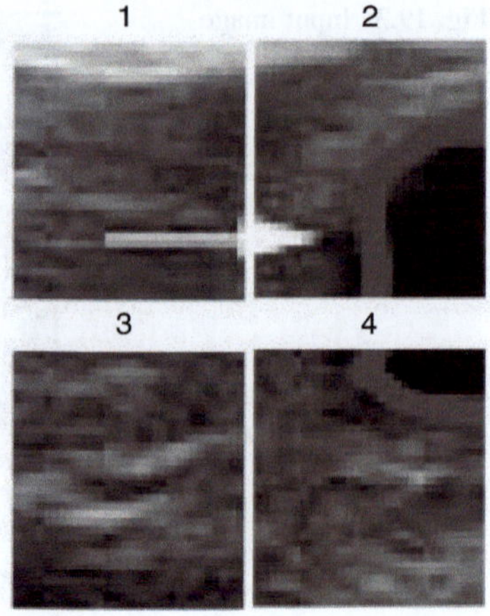

Fig. 19.5 Second level binning

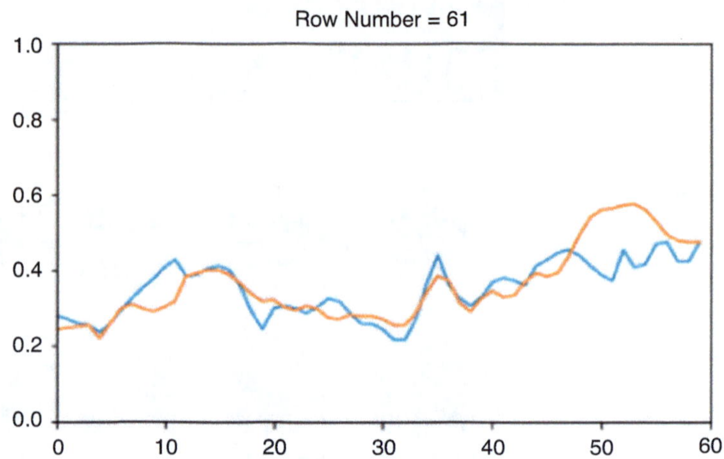

Fig. 19.6 Reflection coefficient Plot 61

The clarity of these photos had first been improved by enhancing the margin of each yogurt particle by changing contrast. After thresholding, the image in Figs. 19.9 and 19.10 was divided into the foreground and background elements. The edge detection procedure was tailored for each shot by taking into consideration the borders of the RoI region because the levels of intensity in the region of interest were not uniform. Each granule with a boundary that could be easily seen or that was clearly delineated from the others was chosen. Prior to determining the particle diameter and shape, every selecting area change was examined.

By decreasing the logical distance out over a set of M sample points in such a fewest sense, one can fit an elliptic to a general conic. The finest ellipse for the given collection of points is then represented by the solution of the minimization problem. For each elliptical fitting, six edge samples were chosen at random from a list of

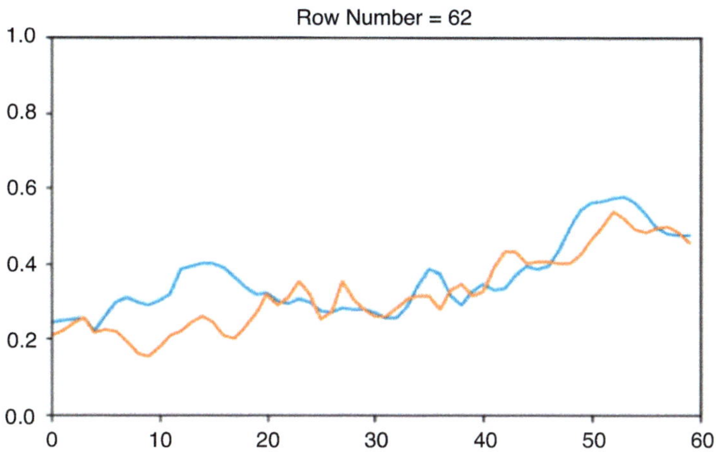

Fig. 19.7 Reflection coefficient Plot 62

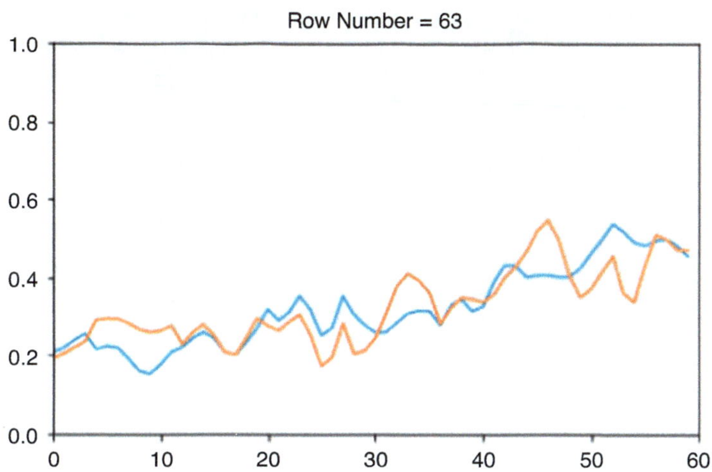

Fig. 19.8 Reflection coefficient Plot 63

sorted edge points. Figure 19.10 displays the end result of obtaining fit ellipses. The mathematical specifics of the ellipse fit application have been reported by picture. Following that, all of the objects in the image had their ellipse properties determined, including rotation, minor axis length, and centroid. Table 19.1 displays the quantitative analysis of mass densities obtained from RoI at different levels and Fig. 19.11 depicts these parameters. Owing to their size being below limits, the remaining smaller spheres within the image were disregarded.

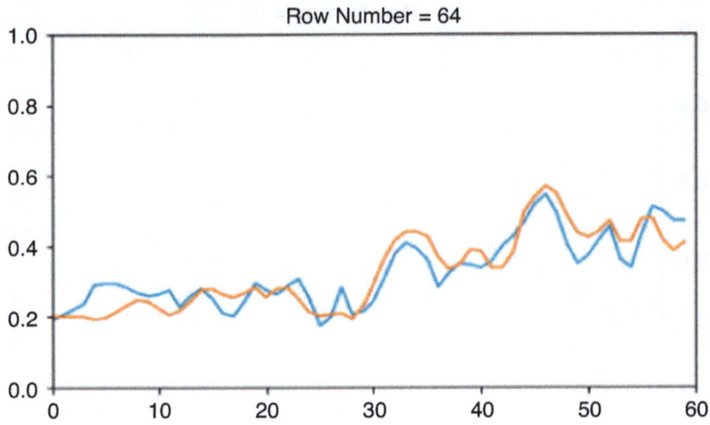

Fig. 19.9 Reflection coefficient Plot 64

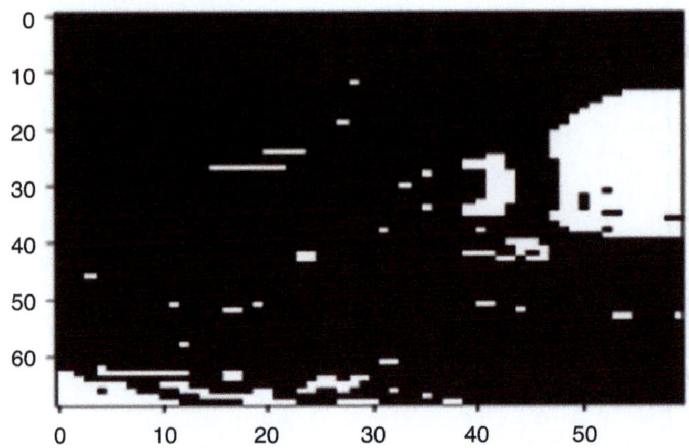

Fig. 19.10 Identifying the region of interest by thresholding

Table 19.1 Comparison of mass densities at different levels

Substantial	Sequential	Eternity	Rational
2.32 T	2.52 T	2.56 T	2.53 T
2.43 T	2.56 T	2.62 T	2.72 T
9.57 A/m	5.86 A/m	4.63 A/m	6.75 A/m
1.8 A/m	5.65 A/m	6.71 A/m	6.84 A/m
274.96 emu/g	2 78.21 emu/g	231.42 emu/g	267.72 emu/g
554 °C	314 °C	528 °C	372 °C

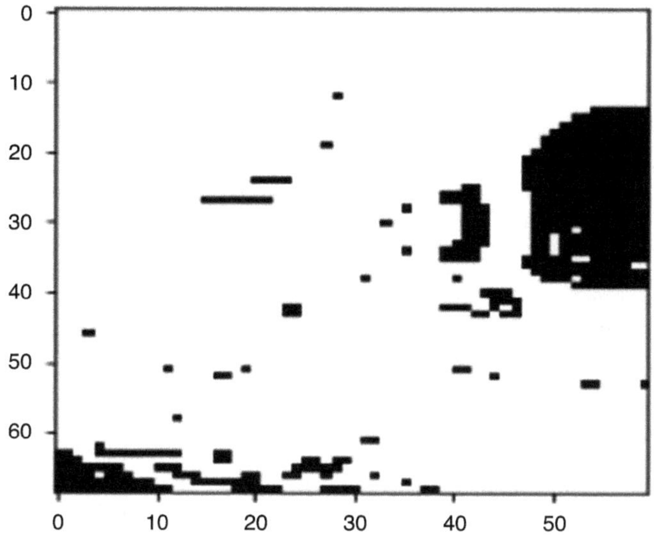

Fig. 19.11 Exact region of interest by mapping

19.5 Conclusion

The proposed approach appears to be able to address the many problems that can arise while automating biological processes. It has not been able to evaluate the suitability of these strategies because there have been insufficient observations from the field or metadata. The generalization of this framework has been the subject of research in the field of health, and it has been demonstrated to be an effective instrument for the characterization of infections. According to what is described in the paper, it is feasible to project the RoI in 3D view by using only two physical factors. This will be more helpful for the physician to analyze and predict the diseased region further in an effective manner. This algorithm is effective in segmenting the cyst with the assistance of the reflection coefficient, which has a range of 0.02–0.225, and mass density measurement (0.92–1.14 g/cm^3), which is a novel concept to increase the true positive rate. Together, these two factors help to increase the true-positive rate. The RoI will be projected in three dimensions in terms of its size as part of a future investigation, and this projection will be utilized to precisely estimate the size of the cyst.

References

1. Freer, T. W., & Ulissey, M. J. (2001). Screening mammography with computer-aided detection: Prospective study of 12860 patients in a community breast center. *Radiology, 220*, 781–786.
2. Obenauer, S., Sohns, C., Werner, C., & Grabbe, E. (2006). Impact of breast density on computer-aided detection in full-field digital mammography. *Journal of Digital Imaging, 19*(3), 258–263. https://doi.org/10.1007/s10278-006-0592-x. PMID: 16741664; PMCID: PMC3045151.

3. Brem, R. F., Hoffmeister, J. W., Rapelyea, J. A., Zisman, G., Mohtashemi, K., Jindal, G., Disimio, M. P., & Rogers, S. K. (2005). Impact of breast density on computer-aided detection for breast cancer. *American Journal of Roentgenology, 184*(2), 439–444. https://doi.org/10.2214/ajr.184.2.01840439. Erratum in: AJR Am J Roentgenol. 2005;184(6):1968. PMID: 15671360.
4. Wolfe, J. N. (1976). Risk for breast cancer development determined by mammographic parenchymal pattern. *Cancer, 37*, 2486–2492.
5. Taylor, P., Hajnal, S., Dilhuydy, M. H., & Barreau, B. (1994). Measuring image texture to separate "difficult" from "easy" mammograms. *The British Journal of Radiology, 67*(797), 456–463. https://doi.org/10.1259/0007-1285-67-797-456. PMID: 8193892.
6. Muhimmah, I., Oliver, A., Denton, R. E., Pont, J., Pérez, E., & Zwiggelaar, R. (2006). Comparison between Wolfe, Boyd, BI-RADS and Tabár-based mammographic risk assessment. In *Proceedings of the 8th international conference on Digital Mammography (IWDM'06)* (pp. 407–415). Springer-Verlag, Berlin, Heidelberg. https://doi.org/10.1007/11783237_55
7. Varjonen, M. (2006). Three-dimensional digital breast tomosynthesis in the early diagnosis and detection of breast cancer. *Lecture Notes in Computer Science, 4046*, 152–159.
8. Dobbins, J. T., & Godfrey, D. J. (2003). Digital x-ray tomosynthesis: current state of the art and clinical potential. *Physics in Medicine and Biology, 48*(19), R65–R106.
9. Niklason, L. T., Christian, B. T., Niklason, L. E., Kopans, D. B., Castleberry, D. E., Opsahl-Ong, B. H., Landberg, C. E., Slanetz, P. J., Giardino, A. A., Moore, R., Albagli, D., DeJule, M. C., Fitzgerald, P. F., Fobare, D. F., Giambattista, B. W., Kwasnick, R. F., Liu, J., Lubowski, S. J., Possin, G. E., Richotte, J. F., Wei, C. Y., & Wirth, R. F. (1997). Digital tomosynthesis in breast imaging. *Radiology, 205*, 399–406.
10. Van Gils, C. H., Otten, J. D., Hendriks, J. H., Holland, R., Straatman, H., & Verbeek, A. L. (1999). High mammographic breast density and its implications for the early detection of breast cancer. *Journal of Medical Screening, 6*(4), 200–204. https://doi.org/10.1136/jms.6.4.200. PMID: 10693066.
11. Raba, D., Oliver, A., Martí, J., Peracaula, M., & Espunya, J. (2005). Breast segmentation with pectoral muscle suppression on digital mammograms. In J. S. Marques, N. Pérez de la Blanca, & P. Pina (Eds.), *Pattern recognition and image analysis. IbPRIA 2005* (Lecture Notes in Computer Science) (Vol. 3523). Springer. https://doi.org/10.1007/11492542_58
12. Ojala, T., Pietikainen, M., & Maenpaa, T. (2002). Multiresolution gray-scale and rotation invariant texture classification with local binary patterns. *EEE Transactions on Pattern Analysis and Machine Intelligence, 24*(7), 971–987.
13. Arai, K., Abdullah, I. N., & Okumura, H. (2012). Automated detection method for clustered microcalcification in mammogram image based on statistical textural features. *International Journal of Advanced Research in Artificial Intelligence, 1*(3). https://doi.org/10.14569/IJARAI.2012.010304
14. Kim, J. K., & Park, H. W. (1999). Statistical textural features for detection of microcalcifications in digitized mammograms. *IEEE Transactions on Medical Imaging, 18*(3), 231–238.
15. Jothilakshmi, G. R., Raaza, A., Rajendran, V., Varma, S., & Guru Nirmal Raj, R. (2018). Pattern recognition and size prediction of microcalcification based on physical characteristics by using digital mammogram images. *Journal of Digital Imaging, 31*, 912–922.
16. Raajan, N. R., Vijayalakshmi, R., & Sangeetha, S. (2013). Analysis of malignant neoplastic using image processing techniques. *International Journal of Engineering and Technology, 5*(2), 1755–1762.
17. Dheeba, J., & Wiselin Jiji, G. (2010). Detection of microcalcification clusters in mammograms using neural network. *International Journal of Advanced Science and Technology, 19*, 13–22.
18. Jemila Rose, R., & Allwin, S. (2013). Computerized cancer detection and classification using ultrasound images. *International Journal of Engineering Research and Development, 5*, 36–47.
19. Qian, Z., Hua, G., Cheng, C., Tian, T., & Yun, L. (2005). Medical images edge detection based on mathematical morphology. *Engineering in Medicine and Biology*, 1–4.

Chapter 20
Contrast Enhancement of Digital Mammograms Based on High Contrast-Limited Adaptive Histogram Equalisation

K. K. Kavitha and A. Kangaiammal

20.1 Introduction

Medical image processing is the greatest solution for a variety of problems, especially in the medical industry [1]. Breast cancer is widely acknowledged to be the most important cause of casualty among women. Screening for cancer early in its development increases the likelihood that the disease can be successfully treated. Radiologists frequently employ mammography for the screening and diagnosis of breast cancer [2]. Due to the high volume of digital mammograms produced annually, accurate and rapid image interpretation is essential. Malignant tumours may go undiagnosed, whereas non-cancerous growths may be misdiagnosed. Therefore, radiologists overlook breast tumours anywhere from 10% to 30% [3].

The low exposure factors utilised in digital mammograms, on the other hand, result in low-contrast images. As a result, to enhance the current image quality, the image enrichment approach is required [4]. The existence of diverse elements inside an image is distinguished by contrast, which is an important characteristic of an image. Histogram equalisation is a generally employed technique for contrast improvement; however, it can sometimes have the unintended consequence of lowering image quality. The proposed histogram technique is used to solve this problem [5]. Preprocessing is a crucial stage in medical image processing that improves image quality [6]. Preprocessing aims to improve the quality of the mammography image by bringing out the details of the lesion location and making

K. K. Kavitha (✉)
Selvamm Arts and Science College (A), Namakkal, Tamil Nadu, India

A. Kangaiammal
Government Arts College (A), Salem, Tamil Nadu, India

F. J. J. Joseph et al. (eds.), *Computational Intelligence for Clinical Diagnosis*,
EAI/Springer Innovations in Communication and Computing,
https://doi.org/10.1007/978-3-031-23683-9_20

the image more visually appealing [7–9]. Thus, the accuracy of early breast cancer detection is much enhanced by the proposed preprocessing approaches for mammographic images.

20.2 Literature Review

For the clinical diagnosis of cancer, a range of image processing and preprocessing methods have been developed. Histogram equalisation [10, 11] is a posterior technique that produces an output image with a uniformly distributed probability distribution for each grey level by representing the input grey levels as a grey level compared to its cumulative density. The result is unnatural-looking, processed images due to the excessive contrast augmentation [12]. Low-contrast photos are improved using a variety of contrast enhancement techniques. The CLAHE is useful for increasing visual contrast. These strategies assist doctors and radiologists in making an accurate diagnosis of diseases as soon as possible [13].

An approach based on the Laplacian-Gaussian transform, morphology, and contrast-limited adaptive histogram equalisation is used to enrich mammographic images with features and contrast; this method employs penalty terms to regulate the various components of contrast enrichment [14]. As a result, the proposed strategy improves image contrast while also significantly reducing increased noise. The suggested system was evaluated on mammograms and compared to available methods such as histogram equalisation and adaptive histogram equalisation, as well as the wavelet transform and morphology-based method. In addition, the evaluated results demonstrate that the proposed strategy appears to be more appropriate for improving mammographic images in terms of both visual quality and qualitative estimation [15].

In this work, the proposed approach improves the picture contrast quality of the mammography in order to better view breast cancer. Histogram equalisation and a Gaussian filter are used to improve image contrast. According to the premise, the Naïve Bayes Classifier (NBC) approach is 90% accurate, whereas the K-Nearest Neighbor (KKN) method is 87.5% accurate. As a result, the mammography image contrast enhancement is excellent [16].

In this study, we use contrast-limited adaptive histogram equalisation (CLAHE) and an entropy-based fuzzy approach to increase the contrast of digital mammography images [17]. Using the publicly accessible Mammographic Image Analysis Society (MIAS) database, we perform qualitative, quantitative, and graphical analyses of the proposed method to compare it to type II fuzzy set-based strategies and determine its potential for improvement. The projected method produces superior visual quality, according to the findings of the experiments. In terms of subjective and quantitative criteria, it outperforms a variety of state-of-the-art algorithms [18].

Increasing the Contrast of a Picture and Providing a Unique Input to the Output Contrast Transfer Function Are Two Common Uses for Histogram Equalisation (HE) [19]. When Applied to an Image, HE Has a Flattening and Spreading Effect on the Histogram of the Number of Pixels at each Grey Level Value [20]. Sharing Histograms throughout the Local Window and Combining them with Global Histogram Distribution Is the most Crucial Part of Adaptive Histogram Equalisation (AHE) [21]. Unlike the Traditional HE Algorithm, the Modified CLAHE Approach Has Been Altered [22]. CLAHE Works by Redistributing the Brightness Values in an Image by First Generating a Set of Histograms, each of which Corresponds to a Different Slice of the Image [11, 23, 24]

20.3 Research Methodology

20.3.1 CLAHE

Contrast-limited adaptive histogram equalisation (CLAHE) is a variant of adaptive histogram equalisation (AHE). Instead of processing the whole image, CLAHE processes it into smaller, manageable chunks called tiles [25]. Bilinear interpolation is used to smooth out the tiles in the vicinity, effectively dissolving the illusion of borders. Using this method, image contrast can be enhanced [26].

Clip Limit – The contrast threshold can be adjusted here. The default value is 40.

Tile Grid Size – This is how we count the number of tiles in each row and column. By default, this is set to 88%. It's for using CLAHE on a tiling representation of a picture.

20.3.2 Proposed HCLAHE Method

The recommended and revised method is intended to enhance contrast and intensity in images. To do this, the image is first segmented into many non-overlapping regions of roughly the same size, and then a 3×3 mask is applied to each of these regions. The histogram should then be calculated for each region (Figs. 20.1 and 20.2).

The updated algorithm improves the image contrast and intensity. HCLAHE increases contrast across an image by adjusting the contrast of every pixel in relation to its immediate surroundings. This procedure improves the contrast in the original image at all levels of contrast. Histograms are deliberate for minute regional areas of pixels, providing local histograms for contrast adaptive histogram equalisation to boost local contrast [27]. Then a 3×3 mask for every region is included. The region size parameter determines how big the neighbour region is. Smaller regions can improve the contrast between smaller spatial scale structures. Lesions seem an obvious relative to the backdrop in digital mammograms produced with HCLAHE, and the image detail is excellent. The images, however, have a noticeable graininess. The algorithm's increased visibility of both image signal and noise causes graininess. Again, this approach could aid radiologists in detecting delicate edge information such as speculation.

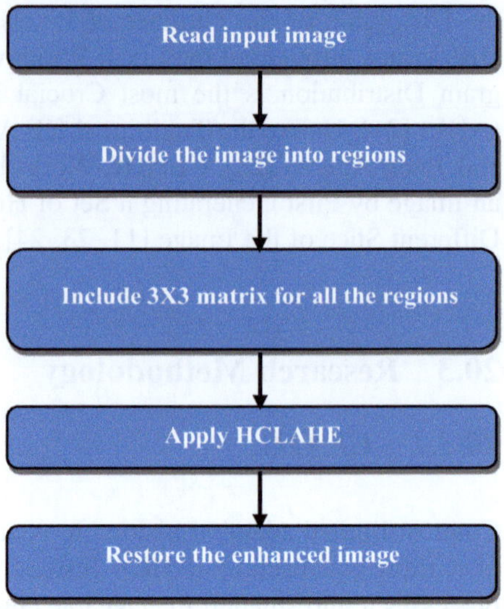

Fig. 20.1 The flow diagram of the proposed system

HCLAHE Algorithm

Step 1: Image-read

Step 2: Identify the histogram variable

Step 3: Split image into regions

Step 4: Every region needs a 3x3 mask.

Step 5: Calculate the intensity

Step 6: Restrengthen the image

Step7: Evaluate using MATLAB

Fig. 20.2 HCLAHE algorithm

20.3.3 Performance Criteria

Existing and prospective mammography image preprocessing methods are compared using two evaluation methods.

Parameters: These metrics measure image quality.

20.3.4 Absolute Mean Brightness Error (AMBE)

The AMBE is employed to assess how well a processed image retains its brightness [28].

AMBE is defined as

$$\text{AMBE}(X, Y) = \mid X_M - Y_M \mid$$

where X_M denotes the input image's average brightness $X = \{x(i, j)\}$ and Y_M denotes the output image's average brightness $Y = \{Y(i, j)\}$.

20.3.5 Entropy

Entropy is a metric for determining how rich the features in the output image are. Entropy: The probability density function (PDF) p [29].

$$\text{Entropy } [p] = -\sum k = 0 \text{ to } L - 1\ p(Xk)\ \log 2\ p(Xk),$$

where $p(Xk)$ is the probability mass function of the picture histogram.

20.4 Dataset

20.4.1 Image Acquisition

This study improves CLAHE to boost image intensity. Mammography case samples were gathered from MIAS [30]. MIAS is a UK research consortium that has built a digital mammography database. It includes 3,221,024 × 1024 mammography photos, such as the type of cancer and severity of the diagnosis.

20.5 Experimental Results

The digital mammograms employed in the projected methodology are obtained from the MIAS database, which includes a different group of images for cancer abnormalities. To determine the degree of brightness preservation, AMBE is used. Based on AMBE, brightness preservation is compared using distinct methods such as HE, AHE, CLAHE, and the proposed high contrast-limited adaptive histogram equalisation. However, the results obtained for the ten images are presented here for better visualisation and understanding. Table 20.1 shows the AMBE value is

Table 20.1 AMBE of different histogram techniques

Image	AMBE			
ID	HE	AHE	CLAHE	HCLAHE
mdb001	39.85	35.34	31.9	26.77
mdb002	45.21	42.78	37.7	31.98
mdb003	52.65	49.24	47.34	41.65
mdb004	42.78	40.19	39.52	34.03
mdb005	58.34	57.26	55.23	44.56
mdb006	37.45	35.11	33.05	29.92
mdb007	49.82	45.7	42.6	34.56
mdb008	55.32	52.61	50.4	30.05
mdb009	41.54	40.07	38.31	33.21
mdb010	53.83	51.47	49.2	31.56

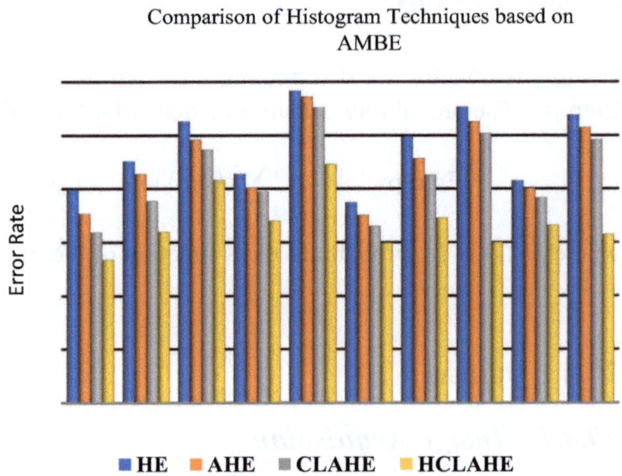

Fig. 20.3 Comparisons of histogram techniques (AMBE)

minimum and consistently reduced compared to the existing techniques HE, AHE, and CLAHE. The AMBE, which is the dissimilarity between the average initial image intensity and the resulting image, has a lower value where it is necessary to preserve brightness. It is portrayed in Table 20.1 and Fig. 20.3.

The histogram and the optimising entropy theory have the same purpose of preserving as much information as possible. Entropy in a random variable is the indicator of uncertainty. The purpose of any histogram is to collect as much data as possible from the information, which is the task of maximising entropy. To improve the accuracy of the estimation of conjunctive predicates, a maximum entropy method is employed. The main aim of this observation is that the maximisation of histograms and entropy has the same purpose of optimising knowledge. The HCLAHE entropy values are compared with the existing methods such as HE, AHE, and CLAHE. That has been depicted in Table 20.2 and Fig. 20.3. The challenge of noise enhancement is solved by HCLAHE used in the proposed technique.

Table 20.2 Entropy of different histogram

Image	Entropy			
ID	HE	AHE	CLAHE	HCLAHE
mdb001	0.04	0.05	0.09	0.13
mdb002	0.18	0.16	0.12	0.19
mdb003	0.13	0.15	0.19	0.28
mdb004	0.19	0.2	0.25	0.39
mdb005	0.22	0.24	0.3	0.37
mdb006	0.15	0.16	0.11	0.18
mdb007	0.08	0.09	0.14	0.21
mdb008	0.19	0.21	0.25	0.39
mdb009	0.14	0.15	0.17	0.22
mdb010	0.21	0.2	0.23	0.26

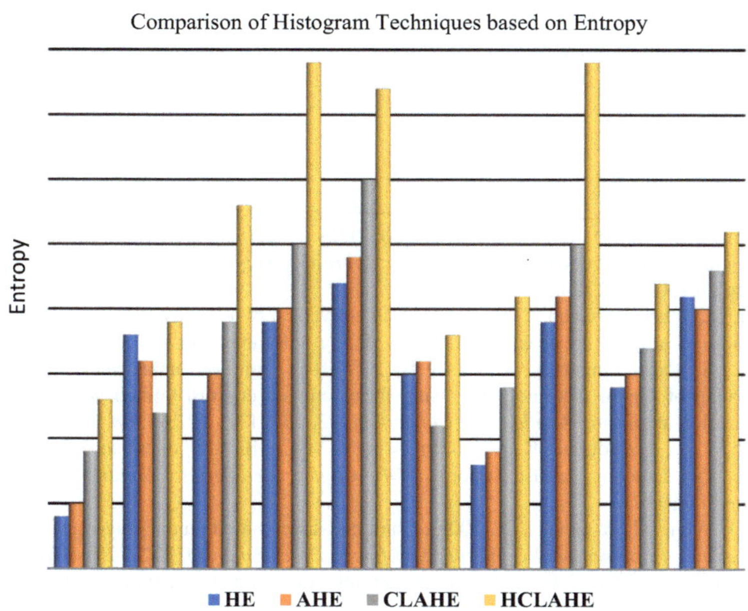

Fig. 20.4 Comparison of entropy techniques

As shown in Fig. 20.4, when compared to the HE, AHE, and CLAHE, our proposed HCLAHE method demonstrates outperformance. On average, HCLAHE processes contain the largest amount of data. Due to its highest entropy value range of 0.13 to 0.39, in the output image, the richness and detailed information can be well kept.

20.6 Conclusion

This publication proposes a high contrast-limited adaptive histogram equalisation picture enhancing technique for mammograms. Experiments suggest the proposed technique can enhance digital mammography contrast. This study shows how to boost entropy to extract more information from variables and improve mammogram viewing. The recommended HCLAHE enhances contrast while keeping local image data. This study evaluates absolute mean brightness error and entropy using the HCLAHE image processing platform. The results are better without losing contrast or data integrity. Compared to the previous methods, the suggested method improves contrast. HCLAHE is optimal for enhancing contrast in fatty, fatty-glandular, and dense-glandular mammograms. Its effectiveness is evaluated for all MIAS mammography pictures. This research could be explored to test how well it works on noisy mammograms and as a preprocessing step to discover micro-calcification. It works for coloured images.

References

1. Hesamian, M. H., Jia, W., He, X., et al. (2019). Deep learning techniques for medical image segmentation: Achievements and challenges. *Journal of Digital Imaging, 32*, 582–596. https://doi.org/10.1007/s10278-019-00227-x
2. Tabár, L., Vitak, B., Chen, T. H., et al. (2011). Swedish two-county trial: Impact of mammographic screening on breast cancer mortality during 3 decades. *Radiology, 260*, 658–663.
3. Jenifer, S., Parasuraman, S., & Kadirvelu, A. (2016). Contrast enhancement and brightness preserving of digital mammograms using fuzzy clipped contrast-limited adaptive histogram equalization algorithm. *Applied Soft Computing, 42*, 167–177. ISSN 1568–4946.
4. Suradi, S. H., & Abdullah, K. A. (2021). Using FC-CLAHE-ADF to enhance digital mammograms for detecting breast lesions. *IOP Conference Series: Materials Science and Engineering*, 1173.
5. Van De Weijer, J., & Gevers, T. (2005). Color constancy based on the grayedge hypothesis. In *Proceeding of International Conference on Image Processing* (pp. 722–725). ICIP.
6. Makandar, A., & Halalli, B. (2017). Mammography image enhancement using linear, nonlinear and wavelet filters with histogram equalization. *International Journal of Computer (IJC), 25*(1), 8–17.
7. Rahmati, P., et al. (2010). A new preprocessing filter for digital mammograms. In *International Conference on Image and Signal Processing*. Springer Berlin Heidelberg.
8. Dehghani, S., & Dezfooli, M. A. (2011). A method for improve preprocessing images mammography. *International Journal of Information and Education Technology, 1.1*, 90.
9. Maitra, I. K., Nag, S., & Bandyopadhyay, S. K. (2012). Technique for preprocessing of digital mammogram. *Computer Methods and Programs in Biomedicine, 107*(2), 175–188.
10. Pisano, E. D., Cole, E. B., Hemminger, B. M., Yaffe, M. J., Aylward, S. R., Maidment, A. D. A., Johnston, R. E., et al. (2000). Image processing algorithms for digital mammography: A pictorial essay 1. *Radiographics, 20*(5), 1479–1491.
11. Pisano, E. D., Zong, S., Hemminger, B. M., DeLuca, M., Johnston, R. E., Muller, K., Braeuning, M. P., & Pizer, S. M. (1998). Contrast limited adaptive histogram equalization image processing to improve the detection of simulated spiculations in dense mammograms. *Journal of Digital Imaging, 11*(4), 193–200.

12. Sundaram, M., Ramar, K., Arumugam, N., & Prabin, G. (2011). Histogram based contrast enhancement for mammogram images. In *Signal Processing, Communication, Computing and Networking Technologies (ICSCCN), 2011 International Conference on* (pp. 842–846). IEEE.
13. Makandar, A., & Halalli, B. (2015, April). Breast cancer image enhancement using median filter and CLAHE. *International Journal of Scientific & Engineering Research, 6*(4).
14. Namdeo, A., & Bhadoriya, S. S. (2016, May). A review on image enhancement techniques with its advantages and disadvantages. *IJSART, 2*(5).
15. Wu, S., Yu, S., Yang, Y., & Xie, Y. (2013). Feature and contrast enhancement of mammographic image based on multiscale analysis and morphology. *Hindawi Computational and Mathematical Methods in Medicine*, 716948, 8 pages.
16. Liantoni, F., Sukmagautama, C., & Myrtha, R. (2020). Increased mammogram image contrast using histogram equalization and gaussian in the classification of breast cancer. *Journal of Information Technology and Computer Engineering, 04*(01), 40–44.
17. Fan, R., Li, X., Lee, S., Li, T., & Zhang, H. L. (2020). Smart image enhancement using CLAHE based on an F-shift transformation during decompression. *Electronics, 9*, 1374. https://doi.org/10.3390/electronics9091374
18. Dabass, J., Arora, S., Vig, R., & Hanmandlu, M. (2019). Mammogram image enhancement using entropy and CLAHE based intuitionistic fuzzy method. In *6th Internwational Conference on Signal Processing and Integrated Networks (SPIN)* (p. 24). IEEE.
19. Ali, S. S. E., & Dildar, S. A. (2020). An efficient quality inspection of food products using neural network classification. *Journal of Intelligent Systems, 29*(1), 1425–1440.
20. Christian, S. (2011). *Analysis of contrast enhancement methods for infrared images*. Master. Thesis, Faculty of California Polytechnic State University.
21. Singh, P., Mukundan, R., & De Ryke, R. (2020). Feature enhancement in medical ultrasound videos using contrast-limited adaptive histogram equalization. *Journal of Digital Imaging, 33*(1), 273–285.
22. Maurya, L., Lohchab, V., Mahapatra, P. K., & Abonyi, J. (2021). Contrast and brightness balance in image enhancement using Cuckoo Search-optimized image fusion. *Journal of King Saud University – Computer and Information Sciences*.
23. Zuiderveld, K. (1994). *Contrast limited adaptive histogram equalization*. Academic Press.
24. Jintasuttisak, T., & Intajag, S. (2014). Color retinex image enhancement by Rayleigh contrast limited histogram equalization. *International Conference on Control, Automation and Systems, 10*, 692–697.
25. Campos, G., Mastelini, S., Aguiar, G., et al. (2019). Machine learning hyperparameter selection for contrast limited adaptive histogram equalization. *Journal on Image and Video Processing, 2019*(59).
26. Dhamodharan, S., & Shanmugavadivu, P. (2018, May). Brightness preserving contrast enhancement of digital mammogram using modified-dualistic sub-image histogram equalization. *International Journal of Computer Sciences and Engineering, 6*(Special Issue-4).
27. Liu, C., Sui, X., Kuang, X., Liu, Y., Guohua, G., & Chen, Q. (2019). Adaptive contrast enhancement for infrared images based on the neighborhood conditional histogram. *Remote Sens, 11*, 1381.
28. Mzoughi, H., Njeh, I., Ben Slima, M., Ben Hamida, A., Mhiri, C., & Ben, M. K. (2019). Denoising and contrast-enhancement approach of magnetic resonance imaging glioblastoma brain tumors. *Journal of Medical Imaging (Bellingham), 6*(4), 044002. https://doi.org/10.1117/1.JMI.6.4.044002
29. Li, P. (2019). EZ Entropy: A software application for the entropy analysis of physiological time-series. *Biomedical Engineering Online, 18*, 30.
30. Anand, S., Murugachandravel, J., Valarmathi, K., Mano, A., & Kavitha, N. (2019, November). Contrast enhancement of mammograms and microcalcification detection. *International Journal of Recent Technology and Engineering*, ISSN: 2277-3878,, *8*(4).

Chapter 21
A Pipelined Framework for the Prediction of Cardiac Disease with Dimensionality Reduction

G. Shobana and Nalini Subramanian

21.1 Introduction

Heart disease is a non-contiguous health problem that disturbs enormous numbers of humans around the world without exhibiting any initial symptoms. There are numerous types of heart diseases. Congestive cardiac failure is commonly called heart failure. Due to heart failure, the body's requirement for oxygen is not sufficiently met. Atherosclerosis occurs when there is a block in the arteries. Sometimes, blood clot formation occurs that interrupts the normal flow of the heart blood. Cardiac stroke may be the result of this condition. When there is an irregular rhythm of the heart, then the condition is termed arrhythmia. A heartbeat rate of fewer than 60 beats per minute, which is slow, is known as bradycardia, while a heartbeat rate of 100 beats per minute, which are fast, is known as tachycardia. Stenosis is a condition that arises due to improper functioning of the valves of the heart. Other heart diseases occur due to genetic and birth deformities [1]. 805,000 US people were found to have a heart attack every year. An unhealthy diet and an inactive lifestyle are the main reasons for a heart attack [2]. Various examinations are conducted on the affected patients to determine the cause of the occurrence of the disease. Diagnostic tests and advanced procedures accurately identify and classify the disease. Manual analysis of the large population of affected patients becomes a major challenge for physicians. Machine learning is the perfect technique to be employed to classify healthy and unhealthy patients. In this paper, all the conventional and ensemble machine learning algorithms were applied to the heart disease-related dataset,

G. Shobana (✉)
Department of Computer Applications, Madras Christian College, Chennai, Tamil Nadu, India

N. Subramanian
Department of Information Technology, Rajalakshmi Engineering College, Thandalam, Tamil Nadu, India

F. J. J. Joseph et al. (eds.), *Computational Intelligence for Clinical Diagnosis*, EAI/Springer Innovations in Communication and Computing,
https://doi.org/10.1007/978-3-031-23683-9_21

obtained from The University of California Irvine (UCI) open repository with 1025 observations and 14 attributes, using Scikit learn [3]. The training and the testing data were taken in the ratio of 70:30. Three hundred eight samples were used for the testing. By implementing the proposed methodology, random forest (RF) achieved a high and perfect prediction accuracy of 100%, and extreme gradient boosting achieved an accuracy of 99.02%. Another significant advantage of this methodology is that it efficiently manages the overfitting problem.

21.2 Related Work

The World Health Organization (WHO) reports state that approximately 17.9 million humans across the earth die due to heart ailments or cardiovascular diseases (CVDs) [4]. High cholesterol levels, lack of exercise, diabetes, smoking, and obesity are some of the factors that contribute to the development of this disease. In the past several decades, there has been a significant rise in cardiac diseases among the Indian urban population. The annual death rate due to cardiovascular diseases is around 4.77 million in 2020 and is expected to rise in the coming years [5]. The major factors that cause CVDs in India are the consumption of alcohol and excessive use of tobacco products. The other factors include hypertension and diabetes. 80% of CVD-related deaths occur in developing countries [6].

Savita et al. [7]. analyzed the performance of six machine learning methods like support vector machine (SVM), decision tree, multilayer perceptron, linear regression, naïve Bayes, and K-nearest neighbor (KNN). They performed K-fold cross-validation with 5 and 10. They investigated Switzerland, Hungarian, and Cleveland datasets from the UCI repository. They concluded that SVM and KNN performed better than other models.

Saumendra et al. [8] classified cardiac disease using support vector machines. They drew the Cleveland heart disease dataset from the UCI repository. They took 303 observations with 13 attributes for the experiment, and the training-testing ratio was 90:10. They investigated the performance of four types of SVM polynomial kernels, RBF, linear, polynomial and sigmoid with the dataset. They found that SVM with a polynomial kernel achieved a higher accuracy of 87.5%.

Deepak Kumar et al. [9] identified non-contagious heart disease using three supervised machine learning techniques, SVM, RF, and KNN, with ten-fold cross-validation. They used a South African dataset for heart diseases and found that RF achieved a high accuracy of 95%.

Hiteshwar et al. [10] compared the performance of naïve Bayes, K-nearest neighbor, and random forest on the Cleveland and Starlog dataset obtained from the open UCI repository. Random forest achieved higher accuracy than the other two models with 93.02%, while KNN and naïve Bayes achieved 90.69% and 83.72% of prediction accuracy.

Muhammad Saqib Nawaz et al. [11] have predicted cardiovascular diseases using the gradient descent optimization (GDO) technique. This method has achieved an accuracy of 99.43%. They performed a detailed study and found that random forest achieved an accuracy of 90.16%. Boosting algorithms and extreme machine learning technique obtained 92.45%. Kernel-based support vector obtained 93.33%. Fuzzy systems achieved 94.50%, while advanced neural networks produced 83.67%, and the gradient descent optimization method obtained 98.54%.

Sibo et al. [12] proposed a novel optimized algorithm to predict cardiac disease. They utilized the heart disease dataset from the UCI repository. They explored ML models like naïve Bayes, KNN, Bayesian optimized SVM (BO-SVM), and salp swarm optimized neural network (SSA-NN). BO-SVM achieved a higher accuracy of 93.3%, while SSA-NN produced an accuracy of 86.7%.

Dengqing zhang et al. [13] predicted cardiac disease using their proposed model, which achieved an accuracy of 98.56%. They proposed a methodology that incorporated linear support vector classifier (SVC) with feature selection technique and obtained the dataset from Kaggle [14].

Rohit et al. [15] predicted heart disease by exploring various machine learning algorithms like random forest, conventional decision tree, logistic regression (LR), boosting algorithms like XGBoost, kernel-based support vector machine, and optimized deep learning techniques. They used the heart disease dataset with 14 attributes from the UCI open repository. They achieved 94.2% accuracy by implementing a deep learning technique.

Women in the postmenopausal stage are also likely to have heart failure. Machine learning approaches can be efficiently used to diagnose the occurrence of heart failure [16]. Chayakrit et al. [17] predicted cardiovascular diseases and investigated various ML models. They concluded that SVM and boosting algorithms performed well with more than 92% prediction accuracy.

21.3 Proposed Methodology

21.3.1 Attribute Description and Dataset

The cardiac or heart disease dataset was obtained from the UCI open and vast repository with 1025 instances and 14 features. There were 499 samples with class 0 in the target feature and 526 samples with class 1 in the target feature. The binary classification classifies the patients with and without heart disease. The features define the age, sex (male 1, female 0), type of chest pain, blood pressure, blood sugar while fasting, level of serum cholesterol, other cardiac parameters during exercise, and information on major vessels.

21.3.2 Proposed Framework

Several researchers have employed varieties of procedures to classify heart disease. Both data and images were used in the medical field for classification and prediction purposes. The proposed methodology has four major phases, namely, the acquisition of the dataset from the repository, pre-processing, designing an efficient pipeline, and selecting the best model.

Procedure:

Step 1: Acquire the cardiac disease dataset from the UCI repository.
Step 2: Pre-processing involves identifying missing values and filling them.
Step 3: Create a pipeline that performs three different steps.

- Normalize the data since the data might fall into different ranges.
- Apply feature extraction technique kernel PCA and select the important features.
- Apply conventional, ensemble, and boosting algorithms to the dataset.

Step 4: Compare and observe the result of all the pipelines.
Step 5: Select the best performing machine learning model.

The proposed methodology is given in Fig. 21.1. The structured pipeline helps to overcome data leakage. The pipeline with ensemble technique, random forest, produces 100% prediction accuracy compared to other machine learning models. Among the boosting algorithms, extreme gradient boosting achieved the highest accuracy of 99.02%.

21.4 Results

With the proposed methodology, random forest obtained the perfect prediction accuracy of 100%. The dataset was split into 70% for training and 30% for testing, respectively. Figure 21.2 shows the output generated by the random forest classifier.

The parameters used for the kernel PCA were n_components = 2, Kernel = 'rbf', and gamma = 0.01. The ideal accuracy score of 100% was attained when a pipeline was set up with a scaling of the data, followed by the feature extraction process of kernel PCA and then applying random forest. Figure 21.3 shows the confusion matrix where the diagonal elements were the correctly identified elements 145 and 163, respectively, while there were no misclassified elements. Figure 21.4 shows the training and testing accuracy. Figure 21.5 shows the receiver operating characteristic (ROC) curve generated by random forest.

The boosting algorithms also produced high prediction accuracy above 94%, with the XGBoost classifier achieving 99.02% accuracy as shown in Fig. 21.6. Figure 21.7 shows the confusion matrix of the XGBoost classifier where 145 and 160 are correctly classified elements, while 3 elements were misclassified. Light gradient boosting machine classifier obtained 98% accuracy.

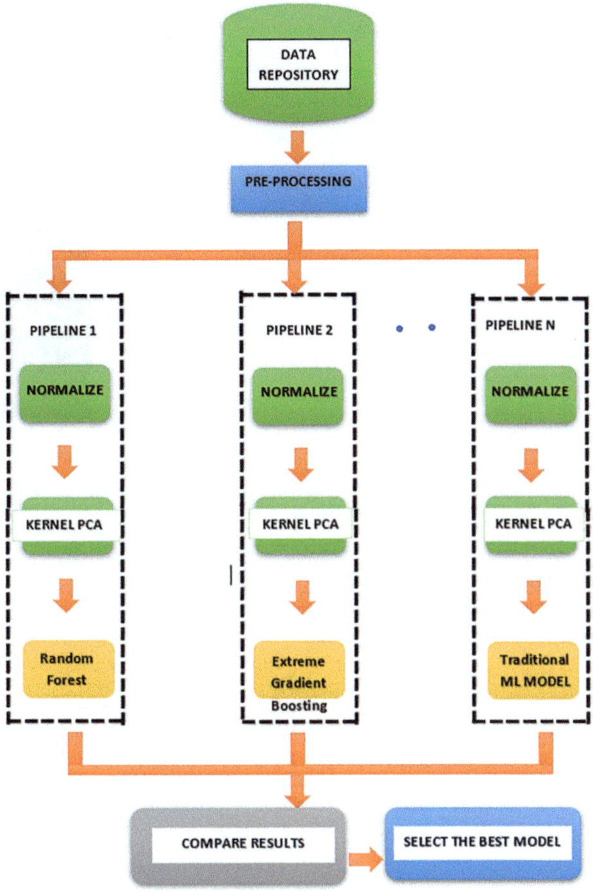

Fig. 21.1 Proposed methodology

```
Test Accuracy: 1.000
              precision    recall  f1-score   support

           0       1.00      1.00      1.00       145
           1       1.00      1.00      1.00       163

    accuracy                           1.00       308
   macro avg       1.00      1.00      1.00       308
weighted avg       1.00      1.00      1.00       308

[[145   0]
 [  0 163]]
accuracy is 1.0
Accuracy on training set: 1.000
Accuracy on test set: 1.000
```

Fig. 21.2 Output generated by random forest

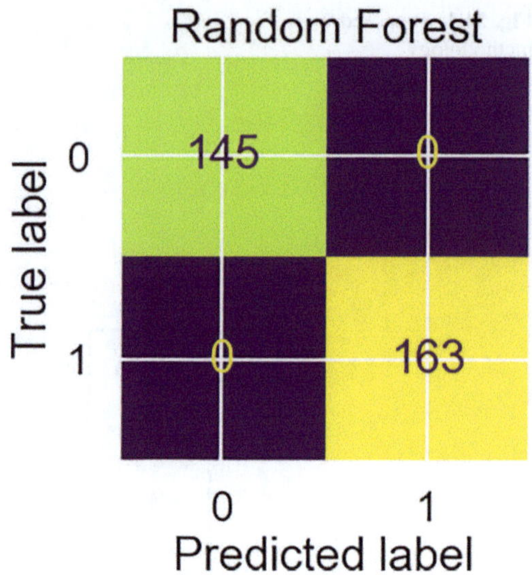

Fig. 21.3 Confusion matrix generated by random forest

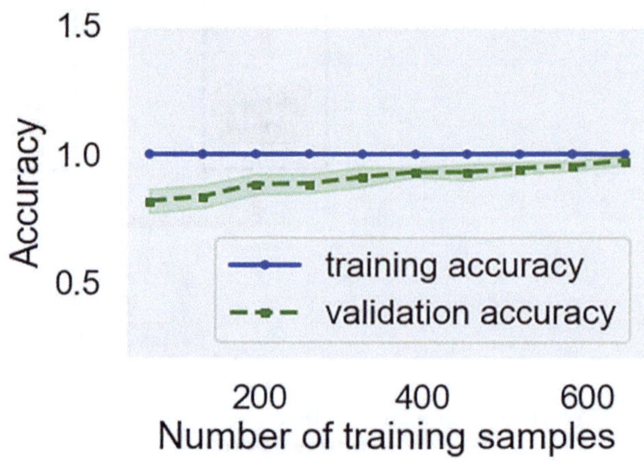

Fig. 21.4 Training and testing accuracy by random forest

Figure 21.8 shows the training and testing accuracy generated by the XGBoost classifier. The curve clearly shows that the proposed methodology has overcome the issue of overfitting. Figure 21.9 shows the ROC generated by the XGBoost classifier.

Figure 21.10 shows the accuracy obtained by the machine learning models applied to the dataset. From the bar chart, it is understood that random forest and the boosting algorithms perform better compared to other models.

Table 21.1 shows various machine learning methods and their metrics. It is also observed that the training and testing have been performed efficiently without overfitting problems. Various metrics like precision, recall, and F1-score were computed for the models. Table 21.2 shows the prediction accuracies of the boosting algorithms. All the boosting algorithms perform well with prediction accuracies above 94%, while XGBoost achieved the highest with over 99%.

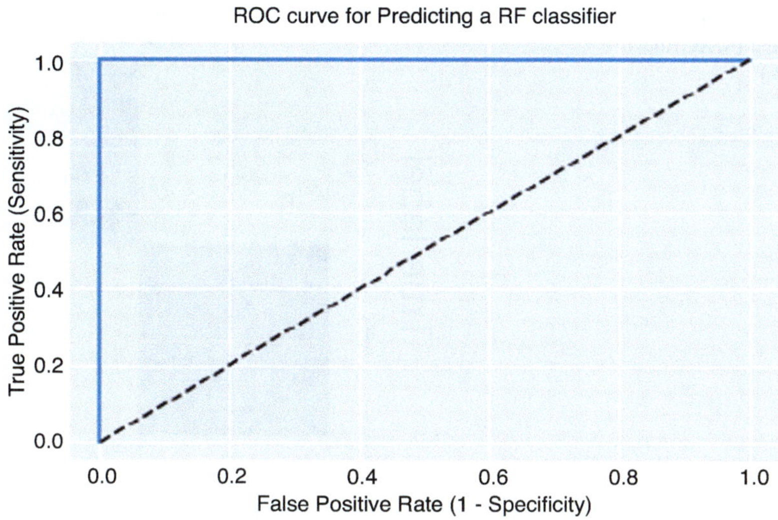

Fig. 21.5 ROC curve by random forest

```
Test Accuracy: 0.990
              precision    recall  f1-score   support

           0       0.98      1.00      0.99       145
           1       1.00      0.98      0.99       163

    accuracy                           0.99       308
   macro avg       0.99      0.99      0.99       308
weighted avg       0.99      0.99      0.99       308

[[145   0]
 [  3 160]]
accuracy is 0.9902597402597403
Accuracy on training set: 1.000
Accuracy on test set: 0.990
```

Fig. 21.6 Output generated by XGBoost classifier

21.4.1 Comparative Study

Several researchers have explored different datasets of heart diseases from the vast and open UCI repository. Cleveland, Long Beach, VA, Starlog, Switzerland, and Hungarian datasets are the popular datasets. In this paper, we have drawn the heart disease dataset from the UCI repository with 1025 observations and 14 features. Figure 21.11 compares the result produced by other researchers and our proposed methodology.

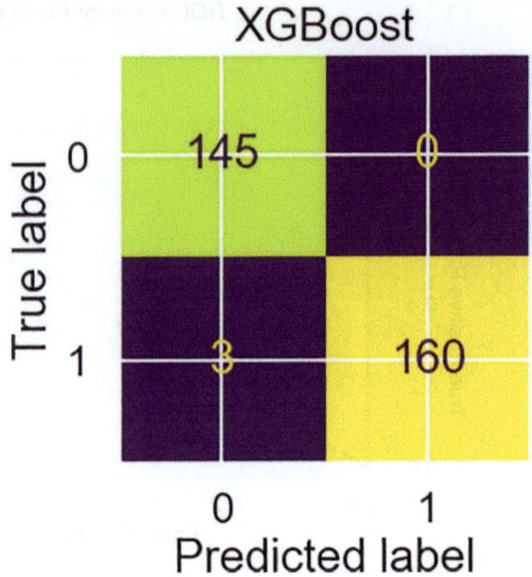

Fig. 21.7 Confusion matrix generated by XGBoost classifier

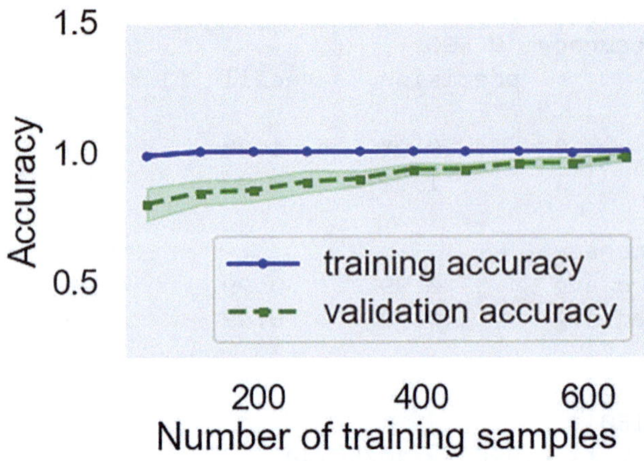

Fig. 21.8 Training and testing accuracy by XGBoost classifier

The researchers have incorporated several techniques like reduction feature elimination, principal component analysis, Pearson correlation, gradient descent optimization, and Lasso regularization to enhance the prediction accuracy. They explored the efficient computation of machine learning algorithms like support vector machines, random forest, M5P, neural networks, reduced error pruning, and other traditional and boosting classifiers. They achieved a maximum prediction accuracy of 99%. The proposed methodology has produced a higher prediction accuracy of 100%, as shown in Fig. 21.11. Random forest obtained the accurate result, while extreme boosting machine (XGBoost) achieved an accuracy of 90.06%.

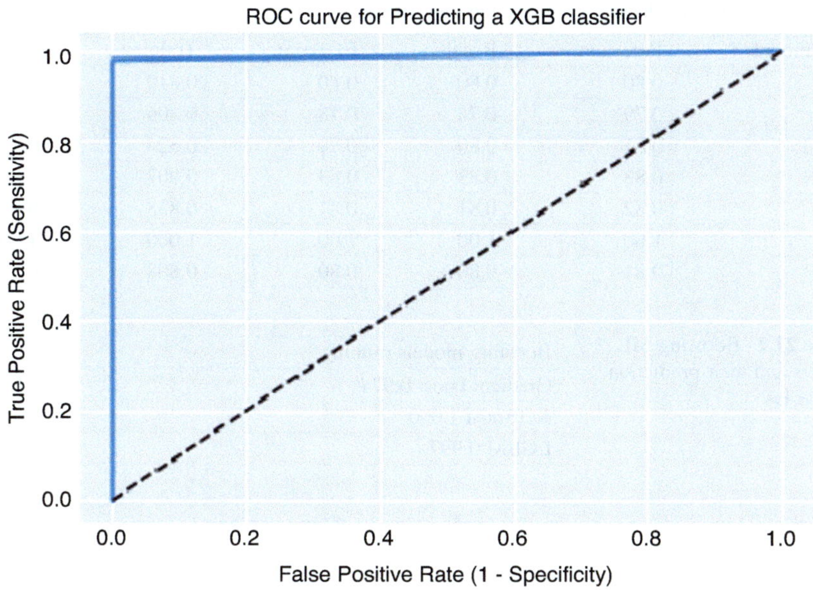

Fig. 21.9 ROC curve by XGBoost classifier

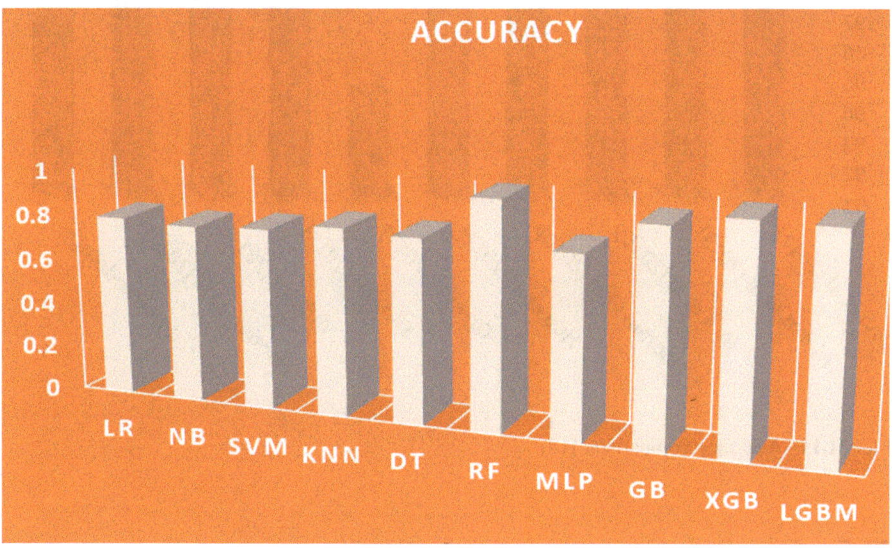

Fig. 21.10 Accuracy obtained by ML models

Table 21.1 Machine learning models and their metrics

ML models	Precision	Recall	F1-score	Training	Testing
LR	0.80	0.80	0.80	0.810	0.795
NB	0.79	0.78	0.78	0.806	0.782
SVM	0.81	0.80	0.79	0.824	0.795
KNN	0.83	0.83	0.83	0.907	0.828
DT	0.82	0.81	0.81	0.838	0.812
RF	1.00	1.00	1.00	1.000	1.000
MLP	0.81	0.80	0.80	0.808	0.802

Table 21.2 Boosting ML models and their prediction accuracies

Boosting models training	Testing
Gradient boost 0.974	0.942
XGBoost 1.000	0.990
LGBM 0.997	0.984

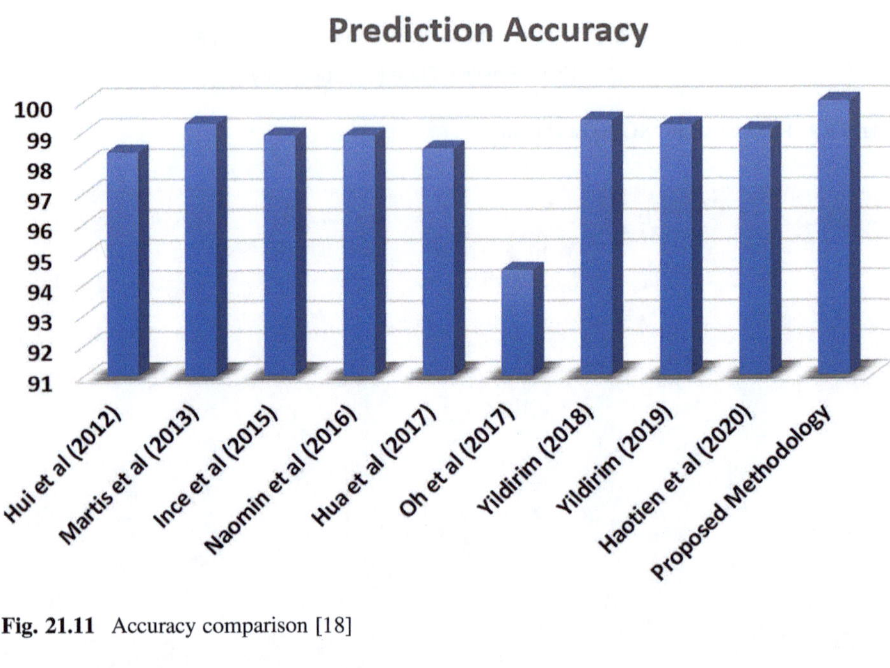

Fig. 21.11 Accuracy comparison [18]

21.5 Conclusion

Cardiovascular diseases affect enormous numbers of people across the world regardless of age. A sedentary lifestyle with high calorie-based food intake is one of the main causes or reasons for this disease. Identification of this disease at an early stage is most challenging, and manual examination of patient history is very tedious and might not produce accurate prediction results. Researchers have explored several machine learning techniques and optimization methodologies to enhance prediction accuracy. In this paper, we have proposed an efficient methodology that accurately classified the cardiac dataset, while other methodologies produced a maximum accuracy of 99%. This technique has proved efficient with a comprehensive dataset. Future work might involve large datasets and other novel ensemble and hybrid methodologies. The performance of this methodology with another similar type of disease dataset may be investigated.

References

1. www.heart.org/en/health-topics/consumer-healthcare
2. www.cdc.gov/heartdisease
3. https://scikit-learn.org
4. www.who.int/health-topics
5. Huffman, M. D., Prabhakaran, D., Osmond, C., Fall, C. H., Tandon, N., Lakshmy, R., Ramji, S., Khalil, A., Gera, T., Prabhakaran, P., Biswas, S. K., Reddy, K. S., Bhargava, S. K., Sachdev, H. S., & Cohort, N. D. B. (2011, April 26). Incidence of cardiovascular risk factors in an Indian urban cohort results from the New Delhi birth cohort. *Journal of the American College of Cardiology, 57*(17), 1765–1774. https://doi.org/10.1016/j.jacc.2010.09.083
6. https://world-heart-federation.org/wp-content
7. Wadhawan, & Maini. (2021). Performance analysis of machine learning techniques for predicting cardiac disease. In *2021 6th International Conference on Communication and Electronics Systems (ICCES)* (pp. 1625–1630).
8. Mohapatra, S. B., & Mohanty, M. N. (2020). A comparative analysis of cardiac data classification using support vector machine with various kernels. In *2020 International Conference on Communication and Signal Processing (ICCSP)* (pp. 515–519).
9. Kumar, D., Verma, C., Gupta, A., Raboaca, M. S., & Bakariya, B. (2021). Detection of cardiac disease and association with family history using machine learning. In *2021 10th International Conference on System Modeling & Advancement in Research Trends (SMART)* (pp. 670–675).
10. Singh, H., Gupta, T., & Sidhu, J. (2021). Prediction of heart disease using machine learning techniques. In *2021 Sixth International Conference on Image Information Processing (ICIIP)* (pp. 164–169). https://doi.org/10.1109/ICIIP53038.2021.9702625.
11. Nawaz, M. S., Shoaib, B., & Ashraf, M. A. (2021). *Intelligent cardiovascular disease prediction empowered with gradient descent optimization* (Vol. 7, p. e06948). Heliyon.
12. Patro, S. P., Gouri, S. N., & Padhy, N. (2021). Heart disease prediction by using novel optimization algorithm: A supervised learning prospective. *Informatics in Medicine Unlocked, 26*, 100696. ISSN 2352-9148.
13. Xiaoqing, G., Zhang, D., Yunyi, C., Yuxuan, C., Shengyi, Y., Wenyu, C., Jiang Junxue, X., Yechuan, Z. G., & Ming, C. (2021). Heart disease prediction based on the embedded feature selection method and deep neural network. *Journal of Healthcare Engineering, Hindawi, 6260022*, 2040–2295.
14. https://www.kaggle.com/johnsmith88/heart-disease-dataset

15. Abd, E.-L. A., Rohit, B., Aditya, K., Mohammad, S., Gaurav, D., Sagar, P., & Parneet, S. (2021). Prediction of heart disease using a combination of machine learning and deep learning. In *Computational Intelligence and Neuroscience, Hindawi* (Vol. 8387680, pp. 1687–5265). https://doi.org/10.1155/2021/8387680.
16. Tison, G. H., Avram, R., Nah, G., Klein, L., Howard, B. V., Allison, M. A., Casanova, R., Blair, R. H., Breathett, K., Foraker, R. E., Olgin, J. E., & Parikh, N. I. (2021, November). Predicting incident heart failure in women with machine learning: The women's health initiative Cohort. *The Canadian Journal of Cardiology, 37*(11), 1708–1714.
17. Krittanawong., Virk, H.U.H., Bangalore, S., et al. (2020). Machine learning prediction in cardiovascular diseases: A meta-analysis. *Scientific Reports, 10*, 16057. https://doi.org/10.1038/s41598-020-72685-1
18. Yadav, D., & Pal, S. (2020). Prediction of heart disease using feature selection and random forest ensemble method. *International Journal for Pharmaceutical Research Scholars, 12*, 56–66. https://doi.org/10.31838/ijpr/2020.12.04.013

Chapter 22
Dispensable Microsystem Technology for Cancer Diagnosis

S. Prasath Alias Surendhar, V. Sowmiya, and R. Sandhiya

22.1 Introduction

According to a population survey, 20% of cancer patients have breast cancer, which is significantly more common than other cancer diagnoses. This may be the most important, delicate, and accurate kind of diagnostic [1]. The mechanical stiffness of breast tissues is the primary biological tool for identifying and researching breast cancer-causing tissues. The elasticity of this feature correlates inversely with the development of cancer cells. The exterior matrix of the cell aids in the connection between the genetic propensity toward tumour growth and the proteins over the matrix, but with there, breast cancer tissues were recognized. According to numerous studies, the outer layer and its elasticity vary between healthy tissue and cancerous tissue. Regular studies on the characteristics of breast cancer cells can help diagnosis by revealing more information. Techniques are vital to ensuring the approximation of the presence of cancer cells in the breast tissues. At the same time, calculating the characteristics of the cancer cells is very few in the progression of research. All bodily areas, both genders, and all ages are affected by cancer. According to statistics, breast cancer was the most prevalent cancer globally in 2014, with death rates being higher in low- and middle-income nations [2]. It is the main global factor in both cancer death and morbidity for females. With an expected 5.3 million new

S. P. A. Surendhar (✉) · R. Sandhiya
Department of Biomedical Engineering, Aarupadai Veedu Institute of Technology, Chennai, Tamil Nadu, India
e-mail: sandhiya.bme@avit.ac.in

V. Sowmiya
Department of Biomedical Engineering, Bharath Institute of Higher Education and Research, Chennai, Tamil Nadu, India

F. J. Joseph et al. (eds.), *Computational Intelligence for Clinical Diagnosis*,
EAI/Springer Innovations in Communication and Computing,
https://doi.org/10.1007/978-3-031-23683-9_22

cases per year, female breast cancer has just eclipsed liver cancer as the most frequently diagnosed cancer [3].

The unchecked growth and division of cells in breast tissue is the basis of breast cancer. Anatomical sites of origin are often used to give cancer its name. The two primary forms of breast tissue are gland tissues and stromal (supportive) tissues. Meanwhile, secretory tissues house the mammary glands (lobules) accompanying channels, whereas stromal tissues consist of the fatty and fibrous connective tissues of the breast [4, 5]. Lymphatic tissue, part of the immune system, is also present in the breast [3]. This tissue drains away waste products and biological fluids.

It is important to note that different types of breast tumors can manifest in a variety of areas. Malignant breast tumors in women are typically brought on by perfectly harmless genetic mutations. Dysplastic change is a noncancerous condition that can cause lumps, thickened areas, discomfort, and sometimes pain in the breasts of women [6–8]. Cancers of the breast typically begin in the lining cells of the ducts. Some cancers (ventricular tumors) begin in the cells that make up the glomeruli [9, 10], but others (the vast majority) arise in other organs. Micro-electro-mechanical systems (MEMS) can range within a small number of microns with mechanical and electrical characteristics. The equipment based upon the MEMS is said to be applicable as sensors or actuators [11]. They are also adjustable and more applicable in the biomedical field. At a very low scale of the activity of the sensor, the cells of the breast are analyzed and palpated with the help of their elasticity, i.e., micro- and nanoscale [12]. The MEMS sensor can be incorporated into the lab on chip devices for the diagnosis. It needs more care, although the MEMS sensor connects with the atmosphere to send and interrelate [13, 14].

Sixty percent of individuals receiving access to health services are women with thick breasts [15]. In these situations, it is less sensitive and produces a higher percentage of false-negative findings [16]. However, despite the fact that the content is is particularly effective for analyzing dense breasts, its overall diagnostic effectiveness is hampered by interpretative problems, including a constrained field of view and a field dependency [2]. Additionally, those types of breast cancers that exclusively manifest as microcalcifications are less sensitive to detection using ultrasound (humans) than with mammograms [17, 18]. Last but not least, imaging is distinguished by greater sensitivity to identify tumor formation by image enhancement than image enhancement of the breast cancers give the outline for affective region. However, a significant percentage of false-positive results worsens the specificity of MRI [14]. The great expense of the appropriate tools and tests, as well as the impossibility of performing MRI on every patient, are additional drawbacks of MRI [19]. All of the primary methods for detecting breast cancer have some drawbacks, including low accuracy and low sensitivity with dense breasts [20], ultrasound operator dependence, and a narrow field of view [21], as well as the frequently untrue results, high cost, and lengthy processing time of MRI [22].

They are more economical and replacements of many method, which is more frequently needed in biomedical applications; at present, the tool is set up to analyze the data by designing itself with button technology to record the electrical connectivity [23]. It has come through many obstacles at a very low-scale level to make this

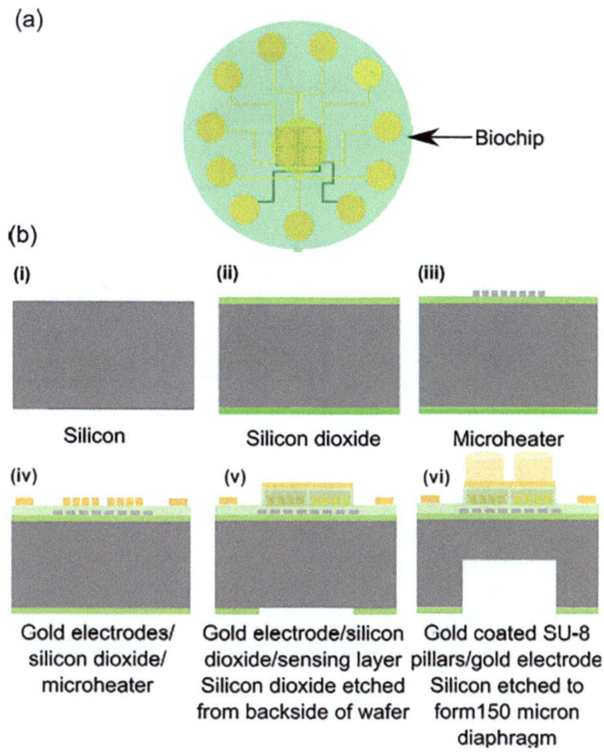

Fig. 22.1 Biochip fabrication

device more convenient and portable. Finally, through the outer connectivity to collect the data and analyze the tissues, a built-in display setup can resolve both the electrical and mechanical properties of the biosystem [24]. To overcome the degradation inside the system a new chip is induced each time during measurement. The functional diagram of the fabrication is described in Fig. 22.1. In the present technique, 12 chips have been introduced, each of which has a 4-inch reliable tool. Through this, the measurement of the properties of the cancerous and normal tissues from the sample of the breast tissues is taken [25]. Until now, the initial set of research in designing and fabricating a set of large functional and portable sensors for the diagnosis has been a remarkable introduction to the cancer diagnosis [26].

22.2 Methodology

22.2.1 Fabrication of the MEMS Sensor

The device incorporates a network of sensors that can withstand a piezoelectric current and a micro-heater, and these sensors are fabricated with the use of a seven-veil silicon oxidation method [20]. The whole width of the device is only 10 mm, yet

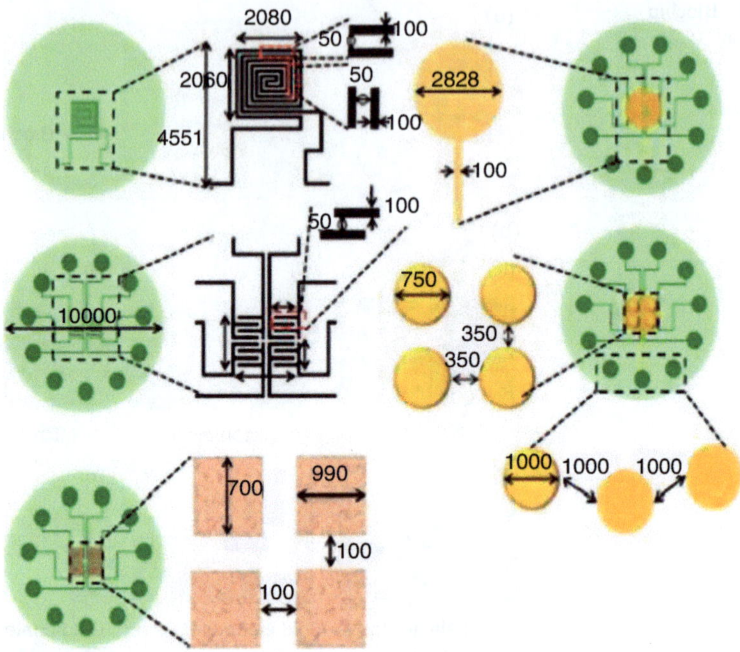

Fig. 22.2 (**a**) Preparation of the breast tissues. (**b**) Images of countable and uncountable tissues of the breast adjacently

the 2000 m × 2000 m sensor array it uses is able to cover the entire area. The fabrication process is as follows (see Fig. 22.2a, b): (i) a silicon (Si) wafer with a thickness of 500 m is used as a substrate; (ii) 1 m of SiO_2 is grown by means of warm evaporation; (iii) a nichrome (NiCr) micro-heater is designed into the oxidized silicon stratum; and (iv) a cell wall-improved concoction vapor testimony on a micro-heater is used to store SiO_2 (0.5 m). Germanium (1.5 m) is kept over Cr/Au terminals using E-pillar dissipation and designed using a lift-off process to frame the detecting part; SiO_2 is scratched from the connection zone of the micro-heater; Cr/Au is preserved via evaporation using an E-pillar; and the middle numbered terminals are fabricated. A layer of SiO_2 is deposited over the sensing layer and scratched off the connecting cushions. The contact cushion for the electrical interaction with the tissue is preserved and designed using a Cr/Au (0.02 m/0.5 m) film. Over this contact cushion, SU-8 columns measuring 100 m in height and 750 m in width are designed to be electrically conductive thanks to their metal covering [27]. These columns fill a double need: (i) they boost the tissue space during the process between the tissues of the breast; (ii) those electrodes are the electrical conductors. Back-to-back placement is utilized for the scratching of silicon to form the baseline. The initiator ship is diced up through micro-automation. Figure 22.3 shows the element die utilized during the initiation of the images of electrodes, sensors, micro-heater, pillars, and the baseline [28].

Fig. 22.3 Micro-automator

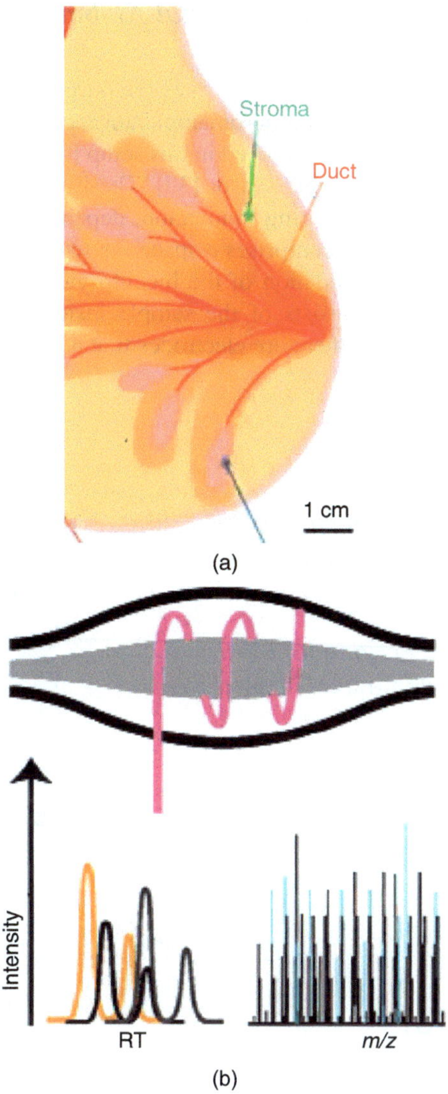

22.2.2 Setting up the Breast Tissues

Larger tissues of the breast have been induced during this process. This is for several reasons: (i) to reduce the complications of diagnosis and to give out a reasonable result; (ii) the simultaneous utilization of more sensors makes the diagnosis easier with the larger tissue samples; (iii) in the previous methods of diagnosis, when the small tissue sampling measurements of the specimen vary during the procedure with the relation of the piezoelectric vibration cause more recertification of stand values; (iv) to increase the sensitivity of the signal, the distance between the sensors of the sample should be increased, and (v) finally, the large tissue samples of the specimen, the area of the tumor, or the tumor portion can be diagnosed [29].

22.2.3 Experimental Ambiance

Figure 22.4a demonstrates the outline of a compact disease conclusion instrument. The chip with micromanipulator module MP-285 and an expendable sensor with an intender are involved in this setup [28]. Figure 22.4b shows the exploded module of the expendable sensor [30]. The framework is a blend of microfabrication innovation, 3D printing innovation, dependable bundling, and various portrayal methods [31]. This comprises a space for setting tissue tests, associating points encouraging the consolidation of the biochip yield to the information-obtaining card [32]. The sensor consists of the sample inside a carrier. In the micromanipulator module, MP-285, there are electrodes that are electrically stable (E1).

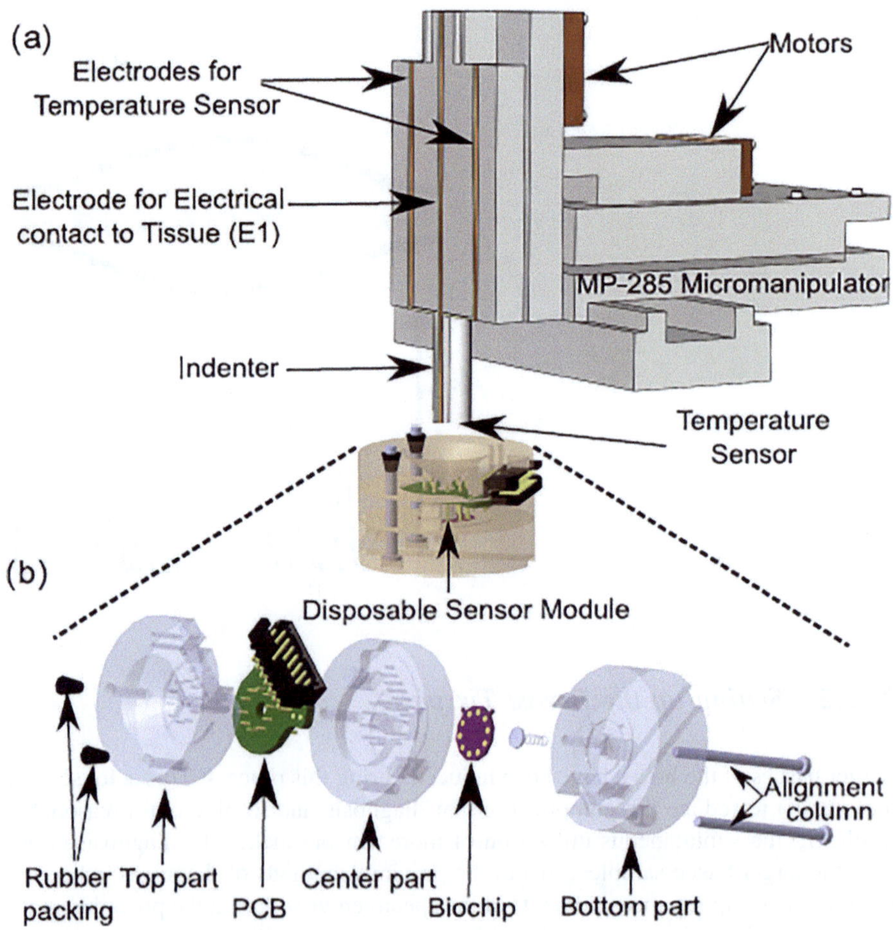

Fig. 22.4 (**a**) Experimental setup. (**b**) Elaborate packaging system diagram

At the bottom of the indenter, there is the temperature sensor. Assume that the tissue samples are uniform in architecture, and the temperature values are transferred into thermal property utilizing:

$$q = kA\Delta T \ (1) \ Lt$$

22.3 Results

A stable voltage is given between the electrodes at the top and the bottom in order to calculate the tissue's electrical conductivity. The electrical activity is finally passed on to the electrode at the bottom through the tissue samples from the electrode at the top. The voltage variation with respect to their tissue's resistance gives an output voltage. Also, this reaction is totally dependent on the tissue type, whether it is cancerous or normal tissue. The main observation is that the tissues normally had a smooth topographic image when compared with the cancer cells that have been observed under the electron microscope and further through scanning. There is a situation of a dilemma: (i) on dependence over the tissue there is a lot of fluctuation in resistance while the tissues are undergoing a current pass; (ii) at the same time, the cancer cells have strong resistance to the current flow compared with the normal tissues.

Figure 22.5 implies that the cancerous breast tissues are more resistant to the electric current than normal tissues. The values of the resistance can differ within the range from 150 to 450 W/cm. Tissues of the breast can be localized as fatty subcutaneous connective gland tissue, unlike other tissues, also causes more

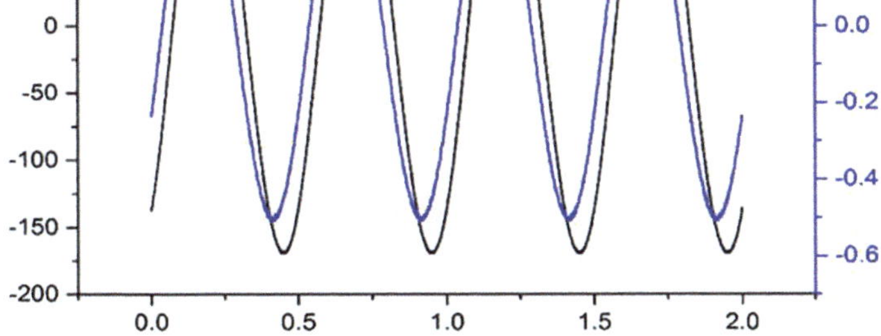

Fig. 22.5 Results are more resistant to the electric current than those of the normal tissues

electrical resistivity due to high current input. Because of the higher resistance, we use this part of the tissues on which to experiment. All the way through the literature review, 08 has gone through several researchers such that the tissues of the cancerous breast cells are more electrically resistive than normal tissues which they are consistently throughout the experiment. Tissues' mechanical properties are measured by placing the tissues in the sensor or the set of the bars used here (SU-8). A force has been transferred to the set of bars. The tissue's elasticity has been measured depending on the force transferred to the sensor.

So the signal changes in the sensor are related to the tissue's elasticity indirectly. A voltage divider connection comprises the sensor. Then the sensor resistance is decreased owing to the artificial compression by which the voltage in the output is also decreased is present in the voltage divider. P-type piezoelectric resistors are used for this kind of applied force procedure. The cancerous tissues and the normal tissues have a large difference up to 220 mm whatever the consequences are, the tissue's difference increases for representation.

Figure 22.6a implies the result of calibration with the economical load cell. The voltage divider just measures the resistance values by applying the force to the voltage where it is gradually in the output.

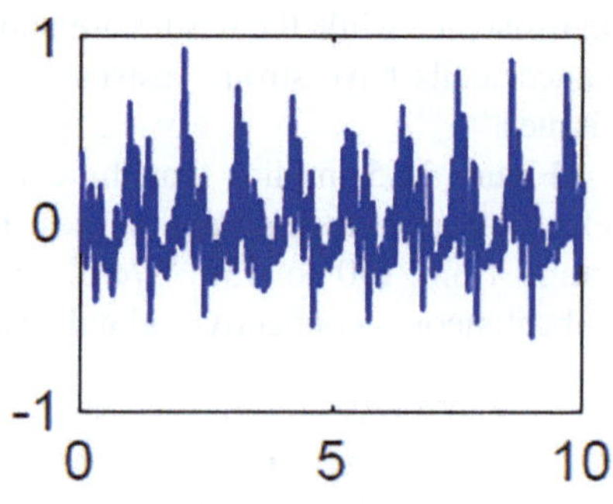

(a)

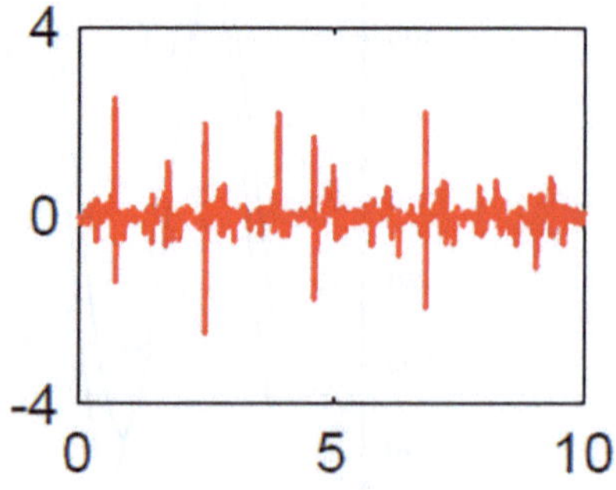

(b)

Fig. 22.6 (**a**) Sensor output voltage (v). (**b**) Tissue indentation depth

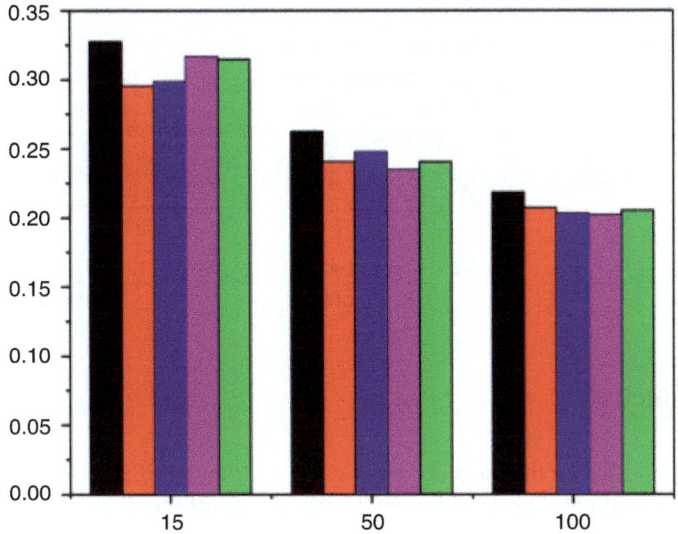

Fig. 22.7 Input voltage and surface temperature

Figure 22.6b implies a FOV analysis taken down during the experiment with a speed of 110 mm/s. At the same time, strain experiment resembles that elasticity between normal and cancerous tissues have higher values comparatively normal tissues.

It has been under observation. There is a difference in the temperature of the surface in the tissues, moreover small in number. These can be taken as thermal conductivity values referring to the value of the temperature measured as in Fig. 22.7.

The tissues of the breast kept on the chip are preheated with an interconnected microheater about 25–50 °C, gradually increasing by 5 °C. With the heat conduction formula, the thermal conductivity of the normal and cancerous tissue is measured. With the help of the thermistor, the temperature of the normal and the cancerous breast tissues is measured and presented over the holder. To determine statistically, two initial examinations were taken up for the cancerous and normal breast tissue for thermal conductivity. All the values of P settle at 0.05 except the initial range of temperature, which is 20–25 °C. The entire calculation of the values of P is statistically an important relation to thermal conductivity. Table 22.1 also indicates the possibilities and occurrence of death according to age. This difference can also be useful in setting as a standard difference of the thermal conductivity of the breast tissues. Thus, it has been noted that in cancerous tissue, there is an increase in thermal conductivity with respect to temperature, whereas the conductivity in normal tissues does not follow the same trend. The thermal conductivity values vary with repeated tests.

Table 22.1 Possibilities and occurrence of death according to age

Present age (years)	Determination of cancer	Death from cancer
35	0.2% (2 out of 2357)	<0.3% (2 out of 26,415)
40	0.7% (2 out of 314)	<0.3% (2 out of 3254)
45	2.7% (2 out of 56)	0.3% (2 out of 738)
50	3.2% (2 out of 35)	0.4% (2 out of 454)
55	4.7% (2 out of 34)	0.6% (2 out of 274)
60	5.2% (21 out of 39)	0.9% (2 out of 243)
65	4.2% (2 out of 42)	2.4% (2 out of 259)
Lifelong risk	23.7% (2 out of 9)	3.4% (2 out of 46)

22.4 Conclusion

Breast cancer is by far the most common cancer to be identified, with most cases of the disease affecting women. Although the prevalence of breast cancer varies greatly by region, it nevertheless accounts for a significant portion of preventable deaths, especially among women in developing nations. To lower incidence and mortality and address the calculated base of the illness, vast international efforts and community health initiatives are required, focusing on the entire span of cancer control, from preventive care to early detection, monitoring, and treatments. The aim of this work is to design and fabricate a complete measuring system of a greater number of tissue measures that can give a stable and informative analysis, analysis for few quantitative characteristics of the breast cancer tissues relating to thermal, electrical, and mechanical characteristics with the diseased tissues as well less than normal tissues. The cancer diagnostic device is a one-way dispensable component and an easier application towards the utilization effects. A micromanipulator has been used for a small-scale representation of the tissue present in the chip in the present work. By calculating the electric, thermal, and mechanical changes, the device could compared the diseased and the normal breast tissues present in the sample. To determine the cancer stage, a wearable device will be developed in the future to undergo negative and positive analysis of the breast tissues.

References

1. American Cancer Society. (2015). *Breast cancer facts & figures 2015*. American Cancer Society. [Online]. Available: https://www.cancer.org/acs/groups/content/@editorial/documents/document/acspc-044552.pdf
2. Deryugina, E. I., & Quigley, J. P. (2011). The role of matrix metalloproteinases in cellular invasion and metastasis. In *Extracellular matrix degradation* (pp. 145–191). Springer.
3. Wegener, J., Keese, C. R., & Giaever, I. (2000). Electric cell-substrate impedance sensing (ECIS) as a noninvasive means to monitor the kinetics of cell spreading to artificial surfaces. *Experimental Cell Research, 259*(1), 158–166. https://doi.org/10.1006/excr.2000.4919. PMID: 10942588.

4. Samani, A., Zubovits, J., & Plewes, D. (2007). Elastic moduli of normal and pathological human breast tissues: An inversion-technique-based investigation of 169 samples. *Physics in Medicine and Biology, 52*(6), 1565–1576. https://doi.org/10.1088/0031-9155/52/6/002. Epub 2007 Feb 16. PMID: 17327649.
5. Sekitani, T., Noguchi, Y., Hata, K., Fukushima, T., Aida, T., & Someya, T. (2008). A rubberlike stretchable active matrix using elastic conductors. *Science, 321*(5895), 1468–1472.
6. Kim, D.-H., Ahn, J.-H., Choi, W. M., Kim, H.-S., Kim, T.-H., Song, J., Huang, Y. Y., Liu, Z., Lu, C., & Rogers, J. A. (2008). Stretchable and foldable silicon integrated circuits. *Science, 320*(5875), 507–511.
7. Someya, T., Sekitani, T., Iba, S., Kato, Y., Kawaguchi, H., & Sakurai, T. (2004). A large-area, flexible pressure sensor matrix with organic field-effect transistors for artificial skin applications. *Proceedings of the National Academy of Sciences, 101*(27), 9966–9970.
8. Someya, T., Kato, Y., Sekitani, T., Iba, S., Noguchi, Y., Murase, Y., Kawaguchi, H., & Sakurai, T. (2005). Conformable, flexible, large-area networks of pressure and thermal sensors with organic transistor active matrixes. *Proceedings of the National Academy of Sciences, 102*(35), 12321–12325.
9. Rusanen, O., & Lenkkeri, J. (1995). Reliability issues of replacing solder with conductive adhesives in power modules. *IEEE Transactions on Components, Packaging, and Manufacturing Technology: Part B, 18*(2), 320–325.
10. Monk, D. J., Maudie, T., Stanerson, D., Wertz, J., Bitko, G., Matkin, J., & Petrovic, S. (1996, June 2–6). *Media compatible packaging and environmental testing of barrier coating encapsulated silicon pressure sensors, solid-state sensor and actuator workshop* (pp. 36–41). Hilton Head, S. Carolina.
11. Pandya, H. J., Park, K., Chen, W., Chekmareva, M. A., Foran, D. J., & Desai, J. P. (2014). Mechanical phenotyping of breast cancer using MEMS: A method to demarcate benign and cancerous breast tissues. *Lab on a Chip, 14*(23), 4523–4532.
12. Pandya, H. J., Park, K., & Desai, J. P. (2015). Design and fabrication of a flexible MEMS-based electromechanical sensor array for breast cancer diagnosis. *Journal of Micromechanics and Microengineering, 25*(7), 075025. https://doi.org/10.1088/0960-1317/25/7/075025. PMID: 26526747; PMCID: PMC4624460.
13. Faes, T. J., van der Meij, H. A., de Munck, J. C., & Heethaar, R. M. (1999). The electric resistivity of human tissues (100 Hz-10 MHz): A meta-analysis of review studies. *Physiological Measurement, 20*(4), R1–R10. https://doi.org/10.1088/0967-3334/20/4/201. PMID: 10593226.
14. Morimoto, T., Kimura, S., Konishi, Y., Komaki, K., Uyama, T., Monden, Y., Kinouchi, Y., & Iritani, T. (1993). A study of the electrical bio-impedance of tumors. *Journal of Investigative Surgery, 6*(1), 25–32. https://doi.org/10.3109/08941939309141189. PMID: 8452822.
15. Lu, P., Takai, K., Weaver, V. M., & Werb, Z. (2011). Extracellular matrix degradation and remodeling in development and disease. *Cold Spring Harbor Perspectives in Biology, 3*(12), a005058. https://doi.org/10.1101/cshperspect.a005058. PMID: 21917992; PMCID: PMC3225943.
16. Mangia, A., Malfettone, A., Rossi, R., Paradiso, A., Ranieri, G., Simone, G., & Resta, L. (2011). Tissue remodelling in breast cancer: Human mast cell tryptase as an initiator of myofibroblast differentiation. *Histopathology, 58*(7), 1096–1106. https://doi.org/10.1111/j.1365-2559.2011.03842.x. PMID: 21707711.
17. Pandya, H. J., Roy, R., Chen, W., Chekmareva, M. A., Foran, D. J., & Desai, J. P. (2015). Accurate characterization of benign and cancerous breast tissues: aspecific patient studies using piezoresistive microcantilevers. *Biosensors and Bioelectronics, 63*, 414–424. https://doi.org/10.1016/j.bios.2014.08.002. Epub 2014. PMID: 25128621; PMCID: PMC4167594.
18. Plodinec, M., Loparic, M., Monnier, C. A., Obermann, E. C., Zanetti-Dallenbach, R., Oertle, P., Hyotyla, J. T., Aebi, U., Bentires-Alj, M., Lim, R. Y., & Schoenenberger, C.-A. (2012). The nanomechanical signature of breast tissue. *Nature Nanotechnology, 7*(11), 757–765.
19. Cross, S. E., Jin, Y.-S., Rao, J., & Gimzewski, J. K. (2007). Nanomechanical analysis of cells from cancer patients. *Nature Nanotechnology, 2*, 780–783.

20. Suresh, S. (2007). Biomechanics and biophysics of cancer cells. *Acta Materialia, 55*(12), 3989–4014.
21. Roy, R., Chen, W., Goodell, L. A., Jun, H., Foran, D. J., & Desai, J. P. (2010). Microarray-facilitated mechanical characterization of breast tissue pathology samples using contact-mode Atomic Force Microscopy (AFM). In *2010 3rd IEEE RAS & EMBS international conference on biomedical robotics and biomechatronics* (pp. 710–715). https://doi.org/10.1109/BIOROB.2010.5625952
22. Lu, P., Weaver, V. M., & Werb, Z. (2012). The extracellular matrix: a dynamic niche in cancer progression. *Journal of Cell Biology, 196*(4), 395–406. https://doi.org/10.1083/jcb.201102147. PMID: 22351925; PMCID: PMC3283993.
23. Keese, C. R., & Giaever, I. (1994). A biosensor that monitors cell morphology with electrical fields. *IEEE Engineering in Medicine and Biology Magazine, 13*(3), 402–408. https://doi.org/10.1109/51.294012
24. Małecka-Massalska, T., Chara, K., Gołębiowski, P., Władysiuk, M., Smoleń, A., Kurylcio, A., Zuchora, B., Zubrzycki, J., Orłowska-Kowalik, G., Lupa-Zatwarnicka, K., & Polkowski, W. (2013). Altered tissue electrical properties in women with breast cancer – preliminary observations. *Annals of Agricultural and Environmental Medicine, 20*(3), 523–527. PMID: 24069858.
25. Jossinet, J. (1996). Variability of impedivity in normal and pathological breast tissue. *Medical and Biological Engineering and Computing, 34*(5), 346–350.
26. Mamishev, A. V., Sundara-Rajan, K., Yang, F., Yanqing, D., & Zahn, M. (2004). Interdigital sensors and transducers. *Proceedings of the IEEE, 92*(5), 808–845. https://doi.org/10.1109/JPROC.2004.826603
27. Swift, J., Ivanovska, I. L., Buxboim, A., Harada, T., Dingal, P. C., Pinter, J., Pajerowski, J. D., Spinler, K. R., Shin, J. W., Tewari, M., Rehfeldt, F., Speicher, D. W., & Discher, D. E. (2013). Nuclear lamin-A scales with tissue stiffness and enhances matrix-directed differentiation. *Science, 341*(6149), 1240104. https://doi.org/10.1126/science.1240104. PMID: 23990565; PMCID: PMC3976548.
28. Rowe, A. C. H. (2014). Piezoresistance in silicon and its nanostructures. *Journal of Materials Research, 29*(6), 731–744.
29. Hvims, H. L. (1996). Conductive adhesives for SMT and potential applications. *Microelectronics Reliability, 36*(4), 554–555.
30. Shahrjerdi, D., Hekmatshoar, B., Rezaee, L., & Mohajerzadeh, S. S. (2003). Low temperature stress-induced crystallization of germanium on plastic. *Thin Solid Films, 427*(1), 330–334.
31. Wellman, P. S., Howe, R. D., Dalton, E., & Kern, K. A. (1999). *Breast tissue stiffness in compression is correlated to histological diagnosis*. Harvard BioRobotics Laboratory. [Online]. Available: https://biorobotics.harvard.edu/pubs/1999/mechprops.pdf
32. Valvano, J. W., Cochran, J. R., & Diller, K. R. (1985). Thermal conductivity and diffusivity of biomaterials measured with self-heated thermistors. *International Journal of Thermophysics, 6*, 301–311. https://doi.org/10.1007/BF00522151

Chapter 23
Segmentation of Attributes of the Skin Lesion Using Deep Ensemble Models

K. Deepasundari and A. Thirumurthi Raja

23.1 Introduction

Deep convolutional neural networks (DCNNs) advances and other scientific challenges on this topic have resulted in a slew of powerful computational methods for dealing with a wide range of problems in this domain [1–3]. When using computer-aided diagnostic (CAD) technology to examine skin lesions, the primary goal is to discover any anomalies or illnesses that may exist inside them. In the literature, it appears that the majority of techniques follow a predetermined analysis path: Lesions are initially segmented so that other computerized algorithms can extract features that can then be utilized to detect the type of lesion [4].

Dermoscopic structures, which is another term for lesion characteristics, are the visible patterns in a lesion texture that may be seen under a microscope. Depending on the type of lesion and the severity of cancer, it is conceivable that the presentation of these symptoms will change. The dermoscopic pattern of some lesions may be nonexistent at all, but the pattern of other lesions may be textural in nature and related to a variety of characteristics. There are several distinguishing qualities in the field of dermatology. Among the most notable clinical findings are globules and dots, milia-like cysts, negative networks, and streaks. In clinical practice, dermatologists look for these characteristics, as well as the general and local appearance characteristics of the lesion, in order to more accurately diagnose the lesion type and the amount of malignancy in the lesion. Because attributes give useful information, CAD systems can also profit from them in order to increase the efficacy of their automated recognition [4].

K. Deepasundari (✉) · A. T. Raja
Department of Computer Science, School of Computing Sciences, Vels Institute of Science Technology and Advanced Studies (VISTAS), Chennai, Tamil Nadu, India

F. J. Joseph et al. (eds.), *Computational Intelligence for Clinical Diagnosis*, EAI/Springer Innovations in Communication and Computing,
https://doi.org/10.1007/978-3-031-23683-9_23

In certain cases, CNNs can extract useful features from raw dermoscopic images and categorize them without the requirement for lesions or a segmentation map of their properties. However, it has been demonstrated that integrating additional information can significantly improve lesion classification. [5] showed in the ISIC2016: Melanoma Recognition competition that the use of a lesion mask improves lesion classification, and they were awarded first place in the competition. In addition to lesion segmentation and attribute probability maps, also [6] proposed a lesion classification framework that was able to produce state-of-the-art results with only one model by incorporating this new information into lesion classification and attribute probability maps [7]. According to this research and its promising outcomes, the lesion mask and its feature segmentation tasks are crucial for diagnostic purposes [8].

The presence of artefacts in the image capture setup and sample preparations and the appearance of the lesion itself present various obstacles in the automatic analysis of dermoscopic images [9–12]. When images are acquired from skin lesion samples using a dermatoscope, a variety of image artefacts may appear, reducing the overall output quality. An image may contain artefacts such as inconsistencies in colour and hair occlusion, to name a couple of examples. Aside from colour charts and ruler marks, other issues include low contrast and sharpness, gel bubbles, uneven illumination, and lens artefacts. In addition, the appearance of skin lesions might differ significantly based on their type and location. In extreme circumstances, it is possible to have a face with a complex or fuzzy texture, low contrast against the skin, and amorphous geometry and a colourful face. As a result, it appears that developing a generic algorithm to circumvent all of these hurdles will be difficult. Given their compact structures and fragile appearance, segmenting attributes is a much more challenging process to perform on them.

23.2 Related Works

A number of different methods for segmenting and classifying skin lesions, both conventional and deep, have been proposed in the literature. According to [10], skin lesion identification and classification using feature selection and probabilistic distribution have been developed and shown. The distribution is then split into smaller segments. A fusion approach is used to extract features from segmented images, which are integrated into parallel, using a fusion approach. Bhattacharyya combines entropy-based approaches with distance and variance formulas to choose characteristics for further investigation.

The author [11] used the ResNet34 layers to train a fully CNN, and they found that it performed well. Pre-training and fine-tuning have been shown to improve the segmentation performance of ResNet34; as a result, these methods have been implemented. For skin lesion classification, pre-trained CNN models were employed. The researchers also tested if image scaling had an impact on the model's capacity to identify skin lesions. It was necessary to examine the categorization results of three CNNs on six different scales in order to reach a conclusion. It was also utilized to create and analyse a multi-scale multi-CNN methodology, which was developed using the ensemble method. This method made use of the three CNN models that had been trained on varying-sized cropped images before being employed. The algorithm correctly predicted 86.2%, which represents a significant improvement over the previous method. It was also determined that cropping rather than resizing is preferred when it comes to attaining the greatest results.

A deep CNN architecture was provided by the researchers in [12] to classify lesions using a deep CNN architecture. For binary classification, the researchers employed GoogLeNet and Inception-V3 software, according to the findings. Using this technique, they were able to improve the accuracy of the multiclass problem by up to 7%. They developed a multiclass classification model for skin lesion classification. Extensive testing of CNN models and their ensembles was carried out over a wide range of scenarios. We used transfer learning to refine these CNN architectures on seven classes of the HAM10000 Dataset in order to fine-tune them.

An innovative hybrid approaches for the categorization and segmentation of numerous skin lesions. The lesion parts were segmented using a full-resolution convolutional neural network to achieve the best results (FrCN). Skin lesions are separated into categories for CNN categorization. They developed a bootstrapping CNN to better detect and categorize skin lesions in order to improve detection and classification Mutual Bootstrapping Deep Convolutional Neural Networks (MB-DCNN) [10]. A coarse segmentation network was used to improve the segmentation, and then the study used a mask-guided network to classify the lesions after they had been classified. The network's features were integrated in order to improve detection and classification.

23.3 Proposed Method

An entirely automated technique for segmentation and classification is proposed, which makes use of relevant deep learning features in conjunction with an entirely automated system. This consists of five basic steps: Further research explored utilizing a deep saliency-based technique to produce an initial map, which would then be refined. After the conversion of images to binary form, the study refines the lesion using morphological approaches. We then install and train our ensemble learning system, which consists of AlexNet, ResNet, and GoogLeNet. This is the final step in the process. An improved Moth Flame Optimization (MFO) approach is employed to make the most of the information gathered from both models. The final classifications are conducted on the fused vectors, which are then validated on a range of datasets to ensure that they are accurate. Figure 23.1 displays a precise, step-by-step procedure that will be explained in further depth later on.

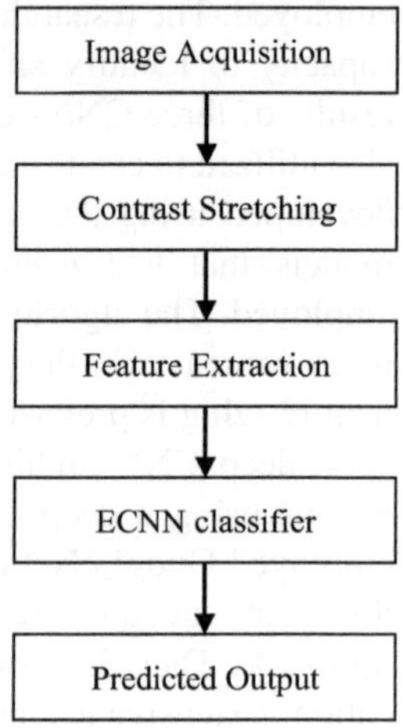

Fig. 23.1 Proposed model

23.3.1 Contrast Stretching

Contrast enhancement is one of the most important aspects of evaluating the overall quality of an image. Improving image clarity can be accomplished in a variety of ways, such as by increasing specific qualities or decreasing the amount of blur in individual pixels. Initially, we wanted to increase the contrast of the lesion region in order to make it easier to identify the region of interest (ROI). A well-known technique, histogram equalization (HE), has been described in a number of academic papers, and it has been applied in a variety of situations. It is possible to create lesion-specific amplification by increasing the number of image pixels within the lower and upper limits.

In order to detect the lesion pixels, we first create an image histogram and then multiply the variance values in order to increase the pixel range of the detection. The use of HE allows for further refinement of the variance value-based image created previously. When using the fitness function, the intensity levels are raised to a level that is appropriate for both the lesion and the surrounding area. The next section provides an explanation of how this technique is carried out.

For example, consider the input dimensions of order $N \times M$. ξ_{xy} is the original image with the same proportions as the resultant contrast-enhanced image, which is seen here. The histogram of the image ξ'_{xy} is initially calculated in the following manner:

$$h_f(k) = Oj \tag{24.1}$$

where

$h_f(k)$ – ξ_{xy} histogram
O_j – grey level occurrence
f_0 – total occurrences

With histogram $h_f(k)$, the infected pixel range is defined as below:

$$h'_f(k) = h_f(k)\left[I_j\right]_{k_1,k_n} \tag{24.2}$$

where

$h'_f(k)$ – infected region
I_j – patch of the infected region
j – value of each pixel

Therefore, the variance is estimated for the entire images ξ_{xy} as below:

$$\sigma^2(\xi_{xy}) = \frac{1}{MN}\sum_{i=0}^{M-1}\sum_{j=0}^{N-1}(\xi_{ij})^2 - \mu^2 \tag{24.3}$$

$$\mu = \frac{1}{MN}\sum_{i=0}^{M-1}\sum_{j=0}^{N-1}(\xi_{ij}) \tag{24.4}$$

The value of the output variance is then multiplied with $h'_f(k) = h_f(k)\left[I_j\right]_{k_1,k_n}$ as given below:

$$H'_f(k) = \left[h'_f(k)\right]\left[\sigma^2(\xi_{xy})\right] \tag{24.5}$$

After that, we produce an infection by splicing together the ξ_{xy} and $H'_f(k)$ genes (k). By employing histogram equalization, it is possible to blend the original and infected images.

$$O\left(\xi_{xy}, H'_f(k)\right) = \left[\xi_{xy}\right]_{N\times M}\left[H'_f(k)\right]_{N\times M} \tag{24.6}$$

When compared to the original images, the infected areas are more easily discernible in this version. However, we are primarily concerned with the use of contrast to isolate the infection from the surrounding tissue, not with the actual contrast itself. Because we establish two fitness functions in a sequential manner, we can acquire more meaningful information on body fitness. This is a mathematical definition of fitness functions as follows:

$$O_1 = O\left(\xi_{xy}, H'_f(k)\right) + L_{(5)} \tag{24.7}$$

$$O_2 = O_1 + L_{(5)} \tag{24.8}$$

Using such a function, the pixel value range can be increased by a factor of one, up to five times, each time by a factor of one. With the utilization of such an objective function, the images are considered beneficial for appropriately segmenting lesions since they contain more information.

23.3.2 Ensemble Voting Classification

The voting classifier for the ensemble classifier will be discussed in detail in this article. We will use the top three classifiers for this voting classification in order to deliver the best execution and output possible.

In cases where the classifiers have been refined, this strategy may be recommended because it anticipates the class names in terms of predicted probabilities p for each classifier.

$$Y = \arg\max{}_i \sum_{j=1}^{m} W_j P_{ij} \tag{24.9}$$

where

$j = [1, 2, \ldots, m]$ and $i \in \{0, 1\}$
W_j – heap doled out to the jth classifier

Listed below are brief descriptions of some of the classifiers that were used to pick the top three candidates for the ensemble:

AlexNet As a result of the competition, AlexNet reduced the top five mistake rates from 26% to 15.3%, outperforming all other competitors. In the second spot, approximately 26.2% of the top 5 errors were made, and this was not due to a CNN fluctuation.

ResNet The design of the ResNet is characterized by skipped connections and robust batch normalization. These gated units, or gated recurrent units, as they are often known, are strikingly comparable to recent successful RNN elements in terms of their structure and function. Using this strategy, a neural network with 152 layers was trained, and it was discovered to be less complex than the VGGNet. Using this dataset, it achieves the lowest error rate in the top five at 3.57%, which is better than human performance.

GoogLeNet During the development of GoogLeNet, the team used a CNN based on the LeNet architecture, but they also included a novel component called an inception module. In the batch normalization procedure, image distortions and Root Mean Square Propagation Algorithm (RMSprop) were used to achieve the desired results. This module makes use of a sequence of extremely small convolutions and acts as an alternative to employing AlexNet 60 million parameters; they employed a CNN with a depth of 22 layers and a parameter count of four million, which was more efficient.

23.4 Results and Discussions

Verification of the system performance has been carried out using other deep learning models, such as convolutional neural networks, fine-tuned neural networks, and extremely deep convolutional networks, among others. On a variety of measures, the accuracy, sensitivity, specificity, f-measure, and percentage error of the model are evaluated in comparison to existing methods, including for the training phase, where we chose a 0.001 learning rate with a batch size of 28. The simulations are conducted using 16 GB RAM on a Matlab simulation tool in this study. The study used a graphics card with a memory of 16 GB to accelerate the execution time of the proposed framework.

23.4.1 Datasets to Evaluate the Effectiveness of Enhanced Convolutional Neural Network (ECNN)

ISBI 2016 Dataset In the ISBI 2016 Dataset, there were 900 for the purpose of training and 379 images for the purpose of testing. In the training images, there are shots of melanoma as well as images of benign lesions. It contains descriptions and features for segmentation, and the other testing images were used to evaluate the ECNN model for segmentation.

ISIC 2017 Dataset This dataset contains 2750 images, which is a significant number. For the purpose of segmentation, 2000 images are used as training images, while 600 images are used for testing and 150 images for validation. There are additional publicly available ground truth samples for this dataset, which were used to validate the segmentation algorithm that was used to create the segmentation results.

ISBI 2018 Dataset This dataset contains information on lesion segmentation, attribute identification, and lesion type classification, among other things. For the purpose of segmentation, 2594 images and ground truth images are provided, while 1000 images are for testing and 100 images are for validation.

HAM10000 Dataset HAM10000 has 10,015 dermoscopy images, which is a significant amount of data. This database has one of the most sophisticated multiclass skin lesion categorization databases available anywhere on the Internet.

The contrast-stretching phase of the original architecture has been abolished, and segmentation has been implemented in its place. The statistics reveal that there is a significant difference in segmentation accuracy when contrast stretching is not used. When this step was left out of our suggested technique, an average accuracy loss of 8% was noticed. For the ISBI 2016 competition, this table had previously achieved an accuracy of 96%. When using the same dataset, our approach had an accuracy of 98%, whereas it had an accuracy of 96% when using the next closest dataset and an accuracy of 98.70% when using the closest dataset.

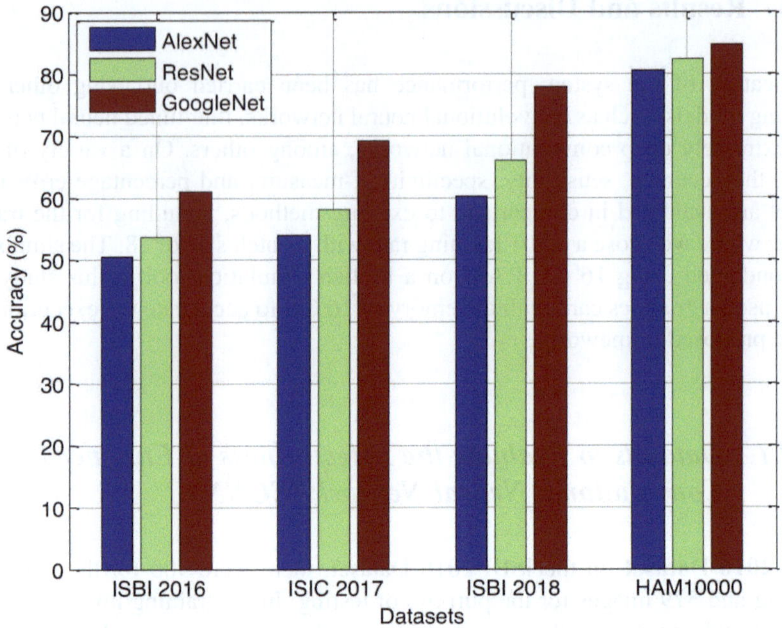

Fig. 23.2 Accuracy of all datasets

This section provides a wide range of classification findings for skin lesions that can be found in the literature and also the computations performed using the proposed framework. Despite the fact that the CNN required less time to test than the ECNN, there was still a statistically significant difference between the two. In addition, we estimated the ECNN sensitivity rate, which is shown in this table as well. On the basis of these calculations, the ECNN sensitivity rate was determined to be 90%. This table also reveals the correct prediction rates for skin classes that include Basal Cell Carcinoma (BCC) with 89%, Benign Keratosis (BKL) with 91%, and Melanoma (MEL) with 90% for the skin classifications in question. In terms of prediction accuracy, Dermatofibroma (DF) had the lowest rate of 85% (Fig. 23.3).

Features retrieved by ECNN using the TL are considered high at a rate of 81% of the time. The ECNN model had the second-best accuracy, with 78% accuracy, but the individual classifier prediction time has increased, which should be considered when using ECNN. The number of recovered features has a considerable impact on the time required to make a forecast (Fig. 23.4).

The classification results obtained after applying the feature optimization are depicted in Fig. 23.2. System performance is improved by an average of 3% through the optimization of features, which results in improved accuracy as well as a reduction in computation time on average. The optimal feature fusion framework we proposed outperformed the individual feature vectors when compared with individual vectors.

The results of Figs. 23.2, 23.3, 23.4 and 23.5 present an evaluation of the methodologies discussed previously. It was found that the proposed model ECNN algorithm improvised the accuracy of the classification process when compared to other methods.

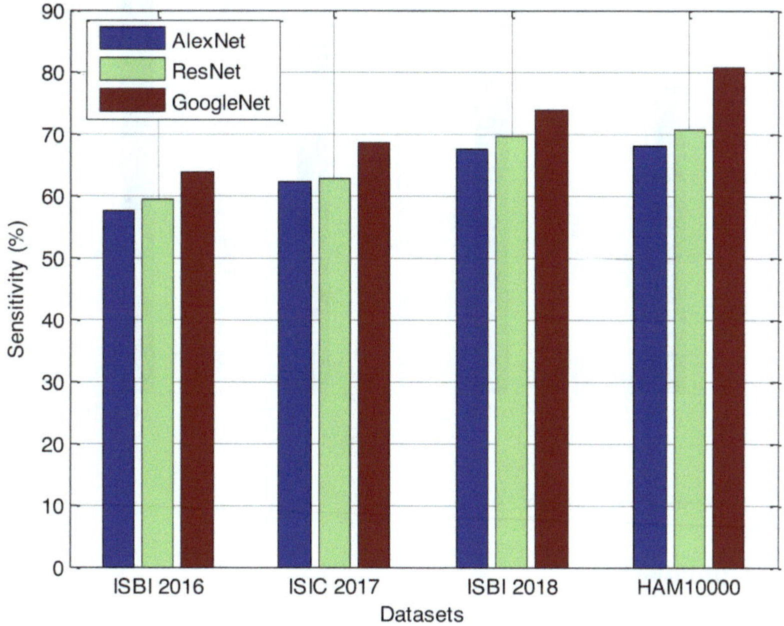

Fig. 23.3 Sensitivity of all datasets

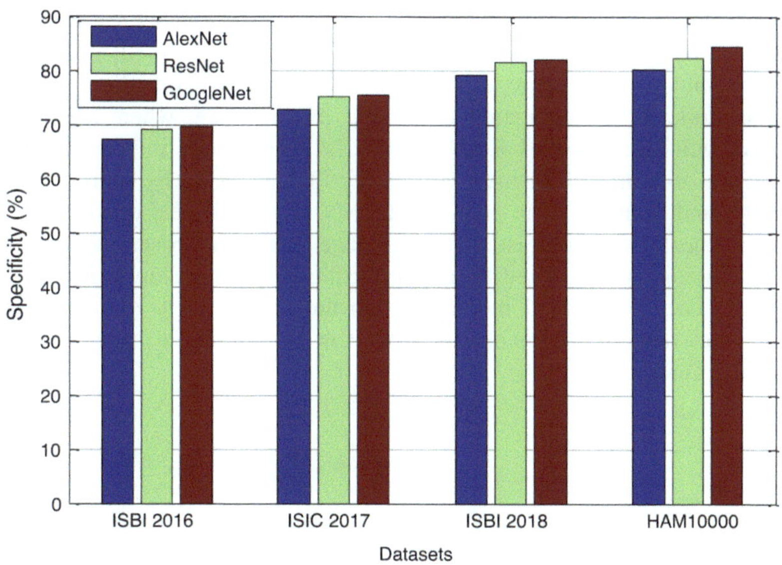

Fig. 23.4 Specificity of all datasets

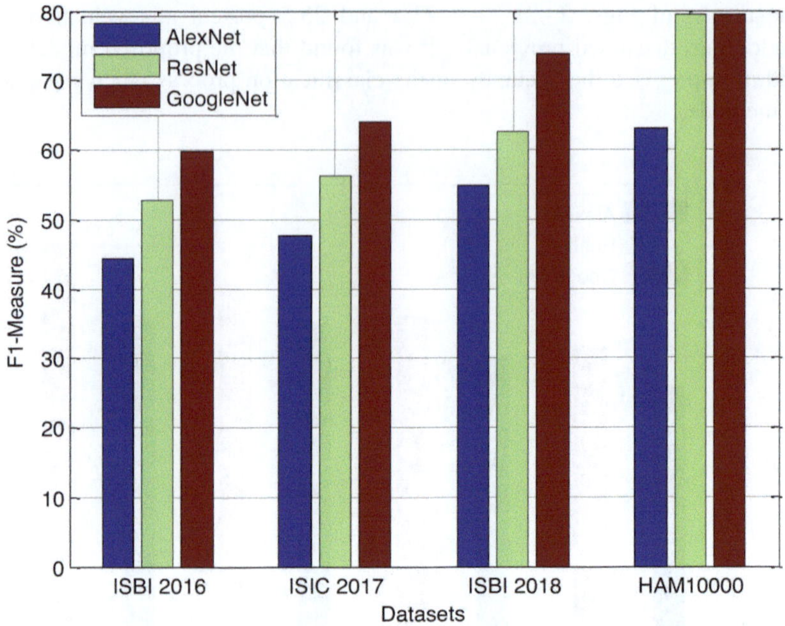

Fig. 23.5 F1 score on all datasets

23.5 Conclusions

The diagnosis of skin cancer is accomplished through the application of a range of deep learning models in the form of ensemble learning. In order to detect artefacts present in skin images, segmentation is carried out using dermoscopic imaging data. More than 15,000 images were taken to prove the performance of the proposed method. All of the final results from each classifier are delivered to the majority voting ensemble, which aggregates the predicted outputs from the convolutional neural network. When compared to current methods, i.e. when GoogLeNet is compared with AlexNet and ResNet, there is a noticeable improvement in the performance of metrics. The metrics used for this study are F1 score, specificity, sensitivity, and accuracy. The proposed ECNN produced great efficiency. This is especially true for the contrast-stretching stage, which increases the accuracy of segmentation and is considered beneficial for the purpose of skin lesion segmentation. Using deep pre-trained models, which are then used to extract significant characteristics from the segmented lesions, it is not possible to achieve high segmentation accuracy.

References

1. Khan, M. A., Akram, T., Zhang, Y. D., & Sharif, M. (2021). Attributes based skin lesion detection and recognition: A mask RCNN and transfer learning-based deep learning framework. *Pattern Recognition Letters, 143*, 58–66.
2. Adegun, A., & Viriri, S. (2021). Deep learning techniques for skin lesion analysis and melanoma cancer detection: A survey of state-of-the-art. *Artificial Intelligence Review, 54*(2), 811–841.
3. Lei, B., Xia, Z., Jiang, F., Jiang, X., Ge, Z., Xu, Y., et al. (2020). Skin lesion segmentation via generative adversarial networks with dual discriminators. *Medical Image Analysis, 64*, 101716.
4. Khan, M. A., Sharif, M., Akram, T., Damaševičius, R., & Maskeliūnas, R. (2021). Skin lesion segmentation and multiclass classification using deep learning features and improved moth flame optimization. *Diagnostics, 11*(5), 811.
5. Yu, L., Chen, H., Dou, Q., Qin, J., & Heng, P. A. (2016). Automated melanoma recognition in dermoscopy images via very deep residual networks. *IEEE Transactions on Medical Imaging, 36*(4), 994–1004.
6. Gonzalez-Diaz, I. (2018). Dermaknet: Incorporating the knowledge of dermatologists to convolutional neural networks for skin lesion diagnosis. *IEEE Journal of Biomedical and Health Informatics, 23*(2), 547–559.
7. Jin, Q., Cui, H., Sun, C., Meng, Z., & Su, R. (2021). Cascade knowledge diffusion network for skin lesion diagnosis and segmentation. *Applied Soft Computing, 99*, 106881.
8. Khan, M. A., Akram, T., Sharif, M., Shahzad, A., Aurangzeb, K., Alhussein, M., et al. (2018). An implementation of normal distribution based segmentation and entropy controlled features selection for skin lesion detection and classification. *BMC Cancer, 18*(1), 1–20.
9. Tschandl, P., Sinz, C., & Kittler, H. (2019). Domain-specific classification-pretrained fully convolutional network encoders for skin lesion segmentation. *Computers in Biology and Medicine, 104*, 111–116.
10. Mahbod, A., Schaefer, G., Wang, C., Dorffner, G., Ecker, R., & Ellinger, I. (2020). Transfer learning using a multi-scale and multi-network ensemble for skin lesion classification. *Computer Methods and Programs in Biomedicine, 193*, 105475.
11. Harangi, B., Baran, A., & Hajdu, A. (2020). Assisted deep learning framework for multiclass skin lesion classification considering a binary classification support. *Biomedical Signal Processing and Control, 62*, 102041.
12. Chaturvedi, S. S., Tembhurne, J. V., & Diwan, T. (2020). A multiclass skin Cancer classification using deep convolutional neural networks. *Multimedia Tools and Applications, 79*(39), 28477–28498.

Chapter 24
The Role of Emotional Intelligence During a Pandemic Crisis

Viney Dhiman and Anupama Bharti

24.1 Introduction

Emotional intelligence (EI) is simply the amalgamation of personal emotions and intelligence, which translates to proper management of every state of mind in crises. It is not a generalized subject and usually differs from person to person, based upon several dependable factors, such as maturity, age, experience, and others. It can also be referred to as a skill set, as the aspect is directly proportional to mental stability and overall peace in one's life. The world is going through a dangerous crisis. In these times, it is necessary to attain a certain level of emotional intelligence to adapt to the ongoing situation. It assists in heightening the personal mental health of individuals.

On the other hand, emotional intelligence can play a crucial role in the maintenance of public health. The capability of a human being is improved with the involvement of emotional intelligence, which is included in this study. Five effective factors are controlled with the help of the emotional intelligence process, and these five factors are self-awareness, empathy, motivation, social skills, and self-regulation. This study explains the response of people towards any pandemic crisis. It is important to maintain the application of emotional intelligence to lead this pandemic crisis. Complex human emotion is evaluated with the help of the emotional intelligence process.

V. Dhiman (✉)
Institute of Medical Education and Research, Chandigarh, India

A. Bharti
Department of Sociology and Social Work, Himachal Pradesh University, Shimla, India

F. J. Joseph et al. (eds.), *Computational Intelligence for Clinical Diagnosis*, EAI/Springer Innovations in Communication and Computing,
https://doi.org/10.1007/978-3-031-23683-9_24

24.2 Literature Review

24.2.1 *Importance of Emotional Intelligence*

The emotion of a leader and manager is adequately maintained with the use of emotional intelligence techniques. Along with this, personal and professional success is maintained by this technological aspect. Self-awareness, self-regulation, social skill, empathy, and motivation are treated as five effective factors of the emotional intelligence process, useful for any organization. Along with this, positive social interactions are maintained with the help of the emotional intelligence process. The self-motivation process is justified with the help of positive social interaction [1]. The emotional intelligence process can help maintain professional success and academic and personal development. Along with this the true potential of an organization is adequately evaluated with the help of emotional intelligence, which can prevent biases in emotions and promote positive emotion in the organization.

In addition, it is observed that employees' social capabilities and job performance are improved with the involvement of the emotional intelligence process. Successful communication is important to maintain the emotional intelligence process, which directly impacts the performance of the organization [2]. To understand and manage employees' emotion, it is important to justify the capacity of the emotional intelligence process. Along with this, good intuition is justified properly by the emotional intelligence process, which directly impacts employees' productivity. The self-confidence of employees, manager, and leader is justified by the emotional intelligence process. Emotional intelligence can play a crucial role in maintaining self-awareness, and maintenance of weakness, strength, drivers, and value is a key aspect of emotional intelligence. This process is important to maintain mental health coverage, and constructive criticism is justified properly by this factor. The involvement of emotional intelligence justifies few effective factors of the organization, and these factors are integrity, comfort with change, and trustworthiness [3].

24.2.2 *Theoretical Approach*

Training and skill in emotional intelligence are important during pandemic situations [4]. Self-awareness and self-control are treated as the main factors for the emotional intelligence process. This process can increase the ability to manage emotions. Training and skill can help to explore the intentions of people. Along with this, interaction with senses is maintained with the involvement of the emotional intelligence process. Emotional intelligence can help people to show attention towards both action and reaction [5]. Personal influence is treated as an effective theory of the emotional intelligence process. Life-based meaning and values are justified with the involvement of the emotional intelligence process. Few effective factors are affected by emotional intelligence, such as decision-making, adaptive behaviour, and people's thinking.

To maintain the efficiency of emotional intelligence, it is important to justify all theories and models properly. Self-management is also justified with the help of all theoretical aspects. To increase the efficiency of the emotional intelligence process, it is important to implement proper and authentic theories. Emotional intelligence is based on high-performing models and theories. Along with this, it is important to maintain a selection of theories and models that can increase the efficiency of emotional intelligence [6]. With the help of various resources, it is observed that Salovey and Mayer are the coiners of the emotional intelligence process. Through this approach inking of a leader is maintained properly. Emotional and intellectual growth is promoted by the emotional intelligence process, which Salovey and Mayer state. The genuine type of emotional intelligence process is maintained with the involvement of the model of Salovey and Mayer.

Both psychological and functional well-beings are justified with the help of emotional intelligence theory. On the other hand, the theory of execution is maintained properly by Daniel Goleman, which is treated as an effective theory of the emotional intelligence process. This theory of execution can play a crucial role in maintaining self-control, self-regulation, and self-motivation. The theory of Goleman is involved in the maintenance of the education world, which is treated as an effective theoretical approach to the emotional intelligence process. Goleman's theory is involved in properly maintaining human relationships, which directly impacts the organization's efficiency. Scientific evidence reveals the emotional intelligence process easily [7]. Five effective components are present in the emotional intelligence process: self-awareness, self-regulation, internal motivation, empathy, and social skill. These five effective factors are evaluated below:

Self-awareness: this component can help to understand personal moods, emotions, and drivers. Self-awareness is conducted with the involvement of realistic self-assessment, self-deprecating sense of humour, and self-confidence. Along with this, identification of emotion is also maintained by this factor.

Self-regulation: the ability of employees is improved with the involvement of the self-regulation process. Along with this trustworthiness and integrity of employees are improved with the help of the self-regulation process. The self-regulation process is involved in the maintenance of comfort and ambiguity and openness.

Internal motivation: the efficiency of an organization depends on the motivation of employees. Internal and external rewards are important to increase the efficiency of internal motivation. Internal motivation can increase the authenticity of workers; the productivity of the organization is increased by this factor of emotional intelligence [8]. High-performing internal motivation processes manage failure and maintenance of organizational commitment.

Empathy: empathy is treated as an effective component of the emotional intelligence process, which can increase the capability of employees. It helps to learn about the emotional makeup of other people. Cross-culture sensitivity, building and retaining talent, and service to clients and customers are maintained with empathy. This component of emotional intelligence maintains the behaviour and

Fig. 24.1 Emotional intelligence [4]

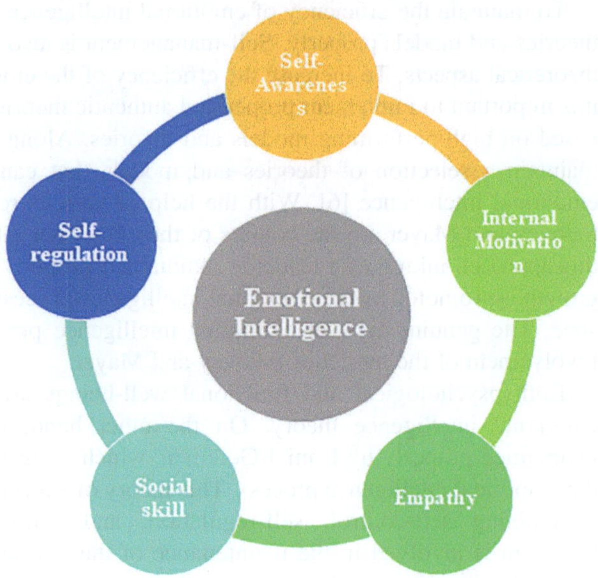

empathetic behaviour of employees. Along with this the educational context of employees is also maintained by this aspect.

Social skill: improvement of social skill is treated as an effective aspect for employees, which directly impacts their efficiency. This component of emotional intelligence can play a crucial role in the maintenance of building rapport and common ground. Managing relationships and building networks are justified properly by social skills [4] (Fig. 24.1).

24.3 Bar-On's EI Competencies Model

The interconnected behaviour of the emotional intelligence process is maintained with Bar-On's competencies model for emotional intelligence. Few effective scales are present in this competencies model, such as self-expression, interpersonal, decision-making, stress management, and self-perception. These scales can increase the efficiency of the emotional intelligence process. Interpersonal relationships, problem-solving, reality testing, impulse control, social responsibility, and assertiveness are maintained properly with the help of the competencies model of the emotional intelligence process. On the other hand, it is observed that optimism and stress tolerances are controlled with the involvement of Bar-On's competencies model for the emotional intelligence process, which is illustrated in Fig. 24.2 [9]. This model can play a crucial role in the maintenance of human behaviour and relationships. Managers of organizations solve many problems with the help of this model of emotional intelligence, which is an effective capability of this model.

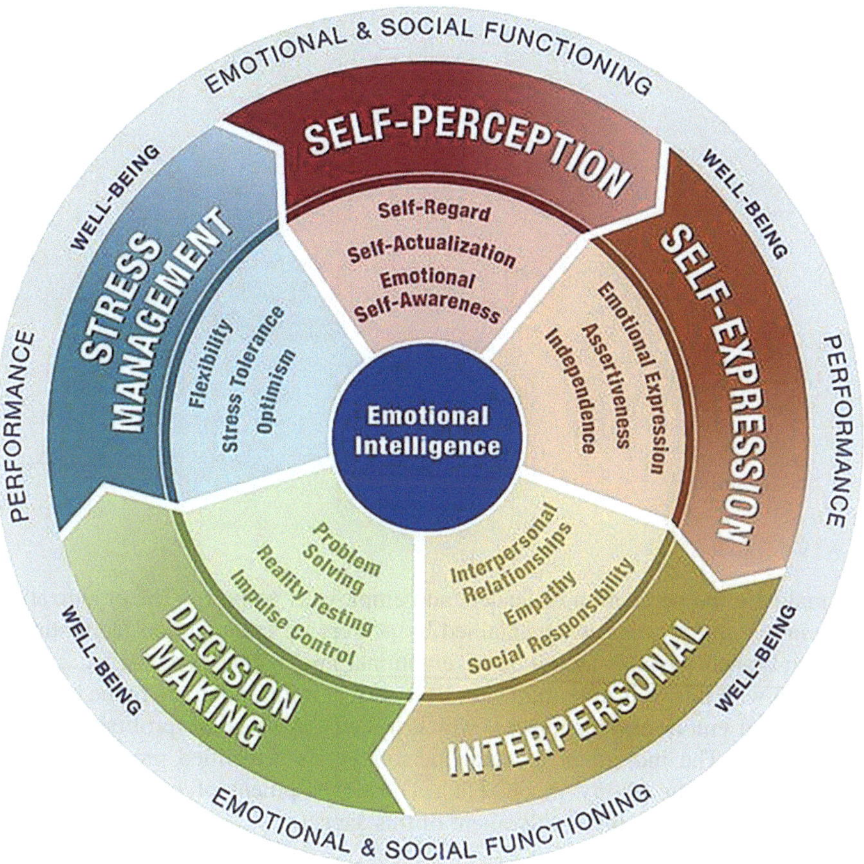

Fig. 24.2 Bar-On's EI competencies model [9]

24.3.1 Mayer, Salovey, and Caruso's EI Ability Model

Thinking of emotional intelligence is maintained properly with the involvement of Mayer and Salovey. Understanding of emotion is maintained using the ability model of Salovey, Mayer, and Caruso. Along with this, it is observed that thinking and decision-making processes are improved properly with the involvement of this ability model. The EI framework emphasizes four branch models of emotional intelligence. These four branch models are conducted with the involvement of perceived emotion, use of emotion to facilitate thought, understanding of emotion, and managing emotion. These four factors can increase the effectiveness of this model, which is illustrated in Fig. 24.3. With proper management, these branches

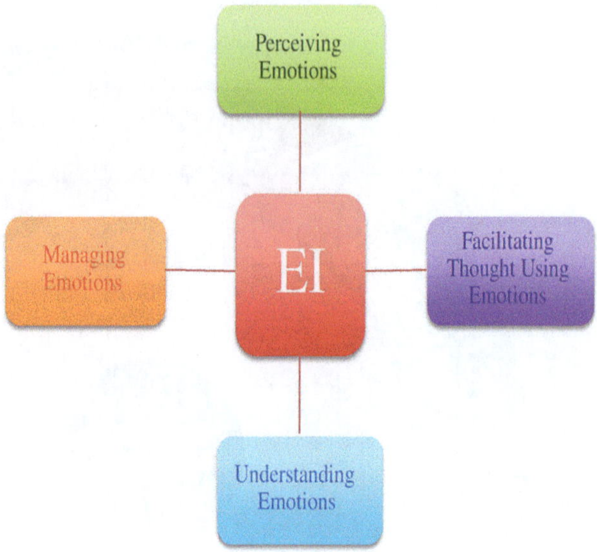

Fig. 24.3 Mayer, Salovey, and Caruso's EI ability model [10]

can maintain the perception of leaders and employees properly. The organization's information and process are maintained by perceiving emotion and facilitating the emotion branches of this model of the emotional intelligence process.

Along with this, it is important to collect correct information about the emotional systems and emotion management, which directly impacts the profitability of the organization. The individual's overall personality is a justified properly with the involvement of the ability model [11]. The development of basic skills is also justified properly with the involvement of this aspect.

24.4 Materials and Methods

Research methods can provide information about the specific procedures and techniques of this study [12]. Process selection, identification, and analysis of information are maintained with the involvement of research methods. Positivism research philosophy has been selected for this research that can maintain all approaches of this study. A descriptive research design has been selected to conduct this study to help researchers provide authentic answers to all research questions. The normal behaviour of research is justified by this research design. The deductive research approach is used widely in this research to fulfil all essential factors of this study. A deductive research approach can develop a hypothesis of this study. All ethical factors are maintained properly in this study [9].

24.5 Research Philosophy

Research philosophy can increase the potentiality of research. Beliefs in data collection, reliability, and analysis are maintained with the help of authentic research philosophy. Positivism, pragmatism, realism, and interpretivism research philosophies are used by nature. Positivism research philosophy has been selected to conduct this study. Data collection and analysis are maintained properly with the help of positivism research philosophy.

24.5.1 Research Design

Research design is an important component of the research methodology, which directly impacts the efficiency of this study. Experimental, survey, semi-experimental, and descriptive design is used normally. This study is conducted with the involvement of descriptive research design. The overall structure of this study and the natural and unchanged natural environments are maintained by this research design [13].

24.5.2 Research Approach

The distinct aspect of research is maintained with the help of a high-performing research approach. Three types of research approaches are observed such as inductive, deductive, and abductive research approach. This research is conducted with the involvement of a deductive research approach and with the help of existing resources; this factor deductive research approach is implemented successfully [10].

24.5.3 Data Collection and Data Analysis

Data collection is an important part of this study, collecting correct information about the emotional intelligence process. Two types of data collection processes are observed such as primary data and secondary data. This study is conducted with the help of secondary data. On the other hand, the qualitative data analysis process is used to analyse the collected information. Secondary data is collected from published articles, journals, books, and other resources. The efficiency of this study is justified with the involvement of this data analysis process [14].

24.5.4 Ethical Consideration

During this study, the researchers observed all ethical considerations to maintain the efficiency of the study. Along with this, it is important also to maintain the confidentiality of the collected data. Data protection is an important factor, which is a crucial ethical consideration for this study. On the other hand, it is important to maintain a conflict of interest, which directly impacts this study. Beneficence and non-maleficence are justified properly by ethical consideration. The researchers maintain all ethical considerations.

24.6 Result and Discussion

Emotional intelligence is treated as an effective factor for the managing of a pandemic situation. It can play a crucial role in human beings with the involvement of the self-awareness process. Self-awareness can help people to recognize emotions such as moods, actions, and others [15]. The balance of thinking and feeling of the brain is controlled with the involvement of the emotional intelligence process. Emotional intelligence can create psychological safety for people that can help them to manage the pandemic crises easily. This process can help people to accelerate performance and meditating variables. Along with this risk of ridicule is decreased with the involvement of the high-performing emotional intelligence process.

According to the evaluation of various secondary data resources regarding emotional intelligence, the baseline description showcased that emotional intelligence is nothing but the determination and monitoring of personal emotions according to the emotional intelligence of the surrounding population, environment, or individual. It also consists of distinguishing between various emotions and visualizing the consequences of reflecting certain actions based on the respective emotion. Gaining expertise or mastery over the aspect of EI or emotional intelligence can prove to be very fruitful for any respective person and individual, and he or she can be a positive influence or example to the others within his/her surroundings. It is not something that can be theoretically explained. The best example would be the feelings of empathy, happiness, love, and anger that one feels when they engage in some form of activity or interaction with their respective families, colleagues, friends, and loved ones. It helps people connect with others on an internal level and lead a prosperous and happy life.

The outbreak and spread of disease across different continents and countries and worldwide are described as pandemic. Usually, they affect the economy, health, and daily workability of the global population negatively. One of the biggest examples of a pandemic is the Covid-19 spread that the world is currently facing. Starting from the city of Wuhan in China, the virus has spread across all the major countries in the world rapidly. It has affected the health of approximately 12% of the global population. That roughly translates to 924 million people all around the world [16]. The examples and reports regarding the infected people showcase various reasons to worry and can cause serious stress in people's minds. The primary stress factor usually includes fear, anxiety, and other strong emotions within the people. A critical evaluation of the stress factors showcases the below-mentioned stress factors:

- Worsening of chronic health problems either due to physical complications or mental anxieties and trauma
- Change of daily life activities like sleeping and eating patterns and other complexities related to concentration in other works
- Increase in addictive substance usages such as tobacco, alcohol, and other illegal drugs
- Misbalanced daily life scales due to the imposed lockdowns and work from home measures

The situation will be far worse for the young and the older adults within the population as their mental health is not within the optimal maturity levels.

The first and foremost step that will help regulate the emotional intelligence and mental health of the people would be periodic consultation with doctors and general physicians. Assurance from doctors helps greatly in boosting the confidence of people. Simple statements from them such as "you are fine" and "you are fit" would prove to be greatly beneficial. Continuation of prescribed medicines should also be among the top priorities among the people, as disregarding them can worsen mental health and anxiety conditions. This pandemic also provides people with an environment where they can stay at home and regularly interact with their family members and engage in collaborative home activities. People should engage in healthy interactions, play indoor games, watch movies, and read books along with their close ones and family members, which will work as a relaxant and way of mental satisfaction [17].

People from the age limit of 18–40 should be the ones who should maintain their emotional intelligence levels the most as they can pose as models and help in balancing the emotional intelligence levels of their respective close ones [18]. The usage of technology can prove to be a huge boon in this situation. People can watch informational contents, videos, and documentaries and discuss them with their peers. The feeling of isolation can also be reduced with the help of video chats and phone calls with peers and family members who are stuck or are situated in far-off places from their home. Being confident is essential, as, in times of crisis like this, one should develop a mindset of dealing with any kind of situation. The intelligent ones among the population should spread positive awareness among their respective peers and loved ones and be ready to emotionally support, empathize, and help others as much as possible [19]. Regular checking of the current status of the crisis or pandemic can also boost confidence within the people, as governments and countries are working upon creating stabilized vaccines against the virus. Following the news and social posts made from governments, medical institutions, and representatives should be practised in this situation. The parents and older adults of the families should not overreact to the crisis as the children and the young ones would imitate their footsteps. The more reassuring and confident the parents, elder brothers, and sister will be, the more beneficial will it be for the teens and the aged ones.

People should talk among themselves, share their feelings, engage in productive activities, and discuss informative and educational information and content. They must be made to realize that it is alright to feel bored, anxious, or down sometimes, as these are nothing but the effects of certain chemical secretions in the body. Speaking about chemical secretions, people should also engage in activities that can enable the secretion of happy hormones within their bodies. These hormones are respectively dopamine, serotonin, oxytocin, and endorphins. They must educate themselves regarding these kinds of technical aspects and find out legitimate and fun ways so that these hormones are secreted within them. Watching videos related to this respective topic can assist further [20]. Lastly, everybody should be aware that they are not alone facing all these kinds of crisis situations, and there are millions of others going through the same. This will help form a "pseudo-connectivity" among the rest of the world and translate to the improvement of the emotional and mental state of the people [21, 22].

24.7 Conclusion

The findings of this study led the researchers to the conclusion that emotional intelligence is a significant factor that can effectively boost the possibility of increasing the levels of self-awareness as well as self-regulation. The process of emotional intelligence helps to preserve the self-censoring tendency, which is one factor that may play a significant part in the ongoing pandemic crisis. According to the findings of this study, the process of emotional intelligence can help individuals maintain personal risk management. The participation of emotional intelligence helps to preserve a variety of thought patterns, as well as constructive disagreement and creative abrasion. This element may be helpful in finding solutions to difficulties. Emotional intelligence may, based on the information in this chapter, recognize all of the essential obstacles posed by a pandemic catastrophe.

References

1. Pool, L. D. (2017). Developing graduate employability: The CareerEDGE model and the importance of emotional intelligence. In *Graduate employability in context* (pp. 317–338). Palgrave Macmillan.
2. Kelly, E. J., & Kaminskienė, N. (2016). Importance of emotional intelligence in negotiation and mediation. *International Comparative Jurisprudence, 2*(1), 55–60.
3. Chandra, Y. (2020). Online education during COVID-19: Perception of academic stress and emotional intelligence coping strategies among college students. *Asian Education and Development Studies, 10*, 229.

4. Soto-Rubio, A., Giménez-Espert, M. D. C., & Prado-Gascó, V. (2020). Effect of emotional intelligence and psychosocial risks on burnout, job satisfaction, and nurses' health during the covid-19 pandemic. *International Journal of Environmental Research and Public Health, 17*(21), 7998.
5. Alonazi, W. B. (2020). The impact of emotional intelligence on job performance during COVID-19 crisis: A cross-sectional analysis. *Psychology Research and Behavior Management, 13*, 749.
6. Paavola, L. E. (2017). The importance of emotional intelligence in early childhood.
7. Miao, C., Humphrey, R. H., & Qian, S. (2017). A meta-analysis of emotional intelligence and work attitudes. *Journal of Occupational and Organizational Psychology, 90*(2), 177–202.
8. Wheeler, R. (2016). Soft skills-the importance of cultivating emotional intelligence. *AALL Spectrum, 20*(3), 28.
9. Abdel-Fattah, H. M. M. (2020). Emotional intelligence and emotional stability in crises. *Journal of Psychiatry and Psychiatric Disorders, 4*(2), 56–62.
10. Norboevich, T. B. (2020). Analysis of psychological theory of emotional intelligence. *European Journal of Research and Reflection in Educational Sciences, 8*(3), 99–104.
11. Newton, C., et al. (2016). Emotional intelligence as a buffer of occupational stress. *Personnel Review, 45*, 1010.
12. Adams, J., Loach, T., & Szomszor, M. (2016). Interdisciplinary research: Methodologies for identification and assessment. *Digital Research Reports, 9*, 1–8.
13. Serrat, O. (2017). Understanding and developing emotional intelligence. In *Knowledge solutions* (pp. 329–339). Springer.
14. Hogeveen, J., Salvi, C., & Grafman, J. (2016). 'Emotional Intelligence': Lessons from lesions. *Trends in Neurosciences, 39*(10), 694–705.
15. Kantor, M. A., et al. (2020). The importance of emotional intelligence when leading in a time of crisis. *Journal of Hospital Medicine, 15*(9), 568–569.
16. Boyatzis, R. E. (2018). The behavioral level of emotional intelligence and its measurement. *Frontiers in Psychology, 9*, 1438.
17. Mestre, J. M., et al. (2016). Models of cognitive ability and emotion can better inform contemporary emotional intelligence frameworks. *Emotion Review, 8*(4), 322–330.
18. Lopes, P. N. (2016). Emotional intelligence in organizations: Bridging research and practice. *Emotion Review, 8*(4), 316–321.
19. Keefer, K., Parker, J., & Saklofske, D. (2018). Emotional intelligence in education. In *Integrating research with practice*. Springer.
20. Miners, C. T. H., Côté, S., & Lievens, F. (2018). Assessing the validity of emotional intelligence measures. *Emotion Review, 10*(1), 87–95.
21. Bacon, A. M., & Corr, P. J. (2017). Motivating emotional intelligence: A reinforcement sensitivity theory (RST) perspective. *Motivation and Emotion, 41*(2), 254–264.
22. Jiménez, M. (2018). Leadership style, organizational performance, and change through the lens of emotional intelligence. *Foundations of Management, 10*(1), 237–250.

Chapter 25
Efficient Maintenance of Hospital Records by Entrusted Proof of Work Algorithm in Block Chain Technology

M. S. Minu, S. S. Subashka Ramesh, Sai Kartheek Reddy Peruru, and N. M. Roshan

25.1 Introduction

Health care is one of the platforms for the organization and operation of huge data transactions. As an example of high data threats that create a stir for a revolution in data organization, secure and sharable records, standardized image recognition, optimized with integrated services, and metadata dependability [1]. Sectoring with the advancement in technologies has made progress for the environment for optimized results in health care. The times of the recent COVID-19 pandemic are a best-case reference. The Contemplation to the era of information and automation placed operability and immutability at the top of the list of demands [2]. The blockchain technology scenario paved the way toward the development cycle with interoperability, decentralization, immutability, and consensus as prime attributes. And we can have the desired quirk, such as computational power or capacity, with the Consensus Protocol. The pressure on the data regimen posed security risks, and the vulnerable methods resulted in ransomware attacks, such as WannaCry in 2017, PYSA in 2019, and a range of 16 health trusts going offline. The average revenue loss of health care per unit of population is US $380. In 2021, there was an infamous ransomware rift, with 15% of breaches synchronizing unauthorized network access and 12% with unrestricted database and server access. The problem of health care breaches worsened in 2021, with the release of PII data on 1.5 billion people [3, 4]. As per the US Department of Health and Human Services, 4.7 million individuals were affected on

M. S. Minu (✉) · S. S. S. Ramesh · S. K. R. Peruru · N. M. Roshan
SRM Institute of Science and Technology, Ramapuram, Chennai, Tamil Nadu, India
e-mail: pk7144@srmist.edu.in; rm1735@srmist.edu.in

F. J. Joseph et al. (eds.), *Computational Intelligence for Clinical Diagnosis*,
EAI/Springer Innovations in Communication and Computing,
https://doi.org/10.1007/978-3-031-23683-9_25

1 January 2018 with a total of 288 total health care data breaches. As of 2020, 32% of individuals were vulnerable to identity theft, with a total of 663 breaches. In 2021, the percentile rose to 2.4% with a total of 679 breaches. However, the attacks increased by 32% from 2020 to 2021.

According to a recent survey conducted by the Department of Health and Human Services (HHS), a data breach claims 6 victims out of 190 global health care organizations, and the breach occurred on 20 November 2021 [5]. Thus, such threats call for the assurance of data confidentiality, i.e., data immutability. With peer-to-peer networks, blockchain technology comes to the rescue, which is a digital ledger to hold transactions between two entities of transfer in the form of immutable blocks that are time-stamped for reliability [1], with the Consensus Algorithm protocol to ensure trust between unfamiliar peers in a distributed decentralized network. Although the interoperability facet is to achieve harmony between blockchains in a network, its true resolve is to facilitate patients' or users' authority over data rather than health care institutions [2]. It is also true that the transfer of possession of blockchain from one to another, which is meant to instigate blockchain, requires extensive legacy systems to be reengineered. In a global health care ecosystem, the legacy blockchain attribute electronic medical records (EMR) or electronic health records (EHR), on the other hand, is based on a centralized architecture. In 2017, health care service providers used EHR at a rate of 67%, up from 40% in 2012. Because EHR is a digital print to share across health care institutions, compared with EMR, digital paper copies are available to the particular organization. Different data sizes and block data compromise blockchain's data storage scalability [22]; the time required to mine a block is included in the database's accessibility and scalability [6–8]. The healthcare data breach ranks at the top in average revenue loss, with a 29.7% increase from 2020 to 2021. A digital signature can be termed as a stamped hash on a document or ledger by using a symmetric key and a private key for authentication and authorization verification.

25.1.1 Interoperability Ascendancy of Blockchain

With the growing use of cases of blockchain-like access control, health care, digital identity, intellectual property, and their applications remain isolated. Blockchain in general is a digital ledger that needs to be operated on the necessity of metadata. Moreover, health care data need to be classified and confined to being public or private. However, authorized personnel need all sensitive data; thus, the disclosure of the data is at stake. Interoperability [9, 10] conceptualizes how to ensure that two or more blockchains work together as a sidechain.

25.1.2 Immutability Ascendancy of Blockchain

The immutability of a blockchain is the ability to be unaltered or indelible. However, this asset of blockchain may not validate its actual data, but it can specify the resistance to tampering that fossilizes the information. Data manipulation is out of the question in the case of blockchain as the data mutation results in the spoiling of the reliability of data in subsequently mined blocks [11, 12]. Immutability can be achieved in many ways, but blockchain provides a hash method that is a unique digital signature that cannot be reverse-engineered. SHA-2 and its variant SHA-64 are predominantly used to generate the hash. Thus, prior speculation of the data is required before packaging in block transitions. In blockchain, incorrect data correction and data reorganization may necessitate higher level access.

25.1.3 Effects of Blockchain in the Health Care Ecosystem

Health care security is of paramount importance to health care providers to help safeguard the privacy of patients' health information [13]. Blockchain technology may turn out to have a doubtful advantage because data in blockchain nodes is immutable, as hit-or-miss usage led to scathing circumstances, which means that if healthcare metadata is not organized well in Blockchain, then there can be deviations in outcomes which will be a potential risk. Large data or volatile data need to be in appropriate files. The other side of using blockchain is safeguarding genomics, tracking diseases and outbreaks, and auditability [14, 15]. The recorded data may be used by research organizations to improve drug refining for diseases. With its widespread connectivity, blockchain can optimize real-world data in health care through data integration, verification, and analysis. It also influences the pharmaceutical industry through the growth of claim management [4].

25.1.4 Recent Breaches Review

Case Study 1: Eskenazi Health has a comprehensive clinical information system that caused the information team to discover suspicious activity on the data. The countermeasures are network operation and taking offline. The personally identifiable information of nearly 1,515,918 records is decoded in previously enciphered files. The attack is supposed to have commenced on 19 May 2021, by a malicious IP address and a data leak occurred on the dark web. Through its review of data, the data leak may consist of patient's information such as name, credit card information, address, insurance information, and social security number. The attack resulted in the bills' payments and the revenue loss of former and current patients. Reported fraudulent transactions of US $370 on a credit card occurred when cyber-attackers accessed a network, resulting in a privacy stake of approximately 1.5 million records of personnel, and former and current patients. The Department of HHS reported the breach as having affected 9851 inpatients and outpatients.

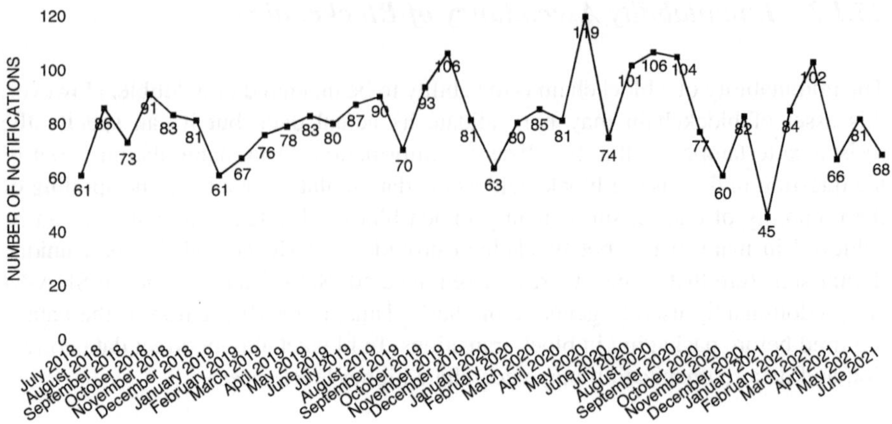

Fig. 25.1 Data breach notification

Case Study 2: Location: Florida, United States; report date: 29 January 2021. One of the most well-known data breaches, the Florida Healthy Kids Corporation (FHKC) Data Breach, affected 3.5 million people. Protected health information (PHI) was endangered. The violation was supposed to have happened on 1 January 2013, but was notified to the FHKC on 29 December 2020. Part of the Florida Kid Care application gave access to an unauthorised third-party and spoiled private and sensitive data. The breach was reviewed by a third-party cybersecurity firm. The investigation reported that vulnerabilities had subsisted since November 2013 as well as significant ones in websites that were unremitted and the vendors failed to provide security patches. Individuals who applied or enrolled in Florida Kid Care coverage between 2013 and 2020 were encouraged to check their insurance plans and sign up for fraud alert notifications. The application has gone offline, although the breachers mutated only subspace data such as addresses and telephone numbers.

Major issues with breach: The long access of the website to the organization's database. The above types of threats are consistently averted by the usage of blockchain and hyperledger technology. Because the data are confiscated in a peer-to-peer network of blocks, the first block encountering the unauthorized data modification may act as a honey trap for the threats (Figs. 25.1 and 25.2).

25.2 Related Work

The blockchain could provide a single transaction layer where organizations can submit and share data through one secure system, by storing a specific set of standardized data on the chain. Tanwar and colleagues [16] point of weighty in cyber-attacks of the ransomware type, which is a form of malware employed by attackers and a key factor in cyber-attacks, health care demands multi-level security

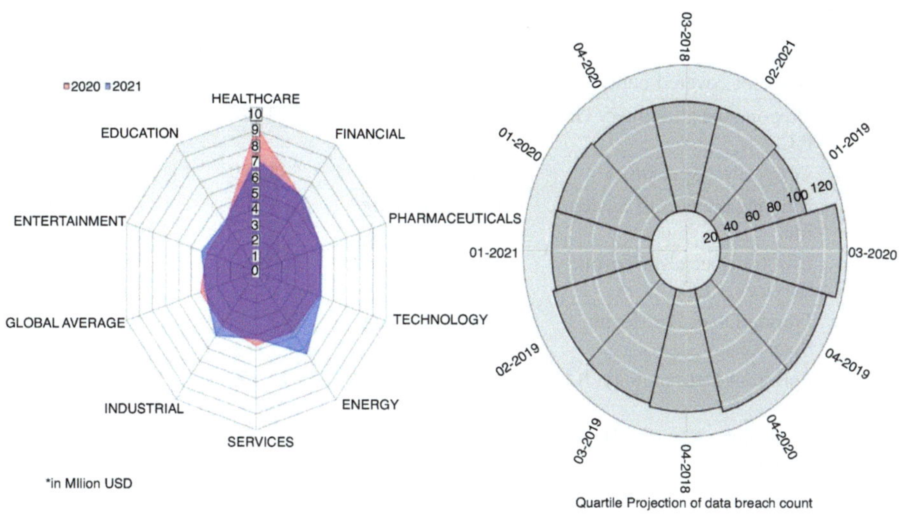

Fig. 25.2 Revenue (average) loss by industry

along with privacy. Hence, a model of blockchain so as with private and symmetric key issues, the authority for sharing an EHR across the network is proposed. All the peers in the blockchain are unknown to each other; hence, all nodes are untrusted nodes. The consensus algorithm helps these nodes to maintain an accord. As a network with one or more blockchains may consider other blockchains to be third-parties and untrusted, the proposed model by Xia et al. [10] is a layered taxonomy of data sharing blockchain model among untrusted parties. The classification of layers puts the user layer, the querying system in the data querying layer, a layer of database infrastructure, along with a layer of smart logic, authentication, and networking [17]. Personal health data may come from wearable devices, and data sharing can overlap with user-centric architecture. As data from real time are dynamic with a need for integrity management of recorded data, linked lists in more specific tree-based scalability are deployed. Thus, the model proposed by Liang et al. help oneself with the Merkle tree, a binary structure variant where hashed records are given as input. In the work presented by Jiang et al. [18], a loosely coupled architectural design of the personal healthcare data (PHD) chain along with the EMR chain is described. Blocks in general have a block header, which taxonomizes the Merkle root, an arbitrary constant called a node [19]. In the loosely coupled architecture of PHD and EMR chains, there is a demand for high and moderate privacy respectively, with latency in a moderate sense, for sharing health care data. The proposed data preserve work by Hongyu et al. [20] is to standardize the transparency of blockchain along with immutability, that is, if the data are packed, then the data cannot be altered. The higher the rate of preservation of data, the greater the mining of nodes. Wang and Yujiao [21] and Bigini et al. [23], propose cloud-based and internet of medical things (IoMT) concepts for interoperability, data perception, integrity, and security, as well as blockchain decentralized design [23]. The security and privacy issues of health care applications involving the IoMT can be solved by using blockchain features (Table 25.1).

Table 25.1 Data breach in health care report 2021

S. no.	Name of covered entity	Cause of breach	No. of records affected	Date breach reported
1	Oregon Anesthesiology Group, P.C	Ransomware	750,500	14-Dec-2021
2	Texas ENT Specialists	Ransomware	535,489	19-Oct-2021
3	Monongalia Health System, Inc.	Email Phishing	398,164	21-Dec-2021
4	BioPlus Specialty Pharmacy Services, LLC	Hacked Network Server	350,000	11-Nov-2021
5	Florida Digestive Health Specialists	Email Phishing	212,509	16-Dec-2020
6	Forefront Dermatology, S.C	Hacked Network Server	2,413,553	07-Aug-2021
7	St. Joseph's/Candler Health System, Inc	Hacked Network Server	1,400,000	08-Oct-2021
8	American Anesthesiology	Email Phishing	1,269,074	01-Aug-2021

25.2.1 *Organization*

The chapter is organised so as to contain related work in Sect. 25.2. Section 25.3 contains the proposed model system architecture, the consensus protocol, and the working model. The performance evaluation is described in Sect. 25.4. Section 25.5 gives a discussion, and Sect. 25.6 is a conclusion, ending with the acknowledgements.

25.3 Proposed Model

As we mentioned, blockchain provides the immutability and security edge, but the metadata that is used does not have a validation point because decentralization destroys central authority over the blockchain network, so that the metadata provided may or may not be trusted. So, in order to evaluate them, consensus algorithms are put into use. The reliability of the data is paramount in the big data and IoT sectors [24, 25]. The consensus protocols are the policies through which all the peers or nodes in the network reach common accord on the current state of the ledger. The consensus protocol makes sure that every new block that is added to the blockchain is the one and only version of the truth that is agreed upon by all the nodes in the blockchain. Reliability can be brought among the unknown nodes by different means; thus, various consensus algorithms are used to win for the entire network. They are:

Proof of work: Entails using computational power to solve a complex math puzzle. The difficulty of the hash is the choice of node. The next block is mined by the block, which attests to the complexity of this algorithm.

Proof of stake: In the algorithm, the block is selected at random with the combination of the block with the lowest hash value and the highest stake, i.e. the one that uses the least amount of energy.

In this algorithm, all the peers are disposed of in a systematic order such that one node becomes the primary one and the rest are backup nodes and they reach an agreement with unity as a source of truth. In practical byzantine fault tolerance, the selected block is final and followed with full integrity.as few complex calculations with low reward variance make it good.

25.3.1 System Architecture

In system architecture, the graphical user interface is deployed as the portal for the collection of metadata. Because the data entered here are transferred to the blockchain, caution must be exercised when administering the data; thus, authenticated individuals are assigned to the Frontend. NextPath's current GUI part is the representational state transfer application programming interface, simply REST API. This REST API helps in aligning the metadata with the data variables in the backend programming. Nodes of a private blockchain are represented in JSON format. The next part is to segment the metadata into two viable components, such as the viewable data and the sensitive data, and make them into the public and private blockchain (Fig. 25.3).

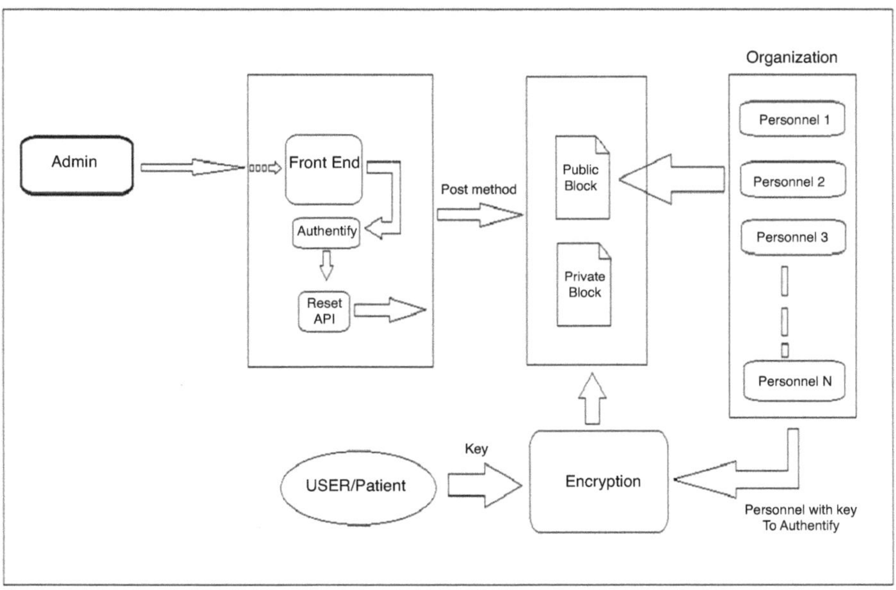

Fig. 25.3 System architecture design

As we know, the immutability and the reliability issues we previously mentioned are involved in the proof of work consensus algorithm. The work of proof of work is done by example. Assume an example network where there is more than one blockchain. We need a hash function for the nodes in those blockchains, but the problem is that the components of one blockchain may match with another blockchain such as serial numbers, data, or in the worst case, all the parameters may match. As a result, the same hash variable may arise. So, we utilize an arbitrary constant or pseudo-random number, coined a "node." Although the data size may vary, the hash value length will be constant throughout the network. Here the miners engage in a fixture to find the node that matches the complexity of the puzzle, and the miner has the highest computational power, and the node is added to the next node. In Finis, the user has the key to access the private blockchain and only authorized personnel may access the user/patient data in the private blockchain.

25.3.2 Module Deployment

Even though blockchain development is effective and efficient by using other programming languages such as those that use ECMAScript, we get the benefit of integrating the blockchain with many other concepts by using Python. In module deployment, we use REST API to render html elements and assign them to the data variables of the main code using the POST method of REST API such as Flask. The frontend can be done using bootstrap or html elements or React software as per resources. Coming to the main code, the data that was obtained from the frontend will be stored in JSON files. The hash value is generated using the _hashlib library and the SHA256 algorithm to give a 64-bit hash value. We use a class and class components in the prior function Object() {[native code]} to initiate a genesis block. The method of creating the block and this generated block will be mined to the genesis block and entities are immutable. As we use SHA256 as basic, we can use SHA512 hexdigest(), which is used to convert our data into hexadecimal format. All entities from the previous block, such as index, node, timestamp, and data, are used to develop the hash. For hash value, we return a utf-8 encoded version of the mathematical puzzle, in string format, which needs to be returned in byte datatype. To make this happen, we use the encode () function from the _hashlib library. We need to check or validate that the chain network is intact, so we create a class method to determine if the previous hash of the current block is the same as the hash of its previous block. Here we need to create another module and we need two modules to channel the metadata gathered into private and public block chains. The private block chain is the access point of the sensitive data. It will be encrypted and only users and authorized personnel have access to it. The third module will be an access point to segregate data, form points, and view data.

25.4 Performance Evaluation

In this part of the chapter, we speculate on the performance of EHR with the proposed blockchain model. Convergence with the proposed model used for technology and other utilities is also achieved.

25.4.1 Graphic Evidence

Our literature review mentioned the reasons that regulated for a blockchain model. Although our study seems to be an effective use of the old vulnerable system, the technology also brings its issues. The proposed model is a two-tier blockchain model. So, the unit testing is done with Python libraries. As we use the two-tier architecture of blockchain, we need to perform analysis of different elements, such as taking the average execution time of dual blockchain individually and also constituently for different records that are higher for proper analysis curvature. If the proposed model needs to possess more than one piece of classified data in its nodes, then the volume of the block chain varies. Thus, in Fig. 25.4, we depicted the error that arises when a block chain uses different volumes and in different cases such as time and space, with the function calls that are executed when the record

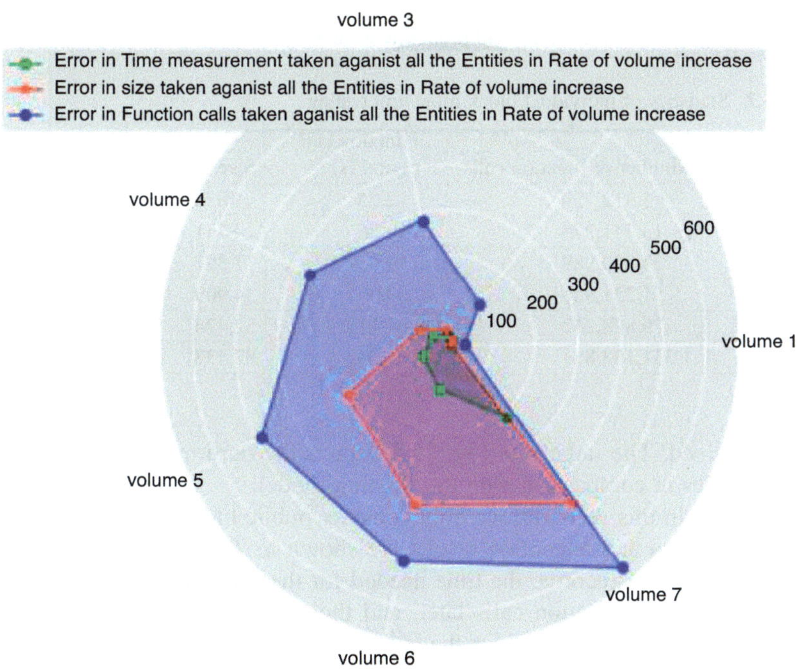

Fig. 25.4 Radar plot of errors in different volumes

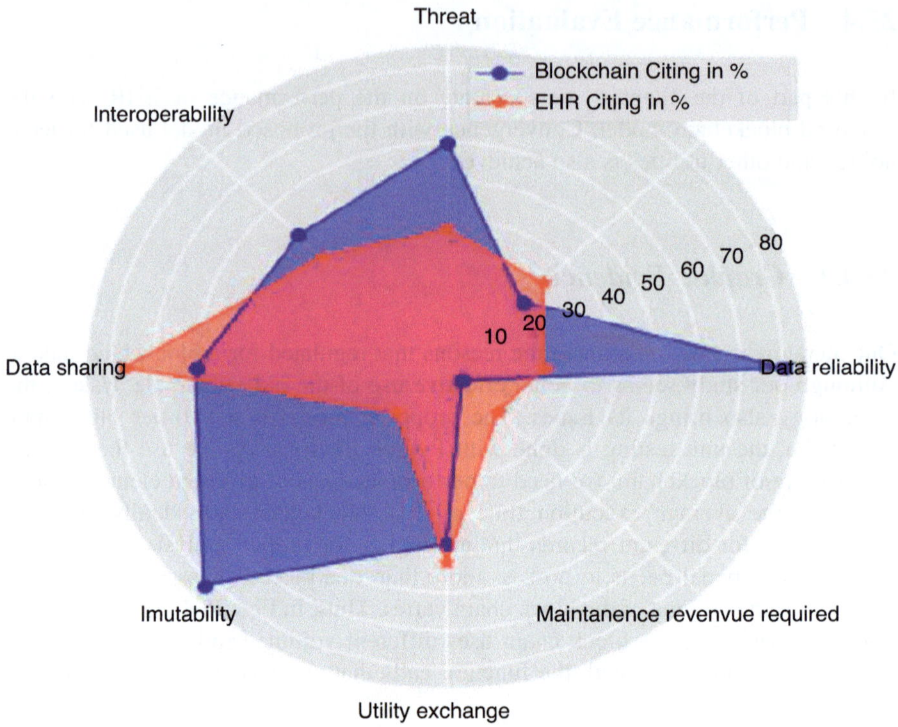

Fig. 25.5 Difference in the existing and proposed system

Table 25.2 Statistics of individual block mine unit testing

Records no	Number of function calls	Function call period (s)	Size of accumulated data (bytes)
10	3,312,759	2.25	1828
50	13,741,275	10.56	8751
100	24,860,989	19.039	17,397
200	51,221,925	39.097	34,909
300	79,828,253	61.119	52,424
500	1,331,138,881	101.042	87,433

nodes are mined. The radar plot Fig. 25.5 depicts the portions that the blockchain model provides in comparison with the existing model.

Scenario 1: In this scenario, we only consider public blockchain as an example, and the input data and execution results are shown in Table 25.2. We considered different numbers of records, the time needed for the function call to be executed, with the number of function calls later, and the size of the JSON file. The main purpose of the execution is to check the individual performance and efficiency of the code.

Table 25.3 Statistics of individual private block mine unit testing

Record no.	Number of function calls	Function call period (s)	Size of accumulated data (bytes)
10	3,150,855	2.98	2013
50	16,460,734	13.132	9626
100	28,491,068	22.589	19,127
200	52,205,328	41.48	38,427
300	75,857,896	60.526	57,721
500	133,543,240	106.024	96,352

Table 25.4 Statistics of dual-tier block mine unit testing

Records no.	Number of function calls	Function call period (s)	Size of accumulated data (bytes)
10	5,962,498	4.650	3667
50	26,151,238	20.178	21,006
100	50,881,060	39.176	35,828
200	100,662,740	77.974	70,017
300	157,630,332	122.545	175,142
500	260,983,412	203.178	350,471

Later, after the public blockchain, we turn to the private blockchain, where the performance analysis is quite complicated because the public blockchain only has data and may or may not be stored in a single file, but the private blockchain is permissioned, so we need the nodes to be in different JSON files as it is difficult to audit. So, for the time being, we mended the data into one JSON file. The question is to check the performance of the code and extract the size of data consumption, because of the private blockchain and semi-decentralized. In this process, the permissioned blockchain or private block chain may also be considered to be the execution of volume2-type entities, where the discussion of volume entities is for another scenario (Table 25.3).

25.4.2 Performance Complexity

Scenario 2: In this scenario, we need to get the dual-tier proposed model for debugging purposes and calculate the performance of the source code of the model. The execution of the code poses the same complexity. The results of execution are depicted in Table 25.4. Traction speed and size are the main parameters of performance.

It is evident that the blockchain may be the most viable alternative in health care in comparison (Fig. 25.6).

Scenario 3: In this scenario we make the model undergo performance.

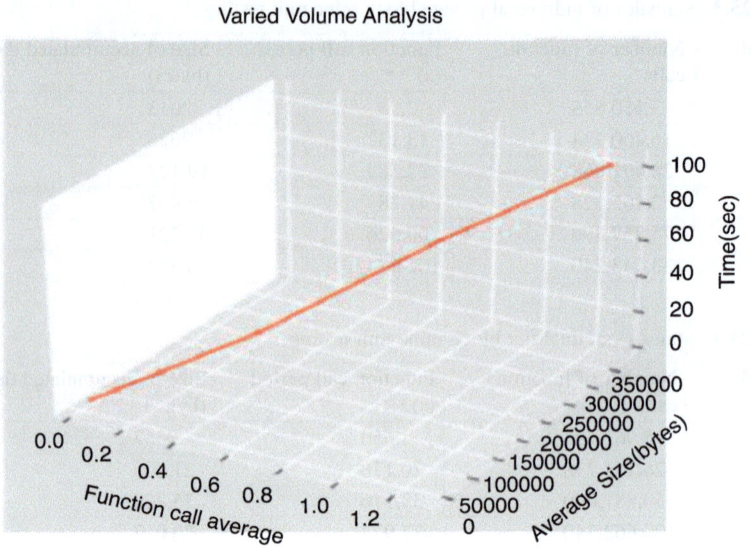

Fig. 25.6 Varied volume analysis

An analysis of change in volume of metadata for many classified datatypes and a huge number of records is administered. The graph depicted represents the change of record from 200 to 2000 to ensure the minimum day of data entry as per the agenda. And we used the worst case for the rival of the least employed method. In general, volume 1 states the type containing the patient data of registration number and name. The volume-2 type is evident to volume-1, along with the encryption key for authorized access. Volume 3 depicts the evidence of volume 2 along with sensitive data such as the doctor's prescription note. Similar to volume 4 where medical equipment is prescribed, volume 5 contains more sensitive data, such as an address, and volume 6 contains credit transaction information. Volume 7 contains other sensitive data. Although the health care blockchain is immutable to data changes, it is not immutable to threats with zero tolerance for breaches of probation and will impose strict penalties. Although the blockchain is generally decentralized, attacks such as distributed denial of service, Sybil attack, and others exist.

As we use the decentralized and consensus algorithm for the model, these are more prone to Sybil attacks – creating fake multiple identities in order to manipulate the peer-to-peer network.

Although we pose dual-tier architecture, there is no object for lifting an electromagnetic switch in the dual-tier blockchain. As a result, the resource is not used to its potential. The revenue model is eligible for lower costs than the current system, but it falls short of the mark. We use the proof-of-work consensus algorithm, which requires more computational power to generate the complex hash for time change reliability.

Table 25.5 The latency

Transaction: difficulty	3	4	5
10	0.098	3.037	49.88
100	1.053	20.23	618.97
1,000	12.79	210.82	2743.63

25.4.3 Analysis of the Proof-of-Work Algorithm

The consensus algorithm of proof of work is a peer-to-peer protocol that relies on the difficulty of entrusting the data. Thus, the latency, which is the difference between the execution time and the deployment time, to get the recession period. The analysis of the algorithm is depicted in Table 25.5, indicating the difficulty, which may be chosen on request.

$$L = E([\sec]) - D([\sec])$$

25.5 Discussion

According to the IBM 2021 report, health care is one of the most vulnerable areas to cyberattacks and has the highest revenue breaches. The EHR is particularly vulnerable to the current methods; thus, the consensus algorithm implementation of the blockchain model reduces and minimizes the breach calls with reliability and immutability of data. As mentioned in this chapter, the dual-tier model boasts reliability with proof of work. Because the block chain is decentralized, with the dual-tier architecture, it may result in semi-centralization. A large-scale implementation that is more resistant to threats is evidence of the use of the proof of work. The primary concern about the EHR system is that denial of service attacks is common. As the proposed model is a permissioned block chain, it answers a primary need and provides a replacement. The next question is whether, in the sense of better interoperability and immutability, the blockchain stands higher in regard to the EHR [14, 15, 26]. The consensus peer-to-peer relay may have better reliability. The latency of the proof of work increases with alteration of the difficulty and transaction rates at a directly proposed rate. The future curve bends to initiate a key shuffling mechanism with machine learning logic, enhancing performance through semi-centralized and decentralized communication.

25.6 Conclusion

Health care includes hospitals, rehabilitation facilities, medications, and genomics. Therefore, actual and dynamic data dominate. For many applications, including research, IoT, and big data, data constitute a digital asset. As dynamic metadata are large, data dependability, security, and interoperability must be improved. "Blockchain adds decentralized specifications. An EHR is an EMR upgrade with data exchange. Digitalization of COVID-19's health care sector is leading to a US $95.9 billion market by 2024. Approximately US $3.2 trillion is invested in artificial intelligence, record quantization, and storage scalability to improve health care. Blockchain's other features must attract consumers' trust and attention and ensure their privacy and comfort. Cloud revenue is excluded from the analysis. Distributed Ledger Technology (DLT) with no central administrator synchronizes large-scale, programmable, disrupted, change-resistant data. With this, patients may access personal data across the network, allowing hospitals to optimize services and treatment. User-encrypted personal data ensure data privacy. Electronic Medical Records (EMRs) and Electronic Health Records (EHRs) are a pack, but cybercrime cost 125 million USD revenue loss in 2015 alone. Blockchains may also be prone to threats but the range of attacks compared to EHR is minimal. We feel that maybe in the future blockchain could be affected because of the following reasons: (1) consensus protocol threats, (2) breach of privacy and confidentiality, (3) compromising of private keys, and (4) smart contract defects. Blockchain technology with DLT Domain can put an influence on feature like track diseases, genomics data integrity, and medicine traceability. Initial implementation is in finance and crypto-assets. Using a consensus mechanism, DLT gives essential critical features for unknown network nodes. The biggest after effect of a cyberattack is offline services, although decentralization allows the reinvocation of offline services on sidelines with the online architecture, as the same blockchain is dispersed across the network. Interoperability and privacy revolutions ensure optimal resource usage in a safe environment.

References

1. Saha, S., Majumder, A., Bhowmik, T., Basu, A., & Choudhury, A. (2021). A healthcare data management system on blockchain framework. In *2021 international conference on smart generation computing, communication and networking (SMART GENCON)* (pp. 1–5). https://doi.org/10.1109/SMARTGENCON51891.2021.9645890
2. Vazirani, A., O'Donoghue, O., Brindley, D., & Meinert, E. (2018). Implementing blockchains for efficient health care: Systematic review. *Journal of Medical Internet Research, 21*(2), e12439.
3. Jmaiel, M., et al. (2020, May 31). The impact of digital technologies on public health in developed and developing countries. In *International conference on smart homes and health telematics* (vol. 12157, pp. 268–276). Springer Nature.
4. Minu, M. S., Aroul Canessane, R., & Subashka Ramesh, S. S. (2022). Optimal squeeze net with deep neural network-based arial image classification model in unmanned aerial vehicle. *Traitement du Signal, 39*(1), 275–281.
5. Butt, G. Q., Sayed, T. A., Riaz, R., Rizvi, S. S., & Paul, A. (2022). Secure healthcare record sharing mechanism with blockchain. *Applied Sciences, 12*(5), 2307.

6. Mamun, A. A., Azam, S., & Gritti, C. (2022). Blockchain-based electronic health records management: A comprehensive review and future research direction. In *IEEE Access* (vol. 10, pp. 5768–5789). https://doi.org/10.1109/ACCESS.2022.3141079
7. Magyar, G. (2017). Blockchain: Solving the privacy and research availability tradeoff for EHR data: A new disruptive technology in health data management. In *2017 IEEE 30th Neumann Colloquium (NC) – Budapest, Hungary.* https://doi.org/10.1109/NC.2017.8263269
8. Arul, R., Alroobaea, R., Tariq, U., Almulihi, A. H., Alharithi, F. S., & Shoaib, U. (2021). IoT-enabled healthcare systems using block chain-dependent adaptable services. *Personal and Ubiquitous Computing*, 1–15. https://doi.org/10.1007/s00779-021-01584-7
9. Lafourcade, P., & Lombard-Platet, M. (2020). About blockchain interoperability. *Information Processing Letters, 161*(2), 105976.
10. Xia, Q., Sifah, E., Asamoah, K. O., & Gao, J. (2017). MeDShare: Trust-less medical data sharing among cloud service providers via blockchain. *IEEE Access, PP (99)*, 1.
11. Wood, G. (2014). Ethereum: A secure decentralised generalised transaction ledger. *Ethereum Project Yellow Paper, 151*(2014), 1–32.
12. Wahsheh, H. A., & Al-Zahrani, M. S. (2021, May). Secure and usable QR codes for healthcare systems: The case of Covid-19 pandemic. In *2021 12th international conference on information and communication systems (ICICS)* (pp. 324–329). IEEE.
13. Wang, J., Han, K., Alexandridis, A., Chen, Z., Zilic, Z., Pang, Y., Jeon, G., & Piccialli, F. (2020). A blockchain-based eHealthcare system interoperating with WBANs. *Future Generation Computer Systems, 110*, 675–685.
14. Saeed, H., Malik, H., Bashir, U., Ahmad, A., Riaz, S., Ilyas, M., Bukhari, W. A., & Khan, M. I. A. (2022). Blockchain technology in healthcare: A systematic review. *PLoS One, 17*(4), e0266462.
15. Tosh, D. K., Shetty, S., Liang, X., Kamhoua, C. A., Kwiat, K. A., & Njilla, L. (2017, May). Security implications of blockchain cloud with analysis of block withholding attack. In *2017 17th IEEE/ACM international symposium on cluster, cloud and grid computing (CCGRID)* (pp. 458–467). IEEE.
16. Tanwar, S., Parekh, K., & Evans, R. (2020). Blockchain-based electronic healthcare record system for healthcare 4.0 applications. *Journal of Information Security and Applications, 50*(10), 102407.
17. Liang, X., Zhao, J., Shetty, S., Liu, J., & Li, D. (2017). Integrating blockchain for data sharing and collaboration in mobile healthcare applications. In *2017 IEEE 28th annual international symposium on Personal, Indoor, and Mobile Radio Communications (PIMRC)* (pp. 1–5). IEEE.
18. Jiang, S., Cao, J., Wu, H., Yang, Y., Ma, M., & He, J. (2018). BlocHIE: A BLOCkchain-based platform for healthcare information exchange. In *2018 IEEE international conference on smart computing* (pp. 49–56). https://doi.org/10.1109/SMARTCOMP.2018.00073
19. Akkaoui, R., Hei, X., & Cheng, W. (2020). EdgeMediChain: A hybrid edge blockchain-based framework for health data exchange. *IEEE Access, 8*, 113467–113486.
20. Hongyu, L., Liehuang, Z., Meng, S., Feng, G., Tao, X., & Liu, S. (2018). Blockchain-based data preservation system for medical data. *Journal of Medical Systems, 42*(8), 141.
21. Wang, H., & Yujiao, S. (2018). Secure cloud-based EHR system using attribute-based cryptosystem and Blockchain. *Journal of Medical Systems, 42*(8), 152.
22. Bharimalla, P. K., Choudhury, H., ShantipriyaParida, Silo, A. I., & Mallick, D. K. (2022). A blockchain and NLP based electronic health record system: Indian subcontinent context. *Informatica, 45*(4), 605–616.
23. Bigini, G., Freschi, V., & Lattanzi, E. (2020). A review on blockchain for the internet of medical things: Definitions, challenges, applications, and vision. *Future Internet, 13*, 61029.
24. Aljassas, H. M. A., & Sasi, S. (2019). [IEEE 2019 2nd international conference on computer applications & information security (ICCAIS) – Riyadh, Saudi Arabia (2019.5.1–2019.5.3)] 2019. In *2nd international conference on computer applications & information security (ICCAIS) – performance evaluation of proof-of-work and collatz conjecture consensus algorithms* (pp. 1–6). IEEE.
25. Chernyshev, M., Zeadally, S., & Baig, Z. (2019). Healthcare data breaches: Implications for digital forensic readiness. *Journal of Medical Systems, 43*, 7.
26. Clim, A., Zota, R. D., & Constantinescu, R. (2019). Data exchanges based on blockchain in m-Health applications. *Procedia Computer Science, 160*, 281–288.

Chapter 26
Promethean Utilization of Resources Using Honeybee Optimization Techniques in Cloud Computing with Reference to Pandemic Health Care

S. Sree Priya and T. Rajendran

26.1 Introduction

The COVID-19 pandemic-related crisis left fewer medical professionals than normal access to care for the usual patient group. Owing to the shortfall, numerous nations took extra measures to deal with the unexpected spike in demand for doctors in health care. Data can now be kept in a virtual location that is accessible from anywhere at any time, thanks to cloud storage [1]. A distributed computing service known as "cloud computing" provides a significant amount of computer power without requiring the user to actively control it. Cloud computing services are being utilized by a variety of organizations, including individuals, hospitals, educational institutions, businesses, and the government. Cloud services are crucial in the health care industry for storing clinical information such as health records, ongoing patient monitoring, patient diagnosis using historical data, infection rate pattern prediction, etc. Cloud data security is on par with data security.

The cloud has one of the most important roles in tracking, tracing, diagnosing, and controlling the transmission of infection in pandemic conditions, like the spread of COVID-19. With the advancement of the cloud and lattices, complete instantaneously distributed processing, made possible by the development of the cloud, gives organizations and society a huge benefit by providing sorts of support that are more affordable and reliable [2]. With framework registering, we have the benefit of processing a greater undertaking within a more modest range of time, yet with cloud computing, any assignment can be figured out effectually a lot quicker by utilizing

S. S. Priya (✉) · T. Rajendran
PG and Research Department of Computer Science, Government Arts & Science College, Kangeyam, (Affiliated to Bharathiar University, Coimbatore), Tiruppur, Tamil Nadu, India

F. J. Joseph et al. (eds.), *Computational Intelligence for Clinical Diagnosis*, EAI/Springer Innovations in Communication and Computing,
https://doi.org/10.1007/978-3-031-23683-9_26

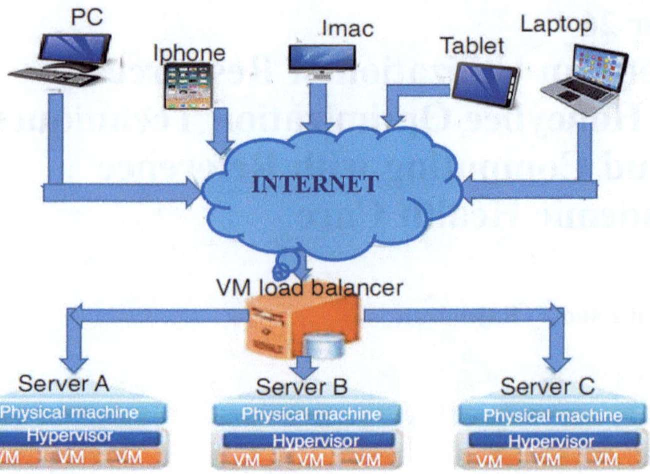

Fig. 26.1 Virtual machine load balancer

the calculation force of workers and in a safer manner. Cloud computing is an excellent illustration of distributed computing. Using a virtualization and hypervisor technology, on-premise workloads that already exist in the cloud can be transferred more rapidly and with a less outlay of time, money, and resources to any cloud computing platform. Load balancing is the most obligatory way of dispersing jobs and cataloguing resources in a cloud computing environment. As the client workload in the cloud computing environment escalates, the interest in shared assets has impetuously expanded. Consequently, load adjusting between these assets for scheduling turns into an important challenge (Fig. 26.1).

It offers all varieties of benefits that are powerful in terms of programming or amenities. Puissance given by the cloud is structured into three categories: software-as-a-service (SaaS), platform-as-a-service (PaaS), and infrastructure-as-a-service (IaaS). SaaS proffers types of assistance over the cloud as far as applications handle information. Cloud IaaS has four essential postures:

- Virtualization
- Elastic registering
- Pay per use
- Cost

26.2 Related Work

Load adjusting accords with decreasing energy utilization and further developing the use of hosts. For the antibacterial ecosystems to flourish sustainably, early incident identification must be encouraged [3]. Building an non-infectious, intelligent city framework in an intergenerational urban setting in light of the post-COVID-19 age is a necessity. Innovative technical solutions based on cloud computing were employed in the context of relief efforts during the pandemic [4, 5]. With the help of our research, we hope to provide wise remedies for full control of the exponential development of increasing infection rates and the creation in this phase of COVID-19 deaths. To deal with unusual circumstances, different technology advancements and response activities have been established [6]. To support trustworthy urban ecosystems and efficient virus defense, it is crucial to build a reference framework [7–9]. To improve integration and adapt to the post-COVID-19 antiviral society, a multiple generational template will be a key step [10]. We can evaluate and forecast increasing infectious cases thanks to basic mathematics, which is essential for comprehending the pandemic's progression [11, 12].

Dalapati and Sahoo [13] envisaged a green scheduling strategy, ameliorating potency utilization in cloud computing. The honeybee technique is cannibalized for rescheduling and domain scheming for power harnessing. Intriguingly, this paper follows the honeybee technique applied for the emplacement of overloaded servers.

Before resolving the multiple needs of jobs removed from densely packed virtual machines (VMs), Babu and Venkata Krishna [14] utilized the heap-adjusting techniques. This approach depends on the conduct of the honeybee searching system, works on the general throughput of handling, and lessens the reaction of the VM seasons. In any case, the authors did not research the controlled rule handling for load balancing.

Anton et al. [15] proposed standards for managing clouds in an energy-efficient manner. In addition, they proposed energy-productive asset assignment contrivances and scheduling strategies. Nevertheless, because of the way in which they utilized fixed usage edges, this methodology may not be effective for distributed computing conditions. In their more progressive work [15], Beloglazov et al. proposed pliable heuristics for active solidification of VMs dependent on sequence data obtained from resource utilization by VMs. This calculation denigrates energy utilization.

Garala and Goswami [3] suggested heap-adjusting components dependent on the ersatz honeybee state assessment. The authors proposed a further developed honeybee stratagem to build the basis throughput. Nevertheless, they did not research energy utilization or contravention of service level agreements.

26.3 Proposed RAHBO Algorithm Implementation

The following steps in the proposed load-balancing resource allocation honeybee optimization algorithm (RAHBO) are as follows:

1. The capitulation of tasks: When an improvised workflow arrives, it succumbs to the pre-processor.
2. Consign volume and generate load balancer, set the number of cloudlets.
3. Allocate the preliminary load VM = "NULL."

4. Propel the first request by cloudlet. Ready tasks aimed at execution send the request to the VM load balancer [16].
5. Fetch the slot for each VM.
6. Eminence information included data on existing consignments. Load point is taken into account while determining the amount of time to spend on distribution of certain tasks.
7. It directs the allocated requests to busy hosts.
8. If it is less than or equivalent to the threshold value, consign chore to contemporary VM, or it sends a scout to catch the new-fangled VM haphazardly.
9. The task imparts overloaded data that gains lot of attention by dissecting tasks administered by VM, contemporarily manipulating the time of the host and checking the status of the host.
10. The VM matches the overloaded data to the servers.
11. Instructs the entire VM.
12. The task owed to a particular VM is initiated.
13. If true, it ascribes the task to the VM that has the least capacity or, if false, it curbs whether the existing load <= threshold.
14. Irrevocably, computation cost, fault rate, average response time, and execution time are carried out with the appropriate predictable outcomes.

26.3.1 The Pseudocode Shows the Core Processes of RAHBO

```
Input- host , VMs, Output- VM(k)
//number (p) of host partaking minimum processing time, p - Number of
quantified hosts

p = 0
minimum(RS) -> Integer(maximum_values)
For nodes(p) each in List nodes:
  If nodes(p) accessible
      If (RS(nodes(p) <minimum(RS))then
          minimum(RS) = RS(nodes(p))
          p -> number of entire existing nodes
      Endif
  Endif
Endfor
//number (q) VM consuming least total of needs, q - Number of indicated VM
q=0
minimum (UV).count← Integer (maximum_value)
For each VM(q) in ListVMhost(q)
  If VM offered:
     If (requiredVM.count(q)< minimum.count) then
        minimum.count = requiredVM.count(q)
        q -> Number of contemporary VM
     Endif
  Endif
Endfor
```

```
21: if (q! = -1) then
22:    Distribute the task to VM(p)
23: else
24:    Join imminent task in expectancy queue in anticipation of one VM
obtainable.
25:    Refurbish owed information indicating that number of tasks
actioned, recent dispensation  time of host and check handiness of VM,
node
26:    Unassigned job from this VM subsequent end of job execution.
27:    Apprise assigned info that number of tasks prosecuted, existing
processing time of nodes and crisscross accessibility of VM and host.
28:    Evaluate Processing cost C(p,q) = minimum(VM(p,q), host)
29:    Compute Fault rate FR(p,q)=f(VM(p,q), Networkload,host)
30:   Assess Average responsetime avg_response(p,q) = min(minimum(UV).
count(VM(p,q)), host)
30: Endif
```

26.4 Experimental Result Consistent with the Effect of the Parameters

The tests instigated in excess of 5 datacenters, 60 VMs, and 200–2000 tasks underneath the simulation tool [17]. Distributing speed, accessible memory space, and bandwidth govern the permissible load of each VM. Parameters of simulation are shown in Table 26.1.

The proposed calculation simulated cannibalization of the Cloudsim simulator system. Clouds naturally employ first-in, first-out computations and chain cost estimation to arrange the allotted and unallocated resources sequentially [18]. Initially, the Cloudsim programming cohort did not stick up for the dereliction rate at the data center. Incipiently, the fault rate was added as a frontier of datacenter responses to foible obscuring at the data center.

Table 26.1 Parameter simulator

Type	Parameters	Value
VM	Total VMs	60
	Speediness of processor	700–2000 MIPS
	Obtainable room for memory in a single VM	556–2055 Mb
	Bandwidth	600–1200
	Cloudlet scheduler	Time ploughshare
	Requirement of processor elements	1–7
Data center	Data centers	5
	Hosts	1–7
	VM scheduler	Time apportioned
Cloudlet	Task length	100–10,000
	Enumerate number of tasks	200–2000

VM virtual machine

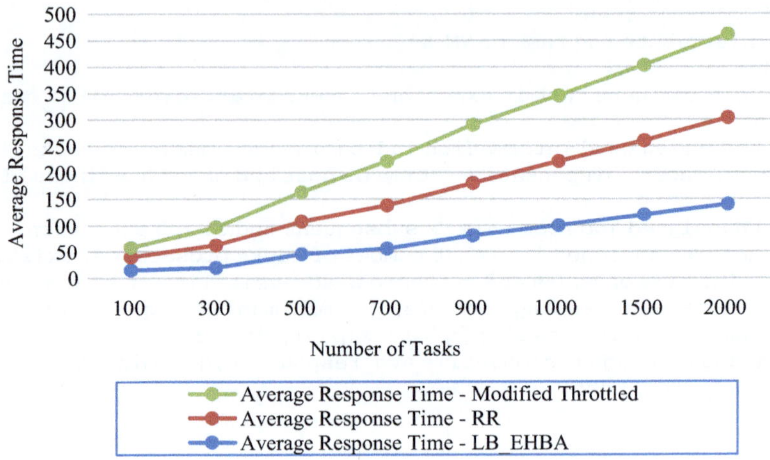

Fig. 26.2 Average response time versus number of tasks

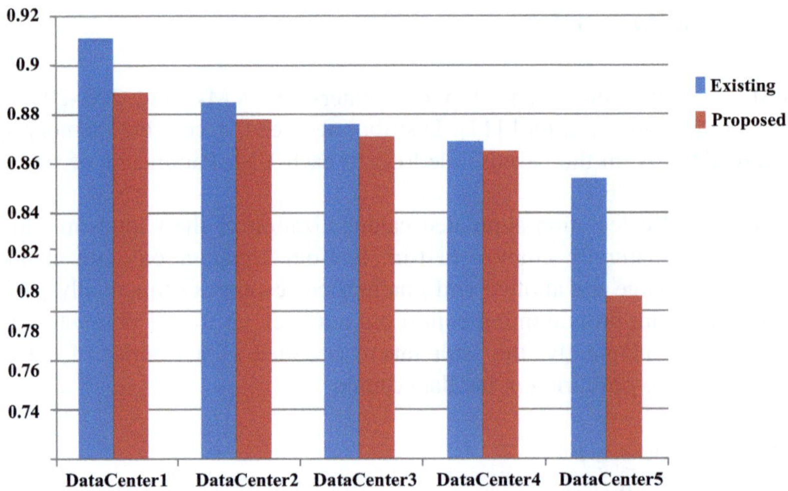

Fig. 26.3 Datacenter requesting serving time for the existing and proposed algorithm

Here, Cloudsim is cannibalized for the simulation of cloud IaaS. It all-encompassing cloud IaaS environment. In Cloudsim, Honeybee replaces the standard round robin algorithm's definitive first-come, first-served inscribing computation. Figure 26.2 shows the comparison chart of the algorithms, such as the round robin algorithm and the modified throttled algorithm, with the proposed load-balancing honeybee algorithm (Fig. 26.3).

Relative reappraisal accomplished between existing techniques with load witting honeybee accords demand on the datacenter owing to a minimal load and proposed calculation (Figs. 26.4 and 26.5). Table 26.2 reveals the average response time of the

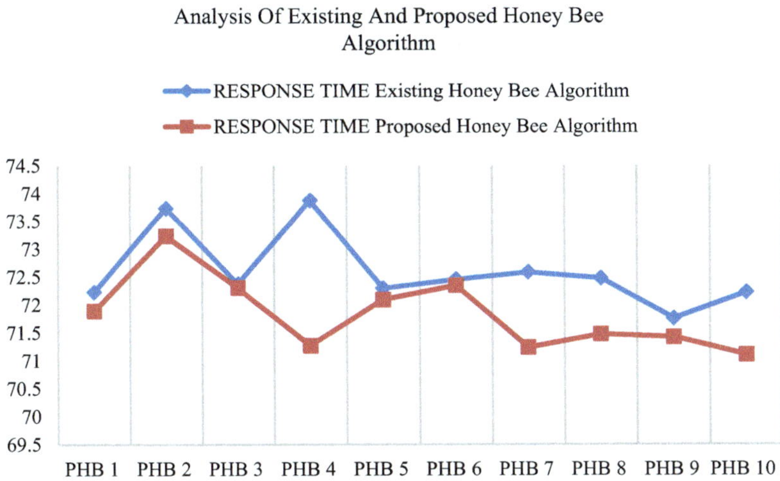

Fig. 26.4 Response time for existing and proposed honeybee algorithm

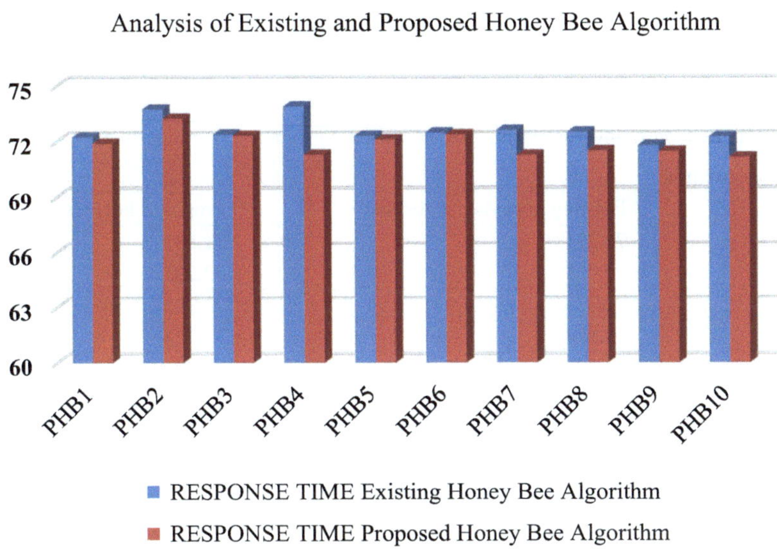

Fig. 26.5 Analysis of existing and proposed honeybee algorithm

modified throttled, round robin (RR) load balancing and RAHBO algorithms. Table 26.3 shows the data center request serving time, and Table 26.4 shows the response time for the existing and proposed honeybee algorithm.

Table 26.2 Average response time of modified throttled, resource allocation honeybee optimization (RAHBO) and round robin (RR) load balancing algorithm

Average response time – modified throttled	Average response time – RR	Average response time – RAHBO	Number of tasks
18	25	15	100
35	42	20	300
55	63	45	500
83	82	56	700
110	100	80	900
124	121	100	1000
143	140	120	1500
158	163	140	2000

Table 26.3 Data center request serving time

Data center	Existing request serving time	Proposed request serving time
DataCenter1	0.911	0.889
DataCenter2	0.885	0.878
DataCenter3	0.876	0.871
DataCenter4	0.869	0.865
DataCenter5	0.854	0.806

Table 26.4 Response time for existing and proposed honeybee (PHB) algorithm

User response time		
	Existing honeybee algorithm	Proposed honeybee algorithm
PHB1	72.231	71.891
PHB2	73.735	73.235
PHB3	72.375	72.305
PHB4	73.874	71.274
PHB5	72.297	72.092
PHB6	72.457	72.351
PHB7	72.582	71.237
PHB8	72.475	71.475
PHB9	71.758	71.427
PHB10	72.218	71.108

26.5 Conclusion

Devices that use cloud-based applications and eHealth have the potential to be very important in this field. On the one hand, they try to prevent or reduce hospital visits for patients by monitoring them online from their homes using smart health care equipment, and on the other, they are aimed at giving doctors more accurate health data before or during virtual consultations. In order to help with diagnosis and treatment, cloud computing-based eHealth devices may typically measure a variety of health factors from the patient's home, including hypertension, heat, blood glucose, and heart rate. For instance, there has been a noticeable increase in the use of instruments such as wearable sensors in COVID-19. To forecast the spread of germs, cloud storage is evaluated. Without the contributions of these technologies, the pandemic situation could get substantially worse. In this paper, the cloud for load-adjusting resource allocation unveils the proposed better energy utilization, response time, cost and processing time. Energy-productive distributed computing invention is behind innovation, and there have been numerous regions that have still not been investigated completely when contrasted with different parameters, and consequently there is a huge, impending need for new technological improvements. The execution results confirm that the VM designation strategy honeybee calculation contributes to better outcomes. In energy production, cloud computing focuses on the efficient use of energy utilization. As a future development, we tried to build this computation with QoS boundaries because it was undesirable when the scope of application transfer on the cloud was entirely defeated, including informal communication on websites or information from web search tools.

References

1. Archer, A., Aydin, K., Bateni, M. H., Mirrokni, V., Schild, A., Yang, R., & Zhuang, R. (2019). Cache aware load balancing of data center applications. *Proceedings of the VLDB Endowment, 12*(6), 709–723. https://doi.org/10.14778/3311880.3311887
2. Gurumurthy, K., & Selvadurai, M. V. (2020). Intelligent resource scheduling with neutrosophic knowledge and optimized cache management using cuckoo search method in cloud computing. *International Journal of Intelligent Engineering and Systems, 13*(3), 327.
3. Garala, K, & Goswami, N. (2015). *A performance analysis of load balancing algorithm in cloud environments* (pp. 45–50). 978-1-4799-6805-3, IEEE. https://doi.org/10.1109/ICCCI.2015.7218063
4. Masadeh, R., Sharieh, A., & Mahafzah, B. A. (2019). Humpback whale optimization algorithm based on vocal behavior for task scheduling in cloud computing. *International Journal of Advanced Science and Technology, 13*(3).
5. Liu, X., Yabing, Z., Yin, Q., Peng, Y., & Qin, L. (2015). Scheduling parallel jobs with tentative runs and consolidation in the cloud. *Journal of System Software, 104*, 141.
6. Neelima, P., & Reddy, A. R. M. (2020). An efficient load balancing system using adaptive dragonfly algorithm in cloud computing. *Cluster Computing, Springer, 23*, 2891. https://doi.org/10.1007/s10586-020-03054-w
7. Kathalkar, P. R., & Deorankar, A. V. (2018). A review on different load balancing algorithm in cloud computing. *International Research Journal of Engineering and Technology, 5*(2), 1–3.
8. Greco, A., Pluchino, A., & Cannizzaro, F. (2019). An improved ant colony optimization algorithm and its applications to limit analysis of frame structures. *Engineering Optimization, 51*(11), 1867–1883. https://doi.org/10.1080/0305215X.2018.1560437
9. Dave, A., Patel, B., & Bhatt, G. (2016). Load balancing in cloud computing using optimization techniques: A study. In *Proceedings of international conference on communication and electronics systems (ICCES)*. https://doi.org/10.1109/CESYS.2016.7889883
10. Mallikarjuna, B., & Venkata Krishna, P. (2018, December). A nature inspired bee colony optimization model for improving load balancing in cloud computing. *International Journal of Innovative Technology and Exploring Engineering (IJITEE), 8*(2S2). ISSN: 2278-3075.

11. Mallikarjuna, B., & Krishna, P.V. (2018, December). A nature inspired approach for load balancing of tasks in cloud computing using equal time allocation. *International Journal of Innovative Technology and Exploring Engineering. 8.*
12. Hashem, W., Nashaat, H., & Rizk, R. (2017). Honey bee based load balancing in cloud computing. *KSII Transactions on Internet and Information Systems, 11*(12), 5694–5711.
13. Dalapati, P., & Sahoo, G. (2013). Green solution for cloud computing with load balancing and power consumption management. *International Journal of Emerging Technology and Advanced Engineering, 3*(3), 353–359.
14. Dhinesh Babu, L. D., & Venkata Krishna, P. (2013). *Honey bee behaviour inspired load balancing of tasks in cloud computing environments, 1568–4946* (pp. 120–131). Elsevier.
15. Anton, B., Jemal A., & Rajkumar B. (2012). Energy-aware resource allocation heuristics for efficient management of data centers for cloud computing. *The International Journal of Grid Computing and eScience, Future Generation Computer Systems (FGCS), 28*(5), 755–768.
16. Mishra, K., & Majhi, S. K. (2021). A binary Bird Swarm Optimization based load balancing algorithm for cloud computing environment. *Open Computer Science, 1*(1), 146–160. https://doi.org/10.1515/comp-2020-0215
17. Kruekaew, B., & Kimpan, W. (2020). Enhancing of artificial bee colony algorithm for virtual machine scheduling and load balancing problem in cloud computing. *International Journal of Computational Intelligence Systems, 13*(1), 496–510.
18. Shahid, M. A., Islam, N., Alam, M. M., Su'ud, M. M., & Musa, S. (2020). A comprehensive study of load balancing approaches in the cloud computing environment and a novel fault tolerance approach. *IEEE Access, 8*, 130500.

Chapter 27
Healthcare Operational Intellectual Ability in Analysing the Factors Affecting Employee Churn

V. Mahalakshmi, D. Chitra, Yabesh Abraham Durairaj Isravel, and B. Lakshmi

27.1 Introduction

In today's firms where specific individuals work, having good mental health at work is a crucial management component. The improvement of workplace culture is made possible by the promotion of excellent mental health, which has a favourable effect on employees and on the outcomes of their job assignments. The significance of having good psychological health at work is growing, particularly at times of abrupt shifts and reorganisation brought on by significant events like the COVID-19 epidemic. The introduction of the coronavirus SARS-CoV-2 sickness brought about a lot of changes in how society and businesses operated. In a number of nations, an epidemic emergency was declared in an attempt to stop the virus's spread.

Attrition rate is calculated using recruitment and termination criteria. Employees resign for several reasons. Turnover and attrition are contradictory business terms. A company's 'turnover' can take several forms. Attrition means staff loss. Manpower data and other measurements for manpower planning can be analysed using these terms. Employee departures cause attrition and turnover. Release, termination, abdication, or occupation relinquishment can cause turnover. Attrition occurs when a worker quits or is laid off. When an employee leaves, the company replaces them. Attrition is when a corporation leaves a post empty or eliminates it, also called employee churn.

V. Mahalakshmi (✉) · D. Chitra · Y. A. D. Isravel · B. Lakshmi
Department of Management Studies, Panimalar Engineering College, Chennai, India
e-mail: mbadean@panimalar.ac.in

F. J. J. Joseph et al. (eds.), *Computational Intelligence for Clinical Diagnosis*,
EAI/Springer Innovations in Communication and Computing,
https://doi.org/10.1007/978-3-031-23683-9_27

Employee analytics focuses on helping organisations determine what matters most to their employees to improve engagement and efficiency and reduce turnover. Analytics on employee attrition focuses on why people departed, what could have stopped them, and how data can anticipate attrition risk [1]. This form of employee prediction analytics can help firms identify and implement ways to reduce undesired turnover [2]. Employee churn (ECn) hurts income and brand image. Many ML-based methods have been developed to solve ECn. They disregard staff categorisation, category-wise turnover forecast, and retention strategy while addressing ECn. To solve these challenges, a MADM-based method incorporating ML algorithms was devised. The proposed technique is called churn prediction and retention (ECPR).

A company's greatest asset is its employees. When people depart an organisation, productivity, project continuity, and growth initiatives suffer, affecting image and turnover. Others leave the company. Hiring new workers is a time-consuming and expensive process. Employee churn (ECn) is a problem that needs a quick solution to remain productive and competitive. In this scenario, machine learning is useful for churn prediction and retention policies (ML). ML algorithms have exploded in popularity in recent years and are used in recommender systems, personal life event prediction, stock price prediction, etc. ML algorithms solve ECn for three reasons. The organisation lacks the resources to estimate staff turnover manually. Second, ECn prediction data is abundant and should be used to make a judgement. Third, the dataset is updated regularly.

In recent years, several machine learning-based ECn solutions have been proposed. A customer turnover problem was solved by constructing and comparing employee churn models – an actionable answer to client attrition. Hybrid clustering technique is used in many research to predict technology staff attrition. Many studies use extreme gradient to predict turnover. Studies predict employee turnover using a weighted quadratic random forest method. None of these studies classify employees into groups, such as those who significantly contribute to turnover. They haven't examined retention rules based on employee types to combat ECn. These facts warrant further study.

This form of analytic activity has grown in the last 2 years. Because of the COVID-19 pandemic, global labour markets have swung substantially, and 55 per cent of Indian workers said they planned to hunt for new jobs in the next 12 months in August 2021. Employee attrition analytics will continue to be vital for firms attempting to retain top personnel as they deal with the ongoing problems of the epidemic and the development of remote work [3]. The ability to develop an employee retention model using predictive analytics allows you to keep these key people engaged and on board [4]. In this article, we are going to determine the important variables that could be considered in churn analytics to estimate the employee engagement level and employee turnover behaviour in the IT sector. Further, the study examines the relationship of existing between employee engagement and employee turnover in the IT sector in Chennai district.

27.2 Literature Review

The significance of enhanced communication in the pandemic-related remote working situations for employee churn was investigated. Employee relationships, in general, represent the constructive interactions among employees in firms [5]. Employee relations have changed as a result of the rise in remote working options and the pandemic's job stress [6]. Employee relations, as well as internal communication methods, are evolving within the firm. Since the findings of the study by [7] indicate that employee relationships affect job satisfaction among academic employees, we predict that they will likewise increase IT employees' feelings of job satisfaction during the COVID-19 pandemic. In order to promote good mental health during the COVID-19 epidemic, this study focuses on a deeper understanding of the elements supporting job happiness. The study's goal is to determine whether employee relations and mutual trust affect job satisfaction when dealing with distant work brought on by a pandemic. Additionally, the inclusion of the idea of trust in this setting permits a thorough examination of underlying interrelationships. In order to increase job satisfaction and encourage good psychological well-being at work, managers can use this to construct precise models that reflect complicated organisational phenomena.

Many CEOs, understandably, zero in on the problem of high turnover when discussing attrition. It costs organisations billions of dollars annually to invest in staff recruitment, recruiting, onboarding, and training. When there is a lot of employee turnover, it hurts a company's productivity and bottom line. It can be difficult and costly to find and hire replacements for exceptional performers [8]. The cost of replacing a single person might be anywhere from half to two times their annual compensation, and this cost rises in direct proportion to the employee's talent. Businesses benefit monetarily and otherwise by retaining valuable personnel and institutional knowledge [9].

Attrition occurs when an organisation loses workers due to natural causes, such as the death rate or the number of people who willingly quit or retire. Employee turnover is the rate at which an organisation's current workforce is replaced by new hires over a certain time frame. Employee turnover is a problem for any company that experiences excessive attrition. Costs associated with human resource activities including hiring, training, and promoting new workers, as well as monitoring their progress and productivity, are inflated as a result. Again, natural selection requires some degree of attrition. By boosting morale and creating a pleasant workplace, we can drastically cut down on this issue.

Lack of attrition can be problematic. The appropriate people leaving at the right moment are preferable [10]. If a low-performing or mismatched person leaves, a high-performing, better-suited replacement can be found. Even if an excellent employee leaves to become a client, it may be a gain if they become a brand ambassador [5]. There may also be transitory positions within the organisation where individuals have a limited tenure before moving on to another position, internally or externally. The goal may not be to maintain personnel in these roles eternally, but rather for a few months longer to avoid turnover costs and disruption [11]. Attrition analytics helps firms establish a balance between retaining top people and knowing that some turnover is healthy.

Employee importance can be measured using a variety of variables, making categorisation challenging. Multi-attribute decision-making (MADM) has shown promise in recent years. MADM approaches have been successfully used in healthcare, marketing, corporate management, and human resource selection. The technique for order of preference by similarity to ideal (TOPSIS) solution has gained popularity due to its many benefits. It's a simple, easy-to-understand concept with good computing efficiency and ability to measure relative performance [6]. TOPSIS compares alternatives to perfect solutions. The best option is closest to positive-ideal solution and farthest from negative-ideal solution. Several approaches have been developed for determining the relative weights of TOPSIS traits. Weighted least squares to determine fuzzy set weights are used. Many research employed analytic hierarchy to rate car seat comfort based on user preferences. The entropy weight approach is often employed since it's sensitive to information entropy or attribute data heterogeneity. It's perfect for separating options. Extended Warehouse Management (EWM) decreases the influence of subjectively used erroneous or fake attribute information [12].

Researchers have studied ECn literature. ECn prediction in HR analysis has been studied extensively. The volume of ECn research based on theoretical ideas has expanded considerably over the previous century due to dynamic and competitive market policy. Employee happiness and organisational loyalty are linked in several research. Highly pleased employees have lower absenteeism rates, make big contributions, and are ready to stay. Perception, cognitive capacity, demographic demographics, expectations, sense of achievement, and contextual factors affect job satisfaction. These studies [7] examine employee churn. Theoretically, these schemes solved the ECn problem. This study examines churn analytics variables.

27.3 Objectives

Healthcare variables are still the focus of several research due to their importance for both the employee and thus the firm. The methods for assessing job happiness and its effects on participation, creativity, business results, and employees' intentions to switch jobs are all covered in surveys. According to studies on teleworking, momentarily carrying out tasks outside of the workplace can improve employee job satisfaction. On the other hand, research undertaken under conditions of social separation and COVID anxiety indicated that distant job satisfaction is negatively affected by isolation.

The objective of the proposed study was to determine the important variables that could be considered in churn analytics to estimate the employee engagement level and employee turnover behaviour in the IT sector. Further, the study examines the existing relationship between employee engagement and employee turnover in the IT sector in Chennai district.

27.4 Methodology

The research made use of a descriptive research design. The data were collected from 196 respondents from 17 IT companies in Chennai district who were adopting churn analytics in the human resource department to investigate the major reason for employee turnover and the reason for reducing employee engagement.

27.4.1 Analysis and Interpretation

The researcher intended to identify the demographic profile of the respondents working with churn analytics in the IT industry in Chennai district (Table 27.1).

Using the percentage analysis conducted from the data collected, it was understood that the majority of the employees working with churn analytics were male, belonging to the age category between 30 and 40 years with 3–5 years of experience.

The analysis depicted below was conducted to identify whether the variables considered for employee engagement can be used in churn analytics as per the opinion of the respondents (Table 27.2).

In the majority of cases, Pillai's trace significance value and the items' significance value were calculated to be larger than 0.05, indicating that the null hypothesis can be accepted. This suggests that there are no significant differences in opinion among the respondents on the elements that affect employee engagement (Table 27.3).

Table 27.1 Percentage analysis – demographic profile

Demographic profile			
		Frequency	Percentage
Gender	Male	119	60.7
	Female	77	39.3
	Total	196	100.0
Age	Below 30 years	53	27.0
	30–40 years	81	41.3
	40–50 years	53	27.0
	Above 50 years	9	4.6
	Total	196	100.0
Experience	Less than 3 years	54	27.6
	3–5 years	85	43.4
	5–7 years	49	25.0
	Above 7 years	8	4.1
	Total	196	100.0

Source: Primary data

Table 27.2 Multivariate test – employee engagement

Multivariate tests						
Effect		**Value**	***F***	**Hypothesis df**	**Error df**	**Sig.**
Gender	Pillai's trace	0.015	.555[b]	5	184	0.734
	Wilks' lambda	0.985	.555[b]	5	184	0.734
	Hotelling's trace	0.015	.555[b]	5	184	0.734
	Roy's largest root	0.015	.555[b]	5	184	0.734
Age	Pillai's trace	0.108	1.383	15	558	0.150
	Wilks' lambda	0.894	1.410	15	508.344	0.137
	Hotelling's trace	0.118	1.436	15	548	0.125
	Roy's largest root	0.107	3.965[c]	5	186	0.002
Experience	Pillai's trace	0.201	2.676	15	558	0.001
	Wilks' lambda	0.801	2.832	15	508.344	0.000
	Hotelling's trace	0.245	2.981	15	548	0.000
	Roy's largest root	0.231	8.588[c]	5	186	0.000
Tests of between-subjects effects						
Source		**Type III sum of squares**	**Df**	**Mean square**	***F***	**Sig.**
D1	Superior support	2.094	1	2.094	1.982	0.161
	Performance appraisal	0.053	1	0.053	0.079	0.779
	Rewards and recognition	0.018	1	0.018	0.024	0.877
	Career support and services	0.305	1	0.305	0.507	0.477
	Organisational environment	0.016	1	0.016	0.017	0.895
D2	Superior support	7.033	3	2.344	2.218	0.087
	Performance appraisal	2.418	3	0.806	1.210	0.308
	Rewards and recognition	4.795	3	1.598	2.186	0.091
	Career support and services	7.072	3	2.357	3.912	0.010
	Organisational environment	2.413	3	0.804	0.871	0.457
D3	Superior support	1.287	3	0.429	0.406	0.749
	Performance appraisal	12.183	3	4.061	6.096	0.001
	Rewards and recognition	24.129	3	8.043	10.999	0.000
	Career support and services	0.537	3	0.179	0.297	0.828
	Organisational environment	3.285	3	1.095	1.186	0.317

Source: Primary data
The opinion of the respondents are categorized into the variable "b" and "c"

Table 27.3 Rank analysis – employee engagement

Rank analysis			
	N	Mean	Rank
Superior support	196	3.7755	5
Performance appraisal	196	4.2194	3
Rewards and recognition	196	4.2653	2
Career support and services	196	4.3010	1
Organisational environment	196	3.9031	4

Source: Primary data

The overall mean score lies between 3.78 and 4.26, meaning the employees working with churn analytics "Agree" that all the variables can be considered for the churn analytics to find employee engagement. Further, using the rank analysis made using the mean score, it was found that career support and service, rewards and recognition, and performance appraisal were the important variables to be considered the most.

The analysis depicted below was conducted to identify whether the variables considered for employee turnover can be used in churn analytics as per the opinion of the respondents (Table 27.4).

The null hypothesis can be accepted because Pillai's trace significance value and the items' significance value were both assessed to be greater than 0.05 in most situations. This means that there are no major differences in opinion among the respondents on the elements examined for determining employee engagement (Table 27.5).

The overall mean score lies between 3.79 and 4.36, meaning the employees working with churn analytics "Agree" that all the variables can be considered for the churn analytics to find the employee turnover. Further, using the rank analysis made using the mean score, it was found that better offer in another company, career opportunity, and low pay are the important variables to be considered the most (Table 27.6).

Also, from the correlation analysis made by consolidating variables of employee engagement and turnover, it can be perceived that employee engagement and employee turnover have a negative relationship, i.e. as employee engagement increases, employee turnover decreases in an organisation.

Having found there is a relationship between the variables, herein we have performed regression analysis to identify whether there is an impact of employee engagement on employee turnover (Table 27.7).

The estimated R-square value is 0.334, meaning the regression equation is 33.4% accurate in forecasting. Further, the ANOVA significance value is less than 0.05, meaning the model is fit. In addition, the coefficient significance value is also less than 0.05; this indicates there is an impact of employee engagement on employee turnover.

Table 27.4 Multivariate test – employee turnover

Multivariate tests						
Effect		**Value**	***F***	**Hypothesis df**	**Error df**	**Sig.**
Gender	Pillai's trace	0.058	2.250[b]	5	184	0.051
	Wilks' lambda	0.942	2.250[b]	5	184	0.051
	Hotelling's trace	0.061	2.250[b]	5	184	0.051
	Roy's largest root	0.061	2.250[b]	5	184	0.051
Age	Pillai's trace	0.185	2.450	15	558	0.002
	Wilks' lambda	0.824	2.464	15	508.344	0.002
	Hotelling's trace	0.203	2.468	15	548	0.002
	Roy's largest root	0.124	4.602[c]	5	186	0.001
Experience	Pillai's trace	0.125	1.612	15	558	0.066
	Wilks' lambda	0.876	1.663	15	508.344	0.055
	Hotelling's trace	0.140	1.711	15	548	0.045
	Roy's largest root	0.134	4.985[c]	5	186	0.000
Tests of between-subjects effects						
Source		**Type III sum of squares**	**Df**	**Mean square**	***F***	**Sig.**
D1	Better offer in another company	2.240	1	2.240	4.352	0.038
	Work hours	3.992	1	3.992	3.760	0.054
	Low pay	0.223	1	0.223	0.256	0.614
	Company culture	0.967	1	0.967	1.034	0.311
	Career opportunity	0.050	1	0.050	0.059	0.808
D2	Better offer in another company	3.629	3	1.210	2.351	0.074
	Work hours	8.141	3	2.714	2.556	0.057
	Low pay	11.478	3	3.826	4.394	0.005
	Company culture	7.121	3	2.374	2.536	0.058
	Career opportunity	14.888	3	4.963	5.911	0.001
D3	Better offer in another company	4.423	3	1.474	2.865	0.038
	Work hours	0.930	3	0.310	0.292	0.831
	Low pay	0.063	3	0.021	0.024	0.995
	Company culture	10.280	3	3.427	3.662	0.013
	Career opportunity	1.060	3	0.353	0.421	0.738

Source: Primary data
The opinion of the respondents are categorized into the variable "b" and "c"

27.5 Findings

Attrition refers to the loss of talent in an organisation as a result of natural causes, such as the departure or retirement of personnel. Employee turnover refers to the rate at which current employees are replaced by new hires over a specified time frame.

Table 27.5 Rank analysis – employee turnover

Rank analysis			
	N	Mean	Rank
Better offer in another company	196	4.3673	1
Work hours	196	3.7908	5
Low pay	196	4.2602	3
Company culture	196	3.8520	4
Career opportunity	196	4.3163	2

Source: Primary data

Table 27.6 Correlation analysis – relationship between employee engagement and turnover

Correlations			
		Employee engagement	Employee turnover
Employee engagement	Pearson correlation	1	−0.578**
	Sig. (2-tailed)		0.000
	N	196	196
Employee turnover	Pearson correlation	−0.578**	1
	Sig. (2-tailed)	0.000	
	N	196	196

Source: Primary data

The low pay is significantly shown as a variable calculated using the rank analysis, hence it is denoted by **

Table 27.7 Regression analysis – impact of employee engagement on employee turnover

Model summary

Model	***R***	**R square**	**Adjusted *R* square**	**Std. error of the estimate**
1	.578[a]	0.334	0.331	0.48181

[a]Predictors: (Constant), employee engagement

ANOVA[a]

Model		**Sum of squares**	**Df**	**Mean square**	***F***	**Sig.**
1	Regression	22.627	1	22.627	97.471	.000[b]
	Residual	45.034	194	0.232		
	Total	67.661	195			

[a]Dependent variable: Employee turnover

[b]Predictors: (Constant), employee engagement

Coefficients[a]

		Unstandardised coefficients		**Standardised coefficients**		
Model		***B***	**Std. error**	**Beta**	***t***	**Sig.**
1	(Constant)	1.653	0.252		6.563	0.000
	Employee engagement	0.602	0.061	0.578	9.873	0.000

[a]Dependent variable: Employee turnover

Source: Primary data

Any business with a high attrition rate will also have a high turnover rate. Consequently, a large amount of money is poured into human resources due to the high costs associated with hiring new staff, providing ongoing education and development, and monitoring employee output. Repeatedly, voluntary attrition is inevitable. Therefore, this employee churn analytics was designed to drastically reduce this problem by boosting morale and creating an environment where people want to come to work.

From the analysis performed and interpretation made, it was understood that the majority of the employees working with churn analytics were male, belonging to the age category between 30 and 40 years with 3–5 years of experience. It was found that there is no significant difference in opinion among the respondents for the variables considered for employee engagement and employee turnover. The employees working with churn analytics "Agree" that all the variables can be considered for the churn analytics to find employee engagement and employee turnover. Further, using the rank analysis made using the mean score, it was found that career support and service, rewards and recognition, and performance appraisal were the important variables to be considered the most. Also, it was identified that better offer in another company, career opportunity, and low pay are the important variables to be considered the most. Furthermore, it can be perceived that employee engagement and employee turnover have a negative relationship, i.e. as employee engagement increases, employee turnover decreases in an organisation.

27.6 Conclusion

Unreported COVID-19 cases have impacted healthcare services. Companies, which are the greatest demography of healthcare professional spend most of the time with patients, are severely harmed during epidemic. This was a high-intention-to-leave occupation before the epidemic. This review compared pre- and post-COVID-19 replacement and intention rates and their drivers in light of COVID-19's psychological effects. Attrition is the loss of personnel who quit or retire voluntarily. Employee turnover is the number of existing employees replaced by new ones over time. High employee turnover results from high attrition. This increases human resource costs for recruitment, training, and performance management. Again, attrition is inevitable. Improving employee morale and creating a pleasant work environment can help decrease this problem. Introducing the employee churn analytics the researchers have explored about ECn literature. ECn prediction in human resource analysis has been studied extensively. Dynamic and competitive market policies have expanded the number of ECn research based on theoretical theories throughout the last century. Numerous studies link employee happiness and retention. Satisfied employees have reduced absenteeism rates, contribute to the firm, and want to stay. Perception, cognitive capacity, demographic demographics, expectancies, sense of accomplishment, and contextual factors affect job satisfaction. Studies on employee turnover proposed a theoretical solution to ECn.

The goal of the study was to identify the key variables that could be used in churn analytics to estimate employee engagement and turnover in the IT industry. A descriptive research design was used in this study. The information was gathered from 196 respondents from 17 IT companies in Chennai district that were using churn analytics in their HR departments to figure out what was causing employee turnover and engagement to drop. The majority of churn analytics' employees were males between the ages of 30 and 40, with 3–5 years of experience, according to the analysis and interpretation. For the variables considered for employee engagement and turnover, it was discovered that there is no significant difference in opinion among the respondents. All variables can be considered for churn analytics to find employee engagement and turnover, according to the employee working with churn analytics. Furthermore, a rank analysis using the mean score revealed that career support and service, rewards and recognition, and performance appraisal were the most important variables to consider. Furthermore, it was discovered that a better offer from another company, a better career opportunity, and low pay are the most important variables to consider. Furthermore, it is possible to believe that employee engagement and employee turnover have a negative relationship, i.e. as employee engagement rises, so does employee turnover.

References

1. Wilkens, M. (2020). Employee churn in after-school care: Manager influences on retention and turnover. *Journal of Youth Development, 15*(1), 94–121.
2. Alamsyah, A., & Salma, N. A comparative study of employee churn prediction model. In 2018 4th international conference on science and technology (ICST) (pp. 1–4). IEEE (2018).
3. Srivastava, P. R., & Eachempati, P. (2021). Intelligent employee retention system for attrition rate analysis and churn prediction: An ensemble machine learning and multi-criteria decision-making approach. *Journal of Global Information Management (JGIM), 29*(6), 1–29.
4. Saradhi, V. V., & Palshikar, G. K. (2011). Employee churn prediction. *Expert Systems with Applications, 38*(3), 1999–2006.
5. Jain, N., Tomar, A., & Jana, P. K. (2021). A novel scheme for employee churn problem using multi-attribute decision-making approach and machine learning. *Journal of Intelligent Information Systems, 56*(2), 279–302.
6. Pekel Ozmen, E., & Ozcan, T. (2022). A novel deep learning model based on convolutional neural networks for employee churn prediction. *Journal of Forecasting, 41*(3), 539–550.
7. Anh, N. T., Tu, N. D., Solanki, V. K., Giang, N. L., Thu, V. H., Son, L. N., et al. (2020). Integrating employee value model with churn prediction. *International Journal of Sensors Wireless Communications and Control, 10*(4), 484–493.
8. Yiğit, İ. O., & Shourabizadeh, H. An approach for predicting employee churn by using data mining. In 2017 international artificial intelligence and data processing symposium (IDAP) (pp. 1–4) (2017). IEEE.

9. Dolatabadi, S. H., & Keynia, F. Designing of customer and employee churn prediction model based on data mining method and neural predictor. In 2017 2nd international conference on computer and communication systems (ICCCS) (pp. 74–77). IEEE (2017).
10. Yadav, S., Jain, A., & Singh, D. Early prediction of employee attrition using data mining techniques. In 2018 IEEE 8th international advance computing conference (IACC) (pp. 349–354). IEEE (2018).
11. Srivastava, D. K., & Nair, P. Employee attrition analysis using predictive techniques. In International conference on information and communication Technology for Intelligent Systems (pp. 293–300). Springer, Cham (2017).
12. Ameer, M., Rahul, S. P., & Manne, S. Human resource analytics using power bi visualization tool. In 2020 4th international conference on intelligent computing and control systems (ICICCS) (pp. 1184–1189). IEEE (2020).

Chapter 28
Impact on Social Work Practice and Research of Technology, Religion, and HIV/AIDS in India

D. Binu Sahayam and C. Joe Arun

28.1 Introduction

> I never worried about anything in life. Even when my husband and in-laws ill-treated me, I didn't bother, but after having HIV, life has changed badly. I have no one to share the pain with, nor is there anyone around to listen to me (Interviewed on 10 May 2015).

The above statement is the cry of a 33-year-old widow who hails from a deprived socio-economic family background. She has been living with HIV/AIDS for the past 11 years. She was thrown out by her own family members. This is the plight of many women getting infected with HIV/AIDS. HIV/AIDS remains one of the world's greatest threats to public health, particularly among women. The World Bank report of 2019 mentioned that "women make up half the world's population but are not treated equally on par with men in society". A study by UNAIDS in the year 2012 revealed the fact that women continue to suffer discrimination and violence in every part of the world, and every minute, one young woman is infected with HIV. Women living with HIV face stigma and discrimination due to their HIV/AIDS status. The study examines the issue from a religious standpoint as well as how technology may aid in the treatment of HIV-affected women.

D. Binu Sahayam (✉)
School of Social Sciences and Languages (SSL), Vellore Institute of Technology, Chennai, Tamil Nadu, India

C. J. Arun
Loyola Institute of Business Administration (LIBA), Loyola College, Chennai, Tamil Nadu, India

F. J. J. Joseph et al. (eds.), *Computational Intelligence for Clinical Diagnosis*, EAI/Springer Innovations in Communication and Computing,
https://doi.org/10.1007/978-3-031-23683-9_28

28.1.1 The Rationale of the Study

Women are more vulnerable than men to HIV infections for biological, social, cultural, and economic reasons such as stigma, discrimination, abuses both verbal and non-verbal, gender inequality, denial of health-care facilities, denial of available resources, etc. While a woman is suffering with a terrible chronic illness like HIV, it is impossible for her to confront society because society blames only women, not men. This study tries to draw attention to the existing situation of women living with HIV and how religious beliefs and the use of technology can serve as a coping mechanism in overcoming their serious illness.

28.1.2 Women and HIV/AIDS

The literature review is presented based on the title of the study: "Women Living with HIV/AIDS and the Role of Religion in Response to Their Status in Society with Implications for Social Work Practice and Research". An extensive literature review is done to gain an in-depth understanding of the existing situation based on the study.

The effects of HIV/AIDS on women, especially those who choose to remain monogamous, are of grave concern. According to a study conducted on the subject, the most common way for HIV to be spread in India is through unprotected intercourse (87.4% heterosexual and 1.3% gay), followed by vertical transmission (5.4%), parent-to-child transmission (1.6%), and injecting drug use (I.D.U.) (1.0 per cent). This study provides more evidence that heterosexual interaction is a major route of HIV/AIDS transmission [1].

Similar to what was seen in NFHS-3 (AOR = 4.9; *p*0.01), the data show that women who have had two or more lifetime partners are more likely to be HIV seropositive (AOR = 2.5; *p*0.01). Possible explanations include the fact that 90% of new HIV infections in India occur within heterosexual partnerships [2] and the widespread stigma associated with HIV testing. The vast majority of persons who engage in sexual activity before becoming engaged do so in the mistaken belief that they would eventually become engaged to the same person with whom they have been having sexual contact. These are the causes of the rapid expansion of the AIDS epidemic. Another study found that marriage was a significant risk factor for HIV transmission among Punjabi women. Overall, the majority of people in Punjab (80.5%) caught HIV/AIDS through heterosexual interaction. Four out of five new infections among married Punjabi women were the result of sexual activity with their spouses. Ninety per cent of AIDS patients in Punjab were not prostitutes but rather monogamous women who caught the virus from their HIV-positive husbands [1]. This demonstrates how women are disproportionately affected by this international health crisis (Fig. 28.1).

Women with HIV/AIDS face different forms of suffering due to their status and are treated indifferently in society by their own family members, relatives, and

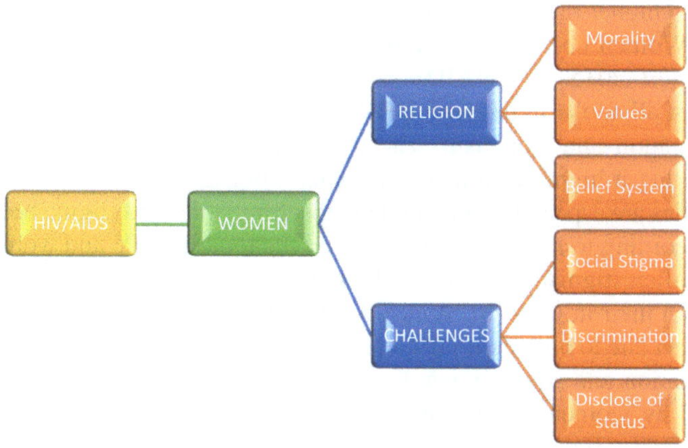

Fig. 28.1 Women with HIV/AIDS and the impact of religion. (Source: Developed by the Researcher)

friends. A study by Bharat of the Tata Institute of Social Sciences (TISS) in Mumbai emphasised that after disclosing their status to their family members, it was men who received care and support [3]. Women with HIV are also subjected to various forms of denial by their family members and carry shameful words. Another study reported that about 20 per cent of positive people face discrimination in their family [4].

HIV/AIDS and women in India: A study [5], highlighted women's heightened susceptibility to the virus. Results from these research have shed light on conditions that place women at a higher risk of contracting HIV: Women are more likely to get HIV than men due to a number of factors, including but not limited to (1) a lack of education, (2) a lack of decision-making power linked to health care, and (3) a lack of access to information and health-care services. Discrimination against women included separate utensils, a ban on sharing meals, and restricted access to public facilities [4]. According to HIV-positive moms, they were refused access to quality health-care facilities and faced discrimination from doctors and health-care personnel [6]. Withholding resources for care and therapy and restricting shares in property and access to children were also documented in qualitative investigations [6, 7].

> *My name is Kani (name changed) from Viluppuram District. I got married to my mother's brother when I was 19 years old. I was diagnosed with HIV when I was pregnant. My husband is a driver, and he keeps travelling. When my husband was asked to do testing, he then said that "He is already aware of his HIV status and is under treatment in some other place". I was totally shocked to hear this and felt cheated. I was taken aback when I was blamed for this illness by my in-laws and villagers, who said that my husband got the illness because of me. Even my parents, siblings, and relatives did not support me. I faced lots of stigma and discrimination (both physically and psychologically).*
>
> (Interviewed on 11 June 2014)

Based on the above case study, HIV/AIDS is often depicted as "a feminised epidemic; the numbers of women infected are greater compared to the numbers of men" [8]. Since the start of the global HIV epidemic, in many regions, women have remained at a higher risk of HIV infection than men. According to the amfAR report 2015 [9], “Women constitute more than half of all people living with HIV”. The statistics report 2015 of UNAIDS revealed that “globally, women account for 51 percent of all adults living with HIV” (Interviewed on 18 June 2014).

Discrimination and ostracism: The joint family system still persists in Indian society, making it highly different from other cultures. Women living with HIV in mixed families are especially vulnerable to discrimination and stigma because of this context. According to a report out of India on the topic of HIV and women, married women are often stigmatised and even blamed of passing the virus on to their sons if they live with their in-laws [5]. Widows with HIV/AIDS in India endure additional discrimination due to both their HIV status and their widowhood. The harshest kinds of discrimination and stigma towards people living with HIV/AIDS (PLWHA) are experienced by women, as shown by this data. The primary response to persons living with HIV/AIDS is a language of blaming [5]. Owen argues that it is tragic because widows are often blamed for their husbands’ deaths and questioned about their own promiscuity, while in most situations it is males who engage in polyamory. Whether or not these widows know they had HIV, a previous study found that those who told their families were shunned, denied access to their children, denied financial support, and sometimes even evicted from the family home [9]. A widow who was living with her in-laws in India was subjected to months of mistreatment before being asked to leave by the family because they feared she was damaging the “marriageability” of one of their sons. This case study was highlighted since it came from real life. The following scenario is also representative of the present:

> I am a widow with three children, and my name is Lakshmi (name has been altered). My third child was in my womb when I found out I was HIV positive; my spouse had died of AIDS before the baby was born. My doctors discouraged me against breastfeeding, and I felt uncomfortable being open about my pregnancy with my mother-in-law. Sharing my status was necessary in order to rescue my child, but it caused me to be discriminated against and eventually blamed for infecting my husband. My in-laws accused me of being sexually promiscuous and urged me to leave the house. Both of my parents rejected me. Three kids and I were out in the street. Later, with the help of another member of the positive network, I joined a nonprofit group for persons living with HIV/AIDS [9].

Depression, disgrace, being unable to accept the fact, isolation, developing low self-esteem, denial, fear, anxiety, guilt, suicidal thoughts, and futureless life are common psychological stress symptoms found in people living with HIV/AIDS, particularly among women. Additionally, research shows that people living with HIV/AIDS who endure stigma and prejudice are more likely to experience melancholy, humiliation, and suicidal thoughts [9]. Similarly, a cross-sectional study was performed on 150 PLWHA (75 men and 75 women) with HIV/AIDS in order to identify the psychosocial elements and depression related with the condition. The study found that the depressive symptoms of female HIV/AIDS patients were substantially more severe than those of male patients (Chi-square $= 12.09$, $df = 1$, p-value $= 0.0001^*$) [10]. Another study stated that depression is one of the most commonly occurring mental disorders among HIV individuals. According to the study findings, 36% of PLWHA screened positive for depression, and 16% of

PLWHA had symptoms of anxiety disorder [11]. This affects the physical, psychological, and emotional status of women with HIV/AIDS.

28.1.3 Impact of Religion

Religious teachings and practices have been historically influential in almost all countries. Religion not only serves as a protective force but also plays a supportive role in a person's development. According to sociologist Max Weber, the purpose of religion is to enhance the wellbeing and long life of their followers, and he also insists that religious experts have the power to interfere with people's everyday lives directly through pastoral care and guidance [12].

Religious leaders of various faiths emphasise social order, ethics, morality, and values. Table 28.1 is based on a chart titled "Religion and Sexual Ethics". The researcher has concentrated on Islam and Christianity from the chart and has taken what is relevant to the study. This table appeared in the *San Francisco Chronicle* in December 1994. It was compiled, according to them, "based on official reports and expert advice" [13].

In this context, it is appropriate to study the role of religion and HIV/AIDS because both have one similarity. Both are connected with morality (moral behaviour). The morality here focuses on sexual issues like pre-marital sex, extramarital sex, homosexuality, bigamy, condoms, and many other practices which are not acceptable by any religion. Religion preaches on morality, whereas HIV/AIDS points out one's moral behaviour. Therefore, studying HIV/AIDS in the context of religion is very important.

In the initial stage of HIV/AIDS, people received less support from their respective faith-based organisations, but now religious institutions are now at the forefront in educating people about the prevention of HIV/AIDS and religious activities

Table 28.1 Sexual behaviour and religions' response

Sexual behaviour	Hinduism	Islam	Christianity (Catholic)
Teenage sex	Not specifically focused [14]	Morally unacceptable in most cases	Condemned
Pre-marital sex	Does not support [15]	Condemned	Condemned
Extramarital sex	Mortal sin [16]	Condemned	Condemned
Divorce	Does not approve [17]	Neutral	Condemned
Masturbation	Not clear	Neutral	Morally unacceptable in most cases
Abortion	Condemned [18]	Neutral	Condemned
Contraceptives	No ban [19]	Condemned	Condemned
Homosexual sex	Controversial [20]	Condemned	Condemned

towards society have gained unprecedented dynamic [12]. Recent HIV/AIDS research has focused on the effect of religion on those living with the virus, and these studies have found that religious beliefs and practices have a significant positive effect on PLWHA's health. Those PLWHA who believed in God, had empathy for others, had inner peace, and practised religion had a higher quality of life and a longer life expectancy than those who did not [21].

Stigma is one of the serious barriers to coping with HIV/AIDS. Mahajan, in his study, argued that stigma is a serious issue because infected people avoid revealing their status and stigma stands as a barrier for HIV testing and treatment. Wolfe's study among 112 HIV patients who are on Antiretroviral therapy (ART) in Botswana revealed that 94 per cent of patients maintained their secret within their community about their HIV status, whereas 69 per cent did not even disclose their status to their family members [22]. The stigma faced by the PLWHA leads to social isolation and stands as a hindrance in prevention aspects. The HIV/AIDS stigma continues to be a barrier for many PLWHA across the globe [23]. This stigma arises from people's attitudes, which have to be changed. People living with HIV/AIDS undergo various forms of psychological distress due to the stigma attached to HIV/AIDS disease. Joshi and Kumari's research [24] demonstrates how people living with HIV experience stigma and guilt, leading some to seek solace in religious practices as a manner of coping with their illness. Depression, shame, and thoughts of suicide have all been documented in the studies of people living with HIV/AIDS who have suffered stigma and discrimination [9].

Religious activism in the fight against AIDS has been the subject of research. The importance of personal behaviour and sexual behaviour in preventing HIV/AIDS is shown by a Brazilian intervention study. The study also stresses that it is the role of religious leaders of different religions to educate their followers on religious norms and practices, which will contribute to a reduction in the HIV/AIDS infection rate [25]. About half of 100 HIV patients surveyed in a study reported feeling more spiritual or religious after receiving their diagnosis [21]. HIV/AIDS is incurable, and this fact may draw people closer to God as they learn to rely on their faith for the strength to face each day. Religious teachings are a powerful source of comfort for individuals in need [21]. Joshi and Kumari, in their own research, found that patients with terminal illnesses who are able to do so turn to religious teachings and practices as a means of alleviating their pain. As HIV progresses to its last stages, a spiritual belief system can assist a person to maintain a positive outlook by easing their anxiety about dying [24]. It is clear from the studies that religion plays a significant role in helping persons who are HIV positive and living with the disease. The literature study demonstrates that religion is an integral component of the lives of persons with HIV, providing them with strength, hope, confidence, satisfaction, inner peace, and the ability to take on life's obstacles.

28.2 Methodology

The study was conducted among 307 women living with HIV/AIDS. In this study, a stratified random sampling method was adopted to collect the data. The study continued with an exploratory qualitative method to draw information from the respondents. The research design used in the study is a descriptive diagnostic design, and to collect the data directly from the respondents, an "interview schedule" was framed consisting of both closed-ended and open-ended questions, and the data was enumerated using the Statistical Package for Social Science (SPSS). The study was conducted based on the responses received from three positive networks functioning in Chennai, Viluppuram, and Tuticorin, which are under Tamil Nadu AIDS Control Society (TANSACS) for data collection.

Inclusion criteria:

- Positive women registered in religious institutions which are part of the positive networks
- Women over the age of 18 living with HIV
- Those who were willing to be interviewed based on informed consent as per Indian Council of Medical Research (ICMR) guidelines

The ethics committee at Loyola College in Chennai's Institute of Dialogue with Cultures and Religions (IDCR) gave their stamp of approval to everything used in the study. All contributors provided their informed consent.

28.2.1 Part I – Quantitative Study

28.2.1.1 Demographic Details of the Respondents

In the study, 87 per cent of the respondents fell into the reproductive and economically active age group of 18–47 years. Sixty-seven per cent of the respondents belong to the Hindu religion. Eighteen per cent of the respondents belong to the Christian religion. Islam constituted a meagre 15 per cent. Out of 307 respondents, merely 19.2 per cent of the respondents were illiterate and the remaining 80.8 per cent were literate. During the interview, the majority (73.6 per cent) of the women revealed that they contracted HIV from their husbands. The nuclear type of family stands at 73.3 per cent of the respondents, whereas 11.1 per cent are from the joint family system. A majority, 76.9 per cent, of the respondents are employed, and they are represented as the breadwinners of the family.

28.2.1.2 Not Disclosing the HIV/AIDS Status

Fear of stigma and discrimination prevents PLWHA from disclosing their status to their immediate circle, which includes family members, relatives, friends, peer groups, and the community with which they are affiliated. The major reasons identified were as follows: fear of discrimination (21.2 per cent), disgrace (4.6 per cent), and rejection (2.9 per cent). The reality is that respondents have not disclosed their HIV-positive status in order to avoid facing any kind of discrimination from family members and outsiders. The respondents also maintained secrecy by not sharing their status because of the shame and negative identity associated with the illness.

28.2.1.3 Acceptance of Family Members After HIV/AIDS Status

The care and support of family members in the lives of HIV/AIDS people plays a crucial role. Acceptance of family members is very important and its absence will lead to psychological stress. A majority, 71.3 per cent, of the respondents said that they were not accepted by their family members after being infected with HIV. The infected person faces indifferent behaviour by their family members on one ground, i.e. social status. The findings of the research study [26] highlighted that 80 per cent of the respondents were isolated at the time of their severe illness by their family members and 30 per cent did not get love and care from their family members [26]. Stigma and discrimination complicate the situation of PLWHA.

28.2.1.4 Involvement in Religious Practices

After being diagnosed, PLWHA face rejection from family members, friends, and close circles. This leads to psychological stress resulting in suicidal thoughts. As far as the religious practices of the respondents are concerned, it is found from the analysis that a majority of 85 per cent of the respondents revealed that after the diagnosis of HIV they were involved in religious practices, whereas 9.1 per cent said they were not involved in any kind of religious practices after their HIV diagnosis. PLWHA turn towards religion as a means of support to lead a peaceful life. Due to his or her HIV status, religion plays a vital role in the life of PLWHA. Religion and its practices strengthen them with strong faith because they often face rejection by their own circle.

28.2.1.5 Respondents Association with Religious Group or Organisations

Religious institutions have presented a variety of responses in addressing the problems faced by PLWHA. Of the 307 respondents, 282 (91.9 per cent) stated that they were part of a religious group or an organisation working for the wellbeing of people living with HIV/AIDS. According to the findings, the respondents believe that belonging to any religious group or organisation is extremely beneficial.

28.2.1.6 Religion Has Given Them the Power to Live in Hope and Face Any Kind of Obstacles

The influence of religion is high among PLWHA. Religion, according to the majority of respondents (78.5 per cent), has given them the ability to live in hope and overcome any obstacle. The respondents who were optimistic spoke about the greatness of religion, whereas those who had drifted away from their religion and its practices spoke in a pessimistic manner.

28.2.1.7 Religion Has the Power to Change Your Wellbeing

Religion has a dynamic role in the wellbeing of PLWHA. It helped PLWHA to view life positively and change their attitudes to lead a better life. PLWHA develop positive ways to cope with their HIV status, increase self-care, and develop positive behaviour toward others [27]. Religion has the power to change people's lives, according to the majority of respondents (77.5%). From the analysis, it is observed that respondents who have faith in their respective religions (Hinduism, Christianity, and Islam) and their preaching indicate that religion plays a dominant role in their wellbeing, i.e. the holistic development of an individual.

28.3 Part II – Qualitative Study

28.3.1 Case Study – 1

Christian Anita (name changed) lost her spouse 3 years ago to HIV/AIDS, and he infected her. She is quite impoverished due to her job as a coolie. She is a mother of two, one of whom is HIV positive and the other of whom is not. The family lives next door to their relatives, but it was these individuals who first exhibited prejudice. Some people avoid her because she has HIV/AIDS. Due to her frequent illness, she rarely shows up for work when she is supposed to. Her goal is to provide her kids a good education. Not only does she have to deal with the social stigma of her situation, but she also cannot afford to send her kids to college. According to Anita, the first steps in preventing the spread of HIV/AIDS are to exercise self-control in sexual matters and to refrain from sharing needles with others.

28.3.1.1 Care System

She was admitted to the TNSACS-operated positive network after being diagnosed with HIV at Kilpauk Medical Hospital in Chennai. Christian Missions Charitable Trust (CMCT), Chennai, was where she was directed. She received help for her mental and spiritual wellbeing as well as therapy and prayer at CMCT. They guaranteed monthly food deliveries and financial assistance for her kids' college tuition. Anita is grateful to CMCT for the preventative guidance, self-awareness training, and spiritual comfort it has provided her. In a time of difficulty, she was able to manage better with the aid of the CMCT. When Anita was finished, she said, "I was in a hopeless situation; I realised that there is no one to help me except God, and so I turned to God and confessed my sins. By the grace of God, I am at peace. I developed guilt feelings because of HIV, which made me attempt suicide, but now I don't feel like it nor do I have guilty feelings".

28.3.2 Case Study – 2

Ayesha (name changed) got married at the age of 18. She is from the Muslim community. There are a total of 12 children in her family tree, and she is the fourth of them. Back in 1999, she entered into an arranged marriage. She's a mother to two young men. Both boys are in school; the older one is 15 and in ninth grade, and the younger one is 13 and in eighth grade. They rushed her eldest kid to Stanley Medical Hospital in Chennai after he complained of a persistent fever. For her son's medical exam, the doctor requested that she complete the entire procedure. She learnt, to her dismay, that her son had become infected with HIV/AIDS. She was tasked with taking the HIV/AIDS test together with her husband and was given specific instructions to do so. Both parents tested positive with HIV in this study. Her spouse found out and promptly beat her up for being unfaithful and then abandoned her. They all turned their backs on her. For safety, she had to approach the mosque's leaders for assistance. In exchange, they provided guidance to her family. She's a housekeeper, and her monthly pay is Rs 3000. She helps support her family by performing menial tasks. Though she wants to send her sons to school, she has a hard time making ends meet each month.

28.3.2.1 Care System

After receiving her HIV/AIDS diagnosis at Stanley Medical Hospital in Chennai, she was instructed to sign up with the TNSACS-run HIV/AIDS network. That connection led her to learn about International alliance for the prevention of AIDS (IAPA) India, a nonprofit group serving those with HIV/AIDS. They help anyone in need regardless of their religious affiliation. She seeks blessings and participates in mosque prayers regularly. The Jamaat, which is an Islamic religious group, met her and her family members personally and requested them to share love and care with her and the children. The Jamaat has been extending all possible support to her by providing spiritual counselling and periodical financial support for treatment purposes. The Jamaat representatives also came forward to support her children's education. According to Ayesha, "My religious teachings, beliefs, and practises played an important part in my life. Disclosing my status to everyone was a difficult move. But religion and religious leaders made me understand the meaning of compassion, which strengthened me to live a meaningful life".

28.3.3 Case Study – 3

Radha (name changed) is aged 25, is illiterate, and belongs to a poor agricultural family. She lives with her husband and son. When they don't have an agricultural job, her husband goes for any kind of unskilled work or travels from one place to another in search of a job, and during his mobility he happened to get infected with HIV/AIDS. Due to his prolonged illness, he was asked to go for a checkup at Tambaram Thoracic Sanatorium, Chennai. The result showed he was seropositive. After hearing this, he lost consciousness and survived for about 4 months. Fortunately, their child tested negative for the virus. When the villagers came to know of their status, they were stigmatised and discriminated against by their community. Due to the social stigma attached to it, they were treated very badly. Even their own family members behaved very rudely. Her child was forced to stay away from other children.

28.3.3.1 Care System

Women face many forms of stigma and discrimination due to their HIV/AIDS status. After being diagnosed with HIV, she was referred to PWN+, an organisation that provides HIV testing, counselling, treatment, and support services to HIV-positive women. A field worker with the positive network, that's what she does. As a devout Hindu, she knows that her misfortunes are a punishment for her previous mistakes. She is devout and follows the Brahmin priest's lead when it comes to doing pujas and making offerings. She's the one who does everything. She also thinks that, because of her faith in God, she will be able to stay in this life. Because of her faith in God, she finds tremendous strength and assurance in herself. NGOs focusing on HIV/AIDS provide cash aid and educational opportunities for her son. On interacting with Radha, the researcher came to know that she practises religious teachings of all faiths. She believes that faith in God will help her to live her life smoothly. Once, when she felt depressed, she attempted to commit suicide, but she was then touched by the testimony of another positive woman and changed her mind to live her life putting all her trust in God.

She goes to temples, does pujas, and does all sorts of rituals so that her child does well and is settled happily. She regularly offers food, as all religions insist on sharing. She offers food now and then. She is involved in these activities just for her own satisfaction. She smiled and said that she went everywhere because only God could answer her pain and suffering.

28.4 Discussion

The results from the study accentuate that irrespective of all interventions, women with HIV/AIDS continue to face multiple forms of discrimination in society. The findings suggest that women need twice as much in the care, prevention, treatment, and support system. The study tries to establish a positive link between religion and HIV/AIDS. Therefore, the inquiry starts with the question of involvement in religious practices by the respondent after the diagnosis of HIV/AIDS status. As far as the religious practices of the respondents are concerned, it is found from the analysis that the majority, i.e. 85 per cent of the respondents, revealed that after their HIV diagnosis they were involved in religious practices, and 78.5 per cent of the respondents shared that religion has given them the power to live in hope and face any kind of obstacle. The respondents felt their religious beliefs and practices helped to increase their faith to lead their lives in this competitive society and to overcome their illness. Religion is a multidimensional construct [28] which can play a vital role in the health status of the respondents.

HIV/AIDS has created an impression that there is no life for an infected person and that it is an illness with no solution. In such cases, those who are infected decide to seek the mercy of their God for greater healing. Religion has given people a faith-based hope for living peacefully. Durkheim [29] argues that religion is a form of social control and it inculcates good values in a person. Religious leaders, through their religious discourse of power and knowledge, need to address the plight of both those infected and affected by HIV/AIDS by showing compassion, care, and support. This will take a positive shape in the community and can make a difference in the lives of PLWHA and further in the prevention aspects of HIV/AIDS. Religious leaders must openly discuss sexual and immoral behaviour, as well as sexual orientation, through their religious discourse of power and knowledge for the good of all, as Foucault [30] insists on an open discussion of sexuality. Religious leaders, through their religious discourse, can break the silence by reaching out to those rejected by society due to their HIV status. It is understandable that the interference of religion in the prevention of HIV/AIDS brings constructive changes in the lives of those infected and affected by HIV/AIDS.

28.4.1 Implications for Social Work Practice

Four decades have passed since the first case of AIDS was identified in 1981; many questions about HIV/AIDS infection, the vaccine to prevent it, and ways and means to stop the spread remain unanswered. This has eventually led to a lot of myths about the spread of the infection, leading to stigma and discrimination within society. HIV/AIDS has not only affected the health of individuals but also their personality and identity. PLWHA have a highly burdensome life that imposes multiple challenges, especially stress, on them.

The social workers are critical as they play a catalyst's role in dealing with the infected ones, their families, and the larger society. Currently, there are social workers engaged in it. However, there is ample scope for appointing more of them in order to deal with the rise in demand and to professionally intervene with those infected and also other stakeholders such as government line departments, educational institutions, the health sector, and the communities to curb the spread of infection and also myths around it as well.

Social workers need to be capacitated and build on their skills to play an effective role. In-depth knowledge of HIV/AIDS (causes, awareness, and prevention), skills to provide emotional support to PLWHA and their caregivers, and training in family-integrated counselling and therapies could all be areas of capacity building. With skills and knowledge acquired, social workers can conduct impactful awareness campaigns and workshops at various educational institutions. A training manual can be drafted and circulated across educational institutions and workplaces as IEC/BCC materials to facilitate enhanced understanding of this epidemic, viz. a platform to break the silence around HIV/AIDS.

The role of social workers appears to be even more important in bringing about behavioural and attitude changes among those affected, their families, and other stakeholders. They may have to advocate for those PLWHA with different fronts for facilitating care, rights, entitlements, and resources from the institutional setup of the government and NGOs working in the sector. Social workers can facilitate the identification and training of women living with HIV/AIDS as peer educators and role models.

There is also a felt need for elective courses on HIV/AIDS such as sexuality and identity, interpersonal care and support, etc., as part of the social work course. Students who enrol in these courses are expected to have a better understanding of HIV/AIDS and its scope for further specialisation, learning, and application for better impact, scale, and sustainable interventions.

28.4.2 Application of Artificial Intelligence

This paper seeks to determine how the use of technology (artificial intelligence) can help people living with HIV/AIDS improve their wellbeing status. AI solutions for HIV prevention could benefit from an experimental, systematic approach that includes qualitative and quantitative assessments and should be developed to reduce HIV infection rates (Fig. 28.2).

AI-based solutions are necessary to help with HIV prevention. Using technology, people living with HIV/AIDS can address their physiological and psychological issues.

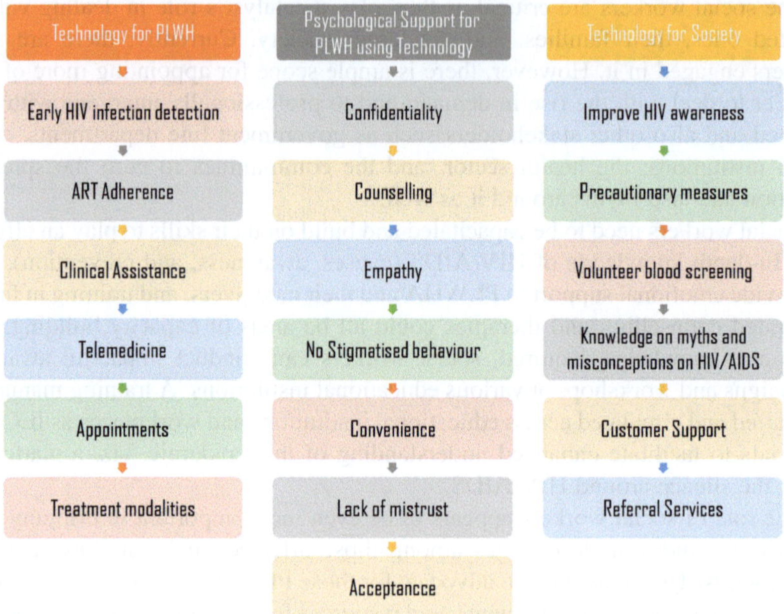

Fig. 28.2 Developed by the researcher

28.5 Conclusion

Globally, the HIV/AIDS epidemic is represented as one of the most important health concerns. It poses social, economic, developmental, religious, and technological challenges to countries globally. Religious institutions act as change agents in addressing the issue of HIV/AIDS. Religious beliefs often help individuals with an HIV infection develop a perspective on the meaning and purpose of their life. Today, directly or indirectly, all religious leaders of various faiths follow Foucauldian theory, which focuses on an open dialogue on sexuality, which leads to removing stigmatised behaviour towards PLWHA and eventually bringing about behavioural and attitudinal change among the general public. The PLWHA are affected in many ways, such as the socio-economic effect, the existence of stigma and discrimination, psychological status, and also taking ART. The findings of this study would undoubtedly facilitate the strengthening of religious and cultural practices that help in the prevention and care of HIV/AIDS. UN organisations like the WHO, UNHCR, UNICEF, WFP, UNDP, UNFPA, UNODC, UNESCO, and the World Bank are working to fight against the spread of HIV infections and to care for people living with HIV. This study is just a starting point towards further study on how religious leaders and the use of technology could help PLWHA cope with the disease and correct their perception of the disease and the ways of eradicating and curing the disease.

References

1. Kaur, A. (2012). *HIV/AIDS stigma and discrimination: A sociological study of amritsar city* (Doctoral dissertation). Retrieved from Shodhganga@INFLIBNET. Available at URL http://shodhganga.inflibnet.ac.in/handle/10603/23455. Accessed on 22 Mar 2016 at 4.00 pm.
2. Singh, S. K., Vishwakarma, D., Sharma, B., & Sharma, S. K. (2020). Inequalities in women's empowerment and prevalence of HIV in India. *International Journal of Community Medicine and Public Health, 7*, 3069–3080.
3. Bharat, S., Aggleton, P., & Tyrer, P. (2001). *India: HIV and AIDS-related discrimination, stigmatization and denial. UNAIDS key material-best practice collection.* UNAIDS. www.unaids.org/publications/documents/
4. Paxton, G. S., Gonzales, K., Uppakaew, K. K., Abraham, S., Okta, C., Green, K. S., Nair, T. P., Merati, B., Thephthien, M. M., & Quesada, A. (2005). AIDS-related discrimination in Asia. *AIDS Care, 17*(4), 413–424. https://doi.org/10.1080/09540120412331299807
5. Hollen, V. C. (2013). *Birth in the age of AIDS: Women, reproduction, and HIV/AIDS in India.* Stanford University Press.
6. Thomas, B., Nyamathi, A., & Swaminathan, S. (2009). Impact of HIV/AIDS on mothers in southern India: A qualitative study. *AIDS and Behavior, 13*(5), 989–996.
7. Bharat, S. (2011). A systematic review of HIV/AIDS-related stigma and discrimination in India: Current understanding and future needs. *SAHARA-J: Journal of Social Aspects of HIV/AIDS, 8*(3), 138–149.
8. Owen, M. 2016. *Widows in third world nations [online] in encyclopedia of death and dying.* Available at: URL http://www.deathreference.com/Vi-Z/Widows-in-Third-World-Nations.html. Accessed on 18 Mar 2016 at 07.30 pm.
9. Abraham, A. D., & Amassoma, D. (2013). Economic implications of stigma and discrimination in Nigeria (case study of clients on antiretroviral treatment at the University Of Abuja Teaching Hospital Gwagwalada Abuja). *IOSR Journal of Humanities and Social Science (IOSR-JHSS), 11*(4), 13–19.
10. Barua, A., Sharma, Y., & Basilio, A. M. (2013). Burning issue of HIV/AIDS: A psychosocial study. *International Journal of Collaborative Research on Internal Medicine & Public Health, 5*(7), 545–551. Available at: URL http://www.iomcworld.com/ijcrimph/files/v05-n07-06.pdf. Accessed on 31 Oct 2016 2.29 pm.
11. Sivagami and Suguna. (2013). A study on stress among HIV/AIDS patients in Tiruchirappalli District. In R. Mangaleswaran (Ed.), *Working with youth, women and children with HIV/AIDS – Strategic interventions for inclusive development* (Vol. 2013, pp. 319–324). Authors Press.
12. Burchardt, M. (2007). *Subjects of counselling: Religion, HIV/AIDS and the management of everyday life in South Africa.* Available at: https://www.unil.ch/files/live/sites/issr/files/shared/colloque_de_recherche/Burchardt_Subjects_of_Counselling.pdf. Accessed on 14 Apr 2020 at 14.41 pm.
13. See: http://www.holyblasphemy.net/sex-and-religion-chart/. Accessed on 12 Sept 2015 at 2.09 pm.
14. See: http://www.hinduwebsite.com/hinduism/h_premarital.asp. Accessed on 21 Sept 2015 at 10.21 pm.
15. See: http://www.hinduwebsite.com/hinduism/h_premarital.asp. Accessed on 21 Sept 2015 at 10.31 pm.
16. See: http://www.hinduwebsite.com/hinduism/h_extramarital.asp. Accessed on 21 Sept 2015 at 10.47 pm.
17. See: http://www.hinduwebsite.com/hinduism/h_premarital.asp. Accessed on 21 Sept 2015 at 10.38 pm.
18. See: http://www.fnsa.org/fall98/murti1.html. Accessed on 8 Oct 2015 at 10.56 pm.
19. See: http://www.bbc.co.uk/religion/religions/hinduism/hinduethics/contraception.shtml. Accessed on 8 Oct 2015 at 11.03 pm.

20. See: http://www.religionfacts.com/hinduism/homosexuality. Accessed on 21 Sept 2015 at 10.31 pm.
21. Ironson, G., et al. (2002). The Ironson-woods spirituality/religiousness index is associated with long survival, health behaviors, less disorders, and low cortisol in people with HIV/AIDS. *Annals of Behavioral Medicine, 24*(1), 34–48.
22. Wolfe, W. R., et al. (2006). Effects of HIV-related stigma among an early sample of patients receiving antiretroviral therapy in Botswana. *AIDS Care: Psychological and Socio-Medical Aspects of AIDS/HIV, 18*(8), 931–933.
23. Simbayi, L. C., et al. (2007). Internalized stigma, discrimination, and depression among men and women living with HIV/AIDS in Cape Town, South Africa. *Social Science & Medicine, 64*, 1823–1831.
24. Joshi, S., & Kumari, S. (2009). Religion and AIDS: An overview. *Indian Journal Social Science Researches* [online], *6*, 46–55. Available at: URL: http://www.ncbi.nlm.nih.gov/pmc/articles/PMC2862135/. Accessed on 30 Mar 2015 at 03.15 pm.
25. Paiva, et al. (2010). Religious communities and HIV prevention: An intervention-study using a human rights-based approach. *Global Public Health, 5*(3), 280–294.
26. Sebastine, Jayabalan, & Richard. (2013). Stigma and discrimination among community people in Chennai Slums affected with HIV/AIDS. In R. Mangaleswaran (Ed.), *Working with youth, women and children with HIV/AIDS – Strategic interventions for inclusive development* (Vol. 2013, pp. 301–305). Authors Press.
27. Lutz, Kremer, & Ironson. (2011). Being diagnosed with HIV as a trigger for spiritual transformation. *Religions, 2*, 398–409.
28. Koenig, K., & Carson. (2012). *Handbook of religion and health.* Oxford University Press.
29. Durkheim, E. (1961). *An elementary form of the religious belief.* George Allen & Unwin.
30. Foucault, M. (1978). *The history of sexuality* (An introduction) (Vol. 1). Pantheon Books.

Chapter 29
Detection of Anomalies in Internet of Things (IoT) Network Using Artificial Neural Intelligence for Healthcare

Gnaneswari Gnanaguru, S. Silvia Priscila, and R. Balamurugan

29.1 Introduction

IoT will lead to an explosion in sensor and stream data, which will be gathered at a rapid pace. It's possible to encounter a variety of anomalous streams in real-time scenarios, such as data that is inconsistent with its usual behaviour or data that jumps abruptly in artificial neural intelligence for healthcare [1].

It is imperative that this anomalous data be captured accurately and timely for further decision-making. The study [2] introduced the Internet of things as a service [3–5] that facilitates stream data processing. In [6–8], the concept of selecting a suitable service or method is discussed. Various data sources should be provided with common functions that can be easily reused and combined to create more complex functions through service composition.

There are a large number of industrialised anomaly detection algorithms (ADAs) available as a service and can be used in a variety of contexts [9, 10]. The work in [11] is used a proactive data service abstraction to properly package up the current ADAs.

In spite of the scenario, capturing anomalous data is still a challenge because of the various circumstances involved. It is tough to find a programme [12] that solves an optimisation technique better than all others in all instances. Statistical

G. Gnanaguru
CMR Institute of Technology, Bengaluru, India

S. S. Priscila (✉)
Bharath Institute of Higher Education and Research (BIHER), Chennai, Tamil Nadu, India
e-mail: silviaprisila.cbcs.cs@bharathuniv.ac.in

R. Balamurugan
Department of Computer Science, Bharath Institute of Higher Education and Research (BIHER), Chennai, Tamil Nadu, India

F. J. J. Joseph et al. (eds.), *Computational Intelligence for Clinical Diagnosis*, EAI/Springer Innovations in Communication and Computing,
https://doi.org/10.1007/978-3-031-23683-9_29

approaches won't work effectively because of situational inconsistencies in a single collection [13]. In terms of the Area Under the Curve (AUC), generative models might perform more effectively than analytical techniques. Depending on how often and constantly the quantity of unique real-time processing emerges, it is easy to ignore part of the abnormal information in artificial neural intelligence for healthcare. An Anomaly Detection System (ADS) can therefore be unable to adjust to various input data structures. Since anomaly detection is both faster and more accurate, dynamically selecting the appropriate service for each stream of data is a requirement.

Each anomaly detection algorithm works better for a specific set of stream collections [14–18]. A stream of data must be accurately and quickly characterised so that IoT services can be computationally selected in a wide range of scenarios [19]. With data from different types flowing in, a range of options can be chosen and customised [20–22].

Following the observation that anomalies are difficult to detect from stream data, an anomaly detection framework was proposed in this paper [23]. In this paper, a machine learning-based framework is developed using artificial neural network (ANN) in intelligence for healthcare [24]. The model preprocesses the input network log data and then the features are extracted from it. The ANN classifier classifies the relevant features required to detect anomalies in a real-time environment in intelligence for healthcare [25–27].

29.2 Background

These methods are primarily used to detect anomalies because of their ability to generalise. For these reasons, supervised methods are not an option for us. There are several challenges with trying to identify anomalies in IoT measurements taken as part of a continuous time series in real time in artificial neural intelligence for healthcare.

In order to quickly deploy ADS, very little or no time is available to train a complex anomaly detection model. Long short-term memory (LSTM) and Autoencoder for transmissions using variable tweaking and training a model are two examples of supervised neural analysis tool techniques for abnormality identification. An increasing number of streams are being launched frequently, which makes it more difficult to determine which service algorithms are best suited for each stream.

A flexible IoT real-time data ADA must keep in mind huge amounts of data type improvements in specific dynamic data vulnerability scanning methodologies. As previously stated, outlier detection at runtime was known to be a problem, but solution formation did not take into account this issue or ignore changes in streaming data. Because of the dynamic nature of IoT data, current methods are ineffective. Using the features gathered in the first phase, we try to build a framework for describing and reshaping the time-series data using deep learning models, which we then apply in the second stage to identify the data patterns in healthcare.

29.3 IoT Stream Data Detection Framework in Healthcare

The full capabilities of the newly added object tracking AD infrastructure: The record includes a tuple that can be used for documentation for the recognition and choice of providers in the process's advanced parts. Through gathering actual instances from abnormality sensing devices or by speaking with subject-matter experts, this material can be enhanced. Typically, the flow input and statistical results are used to construct a technique to choose an ADS for a particular quantity of information. The collected information was used to track the efficiency of new ADAs.

Each stream of information can be expressed as a digital direction by applying a stream feature extraction technique to the stream data. Computational models are trained using the best possible services as practising models for their models. Similar to how we extracted features for our framework's application, an updated stream of data is turned into a feature vector. Using the similarity matrix and the product modelling approach, the most appropriate operation for the current number of bytes is selected, and it is then used in practice to reflect the anomalous data in artificial neural networks for healthcare.

29.3.1 Service Selection Model

To choose the highest quality products for real-time feature extraction, a significant portion of real-time processing must be gathered and their properties extracted. When examining available information, an ADS is the best comparison to the captured processing and data segment and the great quality that satisfies it. In order to find the best service on the market, a small number of common services are put to the test over and over again on these stream data fragments. Reaching a conclusion on an important concern has evolved into a structural precognition challenge due to the flow of numerous types and their highest ADS.

29.3.2 Feature Extraction

The time-series properties are the foundation of our concept. The foundation for anomaly identification is made up of features that are already accessible to the general public and tried-and-true techniques. Using the feature selection strategy that was used, some helpful features for capturing the crucial aspects of stream data were also found. The specified real-time qualities must be used in conjunction with one another in order to select the best treatment for fresh, evolving datasets.

29.3.3 Data Patterns Representations in Intelligence for Healthcare

Given the abundance of modern computing real-time data uses and the diverse properties of real-time processing, the adoption of an ANN approach is practical. The selection of traits to describe sensor information and the choice of suitable technology offerings rank among the most crucial facets of our job. It was necessary to use a feature selection method in order to distinguish between different stream data patterns.

Each feature has its own unique geometric interpretation and statistical significance when used to characterise time-series data from various perspectives. These characteristics can be quantified through the use of computing. In other words, it is possible to tell the difference between these data streams by comparing their characteristics.

Many models are built using different subsets of input features and then handpicked for their best performance based on various performance metrics. This is a part of this approach called "wrapping" feature selection. These approaches may be computationally intensive even though they are not dependent on the type of variables used in artificial neural intelligence for healthcare.

In contrast to procedure objective functions, these properties are particularly well suited for universal pattern recognition tasks, as per the cognitive science field. However, adaptable learning technology might be effective in solving related issues in a vast multitude of distinct domains. Based on the similarities between the two issues, a conclusion can be drawn. Algorithm selection is made easier by the selection of these characteristics. The transfer function is given below:

$$f(a) = 1/(1 + \exp(-a))$$

A classification model can then be trained using these characteristics in order to select a suitable algorithm for a given stream of data. If these characteristics could be calculated in real time, the decision to select the best algorithm service would be made more quickly, and thus more application users would accept it, as previously stated.

No limit exists on how many inputs a neuron can take in anything from one to n. As a result, the inputs can be written as $x1$, $x2$, $x3 \ldots xn$.

$w1$, $w2$, $w3 \ldots$ wn are the weights for the inputs. We can now express the sum of the weights multiplied by the inputs we discussed above in terms of the activation value, which is

$$a = x1w1 + x2w2 + x3w3 \ldots + xnwn$$

To put it another way, the sum of the sum of all of the sums is equal to one.

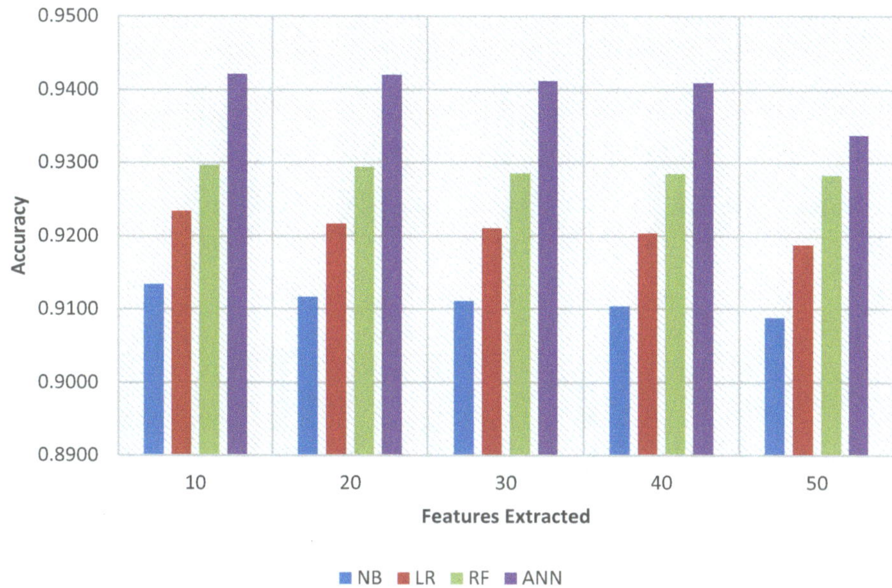

Fig. 29.1 Accuracy

$$a = \sum_{i=0}^{i=n} w_i x_i$$

29.4 Performance Analysis

The method is evaluated in the chart to show the effectiveness of the suggested strategy with a number of alternative approaches, covering ML techniques like randomised trees, Bayesian networks, and categorisation and backsliding trees. Actual and artificial information with three kinds of anomalies—collective, randomised, and focal anomaly—is used to verify the efficiency (Figs. 29.1, 29.2, 29.3 and 29.4).

The outcomes are illustrated in Figs. 29.1, 29.2, 29.3 and 29.4 shows that the suggested procedure has a greater degree of precision when identifying instances from the input set. As a conclusion, it provides better rates of speed and efficiency, memory, and *f*-measure than the current approaches in artificial neural intelligence for healthcare.

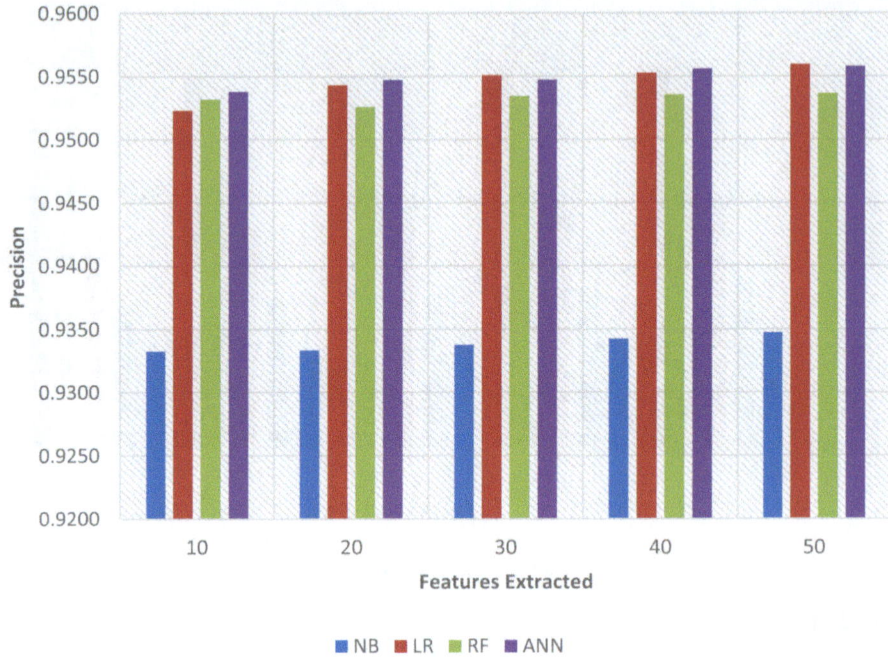

Fig. 29.2 Precision

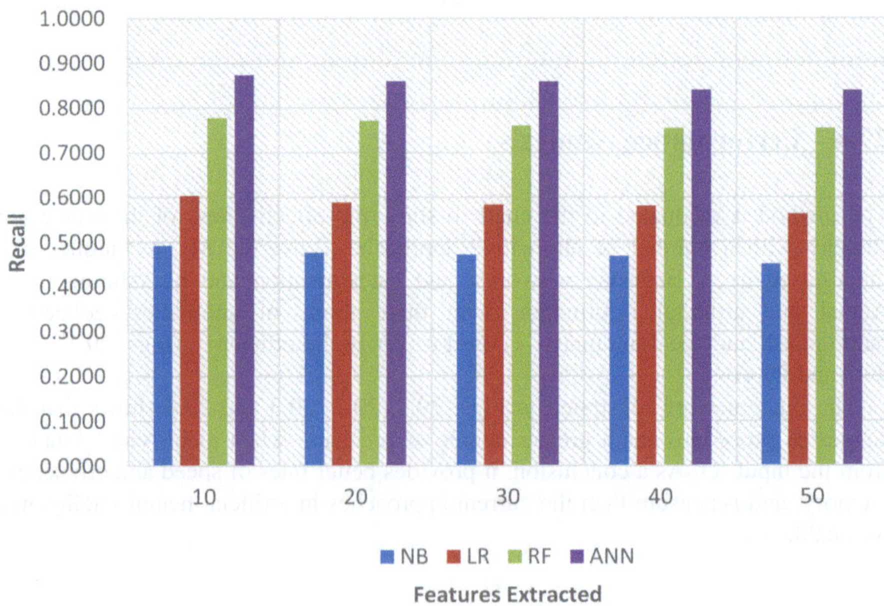

Fig. 29.3 Recall

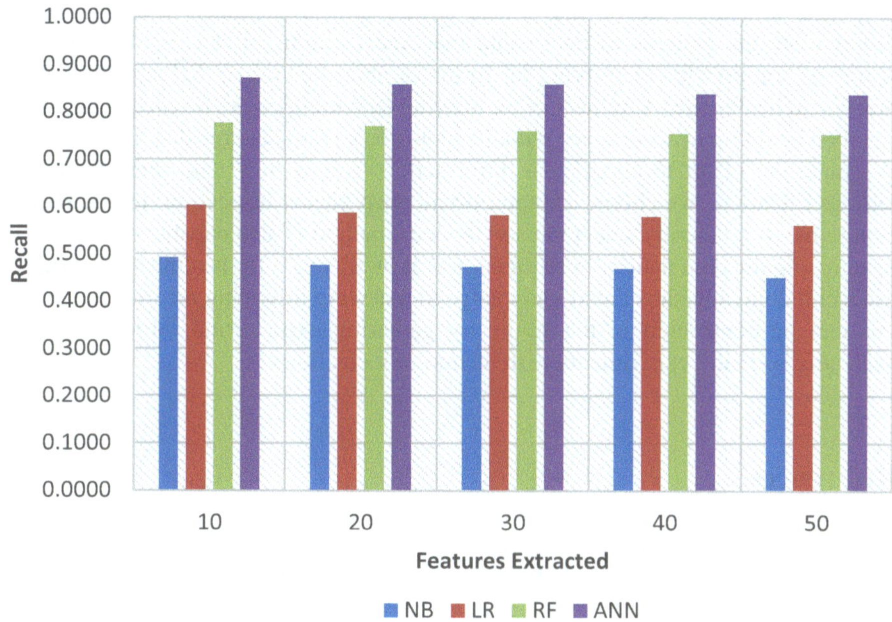

Fig. 29.4 F-measure

29.4.1 Explanation of the Figure and the Findings

In the above illustrated figure, there are four charts, which show four different working fields of the system. Figure 29.1 represents the accuracy, which shows how fast the system compiles the information and provides it. Second, the precise chart comes, which shows how accurate the system works when it's distributing the materials among the structure. However, in total, the method is evaluated in the chart to show the effectiveness of the suggested strategy with a number of alternative approaches, covering ML techniques like randomised trees, Bayesian networks, and categorisation and backsliding trees. Actual and artificial neural Information for healthcare contains three kinds of anomalies—collective, randomized, and focal anomaly—is used to verify the efficiency.

29.5 Conclusion

In this paper, an ANN framework is developed that classifies the relevant features required to detect the anomalies in a real-time environment in intelligence for healthcare. The experiments were conducted to test the efficacy of feature selection and classification. The IoT techniques are reactive, which makes actual-time anomalous characterisation a difficult task. A deep machine-based learning design is proposed, utilising a neural network to allow rapid prediction. We instead try to differentiate the patterns of data using machine learning, as it is hard to create a universal solution for identifying all forms of abnormalities in IoT stream data in practice in healthcare. A number of monitoring technologies can be chosen, and they can then be set up in accordance with the real-time stream patterns that they produce. We make an effort to capture the information from a flow, and then, using the retrieved features, we choose an appropriate deep packet inspection. In addition to being able to efficiently select the service, our method is also capable of efficiently recognising the data pattern in artificial neural intelligence for healthcare. While we use technologically substantial knowledge to make the following recommendations, this can be considered in the future by gathering extra actual information and analysing so many experiments with technology creation.

References

1. Ghazal, T. M., Hasan, M. K., Alshurideh, M. T., Alzoubi, H. M., Ahmad, M., Akbar, S. S., et al. (2021). IoT for smart cities: Machine learning approaches in smart healthcare—A review. *Future Internet, 13*(8), 218.
2. Sara, S. B. V., Anand, M., Priscila, S. S., Yuvaraj, N., Manikandan, R., & Ramkumar, M. (2021). Design of autonomous production using deep neural network for complex job. In Materials today: Proceedings.
3. Sangeetha, S. B., Sabitha, R., Dhiyanesh, B., Kiruthiga, G., & Raja, R. A. (2022). Resource management framework using deep neural networks in multi-cloud environment. In *Operationalizing multi-cloud environments* (pp. 89–104). Springer.
4. Praghash, K., Raja, R. A., & Karthikeyan, T. (2021). An investigation of garbage disposal electric vehicles (GDEVs) integrated with deep neural networking (DNN) and intelligent transportation system (ITS) in smart city management system (SCMS). *Wireless Personal Communications*, 123(2), 1733–1752. https://doi.org/10.1007/s11277-021-09210-8
5. Raja, R. A., Karthikeyan, T., & Kousik, N. V. (2020). Improved privacy preservation framework for cloud-based internet of things. In *Internet of things* (pp. 165–174). CRC Press.
6. Natarajan, Y., Srihari, K., Dhiman, G., Chandragandhi, S., Gheisari, M., Liu, Y., et al. (2022). An IoT and machine learning-based routing protocol for reconfigurable engineering application. *IET Communications, 16,* 464–475 (Open Access).
7. Rahman, M. A., Asyhari, A. T., Leong, L. S., Satrya, G. B., Tao, M. H., & Zolkipli, M. F. (2020). Scalable machine learning-based intrusion detection system for IoT-enabled smart cities. *Sustainable Cities and Society, 61*, 102324.
8. Cheng, J. C., Chen, W., Chen, K., & Wang, Q. (2020). Data-driven predictive maintenance planning framework for MEP components based on BIM and IoT using machine learning algorithms. *Automation in Construction, 112*, 103087.
9. Bhaskaran, P. E., Maheswari, C., Thangavel, S., Ponnibala, M., Kalavathidevi, T., & Sivakumar, N. S. (2021). IoT based monitoring and control of fluid transportation using machine learning. *Computers & Electrical Engineering, 89*, 106899.
10. Arachchige, P. C. M., Bertok, P., Khalil, I., Liu, D., Camtepe, S., & Atiquzzaman, M. (2020). A trustworthy privacy preserving framework for machine learning in industrial iot systems. *IEEE Transactions on Industrial Informatics, 16*(9), 6092–6102.
11. Liu, Y., Pang, Z., Karlsson, M., & Gong, S. (2020). Anomaly detection based on machine learning in IoT-based vertical plant wall for indoor climate control. *Building and Environment, 183*, 107212.

12. Shafiq, M., Tian, Z., Sun, Y., Du, X., & Guizani, M. (2020). Selection of effective machine learning algorithm and bot-IoT attacks traffic identification for internet of things in smart city. *Future Generation Computer Systems, 107*, 433–442.
13. Churcher, A., Ullah, R., Ahmad, J., Masood, F., Gogate, M., Alqahtani, F., et al. (2021). An experimental analysis of attack classification using machine learning in iot networks. *Sensors, 21*(2), 446.
14. Majumdar, S., Subhani, M. M., Roullier, B., Anjum, A., & Zhu, R. (2021). Congestion prediction for smart sustainable cities using IoT and machine learning approaches. *Sustainable Cities and Society, 64*, 102500.
15. Ayvaz, S., & Alpay, K. (2021). Predictive maintenance system for production lines in manufacturing: A machine learning approach using IoT data in real-time. *Expert Systems with Applications, 173*, 114598.
16. Hussain, F., Hussain, R., Hassan, S. A., & Hossain, E. (2020). Machine learning in IoT security: Current solutions and future challenges. *IEEE Communications Surveys & Tutorials, 22*(3), 1686–1721.
17. Priscila, S. S., & Hemalatha, M. (2017). Diagnosis of heart disease with particle bee-neural network. Special section: Computational life sciences and smarter technological advancement. *Biomedical Research*, 1–7.
18. Priscila, S. S., & Hemalatha, M. (2018). Heart disease prediction using integer-coded genetic algorithm (ICGA) based particle clonal neural network (ICGA-PCNN). *Bonfring International Journal of Industrial Engineering and Management Science, 8*(2), 15TO19.
19. Pacheco, J., Benitez, V. H., Felix-Herran, L. C., & Satam, P. (2020). Artificial neural networks-based intrusion detection system for internet of things fog nodes. *IEEE Access, 8*, 73907–73918.
20. Shukla, R. M., & Sengupta, S. (2020). Scalable and robust outlier detector using hierarchical clustering and long short-term memory (lstm) neural network for the internet of things. *Internet of Things, 9*, 100167.
21. An, Y., Yu, F. R., Li, J., Chen, J., & Leung, V. C. (2020). Edge intelligence (EI)-enabled HTTP anomaly detection framework for the internet of things (IoT). *IEEE Internet of Things Journal, 8*(5), 3554–3566.
22. Smys, S., Basar, A., & Wang, H. (2020). Hybrid intrusion detection system for internet of things (IoT). *Journal of ISMAC, 2*(04), 190–199.
23. Derhab, A., Aldweesh, A., Emam, A. Z., & Khan, F. A. (2020). Intrusion detection system for internet of things based on temporal convolution neural network and efficient feature engineering. *Wireless Communications and Mobile Computing, 2020*, Article ID 6689134, 16 p. https://doi.org/10.1155/2020/6689134.
24. Jalali, N., Sahu, K. S., Oetomo, A., & Morita, P. P. (2020). Understanding user behavior through the use of unsupervised anomaly detection: Proof of concept using internet of things smart home thermostat data for improving public health surveillance. *JMIR mHealth and uHealth, 8*(11), e21209.
25. Ramadan, R. A., & Yadav, K. (2020). A novel hybrid intrusion detection system (IDS) for the detection of internet of things (IoT) network attacks. *Annals of Emerging Technologies in Computing (AETiC), 4*(5), 61–74.
26. Chang, T. Y., & Hsieh, C. J. (2018). Detection and analysis of distributed denial-of-service in internet of things-employing artificial neural network and apache spark platform. *Sensors and Materials, 30*(4), 2.
27. Luo, C., Tan, Z., Min, G., Gan, J., Shi, W., & Tian, Z. (2020). A novel web attack detection system for internet of things via ensemble classification. *IEEE Transactions on Industrial Informatics, 17*(8), 5810–5818.

Chapter 30
Evaluation of Antiulcer Potentiality of D-Alpha-Tocopheryl Succinate by Inhibition of Oxidative Stress and Proinflammatory Cytokines

Vikram Nimbalkar, Niraj Vyawahare, Sachin Shinde, and Ganesh Pawar

30.1 Introduction

Gastrointestinal and duodenal ulcers are both a part of the highly common gastric illness known as peptic ulcer (PU) [1–2]. It has just been discovered that PU develops as soon as the physiological equilibrium among harmful and protective components in the gastrointestinal system is upset [3–4]. Among the damaging components include reactive species and peroxides, poor digestion and pepsin production, as well as exogenous substances like ethanol or NSAIDs [5]. Nitric oxide (NO), prostaglandins, acidosis, superoxide dismutase, gastric mucus, and other stomach defence mechanisms also aid in protecting against harmful substances [6]. It has been determined that colonization of the stomach epithelial surface by *Helicobacter pylori* through a predisposing element for the emergence of PU illness, peptic hypertrophy, and rectal cancer is and aerotolerant growing capability and the generation of numerous bacterial pathogens [7].

V. Nimbalkar (✉)
Department of Pharmacology, Dr VVPF's College of Pharmacy, Ahmednagar, Maharashtra, India

N. Vyawahare
Department of Pharmacology, Dr D. Y. Patil College of Pharmacy, Pune, Maharashtra, India

S. Shinde
Department of Pharmacology, Shri R. D. Bhakt College of Pharmacy, Jalna, Maharashtra, India

G. Pawar
Department of Pharmacology, Manohar Naik Institute of Pharmacy, Umarkhed, Maharashtra, India

F. J. Joseph et al. (eds.), *Computational Intelligence for Clinical Diagnosis*,
EAI/Springer Innovations in Communication and Computing,
https://doi.org/10.1007/978-3-031-23683-9_30

Gastric pump antagonists, H2 receptor antagonists, and antibiotics for infection with *H. pylori* are examples of chemical medications used to treat PU [8]. These medications cannot prevent ulcers from recurring, have adverse side effects, and act negatively with a large variety of other substances [9]. Numerous studies on natural supplements were carried out to look into various medications and revolutionary phytochemical brokers for the control of ailments, in line with the Health Institution's focus on the development of traditional indigenous remedies and ethnomedicines [10]. Therefore, this article's objective was to evaluate D-alpha-positive tocopheryl's effects on peptic ulcers. Vitamin E comes in the form of D-alpha tocopheryl. It has been identified for reproduction since 1992 [11]. It has further antioxidants, antiparasitic, and therapeutic properties, according to research [12]. The human body uses D-alpha-tocopheryl succinate to fulfil current nutritional requirements [13]. It is a gastroprotective agent that is naturally occurring. A chromane ring with a side chain, which contributes a hydrogen bond to eliminate an amphipathic chain, as well as oxidants, which facilitates penetration of the biomembrane, make up its structural components [14–16]. It is diffusible, present in several tissues, and metabolized by the body in a wide range of methods. D-alpha-tocopheryl has numerous roles in cellular, molecular, and biochemical processes. It also has a significant impact on lipid homeostasis and total lipoprotein levels [17]. A natural source antioxidant is called alpha tocopheryl succinate. Antioxidants, such as D-alpha-tocopheryl succinate, may be able to shield bodily cells from the harmful effects of free radicals [18]. One of the most popular causes for PU is the development of oxidative stress into the stomach mucosal injury [19–20]. In vitro tests have demonstrated the potency and effectiveness of tocopherol as a free radical scavenger [21].

For the assessment of oxidative stress, glutathione, superoxide dismutase, and catalase are habitually measured as antioxidant enzymes [22]. According to several shreds and pieces of evidence, in vivo studies have suggested that antioxidant enzyme activity in the examination of ulcerogenic chemical substances was greatly reduced and prevented after the administration of tocopherol [23]. Tocopherol has the capability to preserve the antioxidant enzyme itself by scavenging free radicals [24]. Myeloperoxidase, an enzyme, is another source of oxyradicals [25]. Previously reported, the elevation in the myeloperoxidase activity in aspirin, indomethacin, and *H. pylori* induced gastric lesion models [25]. This enzyme activity is reduced after α-tocopherol administration, which further results in a reduction in gastric lesions as well as leukocyte formation [26]. Also, α-tocopherol inhibits neutrophil absorption to lessen the extent of gastrointestinal lesions [27]. According to the literature, D-alpha-tocopheryl succinate shows positive response towards gastroprotective activity. There is a need for more prospective randomized study to be done. In vitro study using cell lines is one of the finest methods to reach the accuracy of results. So, to find D-alpha-tocopheryl succinate useful in gastroprotective studies, in vitro studies using cell line is the most reliable method.

30.2 Resources and Techniques

30.2.1 Chemicals and Tissue Growth

Cells from digestive acids adenocarcinomas were cultured and medium containing 10% FBS, 1.5 ml L-glutamine, and 1% antibiotics (100 U/ml penicillin, 10 mg/ml streptomycin) is described.

The cell viability was cultivated with a dry incubator in the condition of 5% CO_2 at 37 °C → trypsinized cells. According to the requirement, these cells are required. All chemicals as well as cell medium, insecticides, L-glutamine, and trypsin are examples of chemicals (acquired from Gibco), MTT, −alpha-tocopheryl succinate, and indomethacin (procured from Matrix Fine Science Pvt. Ltd).

30.2.2 Test for Treated Cells

For the short-term cytotoxic consequence of d-alpha-tocopheryl succinate in AGS cells, a colourimetric-based MTT sample was carried out.

Following the stimulation of 0.25% trypsin in PBS, the cells were dislodged → suspended growth medium → Approx. 8000–1000 cells seeded into 96 well plates grown 60–70% confluency → cell treated increasing concentration gradients (50, 100, 250, 500, 1000, 1500, 2000 μg/ml) of d-alpha-tocopheryl succinate for 24 hours → remove media →20 μl MTT reagent (5 mg/ml) added → incubate at 37 ° C for 2 hours → purple formazin crystals → in isopropanol, decomposed. A plate reader and a microscope were used to assess the colour intensity (Mithras LB 940, Berthold, Germany).

The % feasibility was determined as follows:

$$\%\text{Viability} = (\text{Measure good absorbency}/\text{Transmittance of untreated control}) \times 100$$

30.2.3 Evaluation of D-α-Tocopheryl Succinate's Anti-Oxidant Properties in Induced Inflammation Cytotoxicity in AGS Cells

Assessment of barrier activity of d-α-tocopheryl succinate in indomethacin-induced damage in AGS cell evaluated via several modifications in MTT assay.

AGS cells drilled in 96-diving properly → for 24 hours → improved with 50, 100, and 250 μg/ml concentrations of d-alpha-tocopheryl succinate → After

24 hours → medium replaced with the fresh medium of indomethacin → for 3 hours → using the procedure outlined above, cell viability was assessed.

30.2.4 Prostaglandins in the Stomach Mucosa Are Measured E2

For the evaluation of the concentration of PGE2, AGS cells seeded in 96-well plates → for 24 hours → cells were handled 50, 100, and 250 μg/ml concentrations of d-alpha-tocopheryl succinate → 24 hours → 800 μg/ml indomethacin → 3 hours for hatching → PGE2 concentrations in the solution were assessed using an ELISA kit (protein immunosorbent assay) (Cayman, MI, USA).

30.2.5 Gastric Oxidative Stress Assessment and Enzymatic Antioxidant Function

In accordance with the package recommendations, the stomach level of glutathione (GSH) was determined after the aforementioned treatments to d-alpha-tocopheryl succinate and indomethacin for the recommended treatment situations. Additionally, as a measure of the enzymatic antioxidant activity, the stomach content of superoxide dismutase (SOD) was determined.

30.2.6 Assessing of Gastric Apoptosis

The caspase-3 ELISA kit was applied to measure the gastric caspase-3 function (ab39401, Abcam, Cambridge, MA, USA). We utilized a spectrophotometer to evaluate the levels of absorbance at 405 nm using a microplate reader (Mithras LB 940, Berthold, Germany). Apoptotic actions were quantified as relative values using the formula below:

$$\begin{aligned}&\%\text{caspase} - 3\ \text{activity}\\&\quad = (\text{Measure good absorbency}/\text{Transmittance of untreated control}) \times 100\end{aligned}$$

30.2.7 Determination of Gastric Cellular Levels of Inflammatory Markers

Oblique ELISA was used in accordance with the procedure to identify pro-inflammatory cytokines (IL-1β, IL-6, TNF-α) as well as generally pro cytokines (IL-10). The antibody antigen (30 μg) combined in partnering buffer was placed onto 96 well plates and incubated (3679, Corning, NY, USA) and left overnight at 4 °C before being washed with 1X phosphate buffered saline tween (PBST) and blocked with super cocktail buffer. 1° antibodies were then added and kept at gradient for 2 hours. The wells were first washed twice with 1X PBST, then incubated with 2° horseradish peroxidase (HRP) coupled antibody for 45 min at gradient. After 10 minutes of dark incubation, the 2, 2′-azinobis (3-ethylbenzthiazoline-6-sulfonic acid) template solution was added, and a retinal reader was used to track the absorbance at 405 nm (Berthold, Germany).

30.2.8 Factoid Evaluation

Statistical software from the USA called Graph Pad Prism 5.0 was used for the descriptive statistics. Results were the average and ± standard deviation of 3 different explorations. One-way ANOVA was used to evaluate the data, and then the Bonferroni multiple comparison test. The variation in the central tendency between the matched controls was deemed to be statistically significant as '*' ($p < 0.05$), '**' ($p < 0.001$) and '***' ($p < 0.0001$).

30.3 Result

30.3.1 Effect of D-α-Tocopheryl Succinate Regarding the Indomethacin-Induced Apoptosis in AGS Cells

To AGS cells were exposed to various quantities of d-alpha-tocopheryl succinate for 24 hours in order to create a spectrum of non-cytotoxic quantities for the intervention. According to Fig. 30.1a, when contrasted to the untreated control, the concentration range of 50–500 μg/ml of D-α-tocopheryl succinate had no effect on cell survival. In addition, up to the treatment concentration of 2000 μg/ml of d-alpha-tocopheryl succinate, the IC50 value was not reached. So, in the following experiments, we have taken 50, 100, and 250 μg/ml occurrences of D-α-tocopheryl succinate. The protective effects of d-alpha-tocopheryl succinate were evaluated versus induced hepatotoxicity cell death. As given in Fig. 30.1b, indomethacin (800 μg/ml), the survival of the cells was drastically lowered by 49.86% especially in comparison to the cell lines that were not treated ($P < 0.0001$) (Fig. 30.1b).

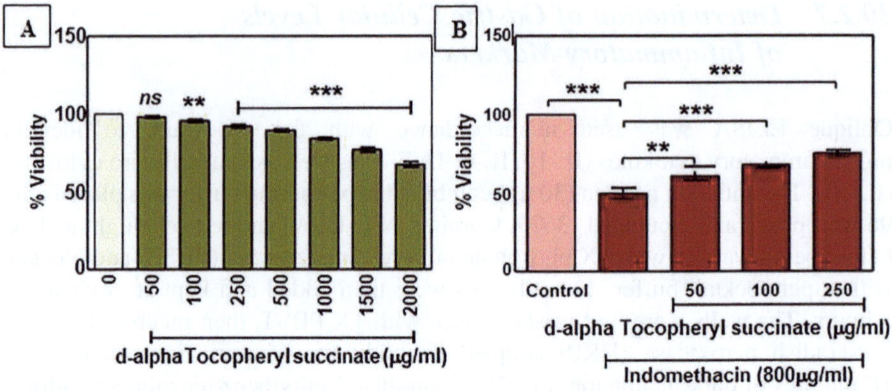

Fig. 30.1 Impact of d-alpha-tocopheryl succinate on the decline in cell viability brought on by indomethacin in AGS cells. (**a**) D-alpha-tocopheryl succinate was applied to AGS cells for 24 hours. (**b**) Cells underwent either a pre-treatment with d-alpha-tocopheryl succinate during 24 hours, followed by an indomethacin incubation (800 µg/ml) for 3 hours. The cell's vitality was assessed using the 3-(4,5- dimethylthiazol-2-yl)-2,5-diphenyl tetrazolium bromide method. Data expressed as mean ± SD ($n = 3$). '**' and '***' indicate statistical significance ($P < 0.001$ and $P < 0.0001$, respectively), where 'ns' indicates statistical non-significance ($P > 0.05$)

Pre-treatment with D-α-tocopheryl succinate at proportions of 50, 100, and 250 µg/ml a mean vitality of substantially reduced treated mice cell death to 60.83% ($P < 0.001$), 67.93% ($P < 0.0001$), and 75.27% ($P < 0.0001$), respectively.

30.3.2 *Effect of D-α-Tocopheryl Succinate on PGE2 Levels in AGS Cells*

As displayed in Fig. 30.2, d-alpha-tocopheryl succinate significantly increased the PGE2 levels. Approximately 3.27-fold decreased level of PGE2 ($P < 0.0001$) was found after the treatment of indomethacin (as compared to control). However, in the pre-treatment conditions (with increasing concentrations of d-alpha-tocopheryl succinate (50, 100, and 250 µg/ml)), approximately 1.1 fold ($P < 0.05$), 2.15 fold ($P < 0.0001$), and 2.63 fold ($P < 0.0001$) elevated level of PGE2 was noted, as opposed to the combination treatment with indomethacin (alone), correspondingly.

30.3.3 *Effects of D-α-Tocopheryl Succinate on Gastric Cellular Level Lipid Peroxides*

Treatment of indomethacin significantly decreased gastric GSH in contrast to the control group, levels (Fig. 30.3a). Treatment with 800 µg/ml indomethacin significantly down-regulated GSH level by approximately 3.55-fold ($P < 0.0001$).

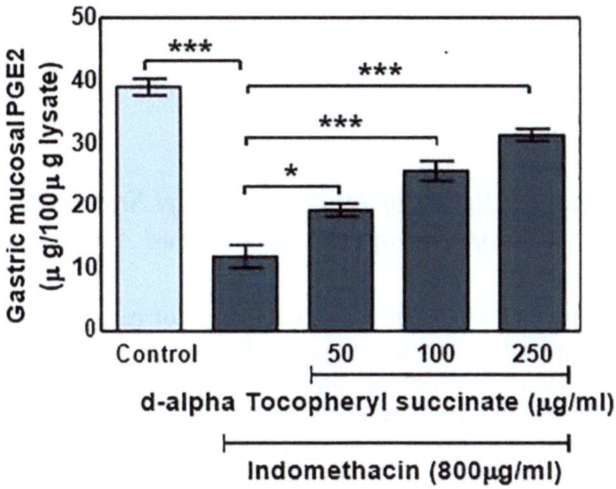

Fig. 30.2 D-α-tocopheryl succinate" influence on the slope of PGE2 in AGS cells. Before being exposed to indomethacin, cells were treated either with d-alpha-tocopheryl succinate for 24 hours followed by indomethacin (800 µg/ml) for 3 hours. Data expressed as mean ± SD ($n = 3$). '*' and '***' significance tests ($P < 0.05$ and $P < 0.0001$, respectively)

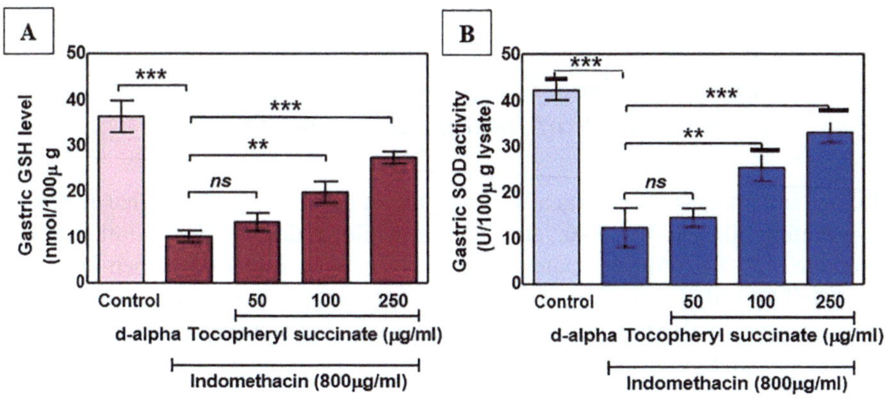

Fig. 30.3 D-α-tocopheryl succinate's influence on the slope of gastric cellular levels of oxidative stress marker, glutathione (GSH) (**a**) and superoxide dismutase activity (SOD) (**b**) in stomach ulcers brought on by indomethacin. The evidence reported as mean ± SD ($n = 3$). '**' and '***' indicate statistical significance ($P < 0.001$ and $P < 0.0001$, approximately), where 'ns' indicates statistical non-significance

However, pre-treatment with d-alpha-tocopheryl succinate produced elevated levels of gastric levels of GSH, along with its increasing treatment concentrations. At 250 µg/ml concentration, D-α-tocopheryl succinate uplifted the GSH level by 2.68-fold (approximately) ($P < 0.0001$), especially in comparison to the group that received indomethacin (Fig. 30.3a). Similarly, cure with indomethacin decreased the gastric SOD activity by approximately 3.42-fold ($P < 0.0001$) as compared to untreated control. Here also, with the increasing pre-treatment concentrations of d-alpha-tocopheryl succinate, elevated SOD levels were documented even after indomethacin treatment. At the treatment concentration of 250 μg/ml, it elevated the SOD level by 2.68-fold ($P < 0.0001$) as compared to the indomethacin treatment group (Fig. 30.3b).

30.3.4 Effect of D-α-Tocopheryl Succinate on Indomethacin-Induced Apoptosis in AGS Cells

In the indomethacin group, expression of caspase-3 was significantly increased as compared to the normal control group. Approximately 4.43-fold ($P < 0.0001$) elevated expression of caspase-3 was measured in the indomethacin-treated group. On the other hand, d-alpha-tocopheryl succinate decreased caspase-3 activity more than that observed in the indomethacin group. Nearly 1.77-fold reduced level of caspase-3 activity was measured in the 250 μg/ml pre-treatment concentration of d-alpha-tocopheryl succinate (Fig. 30.4).

30.3.5 Role of D-Alpha-Tocopheryl Succinate on Gastric Cellular Levels of Inflammatory Cytokines

Taking indomethacin dramatically raised the amount of cytokines that really are aggravating like IL-1β, IL-6, and TNF-α while it decreased anti-inflammatory cytokine, IL-10. Approximately 4.19, 4.7, and 3.15-fold down-regulation ($P < 0.0001$) of IL-1β, IL-6, and TNF-α were measured in indomethacin-treated lysates, respectively (Fig. 30.5a–c). However, with the increasing concentrations of d-alpha-tocopheryl succinate, the elevated expressions of these pro-inflammatory

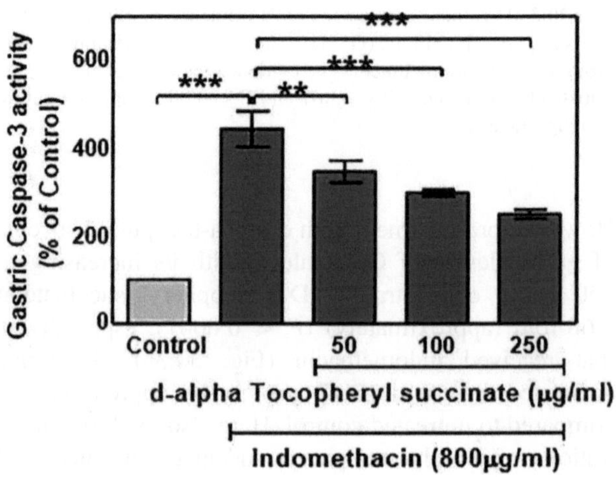

Fig. 30.4 D-alpha-tocopheryl succinate's influence on the level of the gastric cellular level of the apoptotic marker, caspase-3, in stomach ulcers brought on by indomethacin. The evidence reported as mean ± SD ($n = 3$). '**' and '***' indicate statistical significance ($P < 0.001$ and $P < 0.0001$, approximately)

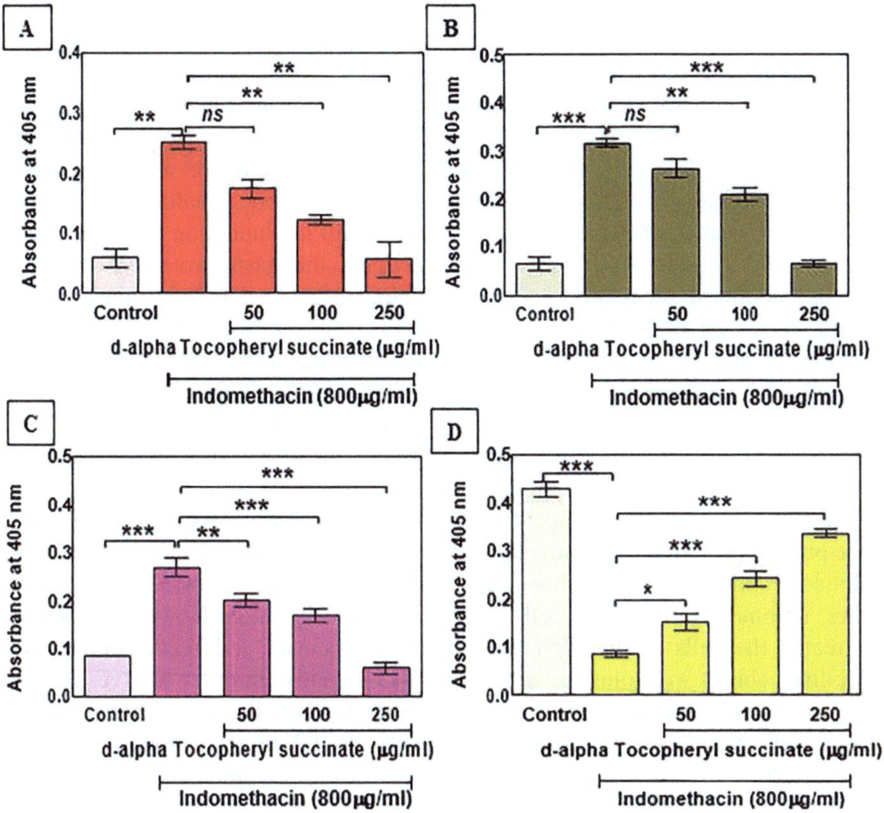

Fig. 30.5 D-alpha-tocopheryl succinate's influence on gastric cellular level cytokines that really are aggravating – IL-1β (**a**), IL-6 (**b**), and TNF-α (**c**) and anti-inflammatory cytokine- IL-10 (**d**) in indomethacin-induced gastric ulcer. The evidence reported as mean ± SD ($n = 3$). '*', '**', and '***' indicate statistical significance ($P < 0.05$, $P < 0.001$, and $P < 0.0001$, approximately), where 'ns' indicates statistical non-significance

cytokines were found to be significantly affected. At 250 μg/ml pre-treatment concentration of d-alpha-tocopheryl succinate, approximately 4.49 ($P < 0.001$), 4.8 ($P < 0.0001$), and 4.6 ($P < 0.0001$) fold decrease in expressions of IL-1β, IL-6, and TNF-α, respectively, were noted (Fig. 30.5a–c).

Further, when we checked for the activation of a cytokine that fights inflammation IL-10 in the above-mentioned treatment condition, it was found that indomethacin treatment decreased the expression of IL-10 by nearly 4.98-fold ($P < 0.0001$), moreover, with the increasing pre-treatment concentrations of d-alpha-tocopheryl succinate, nearly 3.89-fold ($P < 0.0001$) higher expression of IL-10 was measured against just the indomethacin-treated cohort (Fig. 30.5d).

30.4 Discussion

Gastric ulcer, the most common chronic disease of the gastrointestinal tract, is caused mainly due the damage of gastric mucosal by several factors like infection of *H. pylori*, NSAIDs drugs, smoking, alcohol consumption, stress, nutritional deficiencies, etc. [28, 29]. NSAIDs such as indomethacin are widely favoured for its inflammatory-blocking, analgesic, and antipyretic qualities. Moreover, frequent governance of these NSAIDs is linked with the induction of peptic ulcers [30–32]. Our present study seeks to investigate the gastroprotective effect of d-alpha-tocopheryl succinate against indomethacin-induced gastric injury. In the current study, gastrointestinal toxicity is induced by indomethacin via numerous mechanisms like cell inhibition of PGE2 synthesis that results in the regeneration of mucosal cells, antioxidant enzyme inhibition and gastric cell apoptosis. In addition, indomethacin enhances the levels of pro-inflammatory cytokines and has an adverse effect on anti-inflammatory cytokine. Collectively, the treatment with indomethacin in AGS cells showed a perfect model for gastric ulcer [33] (Fig. 30.6).

The IC50 value for the therapeutic concentration of d-alpha-tocopheryl succinate in the present investigation is not attained in the AGS cell line. The data suggest that d-alpha-tocopheryl succinate shows less toxicity in AGS cell lines, as we discussed earlier, indomethacin-induced cell death in the AGS cell line. However, when we pre-treated the cells with d-alpha a-tocopheryl succinate, indomethacin-mediated cell killing ability was found to be affected significantly. In order to investigate d-alpha-tocopheryl succinate mediated gastroprotective activity, we further wanted to check some parameters. According to reports, PGE2 protects both people and animals' stomach mucosa from destruction done by indomethacin [34]. In our

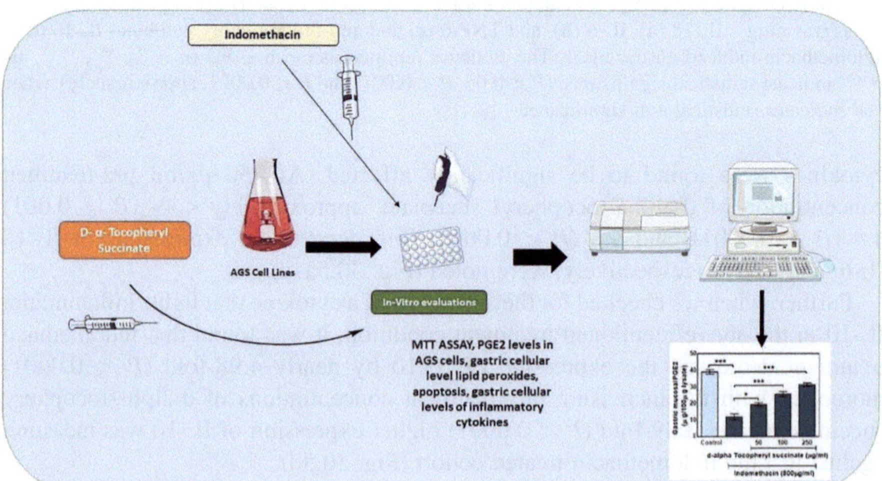

Fig. 30.6 Graphical abstract

current study, enhanced gastric mucosal PGE2 level upon pre-treated AGS cells with d-alpha-tocopheryl succinate appeared to be a protective activity of d-alpha-tocopheryl succinate against gastric ulcer. Further, elevated gastric GSH levels and gastric SOD levels in d-alpha-tocopheryl succinate pre-treated groups supported its gastroprotective efficacy. In order to validate the above observation, we again checked gastric caspase-3 activity. Caspase-3 is a crucial mediator of apoptosis (type I programmed cell death), and pre-treated AGS cells with d-alpha-tocopheryl succinate showed less caspase-3 activity than what we observed in only the indomethacin-treated group, which confirms that d-alpha-tocopheryl succinate is a potent gastroprotective agent in indomethacin-mediated gastric ulcer.

30.5 Conclusion

Literature also suggested that potent gastroprotective agents exhibit a great effect on inflammatory cytokines [35]. In our current study, the incubation of AGS cells with d-alpha-tocopheryl succinate showed indomethacin-mediated lower levels of IL-1β, IL-6, and TNF-α than the indomethacin (alone) treated group. On the other hand, pre-treating AGS cells with d-alpha-tocopheryl succinate showed elevated levels of IL-10 even after indomethacin treatment. Collectively, these data suggested that d-alpha-tocopheryl succinate played an important role in elevating anti-inflammatory cytokines and down-regulating pro-inflammatory cytokines, which further supported its gastroprotective activity.

References

1. Alfahad, M., Jasim, M. H., Qazzaz, M. E., Alassaf, F. A., & Abed, M. N. (2021). Proton pump inhibitors and peptic ulcer management: Antioxidant mechanisms. *Journal of Drug Delivery and Therapeutics, 11*(4-S), 242–246.
2. Salari, N., Darvishi, N., Shohaimi, S., Bartina, Y., Ahmadipanah, M., Salari, H. R., & Mohammadi, M. (2021). The global prevalence of peptic ulcer in the world: A systematic review and meta-analysis. *Indian Journal of Surgery, 9337*, 1–9.
3. Wallace, J. L. (2008). Prostaglandins, NSAIDs, and gastric mucosal protection: Why doesn't the stomach digest itself? *Physiological Reviews, 88*(4), 1547–1565.
4. Bhattacharyya, A., Chattopadhyay, R., Mitra, S., & Crowe, S. E. (2014). Oxidative stress: An essential factor in the pathogenesis of gastrointestinal mucosal diseases. *Physiological Reviews, 94*(2), 329–354.
5. Périco, L. L., Emílio-Silva, M. T., Ohara, R., Rodrigues, V. P., Bueno, G., Barbosa-Filho, J. M., Rocha, L. R. M. D., Batista, L. M., & Hiruma-Lima, C. A. (2020). Systematic analysis of monoterpenes: Advances and challenges in the treatment of peptic ulcer diseases. *Biomolecules, 10*(2), 265.
6. Kwiecien, S., Jasnos, K., Magierowski, M., Sliwowski, Z., Pajdo, R., Brzozowski, B., Mach, T., Wojcik, D., & Brzozowski, T. (2014). Lipid peroxidation, reactive oxygen species and antioxidative factors in the pathogenesis of gastric mucosal lesions and mechanism of

protection against oxidative stress-induced gastric injury. *Journal of Physiology and Pharmacology, 65*(5), 613–622.

7. Molina-Castro, S. (2017). *Study of the hippo/YAP1 signaling pathway in gastric carcinogenesis induced by helicobacter pylori.* Université de Bordeaux.
8. Kapitonova, M., Gupalo, S., Alyautdin, R., Ibrahim, I. A. A., Salim, N., Ahmad, A., Talip, S. B., Nwe, T. M., & Morokhina, S. (2021). Gastroprotective effect of Berberis vulgaris on ethanol-induced gastric mucosal injury: Histopathological evaluations. *Avicenna Journal of Phytomedicine, 12*, 30–41.
9. Mousavi, T., Nikfar, S., & Abdollahi, M. (2021). The pharmacotherapeutic management of duodenal and gastric ulcers. *Expert Opinion on Pharmacotherapy*, 1–27.
10. Khatib, C., Nattouf, A., & Hasan Agha, M. I. (2021). Traditional medicines and their common uses in central region of Syria: Hama and Homs–an ethnomedicinal survey. *Pharmaceutical Biology, 59*(1), 778–788.
11. Prasad, K. N., Kumar, B., Yan, X.-D., Hanson, A. J., & Cole, W. C. (2003). α-tocopheryl succinate, the most effective form of vitamin E for adjuvant cancer treatment: A review. *Journal of the American College of Nutrition, 22*(2), 108–117.
12. Yang, C., Wu, T., Qi, Y., & Zhang, Z. (2018). Recent advances in the application of vitamin E TPGS for drug delivery. *Theranostics, 8*(2), 464.
13. Pitel, M. O., McKenzie, E. C., Johns, J. L., & Stuart, R. L. (2020). Influence of specific management practices on blood selenium, vitamin E, and beta-carotene concentrations in horses and risk of nutritional deficiency. *Journal of Veterinary Internal Medicine, 34*(5), 2132–2141.
14. Sailo, B. L., Banik, K., Padmavathi, G., Javadi, M., Bordoloi, D., & Kunnumakkara, A. B. (2018). Tocotrienols: The promising analogues of vitamin E for cancer therapeutics. *Pharmacological Research, 130*, 259–272.
15. Kiyose, C. (2021). Absorption, transportation, and distribution of vitamin E homologs. *Free Radical Biology and Medicine, 177*, 226–237.
16. Prakash, D., & Gupta, K. (2009). The antioxidant phytochemicals of nutraceutical importance. *The Open Nutraceuticals Journal, 2*(1), 20–35.
17. Rigotti, A. (2007). Absorption, transport, and tissue delivery of vitamin E. *Molecular Aspects of Medicine, 28*(5–6), 423–436.
18. Rowland, D. (2020). Antioxidant therapy to protect against free radical damage implicated in coronary heart disease and cancer. *OSP Journal of Health Care and Medicine, 2*(2), 1–3.
19. Mahmoud, Y. I., & Abd El-Ghffar, E. A. (2019). Spirulina ameliorates aspirin-induced gastric ulcer in albino mice by alleviating oxidative stress and inflammation. *Biomedicine & Pharmacotherapy, 109*, 314–321.
20. Arab, H. H., Salama, S. A., Eid, A. H., Kabel, A. M., & Shahin, N. N. (2019). Targeting MAPKs, NF-κB, and PI3K/AKT pathways by methyl palmitate ameliorates ethanol-induced gastric mucosal injury in rats. *Journal of Cellular Physiology, 234*(12), 22424–22438.
21. Niki, E. (2014). Role of vitamin E as a lipid-soluble peroxyl radical scavenger: In vitro and in vivo evidence. *Free Radical Biology and Medicine, 66*, 3–12.
22. Daud, D. M. A., Ahmedy, F., Baharuddin, D. M. P., Kamalden, T. F. T., & Ngah, W. Z. W. (2021). The effect of exercise intensity and duration on oxidative stress and antioxidant enzymes activity among sedentary healthy adults: A repeated measures study.
23. Huligol, S. V., & Narendar, K. (2012). Evaluation of gastroprotective role of alpha-tocopherol in indomethacin induced peptic ulcer in albino rats. *International Journal of Pharmacology and Clinical Sciences, 1*(2), 39–44.
24. Saral, Y., Uyar, B., Ayar, A., Naziroglu, M., & Yilmaz, S. (2002). Protective effect of topical alpha-tocopherol acetate on UVB irradiation in Guinea pigs: Importance of free radicals. *Physiological Research, 51*(3), 285–290.
25. Kettle, A., & Winterbourn, C. (1997). Myeloperoxidase: A key regulator of neutrophil oxidant production. *Redox Report, 3*(1), 3–15.
26. Odabasoglu, F., Halici, Z., Cakir, A., Halici, M., Aygun, H., Suleyman, H., Cadirci, E., & Atalay, F. (2008). Beneficial effects of vegetable oils (corn, olive and sunflower oils) and

α-tocopherol on anti-inflammatory and gastrointestinal profiles of indomethacin in rats. *European Journal of Pharmacology, 591*(1–3), 300–306.
27. Sugimoto, N., Yoshida, N., Yoshikawa, T., Nakamuara, Y., Ichikawa, H., Naito, Y., & Kondo, M. (2000). Effect of vitamin E on aspirin-induced gastric mucosal injury in rats. *Digestive Diseases and Sciences, 45*(3), 599–605.
28. Dvornyk, V., Ponomarenko, I., Minyaylo, O., Reshetnikov, E., & Churnosov, M. (2021). Association of the functionally significant polymorphisms of the MMP9 gene with H. pylori-positive gastric ulcer in the Caucasian population of Central Russia. *PLoS One, 16*(9), e0257060.
29. Yang, R., Zhao, X., Wu, W., & Shi, J. (2021). Potential of probiotics for use as functional foods in patients with non-infectious gastric ulcer. *Trends in Food Science & Technology, 111*, 463–474.
30. AbdelAziz, E. Y., Tadros, M. G., & Menze, E. T. (2021). The effect of metformin on indomethacin-induced gastric ulcer: Involvement of nitric oxide/rho kinase pathway. *European Journal of Pharmacology, 892*, 173812.
31. Bourgeois, S., Carr, D. F., Musumba, C. O., Penrose, A., Esume, C., Morris, A. P., Jorgensen, A. L., Zhang, J. E., Pritchard, D. M., & Deloukas, P. (2021). Genome-wide association between EYA1 and aspirin-induced peptic ulceration. *eBioMedicine, 74*, 103728.
32. Onadeko, A., & Akinola, O. (2021). Ameliorative effect of Ethanolic extract of Laportea aestuans (L.) chew on gastric oxidative damage in aspirin-induced gastric ulcer in male rats. *World News of Natural Sciences, 39*, 86–94.
33. Chen, Y.-C., Chia, Y.-C., & Huang, B.-M. (2021). Phytochemicals from Polyalthia species: Potential and implication on antioxidant, anti-inflammatory, anti-cancer, and chemoprevention activities. *Molecules, 26*(17), 5369.
34. Elsadek, M. F., Almoajel, A., & Farahat, M. F. (2021). Ameliorative effects of ribes rubrum oil against gastric ulcers caused by indomethacin in experimental models. *Saudi Journal of Biological Sciences*, *29*(1), 30–34.
35. Zhang, Y., Sun, L., Lai, X., Peng, X., Wen, S., Zhang, Z., Xie, Y., Li, Q., Chen, R., & Zheng, X. (2021). Gastroprotective effects of extract of Jasminum grandiflorum L. flower in HCl/EtOH-induced gastric mucosal ulceration mice. *Biomedicine & Pharmacotherapy, 144*, 112268.

Chapter 31
An Intelligent Air Quality During COVID-19 Prediction and Monitoring System Using Temporal CNN-LSTM

S. Anu Priya and V. Khanaa

31.1 Introduction

Recently, air pollution has been increasing vigorously due to the huge volume of automobile usage, and it is becoming a very big issue in the form of various diseases, including asthma, liver problems, and breathing problems. These issues are affecting people seriously with various deadly diseases, but they are not changing the climate [1]. Around 4.2 million people die every year in the world due to air pollution. In addition, it is a very big issue and a life threat for the majority of people due to the presence of heavy air pollution. The developing countries are affected more severely than the developed countries due to the various industries. Because of this, the government has concentrated on this issue and asked research institutes to do more research work and come up with the best solutions for reducing air pollution. On the other hand, the government has taken steps to reduce air pollution by reducing the usage of individual vehicles, instructing people to use public transport, and also trying to give more awareness by updating the pollution level. Even though a good quality air quality prediction and monitoring system is necessary to satisfy the current requirements, many air quality prediction systems have been developed by using machine learning (ML) and deep learning (DL) algorithms by various researchers in the past. These are all the systems that are not fulfilling the current requirements.

S. A. Priya (✉)
Department of Computer Science and Engineering, Bharath Institute of Higher Education and Research, Chennai, Tamil Nadu, India
e-mail: anupriya.mca@bharathuniv.ac.in

V. Khanaa
Department of Information Technology, Bharath Institute of Higher Education and Research, Chennai, Tamil Nadu, India

F. J. J. Joseph et al. (eds.), *Computational Intelligence for Clinical Diagnosis*,
EAI/Springer Innovations in Communication and Computing,
https://doi.org/10.1007/978-3-031-23683-9_31

In the past two decades, ML algorithms have been applied to predict the air quality during COVID-19 frequently. The available prediction systems are developed and tested for the specific cities in the country. For example, the Beijing city in China is considered by many researchers and predicts its air quality by analysing the Beijing air pollution datasets. In addition, the air quality during COVID-19 in prediction systems is classified as data-driven systems and simulation systems, where both apply ML algorithms. In the simulation-based prediction systems, physical and chemical models were used for generating the meteorological details to predict air pollution with the help of transport, emissions, and chemicals [2, 3]. However, the systems are not able to predict the air quality exactly due to the presence of parameter restrictions [4]. Moreover, the time factor is also considered to make a decision on air quality during COVID-19 in records. The ML algorithms are used to predict the future health of the public by applying high-dimensional data with time constraints. Recently, researchers have been applying the DL technique, which is an enhanced version of ML and is also able to learn the input data in depth and identify enough patterns to predict the air quality during COVID-19.

The various DL algorithms, such as deep belief network (DBN), recurrent neural network (RNN), long short-term memory (LSTM), and convolutional neural network (CNN), are available. Of all these DL algorithms, the LSTM is widely applied and also identified as more suitable for handling temporal data and predicting air quality in a better manner. The RNN is also capable of handling temporal data effectively. Moreover, the LSTM is useful for addressing the drawbacks of the RNN and the gated recurrent unit (GRU), which is a simpler model than the standard LSTM. Even though the multi-layered ensemble DL techniques are achieving better results in prediction accuracy in various fields of data, based on this evidence, this work proposes a new ensemble DL technique that combines Bi-LSTM and CNN for predicting the air quality during COVID-19. The important contributions of this work are listed below:

- I propose an intelligent air quality during COVID-19 in prediction model to predict the air quality during COVID-19 in Beijing, China.
- Applies a basic data preprocessing technique and also fine-tunes the exact data.
- To apply a rule-based data grouping algorithm to group the relevant data according to the different seasonal data and group them as various seasonal groups of data.
- To apply the standard Bi-LSTM and the existing T-CNN to learn the seasonal data in depth and also predict the future air quality during COVID-19.
- Conducted the season-wise data analysis to know the air pollution level for the various seasons.

This paper is formulated with four more sections that contain the various things as follows: Section 31.2 explains the contributions, merits, and demerits of the various works that are available in the literature. Section 31.3 describes the workflow of the proposed model diagrammatically. Section 31.4 demonstrates the proposed model with the proposed data preprocessing methods and classification algorithm with necessary background, steps of the algorithms, and equations. The experimental and comparative result analyses are demonstrated in Sect. 31.5 with the reason for achieving significant results. Finally, this work is concluded by highlighting the achievement with possible future direction in Sect. 31.6.

31.2 Literature Survey

There are numerous air quality researchers who have used a wide variety of feature selection algorithms, machine learning, and deep learning methods to construct prediction systems for use during COVID-19. Among these is a new support vector machine (SVM)-based regression model for estimating COVID-19 air quality developed by Suárez et al. [5]. They have considered the Beijing city data as input and conducted many experiments, proving that they are better than other models. José et al. [6] developed a new sigma operator for assessing the air quality during COVID-19 in features by applying their historical data and also determined the negative impact on air quality according to the frequency and deviations [7]. They have introduced a fuzzy inference mechanism for performing the classification process that groups the features as good, regular, excellent, dangerous, and bad.

The work of Metia et al. [8] addressed the issues of enhancing the inverse air pollution emission and prediction in urban areas by applying the air pollution prediction system that includes the transport chemical model with extended Kalman filter. Finally, their system performed better in all the experiments than existing systems [9]. Zhenghua and Zhihui [10] applied a back propagation neural classifier to establish the prediction model to predict the air quality during COVID-19 in index [11]. Their model used the features to solve the problem and accurately predicted the data. Finally, they have achieved around 83% accuracy, which is better than other classifiers. Wang et al. [12] proposed a new air quality prediction method that performs the data preprocessing and classification to address the uncertainties that are involved in the process of future air quality. They have applied fuzzy logic and set theory to handle the uncertainty in the features of an input dataset. Their method outperforms the existing systems in terms of prediction accuracy. Wei and Jingyi [13] presented a new hybrid model that is developed by using principal component analysis and least square SVM that is optimised by Cuckoo Search. In their work, they have adopted the Principal component analysis (PCA) for extracting the necessary features and reducing the dimensionality. Next, they used Least squares support vector machine (LSSVM) to predict the air quality and fine-tuned the result.

Chang et al. [14] developed a new semantic extract transform load framework to predict the air quality during COVID-19 in data. They have achieved better prediction accuracy than other frameworks that are available in the literature. Junshan et al. [15] developed a new ensemble approach that incorporates the spatial and temporal features of LSTM to predict the air quality during COVID-19 effectively. Their approach uses three components, in which the first component uses a partitioning method using weather patterns. Next, they identified the spatial correlation for generating the spatial data. In addition, they have designed a temporal-based

LSTM to predict the air quality. Finally, they have evaluated their model by using Beijing data that has been collected from 35 monitoring stations and proved better than other models. Jianzhou et al. [15] proposed a new early alert method according to fuzzy logic and time series successfully, and it contains three modules such as analysis, assessment, and prediction modules. They have analysed the uncertainties, assessed the relevant features, and predicted the features that are useful for prediction and monitoring the air quality during COVID-19.

Using LSTM, Jiao et al. [16] developed a new air quality prediction model to predict the air quality data using LSTM. They have provided the background, features, development status, and problems of air quality monitoring. Finally, they predicted the air quality index using LSTM and also analysed the errors. Zhang et al. [4] created an improved air quality prediction method that uses the light gradient boosting method to predict PM2.5 air quality data from 35 monitoring stations in Beijing, China. In order to mine the features more thoroughly and hence enhance the dimension, a new window method has been implemented. In terms of accuracy of prediction, their experiments demonstrated that their method is superior than others. Time-varying inertia weights were proposed by Xue et al. [17] as a method that can be used in conjunction with Particle swarm optimization (PSO) and the gravity search algorithm. They have used their method for optimising the penalty parameter using their method and SVM for predicting the air quality with higher accuracy than the various combinations of gradient search, genetic algorithm, and PSO with SVM.

Qiang et al. [18] developed a new image-based model that uses a deep learning technique to predict the air quality. They have used the scene images as input that is preprocessed by extracting the important information and categorising the air quality level. Moreover, they have incorporated a new self-supervision module for performing the feature mapping process for reformulating the features. In addition, they also incorporated the high-quality outdoor air quality dataset for facilitating the training and evaluation processes and also compared their model with SVM and deep residual network and proved it to be better in terms of prediction accuracy. Ying et al. [2] developed a new air quality prediction model that works by considering the multiple features that are selected through ML algorithms. Their model considered the air quality data and meteorological data that were collected in Beijing, China, for 46 days in total. In their model, they have grouped the features according to the time. Finally, their models screened the features and provided input to the gradient boosting decision tree for performing effective prediction, which proved better than other classifiers. Jusong et al. [19] proposed a new hybrid model that combines feature selection, clustering, live decomposition, and deep neural networks for enhancing the prediction accuracy of air quality data. They have performed the time series of air pollutants that are decomposed first. Second, every subset of the data is developed by combining the decomposed components. Then, they applied a deep neural classifier called CNN with the incorporation of three dimensions and Bi-LSTM [20]. They have used Beijing, China, data for evaluating their model and found it to be better than other existing air quality prediction models. Apeksha and Durga [21] developed a new air quality prediction model by using LSTM with the consideration of spatial and temporal constraints, data preprocessing, feature engineering process, and segmentation. The superiority of their approach in terms of prediction accuracy has been demonstrated through a variety of studies.

Chi-Yeh et al. [22] developed a new ensemble learning approach for predicting air quality by using a gated recurrent unit aware deep learning architecture with different models for managing the different space and time-related data. They also proposed an ensemble learning technique called multiple linear regression aware GRU that works based on a multiple linear regression method that integrates with a deep neural network to predict the air quality level effectively and also proved it by achieving better results in all the experiments conducted in the work. Guojian et al. [23] developed a new learning framework that combines the LSTM, fusion deep neural network, Gaussian functionality, and stacked anti-auto encoder network. In their framework, they have incorporated feature extraction according to space and time in the processing layer. Then, they evaluate the weights using a Gaussian function and perform the prediction process using LSTM [24]. Finally, they have proved to be better than their models by achieving better prediction accuracy.

31.3 System Architecture

An overall architecture of the proposed air quality, the COVID-19 prediction model is shown in Fig. 31.1. It consists of eight important components, namely, user query, dataset, user interaction module, decision manager, data preprocessing module, air quality prediction module, knowledge base, and rule manager.

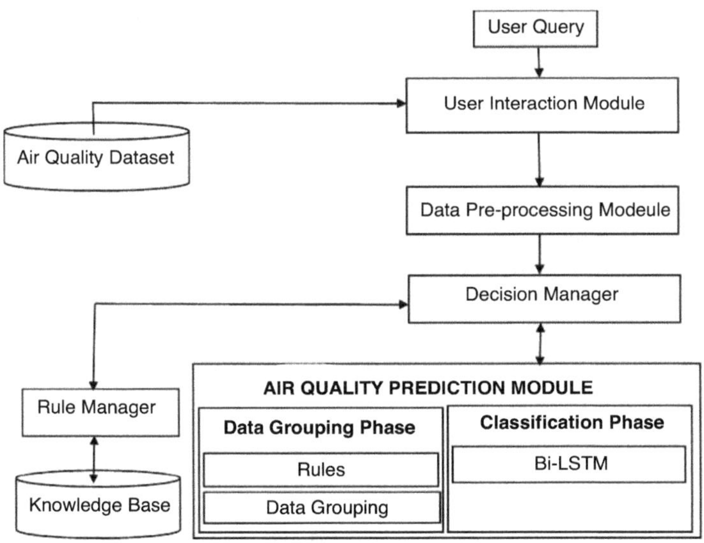

Fig. 31.1 Overall architecture

The necessary data is to be collected from the standard air quality dataset based on the received user query through the user interaction module. The data preprocessing module receives the collected data from the user interaction module and also performs the data preprocessing. The preprocessed data is collected by the decision manager based on the users' requests and it is forwarded to the air quality prediction module, which has two different phases, such as the data grouping phase and the classification phase.

Here, the data grouping phase is helpful for grouping the data seasonally. The grouping phase uses a newly proposed rule-based data grouping algorithm (RDGA) to group the seasonal data. The decision manager received the grouped data from the data grouping phase seasonally and forwarded it to the classification phase for performing classification by applying the standard Bi-LSTM and T-CNN. The rule manager applies the rules that are available in the knowledge base and forwards them to the decision manager for making the final decision. Finally, the decision manager applies the appropriate rules for grouping the data season wise and it also performs the effective classification.

31.4 Proposed Model

This work proposes a new air quality prediction system that incorporates the newly proposed rule-based data grouping method to group the data seasonally and the newly proposed ensemble DL method, which is the combination of Bi-LSTM and CNN with temporal features for predicting the future air pollution level. This section explains the season-wise data grouping process, T-CNN, Bi-LSTM, and the proposed ensemble deep classifier called T-CNN-Bi-LSTM. First, this section explains the data grouping process.

31.4.1 Data Grouping Process

This subsection explains the data grouping process in detail, with necessary steps. The proposed RDGA is used to group the data according to the different seasons such as monsoon, winter, and summer. The proposed RDGA applies the necessary rules for identifying the relevant records that are collected in the different seasons. The steps of the RDGA are as follows:

Input: Air Quality Dataset (ADS)
Output: Season-wise datasets (SAD)
Step 1: Start
Step 2: Read the record set (RS) from ADS
Step 3: Fix the date range between WD_Start and WD_End for winter season.
Step 4: Fix the date range between SD_Start and SD_End for summer season.

Step 5: Fix the date range between MD_Start and MD_End for monsoon season.
Step 6: Load the rules for summer season in to SR.
Step 7: Load the rules for winter season in to WR.
Step 8: Load the rules for monsoon season in to MR.
Step 9: IF SD_Start < RS (Date) < SD_End THEN
        SSD [] = RS // SSD – Summer Season Dataset
    Else
        Read the next record in the dataset.
Step 10: IF WD_Start < RS (Date) < WD_End THEN
        WSD [] = RS // WSD – Winter Season Dataset
    Else
        Read the next record in the dataset.
Step 11: IF MD_Start < RS (Date) < MD_End THEN
        MSD [] = RS // MSD – Monsoon Season Dataset
    Else
        Read the next record in the dataset.
Step 12: Return SSD [], WSD [], and MSD [].
Step 13: End.

The proposed RDGA is used to group the data based on the different seasons such as summer, winter, and monsoon. These are all the groups of data that are analysed by applying predefined methods that are available in the Python programming in this work. The data analysis results are presented in the result section. This data analysis is used to know the density of the data available in the air quality dataset based on the various seasons. Moreover, these different seasonal datasets are used to predict the air quality during COVID-19, the three different seasons in Beijing in the future.

31.4.2 T-CNN

This subsection demonstrates the T-CNN (Sandhiya et al. 2020) workflow with the necessary explanation of all the layers. This temporal CNN model considered the time for making decisions on the input records as "normal", "medium", "danger", and "bad" in the proposed T-CNN. The prediction accuracy depends on the rules that have been generated and applied as knowledge that is forwarded to the CNN for performing an effective training process. Figure 31.2 shows the functionality of the CNN model by applying an architecture that contains four important layers, namely, convolutional, pooling, fully connected, and soft-max layers. In general, CNN is widely used for recognising images through the identified patterns and also recognising speech through the patterns stored in the direction. Even though this T-CNN is used to categorise the numeric and alphabetic data, the standard of air quality datasets for COVID-19 in datasets are available online and used by the T-CNN to perform the prediction process effectively. Generally, the various dense layers were applied like 10 and 50 filters with a rectified linear unit (ReLU)

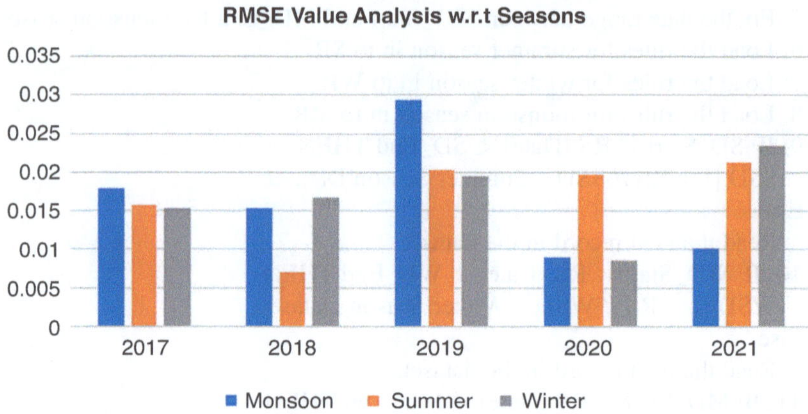

Fig. 31.2 RMSE value analysis w.r.t seasons

activation function. The model is trained and tested using training and testing datasets, respectively.

31.4.2.1 Convolutional Layer

The convolutional layer is applied with 64 and 128 filters to map the features, and the ReLU activation function is helpful for not changing the volume size in every layer. The fully connected layer receives the convolutional layer's output together with the processing unit, bias value, and ReLU function. If you need to determine if a patient is healthy or sick, the completely connected layer can help you with that. In this work, the convolutional function is performed using the formula given in Eq. (31.1):

$$H_j = f\left(h_{j-1} \otimes w_j + b_j\right) \tag{31.1}$$

where is a convolutional function and $f\ (y)$ indicates the ReLU function, *hj* represents the input features, *wj* means the kernel of convolutional layer, and *bj* represents the layer value. After applying the convolutional layer and the feature mapping process with the help of filters and *hj* value is transformed to a vector.

31.4.2.2 Pooling Layer

The pooling layer takes the convolutional layer's output as input for reducing the size of the feature maps by applying non-linear down-sampling such as maximum over non-overlapping subsets of the feature map. Moreover, it enhances the memory usage by reducing the input size. It discards the unwanted attributes for performance enhancement. In addition, the regularisation method like a dropout is included to avoid the overfitting process that improves the prediction accuracy.

31.4.2.3 Fully Connected Layer

The fully connected layer converts the input data matrix from two dimensions to a single dimension and it also passes the network dense layers to prepare it for performing the classification process. The fully connected layer is also considered a classification layer which incorporates an activation function. This layer performs the classification processes such as binary class classification and multiclass classification with the help of activation functions. This model uses a soft-max function with temporal features.

31.4.2.4 Soft-Max Layer

The soft-max layer of the proposed T-CNN plays a vital role, and it performs multiclass classification using temporal features. The soft-max function is applied in this layer to perform classification on input data based on the given condition. This soft-max layer is the last in the CNN. It is used to train data based on cross-entropy, which provides a non-linear variation of multinomial logistic regression. The entropy approach is used to map real number indices and consider index value. Multinomial logistic regression is useful for creating a statistical probability model using the soft-max function Eq. (31.2). It generalises logistic regression to multiclass situations as a classification tool. Soft-max solves multi-class problems:

$$\frac{\partial}{\partial q_k}\sigma(q,i)\ [t_1,t_2] > \ = \ \ldots \ = \sigma(q,i)(\delta_{ik} - \sigma(q,k))[t_1,t_2] \tag{31.2}$$

In the proposed disease prediction system, temporal features are used for prediction with the consideration of time constraints as t_1 and t_2. For the air quality record, the pollution level is taken according to the time constraint of the air quality records. In addition, the activation function is used for the time duration. Finally, the decision can be made on a specific record according to the activation function at a specific time.

31.4.3 *Bi-LSTM*

The RNN is widely applied for resolving the natural language processing – related tasks including translation and recognition that are capable of achieving better performance. Many researchers have identified the RNN contains the benefits of

LSTM. The reason is that the capable of RNN to refer the earlier data to the current tasks. They provided the feature *xt* at *t* time then, the RNN is changed at time by:

$$h_t = f(W_{hh}h_{t-1} + W_{xh}x_t + b_h) \tag{31.3}$$

$$y_t = W_{hy}h_t + b_y) \tag{31.4}$$

where *t* denotes the processing layer's status and output variable. Variables represent the processing layers' and input features' weight matrices. *bh* and *by* indicate processing layer and input feature bias vectors. *f* is a non-linear activation function that uses tanh and sigmoid.

The RNN suffers from the loss of gradient descent in BP and gradient descent approaches, making model convergence more difficult. LSTM helps resolve RNN's gradient vanishing over lengthy sequences. LSTM can only apply forward sequences, not reverse. Consider the mutual constraint between picture sequences and connect Bi-LSTM behind CNN. Bi-LSTM learns pre- and post-data sequences and develops backward and forward RNNs for every training sequence. Bi-x LSTM's *t* at *t* feature modified *t*:

$$S_t = f(U_{x_t} + W_{S_{t-1}}) \tag{31.5}$$

$$S_t' = f\left(U_{x_t}' + W'S_{t+1}\right) \tag{31.6}$$

$$A_t = f(W\,A_{t-1} + U_{x_t}) \tag{31.7}$$

$$A_t' = f\left(W'\,A_{t-1} + U_{x_t}'\right) \tag{31.8}$$

$$y_t = g\left(V\,A_2 + V_{A_2}'\right) \tag{31.9}$$

where *St* signifies forward memory at *t* time and represents backward memory at *t* time. A *t* specifies the backward processing layer at *t* time. Output is Y_t. Non-linear variables and activation functions are also indicated. Bi-LSTM compares with LSTM to estimate poses in picture frames. This model uses 1000 LSTM nodes in each direction and 2000 in Bi-LSTM. Bi-advantage LSTM's is lengthy sequence learning, and CNN's is extracting high-dimensional data features. Transfer CNN and Bi-LSTM characteristics for further learning.

31.4.4 Proposed T-CNN-Bi-LSTM

In this work, a hybrid T-CNN-Bi-LSTM architecture is proposed for forecasting the PM2.5 pollutant in the atmosphere. The features are extracted using three-layered CNN model with temporal, where each layer consists of a convolutional and max-pooling layer in turn. The extracted features are passed on to a Bi-LSTM module consisting of four Bi-LSTM layers stacked in residual fashion. Finally, a dense layer with one neuron is added at the end of the Bi-LSTM module for prediction. The steps of the proposed deep learning model are shown below:

Input: Input data
Output: Dataset with result
Step 1: Read the input record set.
Step 2: Perform the data preprocessing on the input record set.
Step 3: The useful features are extracted by using three-layered T-CNN.
Step 4: Perform the training for the record set that contains only the selected features.
Step 5: Predict the standard air quality dataset and send to the Bi-LSTM.
Step 6: Perform the training for the air quality dataset.
Step 7: Compare the performance of the model on PM2.5 dataset.
Step 8: Return the record set with result column.

In this work, the grouped data can be provided as input record set to the deep learning hybrid model that is the combination of CNN and Bi-LSTM. Here, it performs the convolution and max pooling operations in the respective layers and also performs the initial level filtering process and the Bi-LSTM takes final decision on input data. Finally, it categorises the level of pollution affected on that day record.

31.5 Result and Discussion

This section describes in detail the experimental setup, the PM 2.5 dataset, evaluation parameters, and experimental results. First, it demonstrates the experimental setup that has been adopted for evaluating the proposed air quality prediction and monitoring model.

31.5.1 Datasets

This subsection explains in detail the PM2.5 datasets that were collected from Beijing, China.

31.5.2 Evaluation Parameters

The proposed model is evaluated by using the evaluation parameters such as root mean square error (RMSE), mean absolute error (MAE), and mean absolute percentage error (MAPE):

$$\mathrm{RMSE} = \sqrt{\frac{1}{n}\sum_{i=1}^{n}(y_i - y_i^*)^2} \quad (31.10)$$

$$\mathrm{MAE} = \frac{1}{n}\sum_{i=1}^{n}|y_i - y_i^*| \quad (31.11)$$

$$\mathrm{MAPE} = \frac{1}{n}\sum_{i=1}^{n}\frac{|y_i - y_i^*|}{y_i} \quad (31.12)$$

where, it indicates the observed value of *i*th case and represents the predicted value.

31.5.3 Sub-Headings

The proposed intelligent air quality prediction and monitoring system has been implemented using Python, and the user interface is designed using the Python Flask environment. Here, the PM values in Beijing, China, are used as an input dataset that is divided into two datasets, such as training and testing datasets. In this case, 80% of the dataset is used for training and 20% for testing. Among them, the datasets are grouped into three sub-datasets such as winter, monsoon, and summer according to the various seasons by applying the rule-based data grouping algorithm. Figure 31.2 shows the performance of the proposed Intelligent Air Quality During COVID-19 Prediction and Monitoring System (IAQPMS) in terms of RMSE value with respect to the seasons. Here, we have considered 5 years of data, including the years 2017, 2018, 2019, 2020, and 2021.

From Fig. 31.2, it is observed that the RMSE values in all the 5 years are in three different seasons, such as monsoon, summer, and winter. Here, it is observed that the RMSE value in monsoon seasons in the years 2017, 2018, and 2019 is higher than in the years 2020 and 2021. Moreover, the RMSE value of the summer season of the year 2018 is lower than all other years. The RMSE value of the winter season in the year 2020 is lower than in all other years.

Figure 31.3 illustrates an RMSE comparison between the proposed IAQPMS and existing prediction systems created utilising models such as Autoregressive Integrated Moving Average (ARIMA), LSSVM, Artificial Neural Networks (ANN), RNN, LSTM, Bi directional Long Short Term Memory (BLSTM), CNN-LSTM, Inverse Distance Weighting-Bi directional Long Short Term Memory (IDW-BLSTM), and Zhan et al. [3]. Experiments are conducted using all three seasonal data.

Figure 31.3 shows that the proposed IAQPMS has a lower RMSE than ARIMA, LSSVM, ANN, RNN, LSTM, BLSTM, CNN-LSTM, IDW-BLSTM, and Zhan et al. [3]. The rule-based data grouping algorithm (RDGA) and ensemble deep classifier (EDC), which combines Bi-LSTM and T-CNN, are responsible for the improvement.

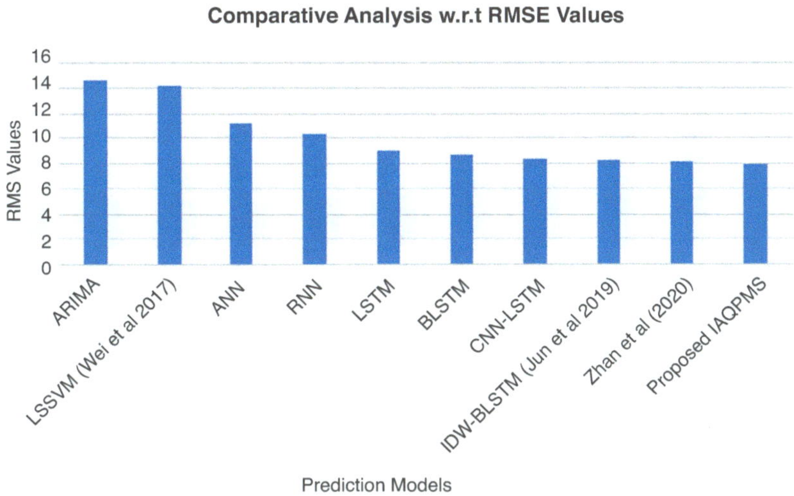

Fig. 31.3 Comparative analysis w.r.t RMSE values

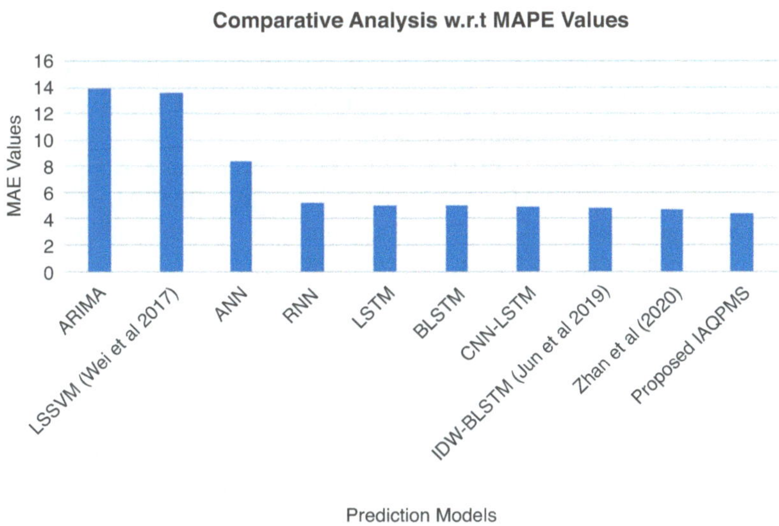

Fig. 31.4 Comparative analysis w.r.t MAE values

Figure 31.4 compares the MAE values of the proposed IAQPMS and existing prediction systems built utilising models such as ARIMA, LSSVM, ANN, RNN, LSTM, BLSTM, CNN-LSTM, IDW-BLSTM, and Zhan et al. [3]. Experiments are conducted using all three seasonal data.

The MAE of the proposed IAQPMS is lower than existing approaches such as ARIMA, LSSVM, ANN, RNN, LSTM, BLSTM, CNN-LSTM, IDW-BLSTM, and Zhan et al. [3]. The RDGA and EDC, which combines Bi-LSTM and T-CNN, are responsible for the improvement.

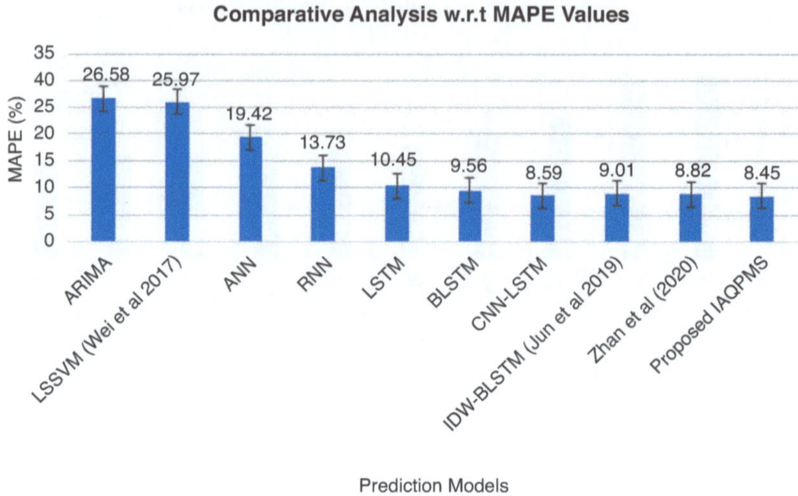

Fig. 31.5 Comparative analysis w.r.t MAPE values

Figure 31.5 compares the MAPE values of the proposed IAQPMS and existing prediction systems built utilising models such as ARIMA, LSSVM, ANN, RNN, LSTM, BLSTM, CNN-LSTM, IDW-BLSTM, and Zhan et al. [3]. Experiments are conducted using all three seasonal data sets.

The MAPE value of the suggested IAQPMS is lower than existing approaches such as ARIMA, LSSVM, ANN, RNN, LSTM, BLSTM, CNN-LSTM, IDW-BLSTM, and Zhan et al. [3]. The RDGA and EDC, which combines Bi-LSTM and T-CNN, are responsible for the improvement.

31.6 Conclusion and Future Works

IAQPMS has been developed to predict and monitor the air quality during COVID-19 and the pollution level in different seasons in Beijing, China. The proposed IAQPMS applies a preliminary data preprocess to get exact data and a newly proposed RDGA to group the data according to the different seasonal data by applying the necessary rules. Moreover, it applies a newly proposed EDC that is a combination of T-CNN and Bi-LSTM to perform effective classification and prediction processes. Finally, the proposed IAQPMS has been shown to outperform existing prediction models in terms of RMSE, MAE, and MAPE values in a variety of experiments. It can be done in this direction with the introduction of a new efficient classifier for predicting the air quality in advance and updating it on time.

References

1. Monteiro, A., Ferreira, J., Ribeiro, I., Fernandes, A. P., Martins, H., Gama, C., & Isabel, A. (2015). Miranda: Air quality over Portugal in 2020. *Atmospheric Pollution Research, 6*(5), 788–796.
2. Zhang, Y., Zhang, R., Ma, Q., Wang, Y., Wang, Q., Huang, Z., & Huang, L. (2020). A feature selection and multi-model fusion-based approach of predicting air quality. *ISA Transactions, 100*, 210–220.
3. Zhan, C., Li, S., Li, J., Guo, Y., Wen, Q., & Wen, W. (2020). Prediction of air quality in major cities of China by deep learning. In *16th international conference on Computational Intelligence and Security* (*CIS*) (pp. 68–72).
4. Zhang, Y., Wang, Y., Gao, M., Ma, Q., Zhao, J., Zhang, R., Wang, Q., & Huang, L. (2019). A predictive data feature exploration-based air quality prediction approach. *IEEE Access, 7*, 30732–30743.
5. Suárez Sánchez, A., García Nieto, P. J., Riesgo Fernández, P., Del Coz Díaz, J. J., & Iglesias-Rodríguez, F. J. (2011). Application of an SVM-based regression model to the air quality study at local scale in the Avilés urban area (Spain). *Mathematical and Computer Modelling, 54*(5–6), 1453–1466.
6. Carbajal-Hernández, J. J., Sánchez-Fernández, L. P., Carrasco-Ocho, J. A., & Martínez-Trinid, J. F. (2012). Assessment and prediction of air quality using fuzzy logic and autoregressive models. *Atmospheric Environment, 60*, 37–50.
7. Ma, J., Ding, Y., Gan, V. J. L., Lin, C., & Wan, Z. (2019). Spatiotemporal prediction of PM2.5 concentrations at different time granularities using IDW-BLSTM. *IEEE Access, 7*, 107897–107907.
8. Metia, S., Oduro, S. D., Duc, H. N., & Ha, Q. (2016). Inverse air-pollutant emission and prediction using extended fractional kalman filtering. *IEEE Journal of Selected Topics in Applied Earth Observations and Remote Sensing, 9*(5), 2051–2063.
9. Qi, Z., Wang, T., Song, G., Hu, W., Li, X., & Zhang, Z. (2018). Deep air learning: Interpolation, prediction, and feature analysis of fine-grained air quality. *IEEE Transactions on Knowledge and Data Engineering, 30*(12), 2285–2297.
10. Zhenghua, W., & Zhihui, T. (2017). Prediction of air quality index based on improved neural network. In *International conference on Computer Systems, Electronics and Control* (*ICCSEC*) (pp. 200–204).
11. Chau, P. N., Zalakeviciute, R., Thomas, I., & Rybarczyk, Y. (2022). Deep learning approach for assessing air quality during COVID-19 lockdown in quito. *Frontiers in Big Data, 5*, 842455. https://doi.org/10.3389/fdata.2022.842455
12. Wang, J. Z., Zhang, X., Guo, Z. H., & Lu, H. (2017). Developing an early- warning system for air quality prediction and assessment of cities in China. *Expert Systems with Applications, 84*, 102–116.
13. Sun, W., & Sun, J. (2017). Daily PM2.5 concentration prediction based on principal component analysis and LSSVM optimized by cuckoo search algorithm. *Journal of Environmental Management, 188*, 144–152.
14. Chang, Y. S., Lin, K. M., Tsai, Y. T., Zeng, Y. R., & Hung, C. X. (2018). Big data platform for air quality analysis and prediction. In *27th Wireless and Optical Communication Conference* (*WOCC*) (pp. 1–3).
15. Wang, J., & Song, G. (2018). A deep spatial-temporal ensemble model for air quality prediction. *Neurocomputing, 314*, 198–206.
16. Jiao, Y., Wang, Z., & Zhang, Y. (2019). Prediction of air quality index based on LSTM. In *IEEE 8th Joint International Information Technology and Artificial Intelligence Conference* (*ITAIC*) (pp. 17–20).
17. Xue, H., Bai, Y., Hu, H., Xu, T., & Liang, H. (2019). A novel hybrid model based on TVIW-PSO-GSA algorithm and support vector machine for classification problems. *IEEE Access, 7*, 27789–27801.

18. Zhang, Q., Fu, F., & Tian, R. (2020). A deep learning and image-based model for air quality estimation. *Science of The Total Environment, 724*, 138178.
19. Kim, J., Wang, X., Kang, C., Yu, J., & Li, P. (2021). Forecasting air pollutant concentration using a novel spatiotemporal deep learning model based on clustering, feature selection and empirical wavelet transform. *Science of the Total Environment, 801*, 149654.
20. Kök, İ., Şimşek, M. U., & Özdemir, S. (2017). A deep learning model for air quality prediction in smart cities. In *IEEE International Conference on Big Data* (*Big Data*) (pp. 1983–1990).
21. Aggarwal, A., & Toshniwal, D. (2021). A hybrid deep learning framework for urban air quality forecasting. *Journal of Cleaner Production, 329*, 129660.
22. Lina, C.-Y., Changa, Y.-S., & Abimannan, S. (2021). Ensemble multifeatured deep learning models for air quality forecasting. *Atmospheric Pollution Research, 12*(5), 101045.
23. Zou, G., Zhang, B., Yong, R., Qin, D., & Zhao, Q. (2021). FDN-learning: Urban PM2.5-concentration spatial correlation prediction model based on fusion deep neural network. *Big Data Research, 26*, 100269.
24. Wang, J., Li, H., & Lu, H. (2018). Application of a novel early warning system based on fuzzy time series in urban air quality forecasting in China. *Applied Soft Computing, 71*, 783–799.

Chapter 32
Implementation of a 'Useful' Information Measure for Healthcare Decision Making

Pankaj Prasad Dwivedi, Dilip Kumar Sharma, and Appaji M. Ashwini

32.1 Introduction to Information Theory

Natural language processing, cryptography, statistical inference, and molecular biology are a few fields where information theory is used. It is a fundamental area of mathematics of the transmission, processing, extraction, and usage of information. One of the most important goals of information theory is to offer a solid foundation for maximizing the quantity of data collected from a given scenario. Many of the findings of information theory research have been applied in various fields such as engineering points of view, ranging from machine learning and artificial intelligence to cybernetics and complexity science. An analysis of scenarios in which one operator (the transmitter) sends a message via a medium to another operator (the receiver) is central to information theory. This is usually accomplished by sending a succession of incomplete signals from the transmitter. The transmission control protocol, for example, outlines how communication might be broken down into packets before being sent over the Internet, allowing the recipient to reassemble the packets in the right sequence. These partial messages may address some of the receiver's ambiguity about the original message's substance. The information content of an incomplete communication measures how much ambiguity it resolves.

Let's begin with a rebuilt diagram of a broad communication system based on Shannon's original article [1].

An information source creates a message or sequence of messages for a recipient. Destination should be far from information source. A transmitter must convert the

P. P. Dwivedi (✉) · D. K. Sharma
Jaypee University of Engineering and Technology, Raghogarh, Madhya Pradesh, India

A. M. Ashwini
IEEE, Bangalore Section, Bangalore, India
e-mail: ashwini.am@ieee.org

F. J. J. Joseph et al. (eds.), *Computational Intelligence for Clinical Diagnosis*,
EAI/Springer Innovations in Communication and Computing,
https://doi.org/10.1007/978-3-031-23683-9_32

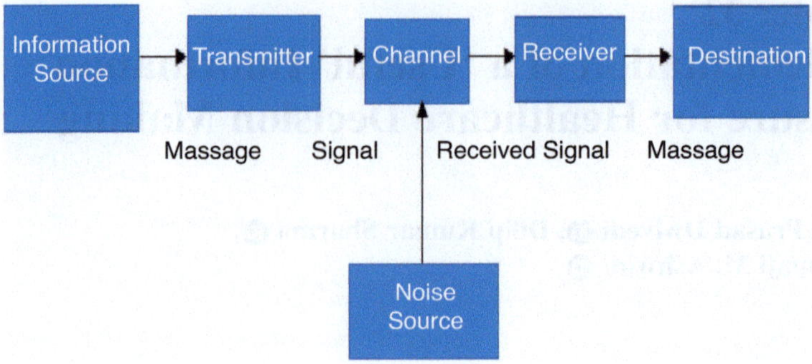

Fig. 32.1 A broad information system diagram [2]

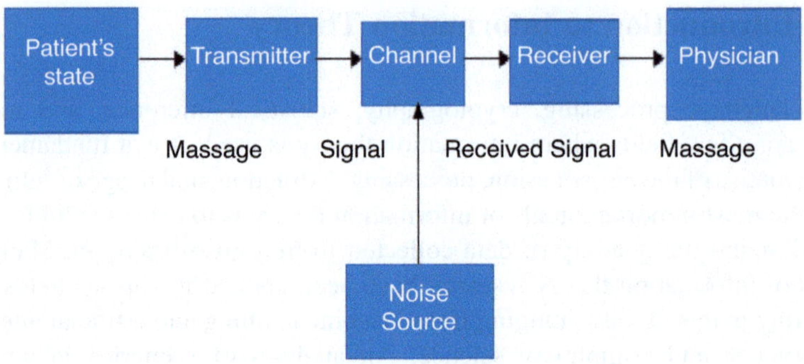

Fig. 32.2 In a clinical setting, the communication system [2]

message into a channel-acceptable signal. A receiver must convert a received signal into a format the destination can understand. The communication system determines how source information can be received and processed by the endpoint. Each message route has a noise source that contaminates the broadcast signal before it is received. Additionally, we cannot be assured that the transmitter and receiver are ideal signal-to-signal and signal-to-signal converters. Each test or action may be viewed as a piece of the puzzle that leads to the desired full message, which contains enough information to validate a diagnosis. Throughout an inquiry, the next test would be chosen to maximize the information gathered. The significant aspect of this viewpoint is that it gives a reasonable foundation for determining which tests to provide at each step of patient interaction. The paradigm in Fig. 32.1 may easily be mapped onto the particular of wireless transmission, radio or broadcast media, and the Internet, for instance. However, in the context of this discussion, it will be more interesting to implement the model in a clinical scenario.

In Fig. 32.2, we've altered nothing from Fig. 32.1: The source of information is now the state of the patient, and the destination is the doctor responsible for making the patient's situation diagnostic. We must continue to keep the model as wide as possible. The transmitter may be as follows: in the patient's meeting; a test on the patient; a qualified doctor analysing the patient; the patient's test report. Differentiate between a patient's abnormal communication and a doctor, nurse, or assessor's indication. We cannot guarantee the indicator's accuracy. For instance, the channel may be, if the sender and the receiver are all in the same room, a vocal utterance, a written communication, an Internet link, or a telephone line.

The recipient's job is to convert the indication to a written or electronic memory. Ultimately, the doctor represents the culmination of a chain of messages that will gradually notify diagnostic testing. There are two important aspects to remember: Information in a message may be lost or distorted when it is carried from its source to the physician at any point in the communication system; every communication will have a limited amount of data to guide candidate diagnoses. We should be able to determine the impact of messages required to get a verified analysis if we can optimize the quantity of information in each message. Making such a reduction assumes that we have a certain measure of relevant information accessible. That's the subject of the next section.

32.2 Information Content and Entropy

Let us look at a basic example to justify the appropriate measure selection when we provide a measure of relevant information. This is a condensed version of the introduction. A more comprehensive lesson, such as that offered in [3], could be a good next step for the interested reader. Consider a set of N binary buttons, where N is any positive numeral bigger than zero. There are two potential states for each button. These can be considered 'on' and 'off' buttons. Suppose there are two possible messages: one showing the button seems to be in the 'on' state, and the other showing the button is in the 'off state. One button stores just 1 'bit' of information: all we prerequisite is one message to identify the status of that button. In an array of two buttons, we can store 2 bits of information in, and we'll need two 1 'bit' messages or one 2 'bit' message to identify the array's state. The content of information of a special communication from the collection of two binary buttons is just the total quantity of the useful details from individual information conveyed from those buttons separately. In general, to identify the internal representation of an arrangement of N buttons, we will require a message that is N bits long. Consider the total number of states in a binary button array. We have four alternative states for two buttons: {off, on; off, off; on, on; on, off}. Similarly, we will also have four potential statements which will inform us of the array's status in a single message. We have 2^N potential conditions and 2^N potential instructions in the generalized form have N buttons in an array. When we consider each button operates independently and that every one of those button's access to the information is equally probable, then every individual communication has a chance of occurrence of $p = 1/(2^N)$.

Look at the example where a message x of length N is received. The preceding reasoning suggests the need for an additive measure of information content.

Furthermore, we have shown that many states in a network grow exponentially. This proposes using a logarithmic function like:

$$h(\mu) = -\log_2 p(\mu) \tag{32.1}$$

Putting our message x into (32.1) with the likelihood of occurrence $p(x) = 1/(2^N)$, we get:

$$h(x) = -\log_2\left(\frac{1}{2^N}\right) = \log_2\left(2^N\right) = N \tag{32.2}$$

Thus, the preceding measure (32.1) returns our tentatively suggested content of the information measure; in fact, it is the description of an outcome's relevant information of Shannon [4].

We must now generalize this. Whenever a patient comes, the patient's condition is not understood with confidence. Consequently, the messages that could be received from a random variable X, with each message $x \in X$ possessing a likelihood of detection, $p(x)$.

Suppose $\Delta_n^+ = \left\{P = (p_1, p_2, \ldots\ldots p_n); p_i \geq 0, \sum_i^n p_i = 1\right\}$ be a set of all conceivable discrete likelihood distributions of an arbitrary variable X having utility distribution $U = \{(u_1, u_2, \ldots u_n); u_i > 0 \,\forall\, i\}$ joined to every $P \in \Delta_n^+$ such that $u_i > 0$ is the utility of an occasion having the likelihood of an event $p_i > 0$. If u_i is the utility of outcome x_i at that point, it is independent of the source image x_i of the encoding probability, that is, p_i. Consequently, the information source can be expressed assumed below:

$$\begin{bmatrix} x_1, x_2 \ldots\ldots\ldots x_n \\ p_1, p_2 \ldots\ldots\ldots p_n \\ u_1, u_2 \ldots\ldots\ldots u_n \end{bmatrix} \tag{32.3}$$

Here, $u_i > 0, 0 < p_i \leq 1, \sum_{i=1}^n p_i = 1$ which is a calculation for the normal amount of information 'useful' in the sequence provided by the source (32.3). Consequently, [5] presented the following qualitative-quantitative information measure:

$$H(P; U) = -\sum_{i=1}^n u_i p_i \log p_i \tag{32.4}$$

The above measure (32.4) is called 'useful entropy' and it reduces to Shannon's information [6] when utilities are ignored, as seen following:

$$H(P) = -\sum_{i=1}^{n} p_i \log p_i \tag{32.5}$$

Many authors have portrayed Shannon’s entropy by utilizing various hypotheses. Shannon entropy is a reliable tool for measuring treatment outcomes in tinnitus, as demonstrated by [7], the broad concept of cell migration introduced by [8] and between two primary groups, Shannon’s entropy was compared and computed by [9]. The uncertainty space technique, proposed by [10], is used to calculate a measurement of average uncertainty in a signal. Discovering how more complex ideas, such as mutual information and conditional entropy, can give deeper insights into possible redundancy in laboratory testing, as described by [2]. Many studies exist in the literature in terms of ‘useful’ information measure which was done by Dwivedi and Sharma [11, 12]. The expression more utilizing significant assumptions which were found by [13], how to measure and quantity of information that anticipates obtaining regarding the illness condition of the examined subject before executing a diagnostic test, entropy, mutual information, and relative entropy are all essential information theory functions that are generally relevant to clinical diagnostic tests.

In this context, the term random variable refers to a statistical group. X is a triple (x, A_X, P) wherein x is a ‘random variable’ that can take in some of several potential entries from an alphabet (a collection of permitted letters) $A_X = \{x_1, x_2, \ldots, x_n\}$ with commensurate likelihoods $P = \{p_1, p_2, \ldots, p_n\}$. In other words, the possibility that $x = x_i$ for any $1 \leq i \leq n$ is p_i. Furthermore, we need $p_i \geq 0$ for every i, and $\sum_{i=1}^{n} p_i = 1$.

The ‘useful’ Shannon information content of a result [14] may thus be defined as a measure $H(P; U)$ on the random variable X:

$$H(P, U) = -\frac{\sum_{i=1}^{n} u_i p_i \log_2 p_i}{\sum_{i=1}^{n} u_i p_i} \tag{32.6}$$

Strictly speaking, this merely gives us the work intended for the ‘useful’ information content of a message x received from the random variable X. Furthermore, the formulation of (32.6) is equivalent to the thermodynamic statistical mechanic’s model for the description of ‘useful’ entropy:

$$S = -\frac{k_B \sum_{i}^{n} u_i p_i \ln(p_i)}{\sum_{i}^{n} u_i p_i} \tag{32.7}$$

The chance of a specific sovereign state of the thermodynamic system under investigation is represented by p_i and u_i is the utility distribution attached to probabilities.

Let $H(P; U)$ be related to as the (Shannon) ‘useful’ entropy of those random variables by similarity with the structure of such a variant of Boltzmann’s formula as

Table 32.1 The contents of 'useful' Shannon information for the outcomes *a* to *z*

X	A_X	P	$H(P, U)$	X	A_X	P	$H(P, U)$
1	*a*	0.0575	0.0136	15	*o*	0.0689	0.0183
2	*b*	0.0128	0.0010	16	*p*	0.0192	0.0021
3	*c*	0.0263	0.0036	17	*q*	0.0008	0.0000
4	*d*	0.0285	0.0042	18	*r*	0.0508	0.0111
5	*e*	0.0913	0.0288	19	*s*	0.0567	0.0133
6	*f*	0.0173	0.0018	20	*t*	0.0706	0.0191
7	*g*	0.0133	0.0011	21	*u*	0.0334	0.0055
8	*h*	0.0313	0.0049	22	*v*	0.0069	0.0003
9	*i*	0.0599	0.0146	23	*w*	0.0119	0.0009
10	*j*	0.0006	0.0000	24	*x*	0.0073	0.0004
11	*k*	0.0084	0.0005	25	*y*	0.0164	0.0016
12	*l*	0.0335	0.0055	26	*z*	0.0007	0.0000
13	*m*	0.0235	0.0030	27	–	0.1928	0.0883
14	*n*	0.0596	0.0145	$H(P,U) = -\frac{\sum_{i=1}^{27} u_i p_i \log_2 p_i}{\sum_{i=1}^{27} u_i p_i} = 0.26$ bits			

well as the notion that the random variable X in some way reflects the various behaviour of systems (an individual in our example) under observation. It, too, has the unit of bits, as does Shannon information content (when using logarithm to the base 2). Before returning to a medical context, let us look to understand better how (32.6) could be employed with a few general-purpose examples. Taking into account the random variable X, picked from an English document where the consequence is just a character randomly. That is, the variable x will be created randomly by picking a letter from an English article as well as A_X is the alphabet defined in Table 32.1. We will not discriminate between lower-case and upper-case characters, but we will utilize a space character, " – ". And P is the corresponding probability p_i for $1 \leq i \leq 27$.

To use Table 32.1 supplied, the result $x =$ "z" has content of 0.0 bits and 'useful' Shannon information, whereas the $x =$ "e" has content of 0.02 bits and 'useful' Shannon information. The total 'useful' Shannon information is 0.26 bits in our English document text [15] has given the contents of the probability table, and we utilize its accompanying metrics to measure 'useful' information content. Now let us take a closer look at this. It is still debatable if Shannon entropy has a clear meaning [6]. Boltzmann's entropy has Joules per Kelvin, whereas thermodynamic entropy has bits. It is inaccurate to say that Shannon's entropy is 'the same thing' as 'entropy' or that they are unrelated. These calculations differ only by a variable (that specifies a measurement scale). Some may even start to explain them by relating the chances of the system's microstates to the possibilities of the symbols created by that system (Table 32.1).

Jaynes, indeed contended persuasively that the theoretic interpretation of information entropy constituted an extension entropy of thermodynamics [16, 17]. In the context of medical assessment, we implicitly promote the same stance. Returning to our document scenario, let us take a fresh document and randomly select a letter, and that letter comes out to be a '*z*' in a typical English document, a letter with one of the lowest likelihoods of occurrence.

Property 1

$$H(P;U) = 0$$

If $p(x_i) = 0$, then $0 \times \log_2 0 = 0$.

On the opposite end of the spectrum, if all scenarios are equally probable, the $H(P; U)$ is maximized. It is 'useful' relatively simple to get an expression for this value. Allow X_e, our random variable, to have n potential outcomes. Then, for any i, $p(x_i)$ must equal $\frac{1}{n}$. Trying to replace this into (32.6) yields:

$$\begin{aligned} H(P_e;U) &= -\frac{\sum_{i=1}^{n} u_i \cdot \frac{1}{n} \log_2 \frac{1}{n}}{\sum_{i=1}^{n} u_i p_i} \\ &= \log_2(n) \frac{1}{n} \left(\frac{\sum_{i=1}^{n} u_i}{\sum_{i=1}^{n} u_i p_i} \right) = \log_2(n) \end{aligned} \tag{32.8}$$

$\log(n)$ is a constant, keep in mind that $\log_2(1/n) = -\log_2(n)$, therefore.

Property 2 $H(P_e; U) = \log_2(n)$ if each of the n possibilities is fairly probable. Throughout the instance of our English document, if the letters were distributed uniformly and u_i are the utilities attached to probabilities, we would get $H(P_{\text{uniform}}, U) = -\frac{2 \times \frac{1}{27} \log_2 \left(\frac{1}{27}\right)}{2 \times \frac{1}{27}} = 0.0065$ bits. That is less than the figure for our typical English language document (0.26 bits). Coming to the implementation of this to clinical analysis, we may understand the following two scenarios: If just one message/positive test result is feasible, $H() = 0$. In other words, a particular diagnosis has been established. When all messages are equally feasible, H reaches its maximum. That is, we are completely unaware of the patient's inside condition. We can see from this also that the task of prognosis is to decrease entropy as near zero as potential and choose the trials such that the consequence of each trial (what we named 'messages' in this) gives a maximum entropy reduction. Before we proceed, two points should be made: To demonstrate the use of the phrase 'entropy', we are trying to equate the likelihood detection of messages with the patient under consideration of the possibility of microstates; we neglect uncertainty and risk in the factuality of a message that may be presented by the information on a wide range depicted in the figure.

32.3 Diagnostic Tests and 'Useful' Relative Entropy

Assume that the state of the diagnostic technique is very precise. A random variable of signals $X = (x, A_X P)$ is connected with a patient's individual internal state. The patient's 'interrogation' usually prompts a message. An inquiry may be a patient question, diagnostic test, or nursing assessment. According to questioning, the signal alphabetic A_X will have a likelihood distribution Q over it. Receiving a signal x_i (for instance, a positive test result) results in a probability model P over the alphabet of signals. We utilize 'useful' Kullback–Leibler divergence or the 'useful' relative entropy between the two probability distributions [15] to calculate the change in entropy:

$$D_{\mathrm{KL}}(P\|Q;U) = \frac{\sum_{i=1}^{n} u_i p_i \log_2\left(\frac{u_i p_i}{q_i}\right)}{\sum_{i=1}^{n} u_i p_i} \tag{32.9}$$

There are two aspects of 'useful' relative entropy worth highlighting. For starters, it meets Gibbs' inequality, which states that equality exists iff $P = Q$:

$$D_{\mathrm{KL}}(P\|Q;U) \geq 0 \tag{32.10}$$

Furthermore, the exchange of the two probability distributions is not symmetric. That is, $D_{\mathrm{KL}}(P\|Q;U) \neq D_{\mathrm{KL}}(Q\|P;U)$. As a result, 'useful' relative entropy does not strictly qualify as a metric (thus the word 'divergence'). Here $D_{\mathrm{KL}}(P\|Q;U)$ is a measurement of the information obtained when a doctor's views are altered from a before Q to a prospective P of some inquiry, described in Bayesian statistics. Thus far, we will use a hypothetical scenario borrowed from [18] to demonstrate the technique. We propose a community of arthritis patients with a previous likelihood dispensation across four potential symptoms. We have two screening procedures under our disposal: t_1 and t_2. Table 32.2 shows the pre-test and post-test probabilities after each of the two tests, which yields a good result. Which of the two tests yields the most information?

By utilizing (32.9), we can easily compute that the information gained from t_1 are 0.75 bits, while the information gained from t_2 would have been 0.35 bits (to 2 d.p.).

Table 32.2 Theoretical example [18]

Candidate diagnosis	Utility (u_i)	Pre-test probability (t_0)	Post-test probability (t_1)	Post-test probability (t_2)
Gout	2	0.25	0.5	0.4
Osteoarthritis	3	0.5	0	0.1
Pseudogout	4	0.125	0.5	0.4
Other possibilities	5	0.125	0	0.1

Remember that we assume that the chances are uniform; therefore, 0. $\log_2(0) = 0$. As a result, throughout the first situation, we have:

$$D_{\mathrm{KL}}(t_1 \| t_0; U) = \frac{2 \times 0.5 \times \log_2\left(\frac{0.5}{0.25}\right)}{2 \times 0.5} + \frac{4 \times 0.5 \times \log_2\left(\frac{0.5}{0.125}\right)}{4 \times 0.5}$$
$$= 0.25 + 0.5 = 0.75 \text{ bits}$$

We have, in the second situation:

$$D_{\mathrm{KL}}(t_2 t_0; U) = \frac{2 \times 0.4 \times \log_2\left(\frac{0.4}{0.25}\right)}{2 \times 0.4} + \frac{3 \times 0.1 \times \log_2\left(\frac{0.1}{0.5}\right)}{3 \times 0.1}$$
$$+ \frac{4 \times 0.4 \times \log_2\left(\frac{0.4}{0.125}\right)}{4 \times 0.4} + \frac{5 \times 0.1 \times \log_2\left(\frac{0.1}{0.125}\right)}{5 \times 0.1}$$
$$= 0.108 - 0.023 + 0.268 - 0.003$$
$$= 0.35 \text{ (to 2 d.p.) bits}$$

The obvious concern is to utilize 'useful' relative entropy rather than the difference between pre-test and post-test entropies (32.6). Early talks on entropy in medical decision-making did suggest the latter. On the other hand, Hershey, Asch, and Patton determined that it 'fails to capture plausible intuitions about the amounts of information offered by diagnostic tests' [4]. The present idea is addressed in [18], demonstrating that relative entropy better efficiently represents these perceptions [19] offer a more formal argument for 'useful' relative entropy as a suitable statistic for distinguishing among pairs of likelihood distributions. Now consider how these information theories and principles could help clinical decision-making.

32.4 Binary Outcomes and Shannon Entropy

Several lab tests are intended to determine the concentrations of a disease condition; this is referred to as a binary result. We may use flip a coin as a point of reference, with the results actuality tails or heads. Suppose that the coins collection is skewed roughly. This seems to be, and every coin will have a chance p that the result is head, with p changing between 0 and 1. Entropy is calculated for a given coin C using (32.6), observing that the possibility of a tail is $(1 - p)$:

$$H(C) = -p \times \log_2(p) - (1-p) \times \log_2(1-p) \tag{32.11}$$

The entropy fluctuates between 0 and 1, with a maximum at 1 whenever $p = 0.5$ (see Fig. 32.3).

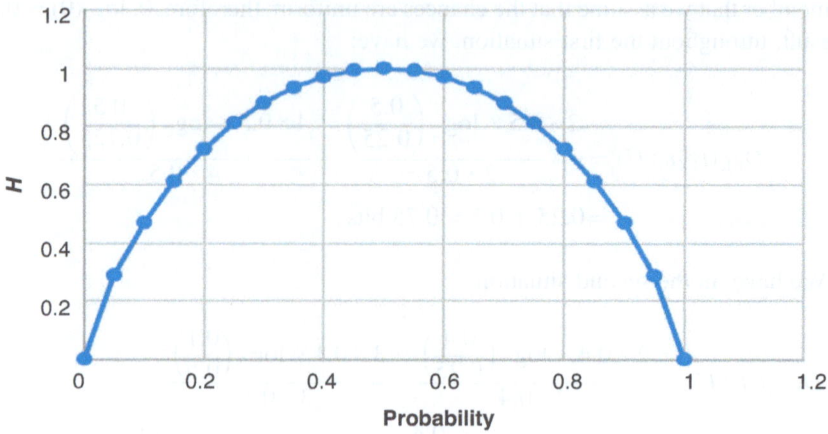

Fig. 32.3 Illustration for a biased coin between entropy vs probability [2]

Flip a coin to determine a patient's health. 'Head' means the patient may have the illness, while 'tail' means not. If the coin is impartial, all internal states are equally plausible. To learn about a patient's interior status, we need a test with low entropy. The use of entropy to assess the information [20] investigated the richness of various test centres. He illustrated how information theory ideas might be utilized to help in the evaluation and comprehension of laboratory test findings. We will utilize Fig. 32.3 as a point of comparison to explain the topic with only one example. For malignant melanoma, Stadelmann et al. [7] stated that using the given formula, the overall chance of 10-year death may be calculated given tumour thickness t:

$$p = 1 - 0.966 \times e^{-(0.2016t)}$$

Figure 32.4 shows a plot between tumour thickness t and entropy H, using (32.11). We can observe that tumor thickness gives modest information regarding the results over a large range of possibilities, with a median of ≈3.5 mm.

32.5 Prioritize Laboratory Tests by Information Theory

We are developing numerous ways to employ strategies in a clinical context to select diagnostic tests. First, we distinguish two candidate tests to employ 'useful' relative entropy. The fluctuation in entropy resulting from certain clinical diagnoses (for a binary decision) was then examined to discover the range of results whereby the test is useful. It should be noted that these are not the exclusive techniques accessible; nonetheless, the documented project to date has argued for their utility as supplementary decision-making. Lee and Maslove [21] proposed that an information-theoretic method may be especially useful in finding duplication in testing in an

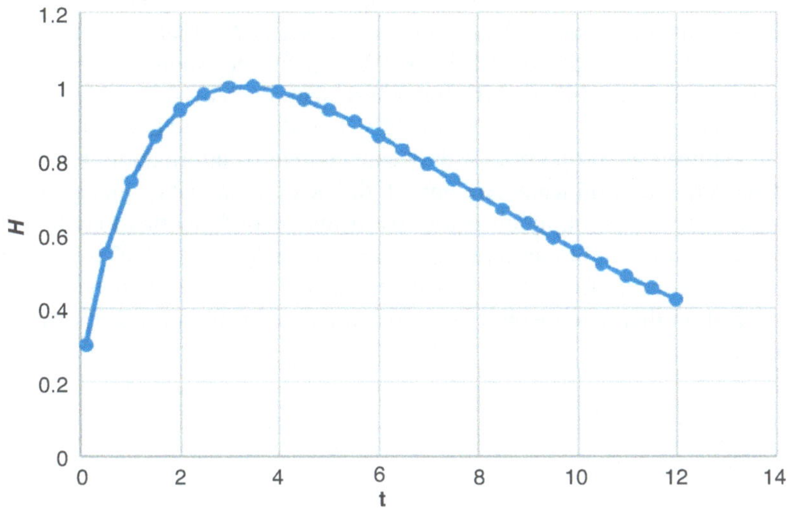

Fig. 32.4 Illustration of entropy of tumour thickness t (in mm) [2]

intensive care unit. The problem, therefore, is to determine whether blood tests are the utmost instructive on a wide system scale. Another fundamental concern for this is that there may be an amount of duplication across laboratory testing; that is, certain tests may contribute less information over earlier tests performed, particularly over time. When we can detect a high level of 'useful' mutual information across assessments (because the similar test is replicated excessively often or because two separate tests rely too much on relevant data), we have an empirical foundation for lowering the number of tests run. Lee and Maslove [21] utilized two more notions. The 'useful' conditional entropy of P provided Q was the first, and U is the utilities attached to probabilities P. This is stated as follows:

$$H(P|Q;U) = \frac{\sum_{xy \in A_X A_Y} u(x,y)p(x,y)\log\left(\frac{1}{p(x|y)}\right)}{\sum_{xy \in A_X A_Y} u(x,y)p(x,y)} \tag{32.12}$$

Returning to the concept of a random variable, A_X is the random variable of X, or the collection of lawful independent ideals of x. Likewise, A_Y is the random variable 's alphabet. An element of 'useful' mutual information among P and Q is a similar notion, and U is the utilities attached to probabilities P. This quantifies the quantity of information sent by x regarding y and is described as:

$$MI(P;Q;U) = H(P;U) - H(P|Q;U) \tag{32.13}$$

It is worth noting that we have adhered to the definitions provided by Mackay [15]. MIMIC-II, a completely anonymized public resource, was used by Lee and

Maslove to extract lab results. They investigated the following lab tests in 29,149 ICU admissions: haematocrit; blood urea nitrogen (BUN); platelet count; glucose; HCO_3; chloride; white blood cell count (WBC); lactate; sodium; creatinine; and potassium. Their data reinforced the hypothesis that much of the ICU blood work is unneeded. It has been described earlier in [22], but Maslove and Lee were potentially viable to estimate the proportion of duplicate content of information. For example, they discovered a significant amount of duplication in data among BUN and creatinine assessments, implying that if one is understood, another may be inferred with fair certainty. Additionally, their findings revealed that BUN would be preferred over creatine if offered the alternative. Nursing diagnosis is often required, but this information-theoretic method provides an empirical framework for making an educated decision.

32.6 Conclusion

In this article, we demonstrated how information theory might be useful in guiding clinical decision-making. To demonstrate this, we used data from multiple kinds of research. However, there is one area in which we vary from most of that research. Some of them use extra terms to lend an accessible interpretation to many of the ideas in information theory, such as 'surprise', 'closeness to a certainty', and possibly a propensity to associate entropy with uncertainties. It is clear. Entropy is one of classical thermodynamics' toughest concepts. However, we have limited our discussion to information and entropy. By linking patient interactions with underlying microstates, we hinted at an equivalency between Shannon entropy and mathematical analysis entropy. The work of [23] and [16, 17] is a good starting point for a more in-depth investigation of Shannon entropy. We think health informatics experts should promote information theory knowledge. Improvements in medical decision-making are waiting to be applied. However, tighter criteria are needed. We have explored numerous methods; it would be helpful to note a common base for them all. In addition, we emphasise network 'noise'. The communication model we outlined at the beginning of the post is an important but often disregarded factor in misdiagnosis risk.

Acknowledgements The authors would like to express their gratitude to Jaypee University of Engineering and Technology, Guna (M.P.), India, for its ongoing assistance.

References

1. Shannon, C. E. (1948). A mathematical theory of communication. *The Bell System Technical Journal, 27*, 379–423.
2. Krause, P. (2019). Information theory and medical decision making. *Studies in Health Technology and Informatics, 30*(263), 23–34. https://doi.org/10.3233/SHTI190108
3. Stone, J. V. (2015). *Information theory – A tutorial introduction*. Sebtel Press.

4. Asch, D. A., Patton, J. P., & Hershey, J. C. (1991). Prognostic information versus accuracy: Once more with meaning. *Medical Decision Making, 11*, 45–47.
5. Belis, M., & Guiasu, S. (1968). A quantitative-qualitative measure of information in cybernetics system. *IEEE Transactions on Information Theory, 14*, 593–594.
6. Pismen, L. (2018). *The swings of science – From complexity to simplicity and back*. Springer.
7. Stadelmann, W. K., Rapaport, D. P., & Soong, S.-J. (1998). Prognostic factors that influence melanoma outcome. In C. M. Balch, A. N. Houghton, A. J. Sober, et al. (Eds.), *Cutaneous melanoma* (3rd ed., pp. 11–35). Quality Medical Publishing.
8. Liu, Y., Jiao, Y., Fan, Q., Zheng, Y., Li, G., Yao, J., et al. (2021). Shannon entropy for time-varying persistence of cell migration. *Biophysical Journal, 120*(12), 2552–2565. https://doi.org/10.1016/j.bpj.2021.04.026
9. Maryam, S., Saeed, T., Mohsen, S., Mehdi, A., & Pourbakht, A. (2021). Shannon entropy measures for EEG signals in tinnitus. *Neuroscience Letters, 762*, 136153. https://doi.org/10.1016/j.neulet.2021.136153
10. Craig Herndon, R. (2021). Determining signal entropy in uncertainty space. *Measurement, 178*, 109336. https://doi.org/10.1016/j.measurement.2021.10
11. Dwivedi, P. P., & Sharma, D. K. (2021). Lower and upper bounds for 'useful' Renyi information rate. In *Communications in computer and information science* (p. 1441). Springer. https://doi.org/10.1007/978-3-030-88244-0_26
12. Dwivedi, P. P., & Sharma, D. K. (2022). Generalized 'useful' converse Jensen's inequality with data illustration. *WSEAS Transactions on Systems, 21*, 62–67.
13. Benish, W. A. (2020). A review of the application of information theory to clinical diagnostic testing. *Entropy, 22*(1). https://doi.org/10.3390/e22010097
14. Bhaker, U. S., & Hooda, D. S. (1993). Mean value characterization of 'useful' information measures. *Tamkang Journal of Mathematics, 24*, 383–394.
15. Mackay, D. J. C. (2003). *Information theory, inference and learning algorithms*. CUP.
16. Jaynes, E. T. (1957). Information theory and statistical mechanics. *Physical Review, 106*, 620–630.
17. Jaynes, E. T. (1957). Information theory and statistical mechanics. *Physical Review, 108*, 171–190.
18. Benish, W. A. (1999). Relative entropy as a measure of diagnostic information. *Medical Decision Making, 19*, 202–206.
19. Kullback, S., & Leibler, R. A. (1951). On information and sufficiency. *Annals of Mathematical Statistics, 11*, 79–86.
20. Vollmer, R. T. (2007). Entropy and Information content of laboratory test results. *American Journal of Clinical Pathology, 127*, 60–65.
21. Lee, J., & Maslove, D. M. (2015). Using information theory to identify redundancy in common laboratory tests in the intensive care unit. *BMC Medical Informatics and Decision Making, 15*(59), 1–8.
22. van Walraven, C., & Naylor, C. D. (1998). Do we know inappropriate laboratory utilization? A systematic review of laboratory clinical audits. *JAMA, 280*, 550–558.
23. Tribus, M., & McIrvine, E. C. (1971). Energy and information. *Scientific American, 225*, 179–190.

Chapter 33
Indian Sign Language Recognition Using Surf Feature Extraction and MDAE for Patient Disability Discussion

Edwin Shalom Soji and T. Kamalakannan

33.1 Introduction

Human life has always depended heavily on communication. A basic human need is the capacity for communication and self-expression. Despite this, regular people have little trouble engaging with one another and expressing themselves through voice, gestures, body language, reading, writing, and talking, all of which are commonly used by them. However, individuals with speech impediments only use sign language, which makes it more challenging for them to interact with the majority of people. This suggests the need for software that can recognise sign language and translate it into vocal or written language. Despite the fact that 17.7% of the world's people call India home, relatively little research has been done in this field, which is quite contradictory when compared to the other nations [1, 2]. The use of sign language is not universal and varies between and within nations, sometimes dramatically. In addition to manual components related to hand positioning and motion, sign languages generally include non-manual elements including body language and facial expressions (Indian Sign Language (ISL)) [3]. This effort is focused on creating a wearable ISL translator using manual components of signing for classification because the bulk of signs can be recognised based on the manual components. One-handed, two-handed, and static or dynamic signs are additional categories for the manual components [4].

The dominant hand, the right hand for right-handed signers and the left hand for left-handed signers, is almost always used by the signer while making one-handed gestures. The dominant hand may be holding itself in a fixed position, such as while

E. S. Soji (✉) · T. Kamalakannan
Department of Computer Science, Vels Institute of Science, Technology & Advanced Studies (VISTAS), Chennai, India
e-mail: KKannan.scs@velsuniv.ac.in

F. J. J. Joseph et al. (eds.), *Computational Intelligence for Clinical Diagnosis*, EAI/Springer Innovations in Communication and Computing,
https://doi.org/10.1007/978-3-031-23683-9_33

signing a number, or it may be moving along a predetermined path while maintaining a fixed or changing position. The dominance condition is when the dominant hand in two-handed signs is more active than the non-dominant hand [5]. The non-dominant hand might then be static, whereas the dominant hand might be active. The symmetry condition [5] is the situation in which both hands are active and have similar hand movements and shapes. The characteristics discussed above are used in this study to develop a multi-label classifier for the initial classification of an isolated sign, subsequent to which the last classification is finished. It makes implementing such a plan exceedingly challenging. Furthermore, there is no standard dataset accessible. These factors demonstrate how intricate ISL is. Recently, authors have considered this topic. The two basic techniques for recognising SL are the sensor-based method and the vision-based approach [6]. A vision-based technique makes use of web cameras toward capturing video or images [7], whereas the sensor-based approach makes use of gloves with the purpose of identifying finger gestures and transferring them into subsequent electrical impulses for sign language recognition (SLR). The three primary processes of the sign language recognition system (SLRS) are preprocessing, feature extraction, and classification. Using skin colour segmentation and a Gaussian filter, the signs are derived from a real-time video during the preprocessing stage. Following segmentation, a suitable feature vector is derived from the gesture sequence. The acquired features are then employed with the mutation denoising autoencoder (MDAE) for classification.

33.2 Literature Review

Dixit and Jalal [8] developed a system which identifies ISL and translates it into regular text. To introduce a new feature vector for sign recognition, combinational parameters of the Hu invariant moment and structural shape descriptors are extracted from the image. To train and detect ISL, a multi-class support vector machine (MSVM) is used for SLRS. The dataset was collected with 720 photos to validate the efficiency of the proposed strategy. The proposed system is able to effectively recognise hand gestures with a 96% recognition rate in the experimentation results.

Otiniano et al. [9] proposed a support vector machine (SVM) classifier and Hu and Zernike Moments-based features for SLR. Using a database made up of 2040 photos for the recognition of 24 symbol classes, the trials compare the offered approaches. The accuracy rate of the approach is increased to 96% via Zernike moments features, which is equivalent to the accuracy rates observed in the literature and suggests that the idea is promising. The results obtained by this method outperform those obtained by the extracted Hu moments features.

Tripathi et al. [10] developed an ISL gesture detection system that can recognise motions made with either one hand or both hands. The frame overlapping method has been used to track gestures in usable frames from continuous frames. A Hidden Markov model (HMM) is then utilised to test probe gestures after a discrete wavelet transform (DWT) is employed to extract features from an image frame. In the robotics and artificial intelligence laboratory, experiments are conducted using a custom continuous ISL dataset that was produced using a Canon EOS camera (IIIT-A). According to the testing findings, the suggested method is effective on a variety of backdrops, including coloured backgrounds and backgrounds with many objects. Additionally, this paradigm offers considerably reduced time complexity and spatial complexity.

Kong and Ranganath [4] adopted a two-layer conditional random field (CRF) technique by effectively recognising continuous sign language texts. CRF is introduced with the lower layer processing the component channels and sending outputs to the upper layer for sign recognition. The outputs of separate CRF and SVM classifiers are fused to create a Bayesian network (BN), which first splits the continuously signed sentences and labels the sub-segments SIGN or ME (motion epenthesis). A new semi-Markov CRF decoding scheme was introduced and tested, where the sub-segments classified as ME are eliminated and the remaining sign sub-segments are combined, and they were recognised by the two-layer CRF classifier.

Elakkiya and Selvamani [11] created a brand-new strategy for subunit sign modelling called enhanced dynamic programming (EDP). In EDP frameworks, dynamic time warping is utilised as a distance measure to compute the distance between two adjacent signs in sign trajectories. Sign language is composed of spatial and temporal feature vectors. For grouping of spatial feature vectors, minimum entropy clustering (MEC) is used for the grouping of these distances. According to experimental findings, the proposed system's lower computation costs and its use of the gesture base space for sign gestures is also extremely lower since it does not involve any modelling toward handling epenthesis movements.

Kumar et al. [12] proposed a multiple intraframe GM for performing temporal matching and spatial matching. Through the use of a motion capture system with eight cameras, a 3D sign language dataset of 200 continuous words in the sign language is produced to evaluate the proposed model. The technique is further confirmed by the HDM05 and CMU benchmark action datasets for 3D motion capture. Results showed that this method improves the precision of identifying signs in continuous phrases. Jayadeep et al. [13] proposed a system to create an ISL hand gesture motion translation tool for banks in order to assist the deaf-mute community in communicating by converting their ideas to text format. A succession of video frames was used to identify actions from larger, prolonged video gestures. To extract the image features, a CNN named Inception V3 was employed in this work for Australian sign language (ASL). These movements were categorised and converted into text using the long short-term memory (LSTM) architecture of the recurrent neural network (RNN). Experimental findings show that this proposed system will give an exact and useful way for the hand gesture motion system to non-signers and signers to engage.

Xie et al. [14] implemented the steps of gesture segmentation and feature extraction in conventional algorithms so that they can be skipped in a tweaked Inception V3 method. To fine-tune the model, a two-stage training technique is used as opposed to typical CNN algorithms. It also creates a feature concatenate layer in the CNN structure by utilising Red, Green, Blue (RGB) and depth images.

The methods are implemented using the American sign language (ASL) recognition dataset. The results achieved the maximum accuracy of 91.35% on the ASL. Bheda and Radpour [15] proposed a method for classifying images of both the letters and numbers in ASL using deep convolutional networks. The actual gesture units that occur in specific gesture contexts have been used in this HMM approach with sequential pattern boosting (SP-boosting), such as capturing the upper-arm movements that come before a particular letter to include that probability weight in the next unit's class.

33.3 Proposed Methodology

The methodology proposed in this system comprises of dataset collection, preprocessing, feature extraction, and classification. Using skin colour segmentation and a Gaussian filter, the signs are derived from a real-time video during the preprocessing stage. Following segmentation, a suitable feature vector is derived from the gesture sequence. The acquired features are then employed with the MDAE for classification. Figure 33.1 depicts the data flows for SLRS at several phases, including dataset collection, preprocessing, feature extraction, and sign classification.

33.3.1 Dataset Collection

The three primary processes of the SLRS are sample preprocessing, feature based extraction, and classification for better analysis. Using various skin colour segmentation techniques and a Gaussian filter, the signs are obtained from a real-time video midst the preprocessing execution. Subsequent to the segmentation process, a suitable feature vector is gathered from the gesture sequence. The collected features are then integrated with the MDAE for further precision result. Datasets for ISL and ASL are gathered from [16, 17]. The second dataset for the study was downloaded from the UCI repository. It is made up of various Indian sign languages that are frequently utilised as a form of communication. A camera was set up, and it recorded various signs, totalling about 232. Both hands have been photographed to improve the accuracy of the predictions. For training purposes, it has 2565 instances and

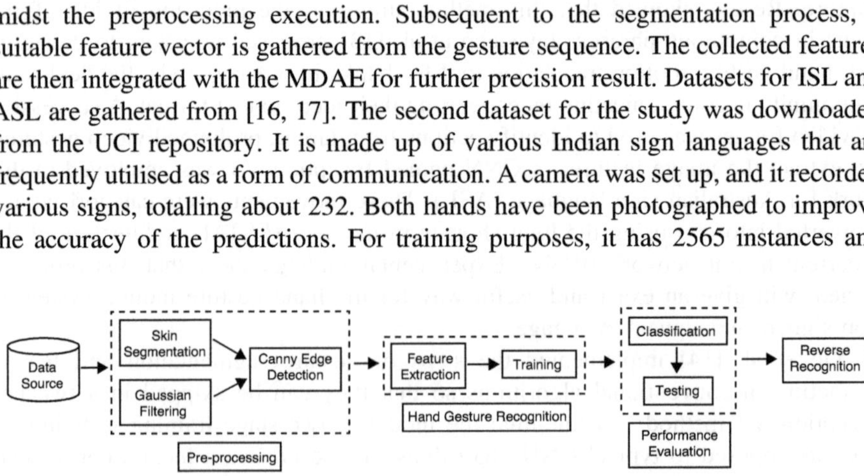

Fig. 33.1 Stages of proposed approach

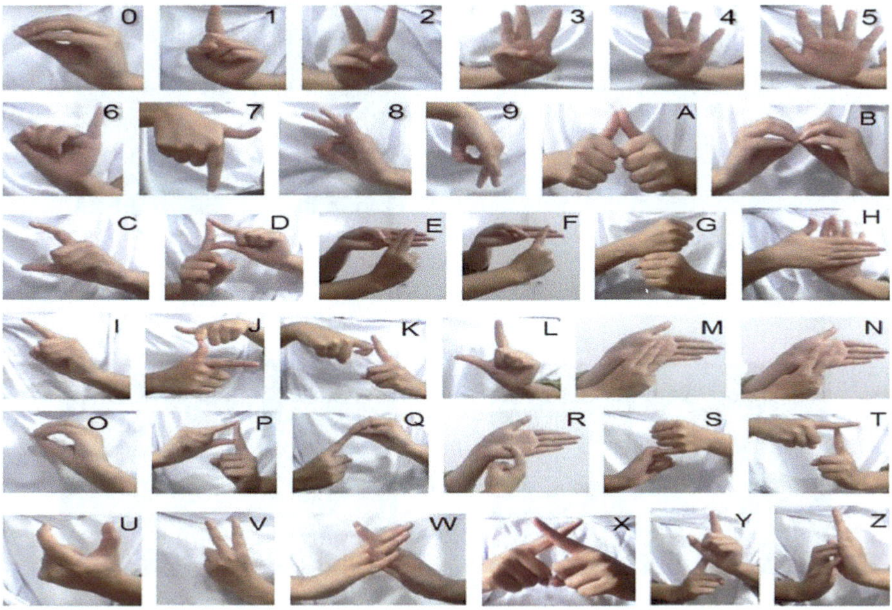

Fig. 33.2 ISL shows patient disability

22 attributes. The important attributes are X position, Y position, Z position, roll expressed, pitch expressed, yaw expressed, thumb bend, forefinger bend, middle finger bend, ring finger bend, and little finger bend (Fig. 33.2).

33.3.2 Preprocessing

At this stage, the image is prepared for feature detection and extraction (see Fig. 33.3). To maintain scale homogeneity, all of the photos have the same dimensions. In the first technique, the video frame that was obtained is translated into the Hue, Saturation, Value (HSV) colour space for the photographs that were taken against a simple background. Since the tint of the skin is distinct from that of the backdrop, it is simple to extract. The frame is then subjected to an experimental threshold that computes hue and removes the pixels with skin tones from the image. Median filter and morphological processes are introduced to further eliminate errors. The foreground portion of the current frame is determined by calculating the absolute difference between the additive total of the preceding 30 frames and the new frame for the remaining frames in the second technique for images with a running backdrop. The photos are first made greyscale, and after that the Gaussian filter is used.

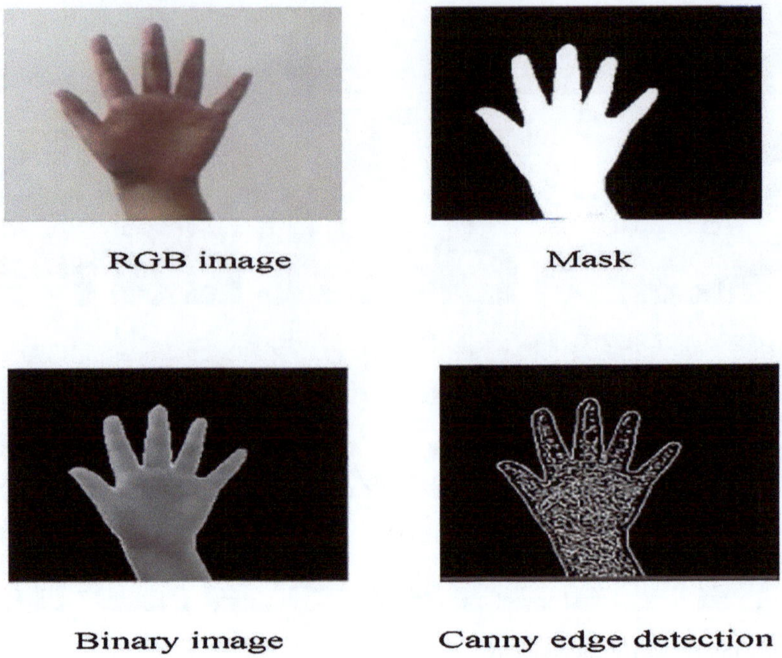

Fig. 33.3 Preprocessing proposed ISL signs patient disability

Extraction of the most linked foreground region creates a hand segmentation mask. After that, the canny function is used to determine the intensity and direction of the images' edges using the gradient of each pixel.

33.3.3 Feature Extraction

Developing a bag of visual words (BOVW) during this step entails feature extraction, feature clustering, building a codebook for the model, and creating histograms. By counting the number of times each word appears in a text, you may determine the keywords from each word's frequency and create a frequency histogram. This concept has been altered such that visual features are used as words in place of actual words. The extraction of descriptors from each image in the collection serves as the first stage in creating a BOVW. SURF, a local feature detector and descriptor, is employed for this. SURF is employed because it offers operators' box filters for quick computing and is resistant to rotation, variation, and point of view occlusion. A set of image descriptors provided by SURF is discussed in Eq. (33.1):

$$I_m = \{d_1, d_2, d_3, \ldots d_n\} \tag{33.1}$$

where n represents all of the picture descriptors and d_i represents the hands' colour, form, etc. The K-means technique can be used to do the clustering. The bag of visual words (BOVW) are Similar to K- means, but they are faster and less memory-intensive. It does not need all the data in memory at once because it uses random, fixed-size batches. In each iteration, a fresh random sample from the dataset is taken and utilised to update the clusters. This process is carried out repeatedly until convergence. The created language can be visualised using Eq. (33.2):

$$v = \{w_1, w_2, w_3, \ldots \mathrm{w}_k\} \tag{33.2}$$

where k is equal to 180, the total number of clusters. Each descriptor is mapped to the closest visual word in accordance with the Eq. (33.3):

$$w(d) = \text{argminDist}(w, d) \tag{33.3}$$

where Dist (w, d_i) denotes the distance between the visual word w and the descriptor d_i, and w (d_i) illustrates the visual word associated with the ith descriptor. The creation of histograms for each image is the final stage, which involves counting the frequency with which each visual word appears in each image:

$$\text{bin}_i = C(D_i) \tag{33.4}$$

$D_i = \{d_j, j\varepsilon 1, \ldots \ldots n \mid w(d_j) = w_i\}$. Here, C (D_i) is the cardinality that represents the count of the elements in set D_i, and D_i is the set of all the descriptors that match to a certain visual word w_i in the image. This is performed for each picture word to produce final histograms, which are delivered to the classifier for recognition.

33.3.4 Mutation Denoising Autoencoder (MDAE) for Classification

For reliable feature extraction and classification, the denoising autoencoder (DAE) is frequently utilised in the construction of deep neural architectures [18, 19]. Figure 33.4 depicts the fundamental DAE processing block. DAE can be thought of as a single-hidden-layer neural associator that uses an image as its input and outputs the sign of the input [20, 21]. For real-valued images, it has one linear decoding stage and one nonlinear encoding stage as follows:

$$h\,(y) = \sigma\,(W_1 y + b_1) \tag{33.5}$$

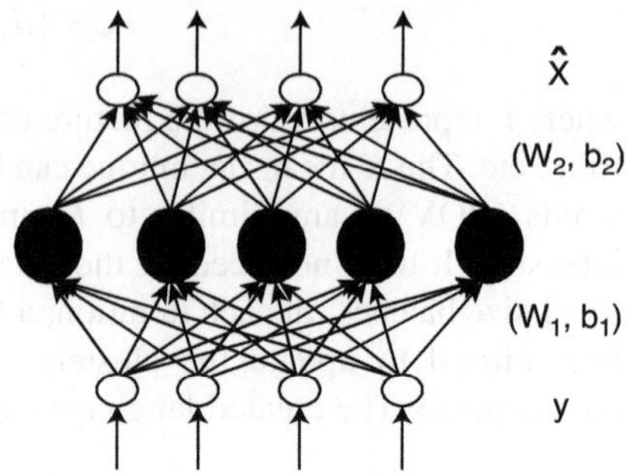

Fig. 33.4 Architecture of DAE

$$\hat{x} = W_2 h\,(y) + b_2 \tag{33.6}$$

where W_1 and W_2 are the neural network connection weights for the encoding and decoding matrices, respectively.

Input picture y and sign detected image x are the two variables, respectively. The bias vectors for the hidden and output layers are b_1 and b_2, respectively. The logistic function $\sigma\,(x) = (1 + \exp\,(-x)) - 1$ is the nonlinear function of the hidden neuron. The following optimisation is used to determine the model parameters:

$$\Theta^* = \arg\min_{\Theta} \left(L(\Theta) + \alpha \left(\|W_1\|_F^2 + \|W_2\|_F^2 \right) \right) \tag{33.7}$$

$$L(\Theta) = \frac{1}{N} \sum_{i=1}^{N} \|x_i - \hat{x}_i\|_2^2 \tag{33.8}$$

N is the total number of training samples, and x_i is the ith training clean sample corresponding to y_i, the noisy sample, where $\Theta = \{W_1, W_2, b_1, b_2\}$ is the parameter set. The mutation parameter is used to optimise the DAE's parameter set.

Mutation: The search mechanisms of five commonly used mutation strategies in DE are represented as follows:

DE/rand/1:

$$Y_i^t = X_{r_1}^t + F\left(X_{r_2}^t - X_{r_3}^t\right) \tag{33.9}$$

DE/rand /2:

$$Y_i^t = X_{r_1}^t + F\left(X_{r_2}^t - X_{r_3}^t\right) + F\left(X_{r_4}^t - X_{r_5}^t\right) \tag{33.10}$$

DE/best/ 1:

$$Y_i^t = X_{\text{best}}^t + F\left(X_{r_1}^t - X_{r_2}^t\right) \tag{33.11}$$

DE/best/2:

$$Y_i^t = X_{\text{best}}^t + F\left(X_{r_1}^t - X_{r_2}^t\right) + F\left(X_{r_3}^t - X_{r_4}^t\right) \tag{33.12}$$

DE/current-to-best/1:

$$Y_i^t = X_i^t + F\left(X_{\text{best}}^t - X_i^t\right) + F\left(X_{r_1}^t - X_{r_2}^t\right) \tag{33.13}$$

where X best denotes that the best individual solution within the DE population is chosen as the target vector; r_1 is the population index of the DE solution chosen as the base vector; r_2, r_3, r_4, and r_5 are DE population indices randomly chosen to produce the mutant vector, and F is a scaling factor used to govern the mutation process. The weighting coefficients' regularisation and reconstruction accuracy are traded off in Eq. (33.8) by the variable, which in this investigation was set to 0.0002. Numerous unconstrained optimisation strategies can be used to solve the optimisation of Eq. (33.8). For learning model parameter, a Hessian-free technique is used in this study.

33.4 Experiment and Results

This section tests the effectiveness of various classifiers using two datasets, including SVM, CNN, enhanced convolution neural network (ECNN), and suggested classifiers (ISL, and ASL). There are two sets of this dataset. Eighty percent of the data is utilised for training, and the remaining 20% is used for testing purposes. Both classifiers (ECNN and MDAE) produced good levels of accuracy for the test images, but MDAE outperformed ECNN with fewer features.

33.4.1 Quantitative Analysis

The performance of the classifiers is assessed in relation to two benchmark datasets using the precision, recall, $F1$-Score, and accuracy metrics. Precision is defined as the proportion of accurately anticipated positive observations to all positive observations. Recall is the proportion of accurately predicted positive labels to all of the positive labels combined. The weighted average of recall and precision is known as the $F1$-score:

$$\text{Precision} = \frac{\text{TP}}{\text{TP} + \text{FP}} \tag{33.14}$$

$$\text{Recall} = \frac{\text{TP}}{\text{TP} + \text{FN}} \tag{33.15}$$

$$F1 - \text{Score} = \frac{2 \times (\text{Recall} \times \text{Precision})}{\text{Recall} + \text{Precision}} \tag{33.16}$$

The simplest performance metric is accuracy, which is just the proportion of properly predicted observations to all observations. True positives (TP), true negatives (TN), false positives (FP), and false negatives (FN):

$$\text{Accuracy} = \frac{\text{TP} + \text{TN}}{\text{TP} + \text{FP} + \text{FN} + \text{TN}} \tag{33.17}$$

33.4.2 *Results Comparison*

This section compares the performance of classifiers using two benchmark datasets and four metrics. In Table 33.1, the metrics of the two datasets are compared. The accuracy attained by SVM, CNN, and ECNN is shown in Table 33.1 and Fig. 33.2. It is evident that the ECNN performs better than other algorithms in terms of accuracy.

Figure 33.5 shows the precision results comparison of classifiers such as SVM, CNN, ECNN, DAE, and MDAE with respect to ISL and ASL datasets. From the results it concludes that the proposed MDAE classifier gives better results of 95.92%, and 96.54% for ISL and ASL dataset. The other methods such as SVM, CNN, ECNN, and DAE give lesser value of 89.18%, 90.62%, 91.98%, and 93.36% for ISL dataset (see Table 33.1).

Recall results comparison of classifiers such as SVM, CNN, ECNN, DAE, and MDAE with respect to ISL and ASL datasets are illustrated in Fig. 33.6. From the results it concludes that the proposed MDAE classifier gives better results of 90.63%, and 92.83% for ISL and ASL dataset. The other methods such as SVM,

Table 33.1 Precision of classification methods vs datasets

Dataset	ISL – Results (%)					ASL – Results (%)				
Iterations/ Classifier	SVM	CNN	ECNN	DAE	MDAE	SVM	CNN	ECNN	DAE	MDAE
20	85.30	87.15	89.13	91.28	93.85	86.51	88.64	90.36	92.00	94.29
40	86.10	88.00	90.00	92.11	94.65	87.09	89.91	91.38	93.48	95.11
60	87.21	88.78	90.21	92.63	95.41	88.25	90.63	91.63	93.91	95.63
80	88.52	90.25	91.51	92.93	95.63	89.63	90.84	91.72	94.42	95.82
100	89.18	90.62	91.98	93.36	95.92	90.56	91.66	92.61	94.91	96.54

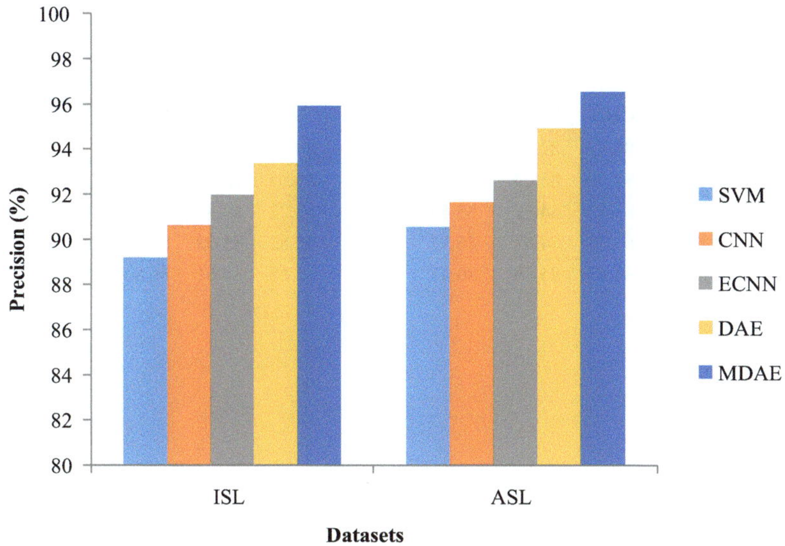

Fig. 33.5 Precision comparison of SLRS classifiers vs datasets

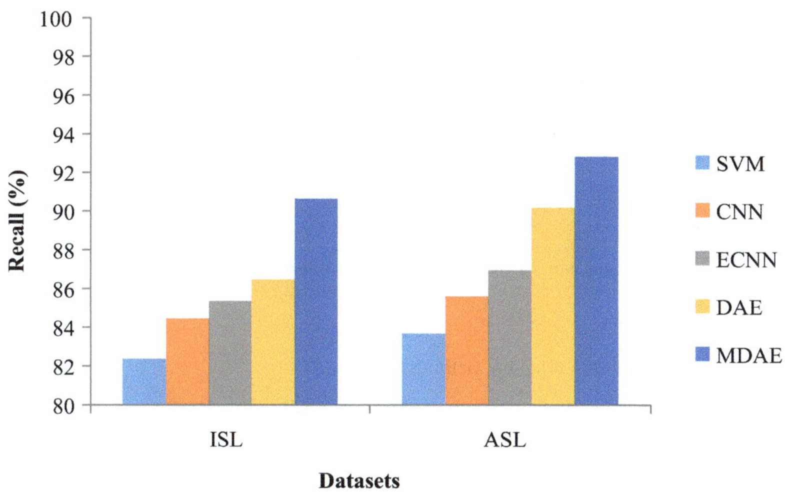

Fig. 33.6 Recall comparison of SLRS classifiers vs datasets

CNN, ECNN, and DAE give lesser value of 82.36%, 84.43%, 85.36%, and 86.47% for ISL dataset (see Table 33.2).

SVM, CNN, ECNN, DAE, and MDAE with respect to ISL and ASL datasets via F1-score results are illustrated in Fig. 33.7. The proposed MDAE classifier gives better results of 93.27%, and 94.68% for ISL and ASL dataset. The other methods such as SVM, CNN, ECNN, and DAE give lesser value of 87.12%, 88.63%, 89.78%, and 92.54% for ISL dataset (see Table 33.3).

Table 33.2 Recall of classification methods vs datasets

Dataset	ISL – Results (%)					ASL – Results (%)				
Iterations/ Classifier	SVM	CNN	ECNN	DAE	MDAE	SVM	CNN	ECNN	DAE	MDAE
20	79.56	81.32	82.94	84.78	86.24	80.66	82.71	84.68	86.28	88.38
40	80.34	82.00	83.64	85.22	87.37	81.05	83.82	85.33	87.46	89.19
60	81.63	83.12	84.32	85.69	88.42	82.22	84.41	85.82	88.63	89.63
80	81.82	83.78	84.93	85.92	89.47	82.82	85.02	86.42	89.41	91.39
100	82.36	84.43	85.36	86.47	90.63	83.68	85.61	86.95	90.18	92.83

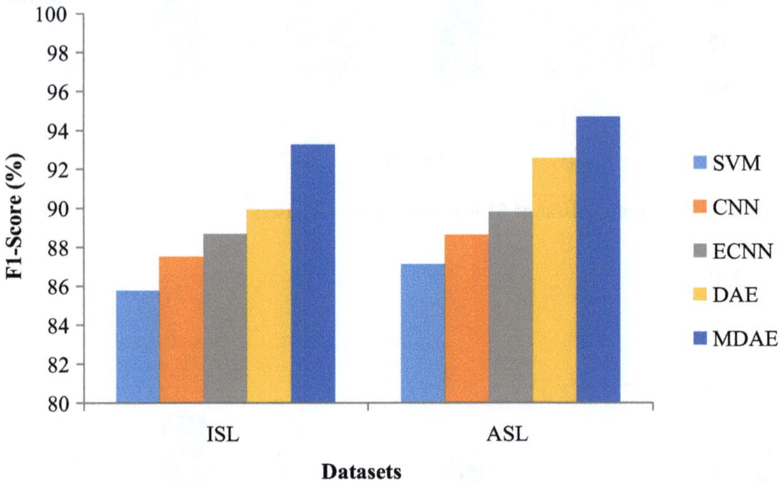

Fig. 33.7 F1-Score comparison of SLRS classifiers vs datasets

Table 33.3 F1-score of classification methods vs datasets

Dataset	ISL – Results (%)					ASL – Results (%)				
Iterations/ Classifier	SVM	CNN	ECNN	DAE	MDAE	SVM	CNN	ECNN	DAE	MDAE
20	82.43	84.23	86.03	88.03	90.04	83.58	85.67	87.52	89.14	91.33
40	83.22	85.00	86.82	88.66	91.01	84.07	86.86	88.35	90.47	92.15
60	84.42	85.95	87.26	89.16	91.91	85.23	87.52	88.72	91.27	92.63
80	85.17	87.01	88.22	89.42	92.55	86.22	87.93	89.07	91.91	93.60
100	85.77	87.52	88.67	89.91	93.27	87.12	88.63	89.78	92.54	94.68

ISL and ASL datasets via accuracy results of SVM, CNN, ECNN, DAE, and MDAE classifiers are illustrated in Fig. 33.8. The proposed MDAE classifier gives better results of 96.78%, and 97.71% for ISL and ASL dataset. The other methods

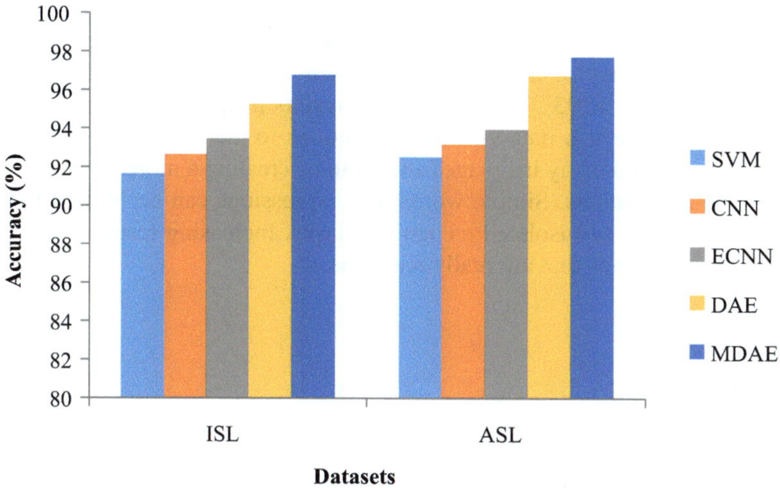

Fig. 33.8 Accuracy comparison of SLRS classifiers vs datasets

Table 33.4 Accuracy of classification methods vs datasets

DATASET	ISL – RESULTS (%)					ASL – RESULTS (%)				
Iterations/ Classifier	SVM	CNN	ECNN	DAE	MDAE	SVM	CNN	ECNN	DAE	MDAE
20	86.85	88.90	90.13	92.19	94.72	87.65	89.49	90.87	92.61	94.91
40	88.02	89.50	91.00	93.29	95.41	88.57	90.21	91.52	93.85	95.77
60	89.25	90.72	92.25	94.32	95.89	89.82	91.55	91.93	94.62	96.45
80	90.18	91.18	93.15	94.69	96.26	90.75	91.92	93.42	95.45	96.95
100	91.63	92.63	93.47	95.28	96.78	92.51	93.17	93.95	96.75	97.71

such as SVM, CNN, ECNN, and DAE give lesser value of 91.63%, 92.63%, 93.47%, and 95.28% for ISL dataset (see Table 33.4).

33.5 Conclusion and Future Work

In this paper, disability in patient discussion is introduced to categorise and identify both ISL and ASL with signs (A–Z) and numbers (0–9) by the MDAE classifier. The proposed SLRS is worked out depending on the SURF features from the image. It has the advantage of rapid computation and it is strong adjacent to rotation, orientation, etc. This proposed SLRS system is also capable of handling the issue of background dependence by continuing the camera at rest. MDAE can be thought of as a single-hidden-layer neural associator that uses an image as its input and outputs the sign of the input with optimised weight and bias from mutation. From the results, it is concluded that the proposed MDAE classifier gives the highest precision, recall, F1-score, and accuracy of ISL and ASL datasets. The proposed MDAE classifier gives 95.92%, 90.63%, 93.27%, and 96.78% results for precision, recall, F1-score, and accuracy for the ISL dataset. Future additions to the collection could include additional signs from many languages and nations, creating a more powerful system for real-time applications. Simple words and expressions can be formed using the method for constant and isolated recognition tasks. Increasing response time is the key to developing apps that are really real-time.

References

1. Bantupalli, K., & Xie, Y. (2019). American sign language recognition using machine learning and computer vision. *Master of Science in Computer Science Theses, 21*, 1–57.
2. Shivashankara, S., & Srinath, S. (2017). A comparative study of various techniques and outcomes of recognizing American sign language: A review. *International Journal of Scientific Research Engineering & Technology, 6*(9), 1013–1023.
3. Pushpa, M., & Karpagavalli, S. (2017). Multi-label classification: Problem transformation methods in Tamil phoneme classification. *Procedia Computer Science, 115*, 572–579.
4. Kong, W. W., & Ranganath, S. (2014). Towards subject independent continuous sign language recognition: A segment and merge approach. *Pattern Recognition, 47*(3), 1294–1308.
5. Theodorakis, S., Pitsikalis, V., & Maragos, P. (2014). Dynamic–static unsupervised sequentiality, statistical subunits and lexicon for sign language recognition. *Image and Vision Computing, 32*(8), 533–549.
6. Nair, A. V., & Bindu, V. (2013). A review on Indian sign language recognition. *International Journal of Computer Applications, 73*(22), 33–38.
7. Athira, P. K., Sruthi, C. J., & Lijiya, A. (2019). A signer independent sign language recognition with co-articulation elimination from live videos: An Indian scenario. *Journal of King Saud University-Computer and Information Sciences*, *34*(3), 771–781.
8. Dixit, K., & Jalal, A.S. 2013. Automatic Indian sign language recognition system. In *2013 3rd IEEE International Advance Computing Conference* (*IACC*) (pp. 883–887).
9. Otiniano-Rodrıguez, K.C., Cámara-Chávez, G., & Menotti, D. 2012. Hu and Zernike moments for sign language recognition. In *Proceedings of international conference on Image Processing, Computer Vision, and Pattern Recognition* (pp. 1–5).
10. Tripathi, K., Baranwal, N., & Nandi, G.C. 2015. Continuous dynamic Indian sign language gesture recognition with invariant backgrounds. In *International conference on Advances in Computing, Communications and Informatics* (*ICACCI*) (pp. 2211–2216).
11. Elakkiya, R., & Selvamani, K. (2018). Enhanced dynamic programming approach for subunit modelling to handle segmentation and recognition ambiguities in sign language. *Journal of Parallel and Distributed Computing, 117*, 246–255.
12. Kumar, D. A., Sastry, A. S. C. S., Kishore, P. V. V., & Kumar, E. K. (2018). Indian sign language recognition using graph matching on 3D motion captured signs. *Multimedia Tools and Applications, 77*(24), 32063–32091.
13. Jayadeep, G., Vishnupriya, N. V., Venugopal, V., Vishnu, S., & Geetha Mudra, M. (2020). Convolutional neural network based Indian sign language translator for banks. In *4th international conference on Intelligent Computing and Control Systems, 2020* (pp. 1228–1232).
14. Xie, B., He, X. Y., & Li, Y. (2018). RGB-D static gesture recognition based on convolutional neural network. *The Journal of Engineering, 2018*(16), 1515–1520.

15. Bheda, V., & Radpour, D. 2017. Using deep convolutional networks for gesture recognition in American sign language. arXiv preprint arXiv:1710.06836.
16. Sonawane, V. *Indian sign language dataset.* Kaggle. https://www.kaggle.com/datasets/vaishnaviasonawane/indian-sign-language-dataset?select=data. Accessed by 25 Apr 2022.
17. https://archive.ics.uci.edu/ml/datasets/Australian+Sign+Language+signs+(High+Quality). Accessed by 25 Apr 2022.
18. Lu, X., Tsao, Y., Matsuda, S., & Hori, C. (2013). Speech enhancement based on deep denoising autoencoder. *In Interspeech, 2013*, 436–440.
19. Li, J., Struzik, Z., Zhang, L., & Cichocki, A. (2015). Feature learning from incomplete EEG with denoising autoencoder. *Neurocomputing, 165*, 23–31.
20. Tagawa, T., Tadokoro, Y., & Yairi, T. 2015. Structured denoising autoencoder for fault detection and analysis. In *Asian conference on machine learning* (pp. 96–111).
21. Lee, W. H., Ozger, M., Challita, U., & Sung, K. W. (2021). Noise learning-based denoising autoencoder. *IEEE Communications Letters, 25*(9), 2983–2987.

Chapter 34
The Security Constructions and Enhancements of Smart Wearable Devices in Modern Technologies and Health Monitoring System

B. Jansi and V. Sumalatha

34.1 Introduction

With smart wearable devices, the concept of health management has become more focused on by the general public. According to a study from Stanford University, data collected by wearable devices can predict diseases, and people improving their health outside of fitness will become a new trend. In the global market, in the first half of 2020, in the wake of COVID-19, global total exports of smart wearables increased by another 20% per year. This shows that after experiencing an infection, people become more focused on their health and on the heart, drastically increasing the need for blood oxygen monitoring, exercise and fitness, and related equipment [1]. Counterpoint, a market research firm points out that the future growth of the smart wearable market will focus on fitness and healthcare applications.

Therefore, monitoring the blood oxygen concentration is seen in the production activities of many innards of smart intercepts this year. In medicine, blood oxygen concentration is an important indicator for diagnosing heart and lung health and overall health. Measurement data of blood oxygen concentration can be used to monitor the health status of patients' lung function. Smart health wearers play a significant role in COVID-19 infections. Koch has developed a "Coronet Data Donation" application that allows users to upload health data monitored by a sports band or smart wearable. Heart rate, sleep, amount of exercise, body temperature, and other physical symptoms monitored by sports innersoles and other devices can change significantly for those with severe respiratory illnesses [2]. The data can

B. Jansi (✉) · V. Sumalatha
Department of Computer Applications, Vels University (VISTAS), Chennai, Tamil Nadu, India
e-mail: sumalatha.scs@velsuniv.ac.in

F. J. Joseph et al. (eds.), *Computational Intelligence for Clinical Diagnosis*,
EAI/Springer Innovations in Communication and Computing,
https://doi.org/10.1007/978-3-031-23683-9_34

reflect the condition of the affected individuals and will assess the development of epidemics in Germany based on this data. As can be seen from the above, the value of health data collected by smart innersoles and other devices is starting to show. But the health data monitored by thousands of smart devices is huge and fragmented, and still worth more to cut. In the future, if smart wearables and other wearable devices offer only one health monitoring service, their competitiveness will not be enough. Only when they are integrated with health management, insurance, and medical ecology can they open up an increasing market for competitive flood health services.

Wearable devices or wearable technologies are accessories or clothing that have specific additional functionality. The main advantage of wearable computers, also called these electronic devices, is their complete integration into the user's daily life [3]. A person and a smart device are constantly communicating, but the gadget itself does not attract much attention and fits in harmoniously with reality. Typically, high-tech wearable devices are controlled by a specific operating system and fitted with several standard technologies that provide their functionality. Classic technologies used include Global positioning system (GPS), Bluetooth, Wi-Fi, Global system of mobile communication (GSM), 3G, accelerometer, compass, thermometer, chronograph, etc. Wearable devices will always multitask. For example, a smartwatch can not only show the time but also count the number of steps taken, announce incoming messages and calls, and track the user's location.

34.2 Literature Survey

In Liu et al. [4], they discussed the sensor-based activity recognition techniques in smart wearable devices. This means that the continuous operation of the sensor systems fitted on the smart devices will constantly monitor the wearer. So, even small changes that occur there will be recorded. Even the small things that are created on a daily basis can be factors that affect their efficiency [5] designed a chemical-based sensor unit for monitoring biofluids and Bandodkar et al. [7] discussed wearable chemical sensors. Different chemicals were identified and different performance matrices were analysed. Here, the chemical reactions are keenly monitored by the given methods. Fang et al. [6] discussed wearable devices for elderly people. It is also important to measure its ability to design and perform radiation functions for adults. This allows adults to wear these devices without fear. Park et al. [8] discussed the heart rate monitoring sensor and wearable devices. Doctors generally advise people with heart disease to be careful not to damage their hearts. These wearable devices can constantly monitor their heart rate by monitoring their heart rate and other cardiac functions. Al Hemairy et al. [9] discussed the health monitoring systems in the smart health care industry. Furthermore, these technologies combine with IoT technology to enable their applications to monitor the patient's activities as if they were a physician.

The key factor here is that wearable devices are commonly worn devices because of their sensors. While their enhanced capability is a combination of all types of inputs and enhances its experiments, small changes in it can have a large impact on the coda. The use of some centres that are highly sensitive to these wearable devices fitted into the body can have some kind of impact on the human body. Thus, it is necessary to meticulously weave some of the tips that occur in its design.

34.3 Wearable Devices

Wearable devices are accessories or clothing with a built-in microcomputer and interfaces and sensors that provide specific functions [10]. The main advantage of such a solution is its full integration into the daily life of the user. One person and wearable devices are in constant contact, but the latter does not attract unnecessary attention and complements reality harmoniously [11]. High-tech wearable devices operate under special operating systems and are equipped with a set of built-in sensors and interfaces. The latter includes a cellular module and wireless adapters for Bluetooth, Near field communication (NFC), and Wi-Fi. Depending on the purpose, the gadget can be equipped with a GPS receiver, accelerometer, electronic compass, thermometer, barometer, heart rate monitor, chronometer, etc. Modern wearable devices are multi-functional [12]. For example, a "smart" watch can not only show the time and date but also calculate the number of steps taken by the user, announce incoming messages and calls to the connected smartphone via Bluetooth, and track the user's location.

34.3.1 SmartWatch

Since the appearance of smartphones, to make them easier to manage, they have a kind of assistant device, an additional device for the smartphone: the SmartWatch. People wanted to make watches rather than toy watches to show time and date. Now "smartwatches" are integrated into mobile devices based on features and software, a notable example of which is the watch. However, the definition of a "smartwatch" is highly controversial [13]. A proper smartwatch is not defined by any international standards. In Japan, the first true "smartwatch" has been released, and it was created by Sony. The Sony SmartWatch acts like a traditional watch and, when linked to a compatible smartphone, offers a plethora of features, including access to real-time information like news and text messages, as well as alerts and reminders [14]. Of course, numerous smaller companies had already come up with their own versions of such devices before Sony unveiled its SmartWatch. Even before the Japanese electronics review [15], Chinese manufacturers had created timepieces that could make phone calls and connect to the Internet. Despite their high quality and dependability standards, these gadgets have already implemented the notion of "smartwatches" [8] that can make and receive phone calls, send and receive text messages, process information, perform computations, and connect to the Internet. In addition, several makers of consumer electronics are wrapping up production on their own versions of this kind of smartwatch. Apple, for instance, has filed for a patent on an "iWatch" in Japan and other countries. In September, Qualcomm plans to release the Zola SmartWatch. Rumour has it that Intel is testing a comparable product. Samsung has revealed they are working on a smartwatch right now. Similarly, Google is rumoured to be working on an Android-powered clock [16].

However, the Android OS–powered smartwatch that can receive calls and take images is reported to be the first of its kind to be introduced to a group of Indian students [17]. The Androiduli is a $150 Indian smartphone that supports Bluetooth. GPS and Wi-Fi are all supported. The Pebble, MotoActv, and WIMM One watches are a few others worth mentioning. The Pebble Watch is a popular Kickstarter project [18]. The 1.26-inch LCD display can provide 144 by 168 pixels. With a 600 MHz OMAP3 ARMv7 processor, 256 MB of RAM, 8 GB of memory, and Bluetooth connectivity, the MotoActv is Motorola's take on the smartwatch. The FM Tuner and Android power this wristwatch. WIMM One has a 220 × 176 pixel [13] display with a screen size of 1.6 inches. They are powered by an altered version of Android and have a see-through display, a magnetometer, an accelerometer, and Bluetooth, Wi-Fi, and USB connectivity [19].

34.3.2 Computer Glasses

Google Glasses introduced a new era of wearable technology. Yes, before "good review", similar devices were offered many times, but none of them. Google Glass seems to have installed a new type of consumer electronics [20]. Glass differs from other similar devices by its small size and many features, such as "augmented reality", a camera, Internet access, and voice-based communication. Google Glass is not only a wearable computer but also an "ubiquitous" computer, meaning that it may be used in both an active and passive capacity. The device has a 5-megapixel camera with a bone transducer sensor, Wi-Fi, Bluetooth, a gyroscope, an accelerometer, a magnetometer, and a touchscreen control panel. Android powers Google Glass, which is powered by a dual-core OMAP 4430 processor. It is believed that more companies, inspired by Google Glass, will soon introduce similar products to the market. Scope Technologies, which has collaborated with Epson on the development of computer glasses, the Spark of Cypriot, whose glasses make it possible to see and study tiny objects, and Innova, which creates breakthrough computer lenses, are all involved in the Vuzix project. Despite claims that it is a major rival to Google Glass, not much is known about this product at this time.

34.3.3 Wearable Computers

Wearable computers are less cumbersome and difficult to operate presently. Small, high-capacity batteries perform well enough to power wearable electronics. Modern devices with high-quality displays make using them much more straightforward. We have greatly improved the system's touch input, so it is much more sensitive to your touches. The CPUs also perform better without getting too hot. They are currently impregnated with dust and even water-proof tiles. The sensors themselves are compact. Who would have guessed that something as thin as 7.9 mm could house an infrared camera, accelerometer, barometer, thermometer, proximity sensor, pedometer, and gyroscope? As battery manufacturers compete to produce the most energy-efficient products, things are looking brighter. For example, the Koreans claim to have created a flexible battery similar to flexible displays. File Sharing can easily be shared outside network via removable media. Offering access to digital information or resources. In addition, hydrophobic technology is so advanced that devices no longer need to be sealed to be waterproof.

34.3.4 Medical Gadgets

A smartphone-sized device that detects cancer and infections within 20 minutes. This gadget is based on the research of the British review Quantum. The Q-Poc Alpha is now in the testing phase, and the finished product will not appear until 2018, as promised by the developers. Drug abuse causes 125,000 deaths a year in the United States. To rectify the situation, US review AdhereTech has developed a tablet box with sensors that read the number of container openings [21]. The smart system reminds you to take medications with sounds, LEDs, phone calls, and text messages sent to the patient's phone. The lipstick level test microscope allows you to independently determine the amount of ovulation by the concentration of salt in the saliva sample. To do this, apply a drop of saliva on the lens, let it dry for 5–-10 minutes, and then evaluate the result on the eyelids. To accurately determine the phase of the cycle, you need to compare what you see with the checklist. An inexpensive miniature device, such as a USB flash drive, connects to the human body using four Velcro electrodes, reads data about the work of the heart, and sends it to a cardiologist via the Android app. Most likely, everything will come to this. Technologies are evolving towards smart clothing. But there are several important technical limitations here. First, direct skin contact is required to accurately capture heart rate and other data. That is, the sensors must fit snugly against the body, which means smart clothing must be tight. It may not be very comfortable to wear such clothes every day. Some techniques will help, which will allow taking data at a distance of 2–3 cm from the body.

On the other hand, even if a person measures his parameters only 2–3 times a day for 5–10 minutes, the data obtained is sufficient to establish a diagnosis and make recommendations. You can take a cardiogram in a relaxed state, and based on this, doctors will tell you whether or not to change your lifestyle. Who is it for? For example, those who have a heart attack, as a rule, have a risk of recurrence. Therefore, they should regularly take a cardiogram and send information to doctors. There are already devices that pierce the fingers in a non-invasive way (laser). In general, insulin pumps are now widespread abroad; they are a box in the body that holds an automatic insulin injection device depending on the blood sugar level. This is a very important device for patients with type 1 diabetes. They are forced to take a basic dose (called long insulin) in the morning and the right dose (short insulin) during the meal. Long-acting insulin is more harmful than short-acting insulin because it raises blood sugar. These pumps allow the short-lived insulin to dispense automatically as the sugar level changes. In Russia, such devices are not made: they are very expensive. Instead, they use insulin injections, which are provided free of charge by the Ministry of Health. All automatic injectors must be imported.

34.4 Modern Technology

It has become customary to see people wearing smart devices that can be worn. Typically, these smartwatches or electronic straps are used to monitor fitness. Due to the advanced technology of sensors, wearable devices are starting to encourage more people to be more active. They help people set and achieve goals, as well as provide a sense of motivation and reward when achieving these goals. As technology has advanced so much, new limitations on wearable devices are helping people improve their fitness. Here is a range of wearable accessories that can get you started on a healthy lifestyle.

34.4.1 Fitbit Smart Wearable

Fitbit dominates the wearable device market. Its simple design, usability, and affordability make it an impressive wearable device. Continuous heart monitoring means that your activity is constantly being recorded. Keep track of how many calories you are burning, as well as make sure you are working at the right intensity.

34.4.2 Jawbone Smart Wearable

The Jawbone is a device for fashion-conscious fitness enthusiasts. If you do not want to wear a bold smartwatch and want something that looks beautiful, Jawbone offers a wide variety of stylish and elegant accessories. Jawbone UP2 monitors your activity, sleep, and food intake. The smart trainer provides you with customised insights to help you achieve your fitness goals.

34.4.3 Microsoft Smart Wearable

Microsoft has jumped on the bandwagon of wearable devices and has developed a device that can detect heart rate, exercise, calorie-burning, and sleep quality. Microsoft, as a device, connects the user to email, text, and calendar. The band has 11 sensors, such as a barometer, an ultraviolet monitor, and GPS.

34.4.4 Activated Steel Smart Wearable

The Activated Steel looks pretty cool on this list. If you have always moved but want a sophisticated wearable device, the Activated Steel is the device to buy. It monitors daily activities such as running, walking, sleeping, and how many calories you burn. It is water-resistant up to 50 metres, which means you can use it to monitor your light swimming. This device requires charging as the replaceable battery lasts up to 8 months.

34.4.5 Apple Smart Wearable

Apple has acquired smartwatches for those who want to get a piece of wearable functionality. Apple Watch has released the Sport for fitness enthusiasts. With the silicone band, the Apple Watch Sport is lightweight and comfortable on the wrist while in operation. The clock includes a heart rate monitor and an accelerometer that monitors activity throughout the day. If you are an avid Apple user and want to sync everything with your iPhone, this is the device.

34.4.6 Samsung Smart Wearable

The Samsung Gear S2 is similar to the Apple Watch. It can perform the functions of a regular smartwatch, but this device emphasises fitness within the design. The straps are made of a silicone-like material, which is dustproof and water-resistant up to 3 metres. The application monitors your activity throughout the day and changes the application accordingly. The quick access to information from the gear screen. There is a built-in heart rate monitor to monitor your heart rate before and after the procedure. You can buy the Samsung Gear S2 with leather straps, which will look like a regular watch if not the one that catches your attention. Samsung is proud to be one of the first wearable devices to be compatible with most Android phones.

34.4.7 Moto Smart Wearable

With the success of the first generation of the Moto 360, Motorola has acquired the Moto 360 Sport. It has IP67 dust and water resistance, making it durable for heavy workouts. The Moto 360 Sport has seven sensors, including a heart rate monitor, an accelerometer, and an ambient light sensor. Lightweight silicone pads are available in black, white, and flame orange. Even with high usage, the battery will last for a whole day. You can add your Moto 360 Sport with a wireless charging dock.

34.5 Security Measurements

The increase in the number of smartphones in 2007 is being monitored by various businesses. Security arrangements that began to enter inside in some way have now reached the prime location. Devices that monitor physiological fitness changes, such as the Fitbit and Jawbone UP, are currently in high demand. These are designed to store your health data on smartphones and thereby provide information about your health. In particular, the smartwatches of companies like Apple have the most sophisticated improvements. Its GPS module is capable of tracking anyone from wherever you are. There are security flaws in such sophisticated achievements.

Usually, these wearable devices are connected to your mobile phones. Hence, activities like attacks or hacking on them can also affect the exposure of your wearable devices. The process by which these functions affect the functionality of your wearable devices is called a "weak connection problem". Its problems are going to be left to you alone. Your wearable devices can also affect the product company.

A skilled hacker can even access that company's server settings via your wearable devices. Most wearable devices have a very small design. Also, these can be easily stolen if their data is connected to a smartphone or computer. Hence, start using it only after you know how to handle it before you use the wearable device. Companies are constantly updating data to escape from these problems and often store the data securely on the cloud server and erase the data and temp information on the local server.

34.6 Inference and Discussions

Highly sensitive sensors fitted to enhance your daily life will not only amaze you but also ensure your safety. Scientists have even begun to design clothes made with smart devices. These dresses, which were initially seen as a big deal, are now becoming more commonly available on the market. Its rise is to be loved and worn by everyone, from children to adults. Rather than simply replacing digitally made jewellery, smart sensors are integrated into your body and monitor your entire body. And with the advanced technology in them, you can easily find yourself wherever you go and save yourself in times of danger. Communication will be easier for you if you have wearable clothes instead of jewellery. Wearable devices that are usually traditionally made are upgraded based on certain health benefits. Using it for a short period and throwing it away is a simple process, but jewellery is not like that. You may always be compelled to wear it. Its special feature is that the smart clothes designed in this manner are comfortable to wear and easy to wash. And for some, as a baby gets older, he or she will outgrow this. The needs of elegant fabric designers and technicians will be very important in designing this. This technology is considered feasible in terms of fabric smart sensors and biometric smart sensor speeds.

The detection of certain significant health conditions in most smart clothing technologies is considered to be the key factor in improving their design. Diabetes is considered to be the most important problem at present. Smart devices are designed to constantly monitor this and help keep patients constantly monitored. It also constantly monitors the patient's body changes and conditions of injuries and constantly raises the appropriate conditions to perform medical first aid accordingly. In this process, it is important to test the physical well-being of the diabetic patient in advance. The cause of skin allergies is a rise in elemental temperature. Thus, the increase in the temperature of the feet indicates a large number of ulcers occurring in that area. Smart wearable socks are designed with this in mind. High-pressure sensor devices are attached to these socks. Thus, there is no need to connect any other devices to monitor body temperature and diabetes. The use of these socks alone is sufficient.

The Wearable-Socks are only available for a limited time; in freezing temperatures, they leave you wanting to snooze in style. Intelligent socks would assist wearable electronics to move toward digital human for diversified applications. The submission gives foot cleanliness marks and warns the client to correct the occupation and/or consult a health-care expert if desired. Clients who are equipped with this novel knowledge can change their utility by self-surviving their skin warmth. This procedure can be included in the daily routine to make sure glucose stage.

34.7 Future Work

We discovered how to build Wearable 2.0 to be good-looking and functional. For example, OM-signal from Canada has designed a game spinner for women that can detect heartbeat and inhalation and provide personalised flow recommendations. Consumer bio-sensors embedded in the inner lining of clothing collect consumer information at the foundation of movement (rather than wrist measurements) to provide more precise advice. These smart devices are put together with an iPhone application, which over time becomes accustomed to the user's body and allows them to supply more reliable preparation. AIQ-Smart Clothing is considered to be another thing that combines wearable clothes with technological devices. Its sensitivity is further enhanced by the fact that it is sewn directly into fabrics with stainless steel threads. As a result, it does not require plating with copper or silver materials also developing into an advanced technology that further enhances the production of gloves on devices that operate in touch panel mode. In this, a special thread of light-penetrating nature is attached to the fingertips. Its sensitivity is high, so its use in the fashion sector is enhanced. This type of clothing for kids can be designed and styled more elegantly. Some specialised sensor systems can be set up to detect the baby's body temperature and oxygen levels. The baby's heart rate can also be accurately monitored. Thus, the sensor systems will immediately report any discomfort from the child's grief and its safety deficiencies. Based on these measurements, the team plans to make appropriate arrangements for the user to easily use or carry the smart devices we plan to build.

34.8 Conclusion

Generally, the smart wearable device technologies with advanced technology currently being designed should be helpful to most humans. Users will trust and buy those wearable devices only if their functionality is fast and of high quality. In many of the leading companies, these types of wearable device technologies are automatically developed and implemented to the extent that they are given artificial intelligence to collect the data for the given jobs and check and make their own decisions. The only real problems are when it comes to security management. These wearable devices cannot do the right amount of work if data is altered or stolen. And the accuracy of the results makes it difficult for users to choose. Therefore, the size and strength of its security improvements measure not only the buyers but also the value of the companies that make them.

References

1. Lee, H. S., Park, S. W., & Heo, H. (2016). Acute acquired comitant esotropia related to excessive smartphone use. *BMC Ophthalmology, 16*(1), 1–7.
2. Kolodzey, L., Grantcharov, P. D., Rivas, H., Schijven, M. P., & Grantcharov, T. P. (2017). Wearable technology in the operating room: A systematic review. *BMJ Innovations Journal, 3*, 55–63.
3. Anaya, L. H. S., Alsadoon, A., Costadopoulos, N., & Prasad, P. W. C. (2018). Ethical implications of user perceptions of wearable devices. *Science and Engineering Ethics, 24*(1), 1–28. https://doi.org/10.1007/s11948-017-9872-8. Epub 2017 Feb 2. PMID: 28155094
4. Liu, Y., Nie, L., Liu, L., & Rosenblum, D. S. (2016). From action to activity: Sensor-based activity recognition. *Neurocomputing, 181*, 108–115.
5. Matzeu, G., Florea, L., & Diamond, D. (2015). Advances in wearable chemical sensor design for monitoring biological fluids. *Sensors and Actuators B: Chemical, 211*, 403–418.

6. Fang, Y. M., & Chang, C. C. (2016). Users' psychological perception and perceived readability of wearable devices for elderly people. *Behaviour & Information Technology, 35*(1–3), 225–232.
7. Bandodkar, A. J., Jeerapan, I., & Wang, J. (2016). Wearable chemical sensors: Present challenges and prospects. *ACS Sensors, 1*(5), 464–482.
8. Parak, J., Tarniceriu, A., Renevey, P., Bertschi, M., Delgado-Gonzalo, R., Korhonen, I. (2015). Evaluation of the beat-to-beat detection accuracy of Pulse On wearable optical heart rate monitor. In *Proceedings of the 37th Annual International Conference of the IEEE Engineering in Medicine and Biology Society* (pp. 8099–8102), IEEE.
9. Al Hemairy, M., Shani, M., Amin, S., & Alahmad, M. (2018). A comprehensive framework for elderly healthcare monitoring in a smart environment. In M. Dastbaz, H. Arabnia, & B. Akhgar (Eds.), *Technology for smart futures* (pp. 113–140). Springer. https://doi.org/10.1007/978-3-319-60137-3_6
10. Patel, M. S., Asch, D. A., & Volpp, K. G. (2015). Wearable devices as facilitators, not drivers, of health behavior change. *JAMA, 313*(5), 459–460.
11. Chen, M., Ma, Y., Song, J., Lai, C., & Hu, B. (2016). Smart clothing: Connecting humans with clouds and big data for sustainable health monitoring. *Mobile Networks and Applications, 21*, 1–21.
12. Shelgikar, A. V., Anderson, P., & Stephens, M. R. (2016). Sleep tracking, wearable technology, and opportunities for research and clinical care. *Chest Journal, 50*(3), 732–743.
13. Deep, S., Zheng, X., Karmakar, C., et al. (2020). A survey on anomalous behavior detection for elderly care using dense-sensing networks. *IEEE Communications Surveys & Tutorials, 22*(1), 352–370.
14. Shoaib, M., Scholten, H., Havinga, P.J.M. (2013). Towards physical activity recognition using smartphone sensors. In *2013 IEEE 10th international conference on Ubiquitous Intelligence & Computing and 2013 IEEE 10th International Conference on Autonomic & Trusted Computing* (pp 80–87), Sorrento.
15. Demir, E., Demir, K., Odabaşı, S., & Odabaşı, F. (2016). A challenge for higher education: Wearable technology for fashion design departments. *World Journal on Educational Technology, 8*(1), 69–77.
16. Stoppa, M., & Chiolerio, A. (2014). Wearable electronics and smart textiles: A critical review. *Sensors, 14*(7), 11957–11992.
17. Thierer AD (2015) The internet of things and wearable technology: Addressing privacy and security concerns without derailing innovation. In Adam Thierer, The internet of things and wearable technology: Addressing privacy and security concerns without derailing innovation (p. 21).
18. Yang, J., Wei, D., Tang, L., Song, X., Luo, W., Chu, J., Gao, T., Shi, H., & Du, C. (2015). Wearable temperature sensor based on graphene nanowalls. *RSC Advances, 5*(32), 25609–25615.
19. Kim, S., Lee, Y., & Lee, H. (2020). Heating effect on the upper body for developing exothermic smart wear. *Korean Journal of Human Ecology, 29*(3), 371–383.
20. Guesmi, C., Mabrouk, I. B., Had, L., Talb, L., & Gharsallah, A. (2016). G-shaped dual-band wearable button antenna for ISM band applications. *International Journal on Communications Antenna and Propagations, 6*(1), 39–43.
21. Sohn, J. W., Han, G. G., Choi, S. B., et al. (2016). Vibro-tactile actuator for smart wear applications using piezoelectric ceramic transducers. *Transactions of the Korean Society for Noise and Vibration Engineering, 26*(7), 881–887.

Chapter 35
Hinokitiol Attenuates LPS-Induced Arthritic Inflammation: A Preclinical Perspective

S. M. Gunjegaonkar, S. L. Nargund, A. A. Joshi, and A. V. Bhalerao

35.1 Introduction

In 1936 a Japanese chemist Tetsuo Nozoe discovered hinokitiol (β-thujaplicin) and isolated the essential oil as a monoterpenoid from Taiwanese hinoki heart wood belonging to the family Cupressaceous [1]. In Japan, "Hinoki" is referred to as a slow-growing tree that mainly contains tropolone hence the name Hinokitiol (Hinoki + tropolone) [2]. Hinokitiol is commonly incorporated in oral, skin care products, and food additives. It is also used as construction wood for long-standing buildings and temples. Hinokitiol plays a crucial role in plant survival by its ability to repel insects, pests, and moulds for years. In recent years hinokitiol has been profoundly considered and revealed its noteworthy broad-spectrum activities. Hinokitiol has been reported for its various in vivo and in vitro activities like antimicrobial and anticancer activity [3], antifungal [4], antiviral [5], antiproliferative [6], anti-inflammatory [7], and antiplasmodial activity [8]. Hinokitiol did not show any carcinogenic effect on rats [9]. Arthritis is highly prevailed in developing and developed countries. Studies have advocated that joint diseases are one of the greatest reasons for work disabilities and compromised performance [10]. Furthermore, these lead to mental stress and economic burden on the patient and caretaker [11]. The patient seeks pharmacotherapy as the symptoms like pain, inflammation, swelling, stiffness, and redness of joints become

S. M. Gunjegaonkar (✉) · A. A. Joshi
ASPM's KT Patil College of Pharmacy, Osmanabad, Maharashtra, India

S. L. Nargund
Nargund College of Pharmacy, Bangalore, Karnataka, India

A. V. Bhalerao
JSPM's Charak College of Pharmacy and Research, Pune, Maharashtra, India

F. J. J. Joseph et al. (eds.), *Computational Intelligence for Clinical Diagnosis*, EAI/Springer Innovations in Communication and Computing,
https://doi.org/10.1007/978-3-031-23683-9_35

unbearable and limit day-to-day activities. The current pharmacotherapy involves symptomatic treatments through NSAIDs, corticosteroids, and disease-modifying antirheumatic drugs (DMARDs) [12]. However, these drugs are providing relief to a certain extent and need to be taken chronically. Several studies reported that long-term consumption of NSAIDs is associated with hepatic and nephrotoxicity, GI bleeding, etc. [13]. Corticosteroids cause suppression of immunity and provoke chances of acquired infections, hyperglycaemia, fluid retention, hypertension, and disturbed hormonal balance [14]. DMARDs are advised in rheumatic arthritis with caution as their chronic consumption leads to liver and kidney damage and GI disturbances [15]; taking into consideration the limitations of currently available pharmacotherapy for arthritis, it is considered extremely necessary to find out the more effective and safe anti-arthritic candidate. Hence, the present research was carried out to tap the prospective anti-arthritis effect of hinokitiol in experimental animals [16].

35.2 Material and Methods

35.2.1 Chemicals, Pieces of Equipment and Instruments Used

Hinokitiol was procurement from Sigma Aldrich, Shimadzu UV-1800 spectrophotometer was used for assay readings, and semi-auto-analyser was used for marker enzyme estimation using marketed kits (Asritha Diatech). All chemicals used for experimental work were of analytical grades.

35.2.2 Preparation of Hinokitiol

The selection of dose and preparation of hinokitiol was performed by referring to earlier studies. As hinokitiol was provided in the form of a solid in the quantity of 5gm considering the same, the stock of it was prepared in dimethyl sulfoxide (DMSO). The dose of hinokitiol dose was reported in the range of 0.1–0.5 mg/Kg in the rat, and based on that, two doses of it were selected. The 0.2 and 0.4 mg/kg of hinokitiol was designated as H-1 and H-2, respectively [17].

35.2.3 Preparation of Lipopolysaccharide (LPS)

Phosphate-Buffered Saline (PBS) buffer (pH 7.4) was prepared and sterilized by autoclaving (20 min, 121 °C). The LPS was dissolved in PBS buffer to get a concentration of 5 mg/ml. 1 mg/Kg LPS doses were selected for arthritis induction. The LPS was stored in a deep freezer at −20 °C temperature when not required [17–19].

35.2.4 *Preparation of Indomethacin*

The standard drug (indomethacin) was obtained from the institutional store. 1% acacia was prepared, and indomethacin was added to obtain a 100 mg/ml concentration. A dose of 30 mg/Kg orally was used for the study [18, 19].

35.2.5 *Experimental Protocol*

Before the commencement of animal experimentation, the Intuitional Animal Ethical Committee (IAEC) approval for the said study was obtained (Ref. No. JSPM/CCOPR/2018-19/04). After a specified period, the animals were indiscriminately allocated into 5 groups of 6 animals. Each experimental group has 6 animals, and the allocation of animals is carried out by random method. Vehicle control group animals received water orally. Arthritic control animals received LPS 1 mg/ml/Kg intra-plantar on day 0. Standard treated animals received indomethacin 30 mg/Kg orally for 7 days and LPS 1 mg/ml/Kg intra-plantar on day 0. H-1 treated animals received hinokitiol 0.2 mg/Kg IP for 7 days and LPS 1 mg/ml/Kg intra-plantar on day 0. H-2 treated animals received hinokitiol 0.4 mg/Kg IP for 7 days and LPS 1 mg/ml/Kg intra-plantar on day 0.

35.2.6 *In Vivo Evaluation of the Severity of Arthritic Inflammation*

35.2.6.1 Change in Paw Volume and Arthritis Index

A mercury plethysmometer was used to measure the change in paw volume. The circular mark was made with the permanent marker on the right hind paw at the tibiotarsal junction. The change in paw volume was noted before treatment and after treatment in respective groups with intervals of 7 days for a period from 0 to 28 days. The change in paw volume was expressed in millilitres of mercury [20]. The change in the arthritic index is directly proportional to the severity of arthritis. The arthritic index was determined per day using the following formula [19]:

$$\text{Arthritis Index} = \text{Hind paw vol.(Final)} - \text{hind paw vol.(Initial)} / \text{Hind paw vol.(Initial)} \times 100$$

35.2.6.2 Change in Paw Thickness

The arthritis severity was investigated by measuring alters in paw thickness using calibrated Vernier calliper [19]. The ipsilateral paw thickness was measured before and after treatment with intervals of 7 days for a period from 0 to 28 days. The percent change in paw thickness was determined on the 7th, 14th, 21st, and 28th day using the following formula [19, 21]:

$$\text{Final paw thickness} - \text{Initial paw thickness}/\text{Initial paw thickness} \times 100$$

35.2.6.3 Change in Body Weight

The calibrated digital weighing balance of 1Kg capacity was used to determine the change in animal weight in all the groups [22]. The weighing of all animals was carried out on 0 and 7 days of treatment protocol between 9:00 am and 10:00 am. The following formula was used to determine the change in body weight [19, 22]:

$$\begin{aligned}\text{Change in mean body weight} = {} & \text{Animal weight in gms(Final)} \\ & - \text{Animal weight in gms(Initial)}/ \\ & \text{Animal weight in gms(Initial)} \times 100\end{aligned}$$

35.2.7 Estimation of Serum Marker Enzymes

The blood was collected from the eye (orbital plexus) by retro-orbital plexus on the 28th day. About 1 ml of blood sample was collected in the clean and sterilized in Effendroff's tubes and kept aside for clotting. The collected blood sample was subjected to centrifugation for 15 min at 3000 g. The serum was separated using a micropipette and kept in the refrigerator for further investigation of serum marker enzymes, namely, serum glutamic-oxaloacetic transaminase (SGOT), alkaline phosphatase (ALP), serum glutamic pyruvic transaminase (SGPT) and antioxidant enzymes. The estimation was carried out using a semi-autoanalyzer as per the procedure given by the manufacturer.

35.2.8 Tissue Preparation

As per the previously reported method, the articular tissue was prepared briefly as on the 28th day of the treatment protocol, animals were subjected to scarification using the cervical dislocation method, and the tibia-tarsal bones were gently removed. The tissue was cut into small pieces and subjected to homogenization with Tris-HCl buffer (50 mM) pH 7.4. Further, the homogenate sample was triturated with NaCl (0.1 M) Triton X-100(0.1%) using a conventional mortar and pestle and put for sonication for 5 min. The resulting sample was subjected to homogenization at 3000 g for 5 min. The resulting aliquots were used for the estimation of superoxide dismutase (SOD), catalases (CAT), glutathione Peroxidase (GPx), myeloperoxidase (MPO), cathepsin D (CAT D), and elastase (ELA) enzyme activities [18, 19, 23].

35.2.9 Estimation of Antioxidant Enzyme Activity

The activity of SOD is measured by inhibition of auto-oxidation of pyrogallol by measuring absorbance at 420 nm. The sample contains 50 mM Tris-cacodylic acid buffer with pH 8.5 with 0.2 mM pyrogallol and 1 mM diethylene-triamine penta acetic acids. The reaction mixture was subjected to incubation for 90 s at 25 °C. The rate of inhibition of pyrogallol auto-oxidation by 50% by SOD is used for the estimation of enzyme activity [19, 24]. The CAT activity was estimated using the method reported by Gunjegaonkar 2018 & Nam et al. 2006 [19, 25]. The method involves the rate of decomposition of a substrate (H_2O_2) at 240 nm to determine the CAT activity. The procedure briefly involves a reaction mixture of 10% homogenate (in buffer 0.1 M), phosphate buffer (0.01 M and pH 7.0), and distilled water. The mixture was incubated at 37 C with the addition of H_2O_2 (0.2 M) and terminated with dichromate: acetic acid reagent (1:3) for 1 min. Further, the test mixture was boiled for 15 min and at 1500 g for 10 min [19]. The index of inhibition of lipid peroxidation (GPx) was determined as per previously reported methods. The reaction mixture consists of H_2O_2, an articular sample (prepared in 0.1 M Tris-HCl buffer solution with pH 7.2), 1 mM Glutathione (GHS), and 0.2 mM NADPH. The reaction mixture was kept for 5 min at 25 °C. The consumption of NADPH for peroxidation of GSH was estimated by reading the absorbance at 340 nm [19, 25, 26].

35.2.10 Estimation of Cartilage Degrading Enzymes

The MPO concentration was evaluated after homogenising tissue in 20 mM potassium phosphate buffer (pH 7.0) for 30 min at 20,000 g and 4 °C. The supernatant containing 0.5% hexadecyl-tri methyl ammonium bromide in 50 mM potassium phosphate buffer, pH 6, was isolated. After 60 s of sonication, the reaction mixture was centrifuged at 20,000 g for 30 min at 4 °C. H_2O_2 and o-dianisidine-dihydrochloride were added to the supernatant. MPO activity fluoresced red at 405 nm as U/g of protein [18, 23]. Calculating cathepsin D concentration [18, 27]. A 0.3 ml homogenate and 1 ml buffered substrate were incubated at 45 ° C for 2 h. We stopped the reaction by adding 10% TCA and waiting 30 min at room temperature. The centrifuged reaction mixture was then analysed. After combining supernatant, sodium hydroxide, and phenolic reagent, 620 nm absorbance was measured. The standard curve for CAT-D activity was plotted using 40–200 nanomoles of tyrosine [18, 27]. ELA activity correlates with synovial polymorphonuclear (PMN). Homogenized tissue samples and 20 mM potassium phosphate buffer, pH 7.0, are mixed 1:10 (w/v). Separating the components took 20 min at 10,000 g and 4 °C. Aliquots of each sample were treated in 0.1 M Tris-HCl buffer (pH 8.0) containing 0.5 M NaCl and 1 ml M N-methoxysuccinyl-Ala-Ala-Pro-Val p-nitroanilide at 37 °C for 24 h (specific substrate for ELA). ELA's activity was measured by p-nitroanilide emitted at 405 nm [18, 23].

35.2.11 Estimation of Blood Cell Count and Erythrocyte Sedimentation Rate (ESR)

The numbers of RBCs were determined by using the haemocytometer method reported by Ghai et al. [28]. The Hayme's reagent fluid was prepared, and the blood sample was sucked in the Thoma red cell diluting pipette up to 0.5 marks. The Hayme's diluting fluid was sucked up to the 101 marks to get a 1:200 dilution of a blood sample. The fluid was filled in the numbers counting chamber and viewed under the compound light microscope. The RBC count was expressed as the number of erythrocytes present per cubic mm of the blood. The WBC count procedure was briefly discussed as a blood sample was sucked in WBC diluting pipette to the mark 0.5. HCl acid 1.5% was filled up to mark 11 in the diluting pipette. The resulting dilution is 1:20 of the blood sample. The fluid was filled in the numbers counting chamber and viewed under the compound light microscope. The WBC count was expressed as the number of erythrocytes present per cubic mm of the blood [28]. Measurement of ESR was carried out by the reported Westergren method. The mixture consists of 2 ml of blood mixed with 3% sodium citrate. Westergren-Katz tube was used, and blood was drawn into it to the 200 mm mark. The sample tubes were kept vertically for 1 h. The rate of cell sedimentation was expressed as millimetres per 1 h, which is the ESR [20].

35.2.12 Statistical Analysis

Statistical analysis was performed using the trial version (9) of GraphPad Prism software. One-way analysis of variance (ANOVA) and Dunnett's multiple comparison tests was used to analyse the data. Values were reported using a mean and standard deviation format, and there were (n) six, an asterisk (*) denotes significance at the P 0.05 level.

35.3 Results

35.3.1 Change in Paw Volume and Arthritis Index

The treatment groups did not differ significantly ($P > 0.05$) in terms of the volume of the animals' paws on day 0. Subsequent day increases in paw volume and arthritic index were statistically significant (P 0.05) in LPS-treated animals. The paw volume and arthritis index of H-1 and H-2-treated rat were significantly lower than those of LPS-treated animals on days 7, 14, 21, and 28 ($P > 0.05$) (Fig. 35.1a, b).

35.3.2 Change in Paw Thickness and Percent Change

On the 0th day of the treatment protocol, there was no significant ($P > 0.05$) difference noted for change in paw thickness in all treatment groups. LPS-treated animals show a significant increase ($P < 0.05$) in paw thickness and percent change on subsequent days. Animals administered with H-1 and H-2 showed a significant decrease in paw thickness and percent change ($P < 0.05$) in a dose-dependent manner on days 7, 14, 21, and 28 when compared with LPS (Fig. 35.1c, d).

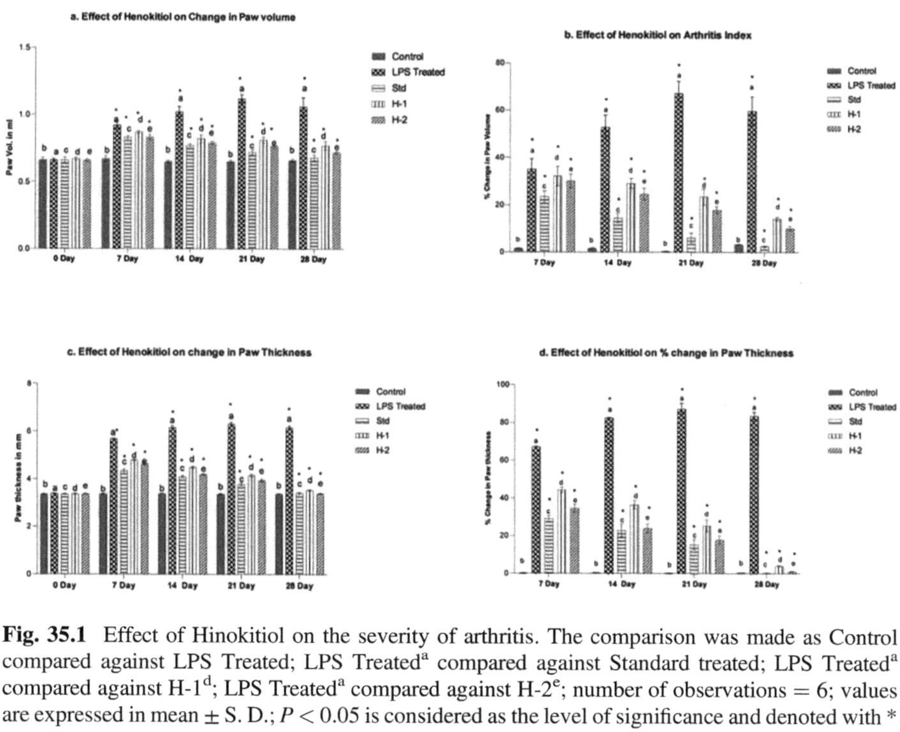

Fig. 35.1 Effect of Hinokitiol on the severity of arthritis. The comparison was made as Control compared against LPS Treated; LPS Treated[a] compared against Standard treated; LPS Treated[a] compared against H-1[d]; LPS Treated[a] compared against H-2[e]; number of observations = 6; values are expressed in mean ± S. D.; $P < 0.05$ is considered as the level of significance and denoted with *

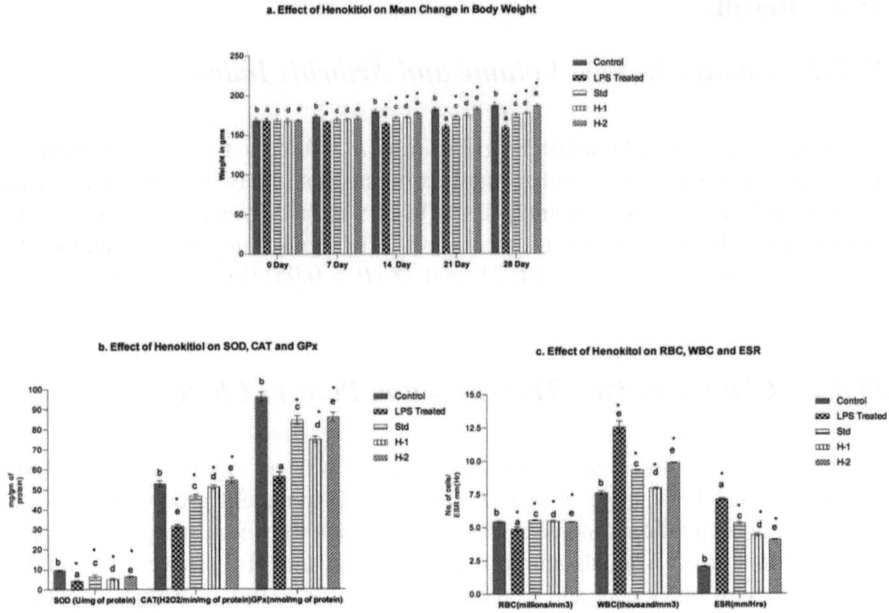

Fig. 35.2 Change in body wt, antioxidant enzymes and haematological parameters. The comparison was made as Control compared against LPS Treated; LPS Treated[a] compared against Standard treated[c]; LPS Treated[a] compared against H-1[d]; LPS Treated[a] compared against H-2[e]; number of observations = 6; values are expressed in mean ± S. D.; $P < 0.05$ is considered as the level of significance and denoted with *

35.3.2.1 Change in Body Weight

Zero-day mean body changes were not statistically significant ($P > 0.05$) across all treatment groups. On future days, LPS-treated rat lose significantly more weight than control group animals (*P* 0.05). On days 14, 21, and 28, animals given H-1 and H-2 had significantly increased body weight compared to LPS-treated rat (*P* 0.05) (Fig. 35.2a).

35.3.3 Serum Marker Enzymes

The levels of SGOT, ALP, and SGPT in the control group are all within the normal range; however, in the LPS group, all three are significantly elevated (*P* 0.05) in comparison to the control group. On day 28, serum marker enzyme levels were significantly lower in the H-1, and H-2 treated group than in the LPS treated group (*P* 0.05) (Table 35.1).

Table 35.1 Effect of H-1 and H-2 on serum marker enzymes

28th Day	Control	LPS Treated	Standard Treated	H-1	H-2
SGOT	60 ± 1.67^{b}	$105 \pm 3.44^{a*}$	$69 \pm 2.99^{ac*}$	$78 \pm 4.42^{ad*}$	$76 \pm 3.7^{ae*}$
ALP	89 ± 4.5^{b}	$167 \pm 7.8^{a*}$	$110 \pm 4.89^{ac*}$	$130 \pm 3.98^{ad*}$	$127 \pm 4.5^{ae*}$
SGPT	55 ± 3.44^{b}	$98 \pm 5.46^{a*}$	$63 \pm 4.5^{ac\$}$	$74 \pm 3.9^{ad*}$	$70 \pm 5.5^{ae*}$

The comparison was made as Control[b] compared against LPS Treated[a]; LPS Treated[a] compared against Standard treated[c]; LPS Treated[a] compared against H-1[d]; LPS Treated[a] compared against H-2[e]; number of observations = 6; values are expressed in mean ± S. D., $P < 0.05$ is considered as the level of significance and denoted with * and $P < 0.005$ is denoted with $

Table 35.2 Effect of H-1 and H-2 on cartilage degradation enzymes

Treatment	Control	LPS Treated	Standard Treated	H-1	H-2
MPO (U/g)	0.45 ± 0.1^{b}	$3.21 \pm 0.5^{a*}$	$0.92 \pm 0.1^{ac*}$	$1.53 \pm 0.1^{ad*}$	$1.20 \pm 0.1^{ae*}$
CAT-D (μmol/ 100 mg)	6.22 ± 0.5^{b}	$23.11 \pm 1.3^{a*}$	$9.05 \pm 0.1^{ac*}$	$13.45 \pm 1.0^{ad*}$	$11.05 \pm 1.2^{ae*}$
ELA (μmol/ 100 mg)	24.11 ± 1.3^{b}	$52.11 \pm 2.4^{a*}$	$29.21 \pm 2.2^{ac\$}$	$33.85 \pm 1.6^{ad*}$	$31.44 \pm 2.1^{ae*}$

The comparison was made as Control[b] compared against LPS Treated[a]; LPS Treated[a] compared against Standard treated[c]; LPS Treated[a] compared against H-1[d]; LPS Treated[a] compared against H-2[e]; number of observations = 6; values are expressed in mean ± S. D.; $P < 0.05$ is considered as the level of significance and denoted with * and $P < 0.005$ is denoted with $

35.3.4 Effect on Antioxidant Enzymes

A significant reduction ($P < 0.001$) in the SOD, CAT, and GPx activity was observed in the LPS-treated animals. Animals treated showed significant restoration of antioxidant enzyme activity and inhibited lipid peroxidation when compared to LPS-treated animals. The effect of Hinokitiol is dose-dependent (Fig. 35.2b).

35.3.5 Effect on Cartilage Degrading Enzymes

The MPO activity of LPS-treated rats was substantially higher than that of the control group (*P* 0.001). Animals given H-1 or H-2 have significantly lower MPO activity (*P* 0.001). This is a significant difference from LPS-treated rat, indicating significantly less neutrophil infiltration at the site of inflammation. A dose-dependent reduction in MPO activity (Table 35.2). Treatment with LPS results in significant increases in CAT-D levels (*P* 0.001), while treatment with H-1 and H-2 results in a significant decrease in CAT-D activity (*P* 0.001) (Table 35.2). As an indicator of PMNs' accumulation at an inflamed site, ELA is a useful metric to track. Animals treated with LPS had significantly higher ELA levels (*P* 0.001), while those treated with H-1 and H-2 had significantly lower ELA levels (*P* 0.001) (Table 35.2).

35.3.6 Effect on Effect on Blood Cell Count and ESR

The LPS-treated animals show significant increases in white blood cell count and ESR (*P* 0.001). When compared to LPS-treated animals, the WBC count and ESR of H-1 and H-2-treated animals are much lower. Compared to animals not treated with LPS, those given H-1 and H-2 have a dramatic rise in their red blood cell count (Fig. 35.2c).

35.4 Discussion

This research was conducted to learn whether or not hinokitiol could mitigate the arthritic inflammation triggered by LPS in rat. Bacterial endotoxins such as LPS [18], monoiodoacetate (MIA) [29], Fraud's adjuvant [30], squalane [31], liquid paraffin [32], quinolones [33], etc., have been proposed as effective tools for inducing arthritis in experimental animals. Still, arthritis triggered by LPS has proven to be a reliable model of inflammation. Pathophysiological alterations comparable to those seen in illness can be induced and mimicked by LPS. In the cell wall of Gram-negative bacteria, you will find lipopolysaccharides that are unlike any other in the living world. The cascades of inflammatory reactions are triggered when LPS is given to a patient because it stimulates their own immune system [34]. Host immune cells, including macrophages and neutrophils, play a key role in mediating these through the elaborate manufacture of inflammatory mediators such as IL, TNF-, and matrix proteases [35].

LPS is also capable of creating oxidative stress by an increased generation of free radicals and contributes to secondary inflammation [36]. The intraplantar injection administration of LPS leads to inflammation and swelling. The assessment of the severity of arthritis can be done using direct measurement of paw volume and thickness [19]. Treatment H-1 and H-2 show a reduction in paw volume, arthritic index, and thickness, possibly due to its anti-inflammatory effect. The arthritic index is related to percent change in paw volume; treatment with H-1 and H-2 shows a significant decrease in the arthritic index. It has been reported that the inflammatory cascades are responsible for the alteration of normal metabolic, absorption of essential nutrients, etc., which pose for inflammation-associated weight reduction [37].

Alteration in the metabolic activities of the diseased group is an underlying cause for a reduction in body weight. Earlier investigations advocated that the decrease in body weight during inflammation is caused due to deprived absorption of essential nutrients through the gastrointestinal tract. The result of the current study revealed that LPS-induced inflammation in rats leads to a significant reduction in body weight as compared to control group animals. However, animals treated with hinokitiol show a significant restoration in body weight which can be correlated with its anti-inflammatory effect. Estimation of MPO activity expresses PMN cell infiltration in the synovial tissues [38]. Administration of LPS initiates the inflammatory events and increases the PMN infiltration, which is in disparity to hinokitiol-treated animals. Cathepsins are a class of lysosomal enzymes and are involved in several inflammatory diseases, including arthritis. They are primarily responsible for cartilage and bone turnover. Elevated levels of CAT-D are found in arthritic patients [39, 40].

The current result indicates that treatment of hinokitiol reduced the CAT-D levels and limited the cartilage damage. ELA from PMN is a class of serine proteinases and is greatly involved in cartilage damage [41]. Increased levels of ELA are found in LPS-treated animals as compared to hinokitiol treated and limit the destruction mediated by ELAase. Clinical investigation of arthritis/joint-related diseases involves the assessment of marker enzymes, specifically SGOT, ALP, and SGPT. The activity of these enzymes indicates the severity of arthritic conditions [42]. In the current study, LPS, inducing inflammation, and associated cartilage damage significantly increase the levels of SGOT, ALP, and SGPT as compared to control group animals. The treatment of hinokitiol shows a significant decrease in marker level activity due to its anti-inflammatory activity. As discussed earlier, LPS induces the synthesis of inflammatory factors as well as oxidative stress through elaborating ROS/free radical generations [18, 19].

Normally these free radicals are eliminated through the endogenous antioxidant system and protect the cellular components from their harmful effects. In an uncontrolled generation of free radicals, the endogenous antioxidant gets deprived and leads to oxidative stress. These free radicals cause interference in normal cellular processes, damage to important cell components, including DNA, peroxidation of lipids, etc., leading to the death of cells [43]. To encounter the effect of free radicals and associated oxidative stress, external antioxidants are useful to protect the cells. In the current investigation, it was found that LPS significantly depletes the store of endogenous antioxidant enzymes like SOD and CAT GPx and induces oxidative stress [18]. Administration of LPS causes the abundant generation of ROS mainly from deference cells like macrophages and infiltration of neutrophils. In the present study, we found that SOD levels of LPS-treated animals are significantly decreased as compared to control animals. SOD, CAT, and GPx are the most important antioxidants present in the joint cartilage, and their scarcity would lead to enhanced free radicals mediated damage to important extracellular matrix components (cartilage, synovial tissue, and subchondral bone) [44].

Studies have revealed that decreased antioxidant enzyme levels were found in arthritic patients [45]. We observed that administration of hinokitiol in experimental animals significantly restores the levels of the antioxidant enzymes. This effect of hinokitiol would be due to its antioxidant and anti-inflammatory action. Several studies reported that haematological investigations are an important consideration for propagating the underlying cause and severity of disease conditions.

The estimation of RBC, WBC, and ESR are important parameters for accessing inflammatory conditions. A fall in RBC count was noted in chronic inflammatory conditions, and it is correlated with iron deficiency and interferes with erythropoietin synthesis, which alternately affects the erythropoiesis process [46]. This fall in RBC is noted in LPS-treated animals, whereas animals treated with hinokitiol show a significant restoration in RBC count, which could be due to a reduction in inflammation. WBCs are prime cells involved in the host defence system. These cells are meant to fight against invaded foreign particles, including viruses, bacteria, and several other microorganisms. Chemotaxis cascades lead to infiltration of WBC, specifically neutrophils, at a site of inflammation which leads to phagocytosis of invaded foreign particles [47]. Enhanced inflammatory events are observed due to the release of interleukins, histamine, prostaglandins, etc. [19]. It was observed that WBC count is significantly increased in LPS-treated animals, which confirms the severity of inflammation. The group of animals treated with hinokitiol shows minimum infiltration of WBC, which can be correlated with the reduction in inflammation induced due to LPS. Assessment of the sedimentation rate of the erythrocyte is a simple, convenient, and reliable method for understanding the severity of arthritic inflammation. Increased ESR is observed in chronic inflammatory conditions [48].

35.5 Conclusion

The result advocated that LPS administration leads to fast sedimentation, whereas the group of animals treated with hinokitiol shows decreased ESR. This effect can be due to a reduction in inflammation induced by LPS. The current investigation reveals that hinokitiol attenuates LPS-induced arthritis by a reduction in paw volume, arthritis index, paw thickness, and improved body weight. Significantly decreased marker enzymes, namely, SGOT, SGPT, and ALP, were observed in hinokitiol-treated animals. Hinokitiol significantly restores the antioxidant enzyme levels and decreases the cartilage damage mediated by MPO, CAT-D, and ELA. The haematological assessment addressed a significant decrease in WBC count and ESR, and RBC count is significantly improved by the administration of hinokitiol. However, additional screenings are essential to identify the consequence of hinokitiol on the expression of inflammatory mediators and the precise underlying mechanism for its anti-arthritic effect.

Acknowledgements ASPM's K. T. Patil College of Pharmacy, Nargund College of Pharmacy, Bangalore, and JSPM's Charak College of Pharmacy and Research, Pune, provided the essential facilities for this research.

References

1. Kaji, M. (2008). Nozoe Tetsuo's chemical research at Taihoku imperial university in Taiwan and its colonial context. *Historia Scientiarum. Second series: International Journal of the History of Science Society of Japan, 18*(2), 132–139.
2. Hirata, R., Ito, S., Eto, K., Sakuta, K., Mizoue, N., & Mitsuda, Y. (2015). Early growth of hinoki (Chamaecyparisobtusa) trees under different topography and edge aspects at a strip-clearcut site in Kyushu, Southern Japan. *Journal of Forest Research, 20*(6), 522–529.
3. Shih, Y. H., Chang, K. W., Hsia, S. M., Yu, C. C., Fuh, L. J., Chi, T. Y., & Shieh, T. M. (2013). In vitro antimicrobial and anticancer potential of hinokitiol against oral pathogens and oral cancer cell lines. *Microbiological Research, 168*(5), 254–262.
4. Inamori, Y., Shinohara, S., Tsujibo, H., Okabe, T., Morita, Y., Sakagami, Y., Kumeda, Y., & Ishida, N. (1999). Antimicrobial activity and metalloprotease inhibition of hinokitiol-related compounds, the constituents of Thujopsisdolabrata S. and Z. hondai MAK. *Biological and Pharmaceutical Bulletin, 22*(9), 990–993.
5. Krenn, B. M., Gaudernak, E., Holzer, B., Lanke, K., Van Kuppeveld, F. J. M., & Seipelt, J. (2009). Antiviral activity of the zinc ionophorespyrithione and hinokitiol against picornavirus infections. *Journal of Virology, 83*(1), 58–64.
6. Yang, P. S., Wang, M. J., Jayakumar, T., Chou, D. S., Ko, C. Y., Hsu, M. J., & Hsieh, C. Y. (2015). Antiproliferative activity of hinokitiol, a tropolone derivative, is mediated via the inductions of p-JNK and p-PLCγ1 signaling in PDGF-BB-stimulated vascular smooth muscle cells. *Molecules, 20*(5), 8198–8212.
7. Lee, J. H., Moon, J. H., Lee, Y. J., & Park, S. Y. (2017). SIRT1, a class III histone deacetylase, regulates LPS-induced inflammation in human keratinocytes and mediates the anti-inflammatory effects of hinokitiol. *Journal of Investigative Dermatology., 137*(6), 1257–1266.
8. El Hachlafi, N., Lakhdar, F., Khouchlaa, A., Bakrim, S., El Omari, N., Balahbib, A., Shariati, M. A., Zengin, G., Fikri-Benbrahim, K., Orlando, G., & Ferrante, C. (2021). Health benefits and pharmacological properties of hinokitiol. *Processes, 9*(9), 1680.
9. Imai, N., Doi, Y., Nabae, K., Tamano, S., Hagiwara, A., Kawabe, M., Ichihara, T., Ogawa, K., & Shirai, T. (2006). Lack of hinokitiol (beta-thujaplicin) carcinogenicity in F344/DuCrj rats. *The Journal of Toxicological Sciences, 31*(4), 357–370.
10. Arden, N., & Nevitt, M. C. (2006). Osteoarthritis: Epidemiology. *Best Practice & Research Clinical Rheumatology, 20*(1), 3–25.
11. Kalia, M. (2002). Assessing the economic impact of stress — The modern day hidden epidemic. *Metabolism-Clinical and Experimental, 51*(6), 49–53.
12. Korotaeva, T. V. (2014). Psoriatic arthritis: Classification, clinical presentation, diagnosis, treatment. *Rheumatology Science and Practice, 52*(6), 650–659.
13. Teoh, N. C., & Farrell, G. C. (2003). Hepatotoxicity associated with non-steroidal anti-inflammatory drugs. *Clinics in Liver Disease, 7*(2), 401–413.
14. Buchman, A. L. (2001). Side effects of corticosteroid therapy. *Journal of Clinical Gastroenterology, 33*(4), 289–294.
15. Albrecht, K., & M ler-Ladner, U. (2010). Side effects and management of side effects of methotrexate in rheumatoid arthritis. *Clinical and Experimental Rheumatology-Incl Supplements, 28*(5), S95.
16. Jayakumar, T., Liu, C. H., Wu, G. Y., Lee, T. Y., Manubolu, M., Hsieh, C. Y., Yang, C. H., & Sheu, J. R. (2018). Hinokitiol inhibits migration of A549 lung cancer cells via suppression of MMPs and induction of antioxidant enzymes and apoptosis. *International Journal of Molecular Sciences, 19*(4), 939.
17. Abu-Ghefreh, A. A. A., & Masocha, W. (2010). Enhancement of antinociception by co-administration of minocycline and a non-steroidal anti-inflammatory drug indomethacin in naïve mice and murine models of LPS-induced thermal hyperalgesia and monoarthritis. *BMC Musculoskeletal Disorders, 11*, 276–282.

18. Gunjegaonkar, S. M., & Shanmugarajan, T. S. (2019). Methyl jasmonate a stress phytohormone attenuates LPS induced in vivo and in vitro arthritis. *Molecular Biology Reports, 46*(1), 647–656.
19. Shanmugarajan, T. S. (2018). Potential of plant stress hormone methyl Jasmonate against lipopolysaccharide attenuated oxidative stress and arthritis in experimental animals. *International Journal of Green Pharmacy (IJGP), 12*(03).
20. Arulmozhi, S., Mazumder, P. M., Sathiyanarayanan, L., & Ashok, P. (2011). Anti-arthritic and antioxidant activity of leaves of Alstoniascholaris Linn. R. Br. *European Journal of Integrative Medicine, 3*(2), e83–e90.
21. Kumar, N., Singh, S., Patro, N., & Patro, I. (2009). Evaluation of protective efficacy of Spirulinaplatensis against collagen-induced arthritis in rats. *Inflammopharmacology, 17*(3), 181–190.
22. Lin, B., Zhao, Y., Han, P., Yue, W., Ma, X. Q., Rahman, K., Zheng, C. J., Qin, L. P., & Han, T. (2014). Anti-arthritic activity of Xanthium strumarium L. extract on complete Freund's adjuvant induced arthritis in rats. *Journal of Ethnopharmacology, 155*(1), 248–255.
23. Sadiq, U., Mishrab, N. K., Kaushal, P., Mir, S., Nehaa, M. A., Sayeed, A., et al. (2012). Protective effect of rutin in attenuation of collagen-induced arthritis in wistar rat by inhibiting inflammation and oxidative stress. *Indian Journal of Rheumatology, 7*, 191–198.
24. Umar, S., Zargan, J., Umar, K., Ahmad, S., Katiyar, C. K., & Khan, H. A. (2012). Modulation of the oxidative stress and inflammatory cytokine response by thymoquinone in the collagen induced arthritis in wistar rats. *Chemico-Biological Interactions, 197*, 40–46.
25. Nam, J. H., Jung, H. J., Choi, J., Lee, K. T., & Park, H. J. (2006). The anti-gastropathic and antirheumatic effect of niga-ichigoside F1 and 23-hydroxytormentic acid isolated from the unripe fruits of Rubuscore anus in a rat model. *Biological & Pharmaceutical Bulletin, 29*, 967–970.
26. Kilimozhi, D., Parthasarathy, V., & Amuthavalli, N. (2009). Effect of Clerodendrumphlomidis on adjuvant induced arthritis in rats: A radiographic densitometric analysis. *International Journal of PharmTech Research, 1*, 1434–1441.
27. Mamatha, K., Rodda, H. C., Ciddi, V., & Bookya, K. (2013). Anti-arthritic activity of root bark of Oroxylumindicum (L.) vent against adjuvant-induced arthritis. *Pharmacognosy Research, 5*(2), 121–128.
28. Ghai, C. L. (2012). *A textbook of practical physiology*. JP Medical Ltd.
29. Nam, J., Perera, P., Liu, J., Wu, L. C., Rath, B., Butterfield, T. A., & Agarwal, S. (2011). Transcriptome-wide gene regulation by gentle treadmill walking during the progression of monoiodoacetate-induced arthritis. *Arthritis and Rheumatism, 63*(6), 1613–1625.
30. Bigoniya, P., Singh, A., & Singh, S. (2013). Analgesic, anti-inflammatory and anti-arthritic activity of Euphorbia thymifolia Linn phytosterol fraction. *Journal of Pharmacy Research, 1*(2), 130–134.
31. Holmdahl, R., Lorentzen, J. C., Lu, S., Olofsson, P., Wester, L., Holmberg, J., & Pettersson, U. (2001). Arthritis induced in rats with non-immunogenic adjuvants as models for rheumatoid arthritis. *Immunological Reviews, 184*(1), 184–202.
32. Sharma, J. N., Srivastava, K. C., & Gan, E. K. (1994). Suppressive effects of eugenol and ginger oil on arthritic rats. *Pharmacology, 49*(5), 314–318.
33. Riesbeck, K. (2002). Immunomodulating activity of quinolones. *Journal of Chemotherapy, 14*(1), 3–12.
34. Ohgami, K., Shiratori, K., Kotake, S., Nishida, T., Mizuki, N., Yazawa, K., & Ohno, S. (2003). Effects of astaxanthin on lipopolysaccharide-induced inflammation in vitro and in vivo. *Investigative Ophthalmology & Visual Science, 44*(6), 2694–2701.
35. Pang, T., Wang, J., Benicky, J., & Saavedra, J. M. (2012). Minocycline ameliorates LPS-induced inflammation in human monocytes by novel mechanisms including LOX-1, Nur77 and LITAF inhibition. *Biochimica et Biophysica Acta (BBA)-General Subjects, 1820*(4), 503–510.

36. Dong, Z., & Yuan, Y. (2018). Accelerated inflammation and oxidative stress induced by LPS in acute lung injury: Inhibition by ST1926. *International Journal of Molecular Medicine, 41*(6), 3405–3421.
37. Granado, M., Priego, T., Martín, A. I., Villanúa, M. Á., & López-Calderón, A. (2005). Ghrelin receptor agonist GHRP-2 prevents arthritis-induced increase in E3 ubiquitin-ligating enzymes MuRF1 and MAFbx gene expression in skeletal muscle. *American Journal of Physiology-Endocrinology and Metabolism, 289*(6), E1007–E1014.
38. Aydin, B., & Akar, A. (2011). Effects of a 900-MHz electromagnetic field on oxidative stress parameters in rat lymphoid organs, polymorphonuclear leukocytes and plasma. *Archives of Medical Research, 42*(4), 261–267.
39. Olszewska-Slonina, D., Matewski, D., Jung, S., Olszewski, K. J., Czajkowski, R., Braszkiewicz, J., Wozniak, A., & Kowaliszyn, B. (2013). The activity of cathepsin D and alpha-1 antitrypsin in hip and knee osteoarthritis. *Acta Biochimica Polonica, 60*(1).
40. Olszewska-Slonina, D., Jung, S., Matewski, D., Olszewski, K. J., Krzyzynska-Malinowska, E., Braszkiewicz, A., & Kowaliszyn, B. (2015). Lysosomal enzymes in serum and synovial fluid in patients with osteoarthritis. *Scandinavian Journal of Clinical and Laboratory Investigation, 75*(2), 145–151.
41. Momohara, S., Kashiwazaki, S., Inoue, K., Saito, S., & Nakagawa, T. (1997). Elastase from polymorphonuclear leukocyte in articular cartilage and synovial fluids of patients with rheumatoid arthritis. *Clinical Rheumatology, 16*(2), 133–139.
42. Srivastava, S., Singh, P., Jha, K. K., Mishra, G., Srivastava, S., & Khosa, R. L. (2012). Evaluation of anti-arthritic potential of the methanolic extract of the aerial parts of Costus speciosus. *Journal of Ayurveda and Integrative Medicine, 3*(4), 204.
43. Sesti, F., Tsitsilonis, O. E., Kotsinas, A., & Trougakos, I. P. (2012). Oxidative stress-mediated biomolecular damage and inflammation in tumorigenesis. *In Vivo, 26*(3), 395–402.
44. Wruck, C. J., Fragoulis, A., Gurzynski, A., Brandenburg, L. O., Kan, Y. W., Chan, K., Hassenpflug, J., Freitag-Wolf, S., Varoga, D., Lippross, S., & Pufe, T. (2011). Role of oxidative stress in rheumatoid arthritis: Insights from the Nrf2-knockout mice. *Annals of the Rheumatic Diseases, 70*(5), 844–850.
45. Taysi, S., Polat, F., Gul, M., Sari, R. A., & Bakan, E. (2002). Lipid peroxidation, some extracellular antioxidants, and antioxidant enzymes in serum of patients with rheumatoid arthritis. *Rheumatology International, 21*(5), 200–204.
46. Olumuyiwa-Akeredolu, O. O., & Pretorius, E. (2015). Platelet and red blood cell interactions and their role in rheumatoid arthritis. *Rheumatology International, 35*, 1955–1964.
47. Santosh, S., Rooke, T. W., Bailey, K. R., McConnell, J. P., & Kullo, I. J. (2004). Relation of markers of inflammation (C-reactive protein, white blood cell count, and lipoprotein-associated phospholipase A2) to the ankle-brachial index. *Vascular Medicine, 9*, 171–176.
48. Brigden, M. L. (1999). Clinical utility of the erythrocyte sedimentation rate. *American Family Physician, 60*(5), 1443–1450.

Chapter 36
Development of Release-Modulated Oxaceprol Topical Niosomal Gel: Assessment of Formulation Parameters and Performance Aspects

Kalyani Patil, Rameshwar S. Cheke, Sachin D. Shinde, and Vikram Nimbalkar

36.1 Introduction

Topical drug delivery is implemented to deliver drugs toward the surface as well as underneath the skin. The main benefit of the topical drug delivery system is that it avoids the negative effects of first-pass metabolism, gastrointestinal pH, gastric enzymes, gastric emptying, etc. [1, 2]. Topical medication delivery systems have several benefits, but the existence of the stratum corneum limits them to the outer layers of the skin. In the case of topical formulations, only a negligible fraction of the medicine is absorbed into the bloodstream after application [3]. To get around these restrictions, a unique drug delivery mechanism is used to regulate medication release within the body. In contrast to the more common direct administration routes, which rely on needle-based injections, topical medication delivery through the skin has become one of the most fully investigated routes of noninvasive drug delivery into the body. In several medical fields, including pain management, hormone therapy, and the treatment of cardiovascular and central nervous system disorders, topical

K. Patil (✉)
Department of Pharmaceutics, Oyster Institute of Pharmacy, Aurangabad, Maharashtra, India

R. S. Cheke
Department of Pharmaceutical Chemistry, Dr Rajendra Gode College of Pharmacy, Malkapur, Maharashtra, India

S. D. Shinde
Department of Pharmacology, Shri R. D. Bhakt College of Pharmacy, Jalna, Maharashtra, India

V. Nimbalkar
Department of Pharmacology, Dr VVPF's College of Pharmacy, Ahmednagar, Maharashtra, India

F. J. Joseph et al. (eds.), *Computational Intelligence for Clinical Diagnosis*,
EAI/Springer Innovations in Communication and Computing,
https://doi.org/10.1007/978-3-031-23683-9_36

medication administration has made a significant impact. It is the goal of novel drug delivery to continue drug activity at a predetermined rate or to maintain a generally constant effective drug level in the body while minimizing undesired side effects [4].

The vesicular drug delivery system shows a firm mechanism to improve the delivery and effectiveness of drugs. Drug-containing vesicles deliver the drugs in a sustained release manner that prolongs in vivo drug action, decreases drug metabolism, and reduces the side effects of the drug. Drug carriers such as microparticles, microcapsules, bicells, lipoproteins, liposomes, niosomes, Nanocochleates, and transferosomes could be formulated by tailoring them to degrade slowly, to be stimuli-responsive, and to target specific sites [5].

When treating diseases, nano-carriers, including liposomes, polymersomes, niosomes, micelles, and polymer-based vesicles, can be employed to transport therapeutic chemicals to specific areas. Nanocarriers are of interest to scientists because of their potential to improve drug delivery in a variety of ways. For example, by optimizing their components or creating a multi-functional surface, nanocarriers can increase the half-life of drugs in serum, prevent their uptake by reticuloendothelial systems (RESs), and lessen the amount of non-specific adsorption. They can also protect the drug from becoming bad while it is being stored or administered to people. Nano vesicles are commonly used as carriers in the delivery (or co-delivery) of chemical medicines, protein drusen, and other therapeutics. Carbopol 934P (CP) is a mucoadhesive polymer that has been studied as a bioadhesive drug delivery adjuvant. However, because the medication release rate from the solid formulation of CP is sluggish, using the polymer's mucoadhesive feature in the oral administration of fast-acting pharmaceuticals is challenging. Between the formulation of CP and the bulk release media, CP produces a swelling gel layer that acts as a drug release barrier.

The model drug Oxaceprol belongs to the class of drugs treating burn infections, as it shows regeneration of tissue in the burned area by stimulating the uptake of 3H-glucosamine and 3H-proline and its incorporation in the macromolecular structure of the matrix of cartilage which is responsible for the activity of regeneration of tissue. It acts as a better candidate for treating first and second-degree type of burns and burns infections [6, 7]. The blood circulation in the burned area is impaired, and if medication is taken orally, the drug will not reach the damaged area in sufficient measure. Hence, niosomal gel can provide a higher and more durable localized drug action as well as prolong retention time at the site of application of the gel. Thus, it could reduce the frequency of dressing, which in turn reduces pain, and discomfort and ultimately increases patient compliance. In addition to this, formulating the niosomal gel is advantageous as it shows an affinity to penetrate through the skin, which acts as a barrier for the permeation of drugs delivered through the topical route.

36.2 Materials and Method

36.2.1 Materials

Oxaceprol was generously gifted by Glenmark Pharma, Sinner, Nashik, India. Carbopol was procured from Choral Pharma, Gujarat. Span (20, 40, 60, 80), cholesterol, chloroform, methanol, potassium dihydrogen phosphate, sodium chloride, and tetra-ethanolamine were purchased from Modern Lab, Nashik; all other chemicals were of analytical grade and used as received.

36.2.2 Method for Preparation

36.2.2.1 Preparation of Niosomal Dispersion

Oxaceprol niosomes were prepared by thin-film hydration technique, and the model drug was loaded using the passive loading method. The method, in brief, involves weighing accurate quantities of surfactant and cholesterol and subsequently dissolving them in chloroform and methanol in a 3:1 ratio in a round bottom flask. At 60 °C and under a vacuum, the resulting dispersion was allowed to evaporate until dry. This video was then maintained under a vacuum for a further 2 h. After drying, the resulting thin film was rehydrated with a drug solution (1 mg/mL) in distilled water, 10% sucrose, or phosphate buffer at 60 °C for 1.5 h while rotating at 120 revolutions per minute. The resulting vesicular suspension underwent an additional 1 h of bath sonication [8, 9].

36.2.2.2 Formulation of Topical Niosomal Gel

The niosomal gel was prepared by the cold method. Wherein, Carbopol 934 (2 g) was dissolved first in 100 mL of cold water and kept for 12 h. for complete soaking of polymer. Formulated niosomal dispersion was added to this gel base as per the quantity calculated based on the entrapment efficiency (%EE) of that niosomal dispersion. Subsequently, a blend of preservatives (Methyl Paraben 0.2 g and Propyl Paraben 0.02 g) was added in the above preparation. A particular ratio of surfactant: cholesterol, and chloroform: methanol, was selected for the processing, as mentioned in Table 36.1.

Table 36.1 Formulation batches of oxaceprol niosomal gel

Formulation code	Drug (mg)	Surfactant	Surfactant (mg)	Cholesterol (mg)	Chloroform (ml)	Methanol (ml)
F1	100	Span 20	80	20	14	6
F2	100	Span 20	60	40	7	3
F3	100	Span 40	80	20	14	6
F4	100	Span 40	60	40	7	3
F5	100	Span 60	80	20	14	6
F6	100	Span 60	60	40	7	3
F7	100	Span 80	80	20	14	6
F8	100	Span 80	60	40	7	3

36.2.3 Analytical Method Development

The analytical UV method was developed and validated as per the ICH guidelines to quantify the drug content in niosomal gel. The drug was initially dissolved in phosphate buffer solution (PBS) of pH 6.8 value and analysed further using UV visible spectrophotometric method (Shimadzu 2450, Japan at 222 nm).

36.2.4 Compatibility Study

Drug and excipient compatibility studies were carried out to establish potential physicochemical interaction between the drug and the excipient used in the formulations. The compatibility was carried out preliminarily using differential scanning calorimetric (DSC) and Fourier transform infrared (FTIR) spectroscopy [10, 11].

36.2.5 FTIR

The FTIR spectrophotometer was utilized to analyse compatibility (Shimadzu, 8400S, Japan). During this experiment, both the unadulterated medication and a physical mixture of the drug and polymers were used. A month's worth of physical mixes was made and stored at 400 degrees Celsius. Oxaceprol, as well as a physical mixture of Oxaceprol and polymers, has its infrared absorption spectrum recorded with KBr from a wavenumber of 4000 to 400 cm^{-1} [12].

36.2.6 DSC

DSC analysis was performed using Shimadzu thermal analyser (DSC 60) by taking a formulation quantity of less than 5 mg of an equivalent amount of the drug. The sample was hermetically sealed in an aluminium pan and heated with a nitrogen gas flow rate of 50 mL/min conducted over a temperature range of 30 to 150 °C under a nitrogen flow of 2 bar pressure. Thermo-gram was obtained by heating the sample at a constant rate of 10 °C/min. A dry purge of nitrogen gas was used for all runs. The melting point and the peak maxima were recorded in the DSC graph [13, 14].

36.2.7 Preliminary Studies for the Preparation of Trial Batches

36.2.7.1 Optimization of Drug Concentration

The niosomes were prepared by using a thin-film hydration method. The amount of drug to be added was a very crucial parameter to be determined. For the determination of the strength of drugs to be incorporated, there was only one way to prepare trial batches of niosomes with different strengths of the drug. Next, it was put through a percent EE estimation, and the drug's strength was chosen accordingly. To do this, seven batches of niosomal dispersion were formulated with drug concentrations of 20, 40, 60, 80, 100, 120, and 160 mg and their percent EE was calculated.

36.2.7.2 Characterization of Oxaceprol Niosomal Dispersion

The influence of surfactant: cholesterol and chloroform: methanol ratio was studied on Oxaceprol entrapment is noisome. For determination of particle size and shape of vesicles, size and scanning electron microscopy (SEM) evaluation were carried out.

36.2.7.3 Physical Appearance

The physical appearance of prepared niosomal dispersion was assessed visually. It was evident that the concentration of lipids could affect the size of the niosomes. The colour of the dispersion was whitish to opaque.

36.2.7.4 Entrapment Efficiency (%EE)

The %EE was determined by using the dialysis method. Wherein a dialysis bag (2–3 cm) was soaked in PBS till the bag gets opened, it was sealed at one end, and 1 mL of niosomal dispersion was placed in the bag, followed by sealing it from another end with the help of thread. This bag was then tied from both ends to the magnetic bead. 50 mL of PBS was added to 250 capacity beakers, followed by placing the magnetic bead in this beaker along with the dialysis bag. This set-up was assembled on a magnetic stirrer and stirred at 120 rpm for 30 min. The bag was withdrawn after 30 min, and 1 mL of an aliquot was collected from the PBS and scanned using UV spectrophotometer; the %EE was calculated by using the formula [9]:

$$\text{EE}\ (\%) = \frac{\text{Total drug} - \text{Free drug}}{\text{Total drug}} \times 100$$

36.2.7.5 Particle Size and Shape Analysis

The formulation batches with high %EE were selected and subjected to their particle size and shape. The mean particle size analysis was determined with the help of a zeta sizer (Malvern). The morphological characteristics of niosomes were observed under SEM [15, 16].

36.2.7.6 Zeta Potential Analysis

An optimized batch was subjected further for zeta potential estimation. Zeta potential helps to determine charges on noisome and its magnitude, which has a significant impact on drug delivery through the skin site. Zeta potential was analysed by using 0.5 to 1 mL of sample diluted by 10 mL of double-distilled water, and then the zeta potential was determined by a laser scattering analyser [8].

36.2.8 Characterization of Gel

36.2.8.1 Physical Parameter

36.2.8.1.1 Clarity and pH

We visually evaluated the clarity of each formulation, and we measured the pH with a digital pH metre. The pH readings were taken soon after the food was prepared.

In order to prevent skin irritation and itching, a tiny amount of tri-ethanolamine was added to the gel (if necessary) to bring the pH level to 5.5–7.4 [17, 18].

36.2.8.2 Rheological Study

36.2.8.2.1 Viscosity

Gel rheological properties were measured by a Brookfield viscometer, spindle LV-64, type DV-II + PRO. At 370 C (room temperature) and for a range of shear speeds, the formulations' viscosity was measured. The viscosity of the gel at respective rpm and torque (shear rate) was determined, and the graph was plotted as shear rate vs viscosity. The gel was evaluated for its flow characteristics, like plastic or pseudoplastic flow [19, 20].

36.2.8.3 Drug Content

For evaluating the drug content, a weighed amount of gel equivalent to 10 mg of drug was placed in a 100 mL beaker; containing 100 mL of PBS of pH 6.8. An aliquot of 01 mL from this solution was diluted up to 10 mL with water to get the final concentration of 10 μg/mL. The absorbance of the prepared solution was measured at 222 nm by using a UV-visible spectrophotometer, and the calculation of the drug content was done using a formula [21]:

$$\text{Drug Content } (\%) = \frac{\text{Practical Yield} \times 100}{\text{Theoretical Yield}}$$

36.2.8.4 Spreadability

They chose two glass slides of the typical size. Slides were used, with gel put to one side and another placed on top. There was a need to displace any air. Therefore, the slides were stacked on top of one another. We balanced the slides on the platform such that the lower slide was held firmly by the opposite fangs of the clamp while the higher slide could freely glide off under the weight of the 125-pound shackle. Spreadability was determined by timing how long it took for the top slide to disengage from the bottom slide [22, 23]:

$$S = m.l/t$$

where S = Spreadability, m = Weight, l = Length of glass, t = Time

36.2.8.5 In Vitro Release Study

It was carried out by using a Franz diffusion cell using a cellulose dialysis membrane. A section of the membrane was cut, measured, and placed on the receiver compartment. The niosomal formulation (1 g of gel) was placed in the donor compartment, and freshly prepared 20 mL of PBS (6.8) was placed in the receptor compartment. The whole assembly was placed on the magnetic stirrer at 37 °C at 300 rpm. A 0.5 mL of sample was withdrawn from the receiver compartment after 1 h up to 12 h and diluted up to 10 mL if necessary, and the same volume of fresh medium was added to maintain a sink condition. The sample was diluted and analysed at 219.50 nm [13, 23].

36.2.8.6 Ex Vivo Permeability Study

A comparative ex vivo permeability study on isolated goat skin was carried out to check the difference in the release rate of the developed niosomal gel and the conventional gel. The study was performed in a Franz diffusion cell. A cm section of goat skin was selected; in one section, noisome gel of 1 g was placed, and in another section, 1 g of conventional gel was placed. Both sections were considered donor compartments. In the receptor compartment, PBS of pH 6.8 value was kept. The whole set-up was done on a magnetic stirrer, and the study was continued for around 12 h. The sample was withdrawn after an interval of 1 h. 0.5 mL of the sample was withdrawn at each time interval, and an equal amount of fresh PBS was introduced to the receptor compartment to maintain the sink condition. The samples were scanned under UV visible spectroscopy, and further, the flux and permeability coefficient was calculated [24, 25].

36.2.8.7 Stability Studies

Physical properties such as colour, clarity, pH, viscosity, and drug concentration were assessed at regular intervals for 1 month for each formulation, following ICH standards [26].

36.3 Result and Discussion

36.3.1 Compatibility Study

36.3.1.1 Fourier Transform InfraRed (FTIR) Spectroscopy

The FTIR spectra of the physical mixture of drug and excipients show similar peaks as that of the drug spectra. The characteristic peaks of the drug were also present unchanged in the spectrum of all drug-polymer combinations, as shown in Fig. 36.1.

Oxaceprol's unique absorption bands are due to the groups contained in its chemical structure. The purity of the donated Oxaceprol sample was confirmed by the existence of absorption bands that matched those of the functional groups found in the molecule's structure. According to Table 36.2, the dominant peaks in the IR spectra of the medications reveal that there was no appreciable interaction between the pharmaceuticals and the polymer.

36.3.1.2 DSC

The DSC curve of Oxaceprol shows a sharp endothermic peak at 131.56 °C, which was near the melting point of the drug. As no significant difference was observed in the melting points of the drug and formulation, we led to conclude that the drug was compatible with the excipients used in the formulation of niosomal gel as well as no

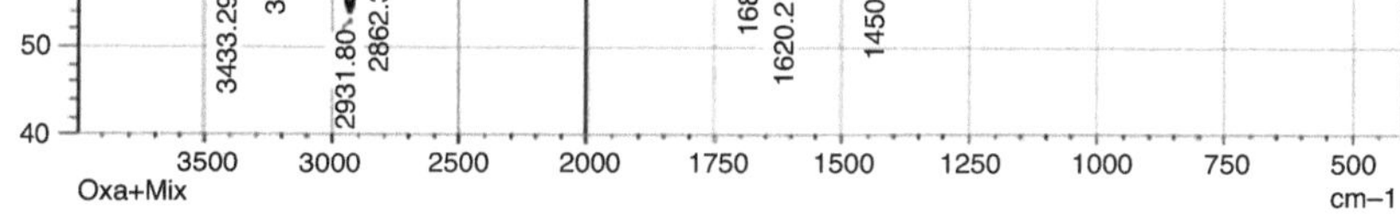

Fig. 36.1 Infrared spectrum of oxaceprol with polymers

Table 36.2 Interpretation of the infrared spectrum of drug and polymer

Sr. no.	Functional group	Peaks	
		Observed frequency cm^{-1}	Stranded frequency cm^{-1}
1	CH_3-C=O (Aldehyde)	2862.36	2900–2700
2	OH-C=O (Carboxylic acid)	2931.80	3400–2400
3	C-N (Amine)	1342.46	1350–1000

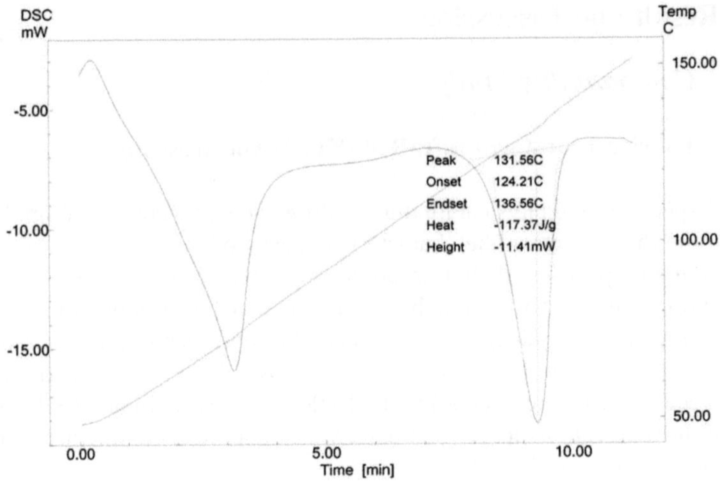

Fig. 36.2 DSC thermogram of oxaceprol niosomal gel

Table 36.3 DSC thermogram data for oxaceprol and oxaceprol niosomal formulation

Sr. no.	Sample	Enthalpy	Onset temperature	Peak temperature	End set temperature
1	Oxaceprol	−224.99 J/g	126.22	133.25	138.68
2	Oxaceprol niosomal formulation	−177.37 J/g	124.21	131.56	136.56

undesired reaction occurred during the formulation process. The DSC thermogram is shown in Fig. 36.2, and the corresponding readings are reported in Table 36.3.

36.3.2 Formulation and Development of Oxaceprol Niosomal Gel

36.3.2.1 Preliminary Studies for the Preparation of Trial Batches

36.3.2.1.1 Optimization of Drug Concentration

The different batches were evaluated for the acceptable concentration of the drug, that is, Oxaceprol; it was observed that a maximum of 100 mg of drug dose could be loaded into the formed niosomes. So, these concentrations were finalized for formulating further batches, which were then evaluated to decide the optimized batch with desired properties. It was observed that batch F5 had the highest %EE (Table 36.4);

Table 36.4 Trial batches for optimization of drug concentration

Batch code	Drug dose strength (mg)	Surfactant	Surfactant (mg)	Cholesterol (mg)	Chloroform: Methanol	Entrapment efficiency (%)
F1	20	Span 20	60	40	7:3	75.96
F2	40	Span 20	60	40	7:3	77.72
F3	60	Span 20	60	40	7:3	78.2
F4	80	Span 20	60	40	7:3	78.43
F5	100	Span 20	60	40	7:3	82.46
F6	120	Spam 20	60	40	7:3	82.66
F7	160	Span 20	60	40	7:3	82.7

hence, a 100 mg dose of the drug can be considered suitable for the formulation of an optimized batch. Batches F6 and F7 also showed an increase in %EE, but it is not up to the desired level. They did not demonstrate a significant increase in %EE as in the case of the F5 batch. The reason behind this might be the vesicles can entrap only 100 mg of the drug in its core, and more amount of the drug cannot be entrapped in the core of the vesicles. Hence, further batches were formulated by taking the drug concentration as 100 mg, which was kept constant for all the batches.

36.3.2.2 Characterization of Niosomal Dispersion

36.3.2.2.1 Physical Appearance

The physical appearance of prepared niosomal dispersion was assessed visually. All the batches obtained were found to be spherical in shape. The shape and size of the particle depend on the concentration of the lipid and cholesterol. As the amount of the lipid gets increased, the particle size was also found to be increased. It was observed that the 80 mg concentration of Span 20 solution could generate a larger size of niosomes than the 60 mg concentration. Therefore, it was observed that as the lipid concentration increases, it could affect the size and shape of niosomes. Furthermore, as the particle size increases, the drug release from that particle could also get affected. As the particle size increases, the drug release is found to be decreased.

36.3.2.2.2 Entrapment Efficiency (%EE)

Oxaceprol %EE was found to be 83.2% and 82.6% of F1 and F2 batches, respectively. Depending on this criterion, they were considered an optimized batch. After preparing niosomal dispersion, the amount of entrapped drug was evaluated from its %EE by the dialysis bag method. The entrapment of drugs in niosomal vesicles depends on the capacity of the vesicle to entrap the drug molecule in its core. As the particle size was increased, the core size of the particle also increased, and the drug

Table 36.5 Entrapment efficiency of oxaceprol niosomes

Batch no.	Entrapped drug %
F1	83.2 ± 0.2
F2	82.46 ± 0.02
F3	79.71 ± 0.06
F4	76.65 ± 0.02
F5	77.19 ± 0.04
F6	79.02 ± 0.02
F7	76.1 ± 0.3
F8	76.2 ± 0.3

oxaceprol, a hydrophilic drug, was entrapped in that core of the vesicle. The particle size depends on the increased concentration of lipids. The results are reported in Table 36.5. The batches showing good %EE were further subjected for evaluation of fit particle size and shape.

36.3.2.2.3 Particle Size and Shape of Vesicles

(A) *Mean Particle Size*

The batches showing the highest %EE were evaluated for their particle size. The F1 and F2 batches were selected for particle size analysis as they revealed the highest %EE. The particle size depends on the concentration of lipids. As the lipid concentration increases, the vesicle size increases, and this can be determined by the %EE. If the lipid concentration is more, then the entrapment of the drug and the particle size will also be more. The mean particle size was done with the help of a zeta sizer. The average mean particle size was calculated. The average mean diameter of F1 and F2 was recorded, and it was found that the F1 batch had a large particle size (shown in Figs. 36.3 and 36.4) than that of batch F2. The reason behind this is the concentration of lipids. The more the concentration of lipid, the more will be the particle size. But the particle size should be in the standard niosomal size range; otherwise, it could demonstrate an undesirable effect on the drug release profile. The F2 batch had an optimum particle size range, that is, within 10 to 1000 nm, which is the standard particle size range of niosomal dispersions. Hence, the F2 batch was selected for the morphological evaluation, that is, SEM studies.

(B) *Particle Shape*

SEM analysis was used to investigate the morphological characteristics of the particles. That brass might be found in the scanning microscope. The needles were dried for a short time in a dryer before being coated in gold using an ion sputter. Noisome images were captured using a random scan of the stab and count. About 30 niosomes were photographed, and their diameters were measured. The final mean diameter of 49 nm was determined. A single membrane is present in each vesicle. Figure 36.5 shows a photomicrograph from a scanning

			Size (d.nm):	% Intensity	Width (d.nm):
Z-Average (d.nm):	1842	Peak 1:	958.3	77.5	102.0
PdI:	1.000	Peak 2:	116.7	22.5	7.938
Intercept:	1.04	Peak 3:	0.000	0.0	0.000
Result quality :	Refer to quality report				

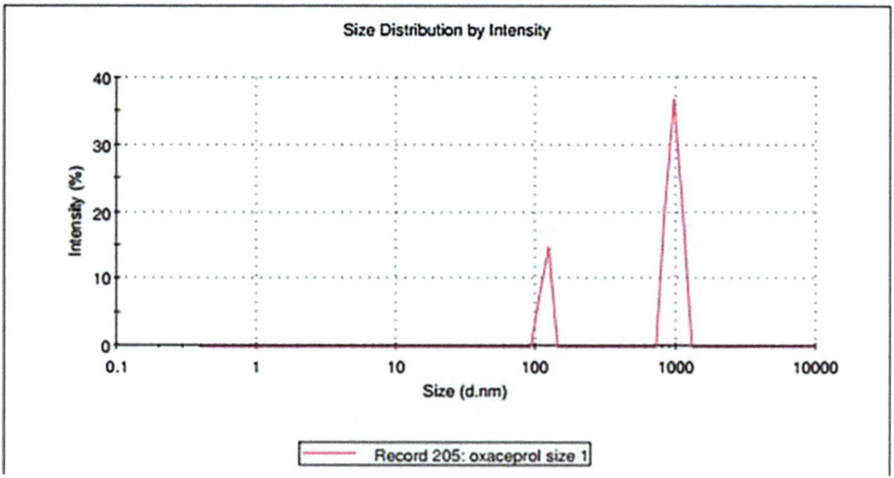

Fig. 36.3 Particle size of F1 batch

			Size (d.nm):	% Intensity	Width (d.nm):
Z-Average (d.nm):	490.0	Peak 1:	142.9	100.0	15.21
PdI:	0.746	Peak 2:	0.000	0.0	0.000
Intercept:	1.14	Peak 3:	0.000	0.0	0.000
Result quality :	Refer to quality report				

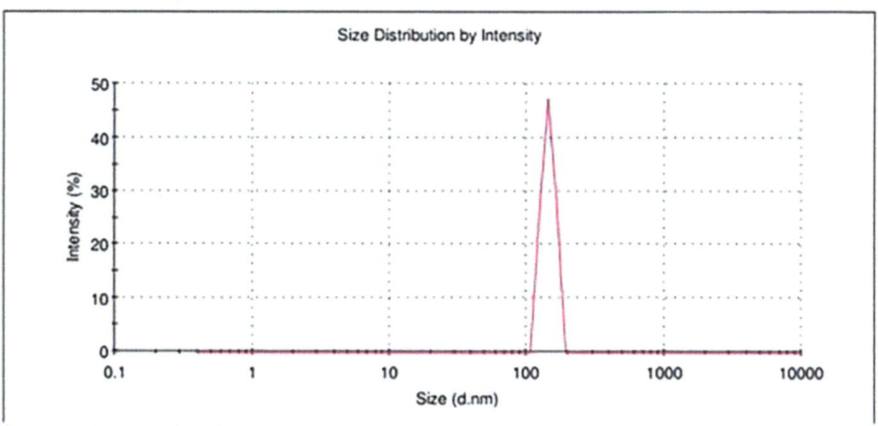

Fig. 36.4 Particle size of F2 batch

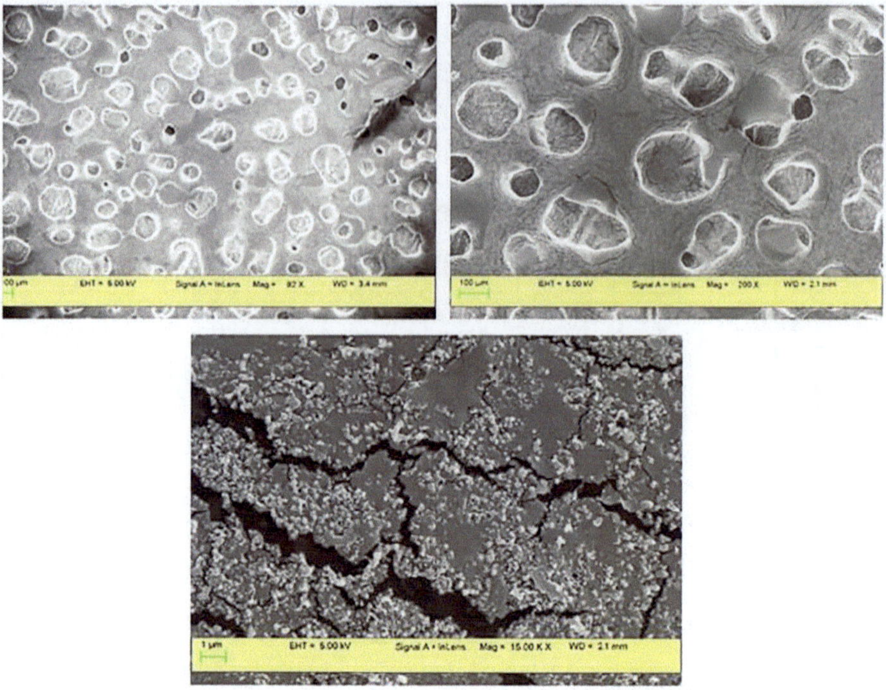

Fig. 36.5 SEM image of noisome of F4 batch

electron microscope (SEM) of the optimized batch (F4 batch), which clearly shows that the niosomes have a round, spherical shape.

36.3.3 Zeta Potential

The zeta potential of the batches of the formulation that achieved the optimal particle size was calculated. The optimized batch had a zeta potential of −34.5. Due to the low likelihood of aggregation, which is reflected in the high zeta potential value, the formulation is stable. Because both the formulation and the skin have negative charges, the net repulsion may be responsible for the reduced aggregation. Drugs delivered topically may be absorbed more effectively through negatively charged formulations because of this. A small negative charge can also be seen in the skin. Since the optimized gel has a negative zeta potential, the electrostatic repulsion between the skin's surface and the gel may contribute to better penetration through porcine skin. Peak zeta potential is shown in Fig. 36.6, and the data may be found in Table 36.6.

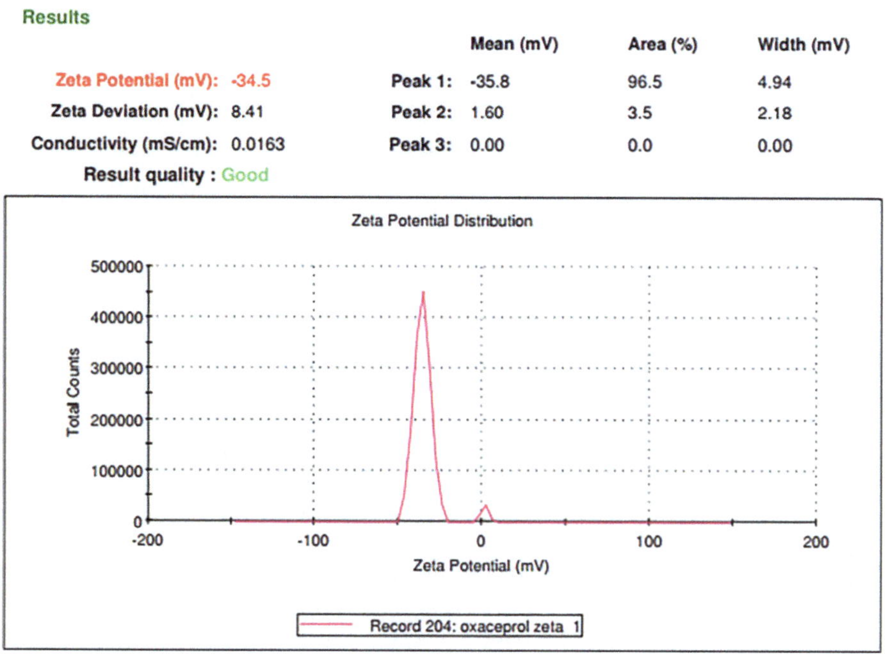

Fig. 36.6 Zeta potential of F2 batch

Table 36.6 Zeta potential and PDI of F2 batch

Formulation batches	Polydispersity Index (PDI)	Zeta potential (mv)
F2	0.746	−34.5

36.3.4 Evaluation of Niosomal Gel

36.3.4.1 Physical Parameter

36.3.4.1.1 Clarity

All of the manufactured topical gel formulations were examined under a microscope against a black and white background and were confirmed to be completely free of dispersed particle matter. Appearance-wise, all of the formulations passed muster. There was no visible particle matter or uneven texture in any of the gels, and the clarity test confirmed that all of the manufactured niosomal gels were clear of microbial contamination.

Table 36.7 pH values of formulations

Sr. no	Formulation code	Observed pH (±S.D.)
1	F1	6.5 ± 0.2
2	F2	6.6 ± 0.2
3	F3	5.9 ± 0.3
4	F4	6.3 ± 0.2
5	F5	5.9 ± 0.2
6	F6	6.1 ± 0.3
7	F7	5.9 ± 0.3
8	F8	6.3 ± 0.3

Table 36.8 Viscosity of formulations at a different shearing rate

		Viscosity (Cp)							
RPM	Torque	F1 batch	F2 batch	F3 batch	F4 batch	F5 batch	F6 batch	F7 batch	F8 batch
15	13.6	5429	5219	3243	4012	1330	3827	4110	1801
20	18	5387	5024	3099	3881	1309	3393	3891	1710
30	28	5379	4961	3047	3610	1240	3010	3808	1680
40	36.3	5340	4482	2929	3325	1215	2945	3328	1692
50	44.9	5249	3133	2915	2825	1161	2919	2831	1545
60	50.8	5049	3325	2879	2582	1103	2799	2530	1440
100	76.2	4577	2813	2834	2132	1032	2513	2146	1400
150	92	3721	2561	2801	1836	1088	2417	1838	820
200	97	3125	2180	2739	1335	922	2328	1337	799

36.3.4.1.2 pH

pH values of formulations were measured, and it was discovered that F1–F8 all have pH values between 6.5 and 6.8. (Table 36.7). The pH of the topical gel needs to be between 5.5 and 8.0 to reduce the likelihood of side effects.

36.3.5 Rheological Study

Gel rheological properties were measured by a Brookfield viscometer, spindle LV-64, type DV-II + PRO. At 370 C (room temperature), a range of shear rates was used to measure the formulations' viscosity. It was found that the gel's viscosity increased with increasing rpm and torque (shear rate). The graph was plotted as shear rate vs viscosity. The gel was also evaluated for its flow properties, that is, plastic or pseudoplastic flow. All the gel formulations showed pseudoplastic behaviour (Table 36.8). From the results, it was observed that as the torque/shear rate increases with rpm, viscosity decreases. Hence, it could be concluded that the prepared niosomal gel has a pseudoplastic flow property.

36.3.6 Drug Content

The % drug content of all the formulations was calculated, and the highest drug content was found to be 95.02 and 92.76% in F1 and F2 batches, respectively. The drug content of each formulation was measured to observe the total amount of drug present in the whole prepared gel formulation, as well as to predict the optimum release pattern at the site of application at the desired time interval. The drug content of Oxaceprol niosomal formulations is shown in Table 36.9.

36.3.7 Spreadability

The spreadability of batches F1 to F8 is shown in Table 36.10; the F1 batch has the highest spreadability, 15 ± 1.5.

36.3.8 In Vitro Drug Release Study

The purpose of this study was to determine the amount of the drug released from the vesicles with respect to the time so that the release of the drug can be studied in a detailed manner. The formulations could be categorized in different releasing dosage

Table 36.9 Percent drug content of niosomal gel

Sr. no.	Batch code	Drug content (%) ± S.D.
1	*F1*	*95.02 ± 0.02*
2	*F2*	*92.76 ± 0.02*
3	F3	86.50 ± 0.04
4	F4	81.01 ± 0.01
5	F5	79.70 ± 0.02
6	F6	82.62 ± 0.03
7	F7	49.97 ± 0.02
8	F8	78.80 ± 0.02

Table 37.10 Spreadability

Sr. no.	Batch code	Spreadability ± S.D. (g.cm^2 /sec)
1	F1	15 ± 1.5
2	F2	11 ± 1.5
3	F3	12 ± 2
4	F4	14 ± 2
5	F5	10 ± 2
6	F6	13 ± 1.5
7	F7	14 ± 1
8	F8	11 ± 1

forms such as sustained release, control release, immediate release, etc. The readings of in vitro drug release are reported in Table 36.11. From the results, it was observed that the F2 batch had a better release pattern than that of other batches. The reason behind his mechanism might be the particle size of the niosomes. The F1 batch had a large particle size; hence it may restrict the release of the drug. The drug release was performed for 12 h of the study, and it was found to be in a sustained manner. From this study, it was observed that the F2 batch had the best-sustained release effect. So, it also helps in increasing the retention time of the dosage form on the skin surface, reduces the frequency of dosing, and is graphically represented in Fig. 36.7.

36.3.9 Optimization

Considering all evaluation data, it was observed that all the niosomal gel formulation batches prepared by using non-ionic surfactants such as Span 20 showed optimum % EE, drug release, and other parameters. The reason behind this could be the Hydrophilic–lipophilic balance (HLB) value of Span 20, which is in the range of 8.6, so it may have better hydrophilicity as well as better lipophilicity. Hence, it might be a deserving candidate for formulating all niosomal gel batches. Moreover, the F1 and F2 batches were compared, and it was observed that the F1 batch containing a high concentration of surfactant and cholesterol had a large particle size and less drug release than that of the F2 batch. The batch showing high entrapment, high drug content, optimum viscosity, better spreadability, as well as optimum particle size and shape was considered to be an optimized batch. As the F2 batch fulfilled the desired criteria of all the evaluation parameters, it was considered to be an optimized batch.

36.3.10 Ex Vivo Permeability Study

This study's results revealed that the conventional gel has a high drug release rate in less time, that is, rapid drug release profile, whereas the niosomal gel could release the drug up to 12 h, that is, it shows the sustained-release effect (Table 36.12). The reason behind this is clear, that is, the vesicles could hold the drug for a longer period in its core and the polymer used to prepare the gel may control the release pattern of the drug. Thus, the formulation is assumed to have a prolonged retention time on the skin surface and may sustain the drug release for localized effect (Table 36.13). Results are graphically summarized in Fig. 36.8.

Table 36.11 The in vitro drug release study of formulation

Time (min)	% Drug release							
	F1	F2	F3	F4	F5	F6	F7	F8
10	7 ± 0.02	4.7 ± 0.02	2.3 ± 0.04	7 ± 0.02	1.3 ± 0.04	7 ± 0.02	1.3 ± 0.04	7 ± 0.02
60	12.2 ± 0.04	10.7 ± 0.02	2.5 ± 0.03	12 ± 0.04	2.3 ± 0.02	12.2 ± 0.04	2.3 ± 0.03	12 ± 0.04
120	16.6 ± 0.02	14.3 ± 0.04	4.7 ± 0.02	16.6 ± 0.02	5.3 ± 0.04	20.15 ± 0.02	5.3 ± 0.02	20 ± 0.02
180	24.5 ± 0.03	19.7 ± 0.03	8.3 ± 0.04	24.5 ± 0.04	8.3 ± 0.02	25.41 ± 0.04	10.76 ± 0.03	25 ± 0.04
240	29.7 ± 0.04	23.32 ± 0.02	13.7 ± 0.04	29.7 ± 0.03	11.3 ± 0.04	40.31 ± 0.02	14.35 ± 0.02	33.3 ± 0.03
300	37.68 ± 0.04	26.31 ± 0.03	19.7 ± 0.03	34.1 ± 0.04	16.7 ± 0.02	47.32 ± 0.04	17.34 ± 0.02	38.5 ± 0.03
360	42.94 ± 0.03	34.0 ± 0.04	23.3 ± 0.02	38.5 ± 0.03	22.7 ± 0.03	57.70 ± 0.03	22.72 ± 0.03	46.4 ± 0.04
420	50.83 ± 0.04	45.45 ± 0.02	26.3 ± 0.03	42.9 ± 0.04	26.3 ± 0.04	59.59 ± 0.03	28.70 ± 0.04	55.2 ± 0.03
480	59.59 ± 0.02	55 ± 0.04	29.3 ± 0.04	47.3 ± 0.02	31.6 ± 0.03	98.36 ± 0.04	32.39 ± 0.02	60.4 ± 0.02
540	64.85 ± 0.04	63.9 ± 0.03	34.6 ± 0.03	58.7 ± 0.03	37.6 ± 0.04	77.12 ± 0.03	35.38 ± 0.03	68.3 ± 0.03
600	68.23 ± 0.03	75.3 ± 0.02	43 ± 0.02	68.3 ± 0.03	41.2 ± 0.02	82.38 ± 0.03	52.63 ± 0.04	77.1 ± 0.04
660	77.12 ± 0.02	84.92 ± 0.03	47.2 ± 0.03	73.6 ± 0.03	46.6 ± 0.03	86.76 ± 0.04	59.21 ± 0.02	82.3 ± 0.02
720	82.38 ± 0.04	93.98 ± 0.02	55 ± 0.02	78 ± 0.04	55.02 ± 0.02	91.14 ± 0.02	84.59 ± 0.02	86.7 ± 0.02

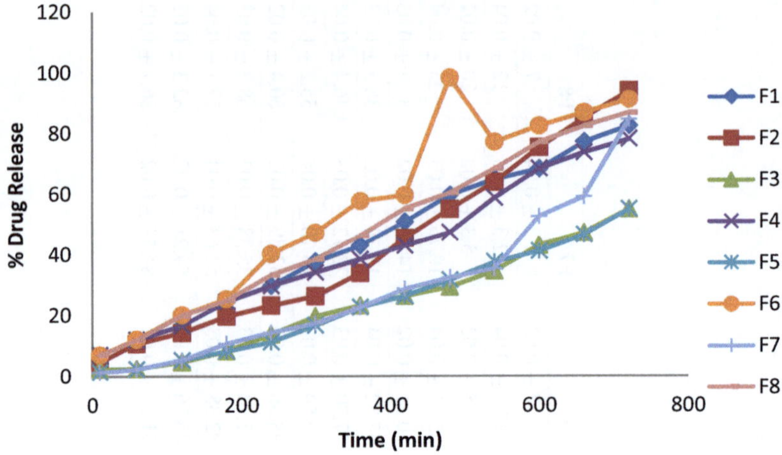

Fig. 36.7 In vitro drug release profile

Table 36.12 % Drug release of oxaceprol gel and oxaceprol niosomal gel

Time (min)	% Drug release	
	Oxaceprol gel	Oxaceprol niosomal gel
0	0	0
60	2.3 ± 0.02	2.30 ± 0.02
120	14.9 ± 0.03	5.38 ± 0.03
180	39.4 ± 0.03	37 ± 0.02
240	54.4 ± 0.02	54.4 ± 0.03
300	66.38 ± 0.04	66.38 ± 0.04
360	78.34 ± 0.03	73.56 ± 0.02
420	85.52 ± 0.02	79.5 ± 0.02
480	98.68 ± 0.02	83.1 ± 0.03
540	98.68 ± 0.04	88.5 ± 0.02
600	98.68 ± 0.04	92.10 ± 0.03
660	98.68 ± 0.03	95 ± 0.04
720	98.68 ± 0.02	98 ± 0.02

Table 36.13 Permeability coefficient of both formulations

Gel	Flux	Permeability coefficient (μg/cm^2/h)
Oxaceprol Gel	0.552	552×10^{-4}
Oxaceprol Niosomal Gel	0.0884	884×10^{-5}

36.3.11 Stability Study

Table 36.14 displays the results of a stability analysis conducted at 25 °C on the optimized F2 batch to determine its shelf life.

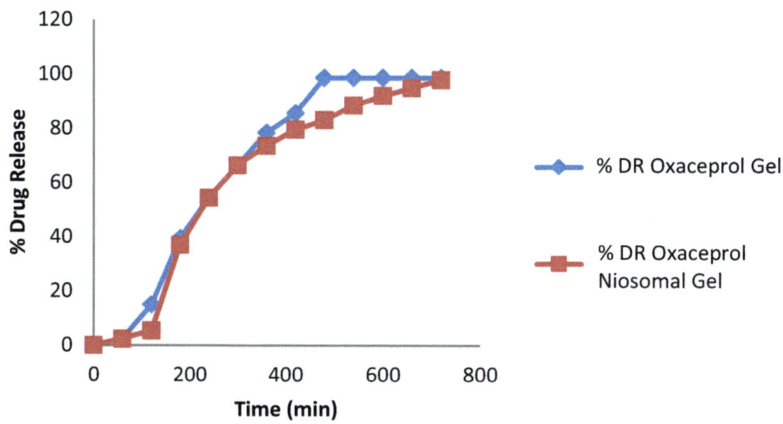

Fig. 36.8 % Drug release of oxaceprol gel and oxaceprol niosomal gel

Table 36.14 Stability study of F2 batch

Sr. no.	Observations	Before stability testing	Stability testing after 1 month
1	Clarity	Clear	Clear
2	Visual Appearance	Transparent	Transparent
3	Ph	6.6 ± 0.02	6.5 ± 0.02
4	Drug Content	92.76 ± 0.02	92.72 ± 0.02

36.4 Conclusion

The present investigation revealed that the niosomal gel could have a better therapeutic potential than conventional dosage forms upon topical application. The fundamental difficulty in using topical medications is that the skin itself acts as a barrier, preventing the majority of pharmaceuticals from penetrating the skin. This research demonstrated that niosomal gel, due to its nanoscale size and elastic nature, can operate as the best vesicles in cutaneous drug administration. Because of the various lipid components, they have the potential to serve as drug carriers by transporting the enclosed drug molecules into or through the skin. They might be more effective at penetrating the stratum corneum and subsequently changing the intercellular lipid lamellae found there. The improved therapeutic efficacy at the afflicted site at lower doses of pharmaceuticals included in the niosomal gel formulation was demonstrated in in vitro and ex vivo trials, providing an intriguing association between the improved permeability capabilities of niosomal gel and conventional dosage forms.

References

1. Bhowmik, D., Gopinath, H., Kumar, B. P., & Kumar, K. P. S. (2012). The pharma innovation recent advances in novel topical drug delivery system. *The Pharma Innovation, 1*, 12–31.
2. Ranade, V. V. (1991). Drug delivery systems. 6. Transdermal drug delivery. *The Journal of Clinical Pharmacology, 31*, 401–418.
3. Akhavan, A., & Bershad, S. (2003). Topical acne drugs: Review of clinical properties, systemic exposure, and safety. *American Journal of Clinical Dermatology, 4*, 473–492.
4. Tiwari, G., Tiwari, R., Sriwastawa, B., Bhati, L., Pandey, S., Pandey, P., & Bannerjee, S. K. (2012). Drug delivery systems: An updated review. *International Journal of Pharmaceutical Investigation, 2*, 2–11.
5. Rizvi, S. A. A., & Saleh, A. M. (2018). Applications of nanoparticle systems in drug delivery technology. *Saudi Pharmaceutical Journal, 26*, 64–70.
6. Ionac, M., Parnham, M.J., Plauchithiu, M., And Brune, K. (1996). Oxaceprol, an atypical inhibitor of inflammation and joint damage. Pharmacological Research 33, 367–373.
7. Harris, A., Schropp, A., & Messmer, K. (1998). Effects of oxaceprol on the microcirculation in ischemia/reperfusion injury. *European Journal of Medical Research, 3*, 182–188.
8. Sohrabi, S., Haeri, A., Mahboubi, A., Mortazavi, A., & Dadashzadeh, S. (2016). Chitosan gel-embedded moxifloxacin niosomes: An efficient antimicrobial hybrid system for burn infection. *International Journal of Biological Macromolecules, 85*, 625–633.
9. Nigro, F., Cerqueira Pinto, C. D. S., dos Santos, E. P., & Mansur, C. R. E. (2020). Niosome-based hydrogel as a potential drug delivery system for topical and transdermal applications. *International Journal of Polymeric Materials and Polymeric Biomaterials*, 1–18.
10. Radmard, A., Saeedi, M., Morteza-Semnani, K., Hashemi, S. M. H., & Nokhodchi, A. (2021). An eco-friendly and green formulation in lipid nanotechnology for delivery of a hydrophilic agent to the skin in the treatment and management of hyperpigmentation complaints: Arbutin niosome (Arbusome). *Colloids Surfaces B Biointerfaces, 201*, 111616.
11. Goyal, G., Garg, T., Malik, B., Chauhan, G., Rath, G., & Goyal, A. K. (2015). Development and characterization of niosomal gel for topical delivery of benzoyl peroxide. *Drug Delivery, 22*, 1027–1042.
12. Budhiraja, A., & Dhingra, G. (2015). Development and characterization of a novel antiacne niosomal gel of rosmarinic acid. *Drug Delivery, 22*, 723–730.
13. Qumbar, M., Imam, S. S., Ali, J., Ahmad, J., & Ali, A. (2017). Formulation and optimization of lacidipine loaded niosomal gel for transdermal delivery: In-vitro characterization and in-vivo activity. *Biomedicine & Pharmacotherapy, 93*, 255–266.
14. Chen, S., Hanning, S., Falconer, J., Locke, M., & Wen, J. (2019). Recent advances in non-ionic surfactant vesicles (niosomes): Fabrication, characterization, pharmaceutical and cosmetic applications. *European Journal of Pharmaceutics and Biopharmaceutics, 144*, 18–39.
15. Sengodan, T., Dubey, A., Rathi, V., & Rathi, J. (2009). Development and characterization of niosomal drug delivery of gliclazide. *Journal of Young Pharmacists, 1*.
16. Kumar, P., & Verma, N. (2021). An overview on niosomes: As an auspesious drug delivery system on the bases of application. *Research Journal of Pharmacy and Technology, 14*, 2896–2902.
17. El-Sayed, M. M., Hussein, A. K., Sarhan, H. A., & Mansour, H. F. (2017). Flurbiprofen-loaded niosomes-in-gel system improves the ocular bioavailability of flurbiprofen in the aqueous humor. *Drug Development and Industrial Pharmacy, 43*, 902–910.
18. Zhou, X., Hao, Y., Yuan, L., Pradhan, S., Shrestha, K., Pradhan, O., Liu, H., & Li, W. (2018). Nano-formulations for transdermal drug delivery: A review. *Chinese Chemical Letters, 29*, 1713–1724.
19. Garg, V., Singh, H., Bhatia, A., Raza, K., Singh, S. K., Singh, B., & Beg, S. (2017). Systematic development of transethosomal gel system of piroxicam: Formulation optimization, in vitro evaluation, and ex vivo assessment. *AAPS PharmSciTech, 18*, 58–71.

20. Waghule, T., Singhvi, G., Dubey, S. K., Pandey, M. M., Gupta, G., Singh, M., & Dua, K. (2019). Microneedles: A smart approach and increasing potential for transdermal drug delivery system. *Biomedicine & Pharmacotherapy, 109*, 1249–1258.
21. Mourtas, S., Fotopoulou, S., Duraj, S., Sfika, V., Tsakiroglou, C., & Antimisiaris, S. G. (2007). Liposomal drugs dispersed in hydrogels. Effect of liposome, drug and gel properties on drug release kinetics. *Colloids and Surfaces. B, Biointerfaces, 55*, 212–221.
22. Kumbhar, D., Wavikar, P., & Vavia, P. (2013). Niosomal gel of lornoxicam for topical delivery: In vitro assessment and pharmacodynamic activity. *AAPS PharmSciTech, 14*, 1072–1082.
23. Alvi, I. A., Madan, J., Kaushik, D., Sardana, S., Pandey, R. S., & Ali, A. (2011). Comparative study of transfersomes, liposomes, and niosomes for topical delivery of 5-fluorouracil to skin cancer cells: Preparation, characterization, in-vitro release, and cytotoxicity analysis. *Anti-Cancer Drugs, 22*, 774–782.
24. Aziz, D. E., Abdelbary, A. A., & Elassasy, A. I. (2019). Investigating superiority of novel bilosomes over niosomes in the transdermal delivery of diacerein: In vitro characterization, ex vivo permeation and in vivo skin deposition study. *Journal of Liposome Research, 29*, 73–85.
25. Ioele, G., Tavano, L., De Luca, M., Ragno, G., Picci, N., & Muzzalupo, R. (2015). Photostability and ex-vivo permeation studies on diclofenac in topical niosomal formulations. *International Journal of Pharmaceutics, 494*, 490–497.
26. Nagalakshmi, S., Krishnaraj, K., Jothy, M., Chaudhari, P. S., Pushpalatha, H. B., & Shanmuganthan, S. (2016). Fabrication and characterization of herbal drug – Loaded non-ionic surfactant based niosomal topical gel. *Journal of Pharmaceutical Sciences and Research, 8*, 1271–1278.

Chapter 37
Using ICT Technologies, Open-Source Software Affects DHH Healthcare Issues

S. Malathi and A. Chitra

37.1 Introduction

When used as a noun, "ICT" (information and communication technology) means that one has acquired the skills necessary to use data and communication systems. The nature of the teaching and the aptitude of the students both influence the content covered. Students are prepared for their future use of ICT in education, work, and civic engagement. ICT [1, 2] functions as a supporting tool for task creation, information collection, documenting, and disseminating and directing research. ICT is a means of educating and learning that also suggests that it is a tool for teaching and learning on its own, serving as a platform for both student and teacher learning. It shows up in various structures, like drill and training, recreations, and instructive organizations. ICT [3, 4] abilities are somewhat important for involving ICT in training. Increased dedication, increased effort, and concise writing is only a few of the many specific benefits [5] that are listed. The main downside of using social networks in the class as a result of integrating the technology into learning including secured concerns, the knowledge curve, managing big groups of students, and it's incapable to manage a variety of advanced systems, including animation videos, text documents, accounting sheets, introductions, and so forth. Its two main components in education are as follows.

S. Malathi (✉)
St. Thomas College of Arts and Science, Chennai, Tamil Nadu, India

A. Chitra
DRBCCC Hindu College, Chennai, Tamil Nadu, India

F. J. J. Joseph et al. (eds.), *Computational Intelligence for Clinical Diagnosis*, EAI/Springer Innovations in Communication and Computing,
https://doi.org/10.1007/978-3-031-23683-9_37

37.1.1 Facilitated Individualized Education

A personalized learning environment that is adapted to each student's unique characteristics, like mobility, interest, pace, and understanding level, may be provided via innovation. Additionally, it engages students to their full potential by giving them the support and challenge they need to stay engaged, convinced, and motivated.

37.1.2 Superior Community Association

Innovation can guide guardians along with local area individuals' association in understudy learning by utilizing strategies, for example, sites, email, sites, text-informing, and so forth, to keep intrigued people mindful and occupied with the framework.

37.1.3 Advantages of Open-Source

- Do not need to reinvent the wheel
- Free as in "freedom"
- Source code are easily available
- Can pick extra support
- Can correct bugs and adapt to changes in requirements and technology
- Costs significantly less than proprietary rivals

37.2 Background

Microsoft, creator of Windows and Microsoft Office, and other software businesses have long backed this economic model, while Microsoft's general manager for interoperability Jean Paoli said in August 2010 that the company "loves open source" and that its anti-open-source stance was a mistake. Trust, acceptance, cooperation, and quality are benefits of such a structure. The FOSS paradigm allows capable persons to examine and edit a product's source code. However, most code is not in the public domain (Fig. 37.1).

Non-free licences limit fundamental liberties, say free software advocates. A copyleft licence protects the "four software freedoms" by explicitly providing them and banning redistributing the package or using its code to produce derivative works without the same licencing restrictions. Some agreements allow redistributors to eliminate the four software freedoms, sometimes called permissive software licencing.

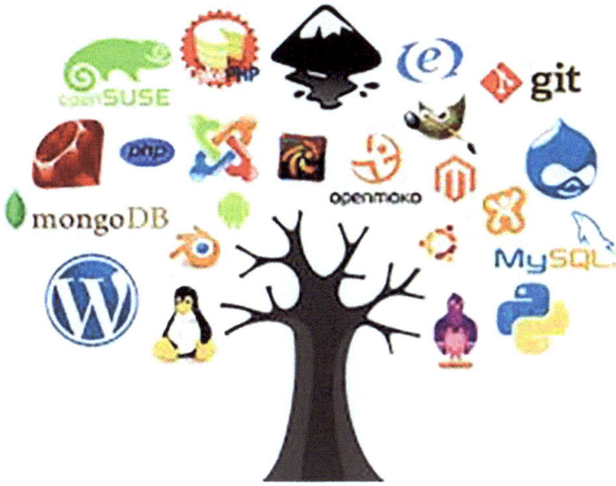

Fig. 37.1 Open-source technologies healthcare issues

The FreeBSD License is an example of such a licence, as it allows for the distribution of derivative software as a closed source so long as the original developers are credited.

37.3 Software from Open Sources for Healthcare Issues

The tools that are frequently used in educational systems include books, teachers, the foundation, and to a lesser extent open-source software (OSS) [6, 7]. In terms of open-source programming, it is becoming increasingly important to prepare for the future. The copyright holder has granted access to and authorization for the use of OSS [8], a PC application that allows anybody, for any reason, to study, modify, and transmit comparable material for free. Individuals or client groups work together to build OSS. According to a Standish Group analysis from 2008, the use of open-source programming techniques has resulted in an annual increase of $60 billion in investment money for purchasers. Researchers Casson and Ryan [9] highlighted a variety of arrangement-based factors, particularly the higher offer from open-source in comparison to constrictive designs in the following classifications: security, moderation, simplicity, endurance, between operability, and adaptability [10].

The GNU General Public License (GPL), which allows designers to freely appropriate their work but imposes the restriction that all future developments and applications be covered by a similar license, is the most well-known example. The source code of a product can be made publicly available through open-source distribution, and licensing provides the developer with the freedom to tweak something comparable.

Software that has been created by and for the user community is known as free and open-source software (FOSS). Developers have fantastic possibilities to collaborate, contribute, and, most importantly, learn through open-source projects. Contributing does not just entail coding; in fact, every project calls for a diverse set of

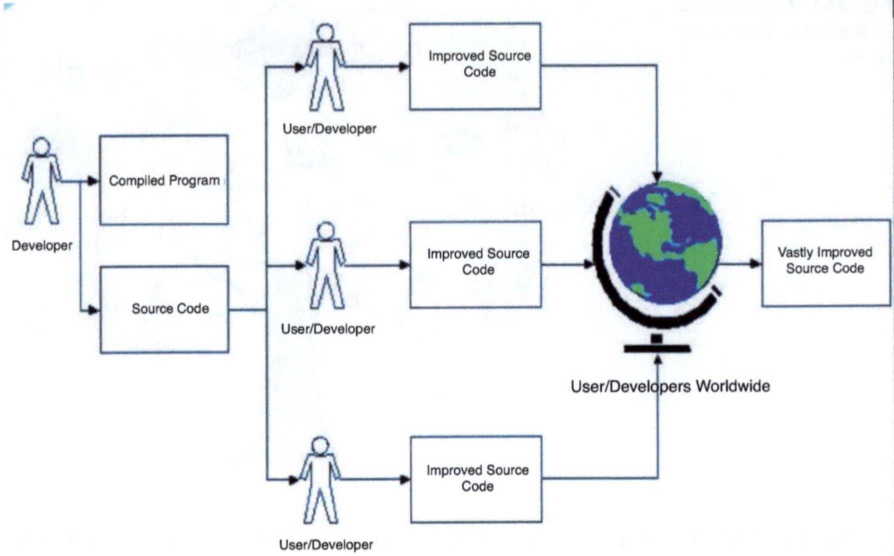

Fig. 37.2 Accessing of open source for deaf or hard-of-hearing (DHH) healthcare issues

abilities. Companies have had to rethink and optimize how they produce, deploy, and use software assets or even rethink their whole IT infrastructure in order to find novel and innovative methods to do business. As a result, open-source ushers in improved quality, more dependability, more flexibility, reduced prices, and an end to proprietary lock-in. Open source is, therefore, ultimately advantageous for business.

The "www.opensourceteaching.org" server, which is secured by a firewall, hosts open-source learning resources.

Subject to a few limitations, anybody may read, copy, or use it. This is known as copyleft.

- Any organization, business, or person may build up a delivery system to utilize any of the information on the websites in any way they see fit, absolutely free of charge, with the exception of copyleft restrictions.

They can only charge for the value contributed, and the cost of distribution; any modifications to the original content must be recognized; and how the material is provided, how much is utilized, or what value is added depends on the end user's intended use (Fig. 37.2).

Use anything you want without breaking pricey contracts, adhering to the vendor's restrictions, shelling out outrageous fees, or working at their pace. You make a choice, not the product's seller. You are free to use whatever version or build of the software and hardware that you require. Anytime you want to improve, you can. In order to work with as many different software products as possible, OSS aims to be as compatible as it can. Many people appreciate having the opportunity to switch between systems and, more crucially, connect to other users, companies, and computers. Everyone can see open-source code.

37.4 Open-Source Government

To allow any interested citizen to participate in the development of policy, like with a wiki document, proponents of open-source governance (also known as open politics) advocate for the merging of democratic principles with the open-source and open-content movements. The general public is democratically given access to legislation, utilizing their pooled expertise to strengthen democracy and the decision-making process. By comparing these methods to software code, some of their proponents call for a "central codebase" in the form of a collection of regulations that are constantly updated in a public registry and infinitely repeatable. Distributions of this policy-base are made available (periodically or dynamically) for usage by locations, where they may be customized using "patches".

- Microsoft's legal method for distributing software source code is known as "shared source". A variety of technologies and licenses are included in Microsoft's Shared Source Initiative, which was introduced in May 2001.
- After completing the necessary requirements, the majority of its source code offers are made available for download.
- The licenses affiliating the offers range from being closed-source, permitting just reading of the code for reference, to permitting it to be updated and redistributed for both commercial and non-commercial reasons.

37.5 Proposed Work

According to the personnel's or the design students' areas of interest, the proposed first stage of hard of hearing preparation/learning would be supplied. Open-source programming that is unavailable in the academic emphasis may be introduced by the certified workforce and design students. They may be viewed as additional courses that return the subject to academic emphasis, allowing for unlimited application of the concept in geological fields. The purpose is that the students will use the video lectures' instructional activities for self-directed learning [11]. If they have any questions after self-learning, they may ask them in the asset community by getting in touch with the staff and the centre's certified design students. This style of teaching combines the instructor's [11] instruction of a class with the students' independent viewing of video lectures, allowing them to grasp the concept more effectively and without the need for outside funding. The several levels of the dynamic learning environment are shown. Thus, the general people will greatly benefit from the educative learning process that makes use of OSS.

Fig. 37.3 Open-source community

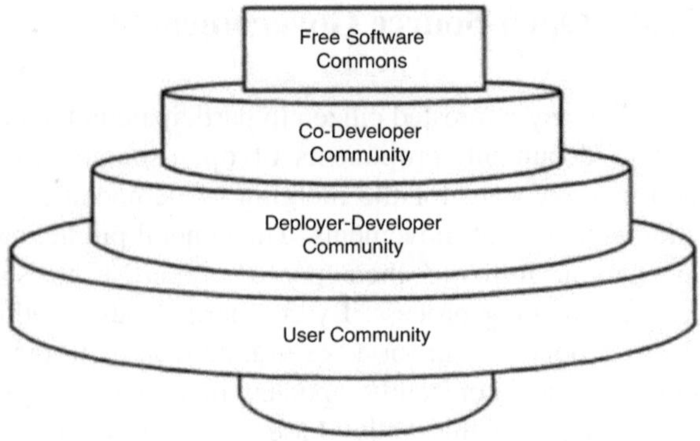

37.6 Design for Open Source

- People with backgrounds in both software and hardware frequently engage in conflicting arguments when debating the merits of open hardware design.
- One reason for this is that the term "software" encompasses both source code and executables, but "hardware" and "hardware design" clearly refer to two distinct concepts.
- The terminology listed below has all been used in discussions on this issue (Fig. 37.3).
- Using the phrase "hardware" as a shorthand for both design and the actual thing is a recipe for misunderstanding.
- It does not mean that the design cannot be sold or that any hardware implementation of the design will be free of charge. Free hardware design refers to a design that may be freely reproduced, disseminated, updated, and fabricated.

37.7 Method for Hard of Hearing

For various client-produced material and innovations, like OSS development, Wikipedia, open access distribution, and so on, the open-source standards have been modified. In order to make the classroom a conducive learning environment, it will be advantageous to think about employing open-source programming. Some of the programming tools and approaches that are available may be used for self-learning, including:

Email, Facebook, Twitter, LinkedIn, Google, and other social media sites, as well as text and video messages.

They called this cycle a studio, and one needs to enlist for something similar at liberated from cost. Following their participation in the online assessment test and receipt of certificates based on the presentation, members who have learned from the video addresses may be eligible to apply for jobs in the relevant industries. For mutants, the method will be as illustrated in Fig. 37.4.

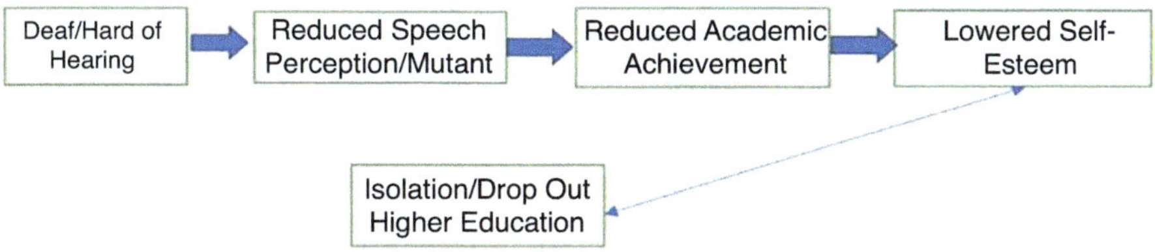

Fig. 37.4 Education among DHH

OSS quickly fixes any bugs, because a larger population will result in quicker response times. The majority of the time, we observe the reverse in the proprietary sector. Patching vulnerabilities frequently take weeks or even months for major corporations like Oracle or Microsoft, for instance. Consider which software suite is most likely the superior one. There is no hidden code. If you want to alter a specific section of the software to suit your needs, you may do so by simply changing, adding, or removing code. A lot of the time, proprietary software bans you from making any modifications at all or makes it extremely difficult to do so. We take this service extremely seriously because it's one of our main lines of business. Make use of all the open-source products' paid support options at costs that are still far less than those associated with purchasing proprietary software. This is frequently erroneously cited as the sole factor, albeit an important one, why a business should convert to OSS. This is because OSS no longer requires required proprietary fees. Most importantly, you get to choose what you need and can obtain it for less money and higher quality.

37.8 ICT for Hearing Impairment

The PC is currently regularly alluded to as a media gadget and can introduce data in an assortment of ways. Disc ROMS use text, still, and moving pictures and sound to pass on data. Word processors permit you to blend text and pictures to give extra importance to composed material. Text can be made from letters, words, and expressions, as opposed to being developed letter-by-letter – this can assist with peopling focusing on the importance and stream of their composition. Video "cuts" of marking can be added to other programming or joined into sight and sound introductions. With overlay consoles and software, for example, Inclusive Writer, Clicker and Writing with Symbols 2000 can interface messages and images to give various composition, spelling, and sentence development exercises (Fig. 37.5).

Pictures and graphics becoming all the more remarkable where many programming includes mixed media approach. Now and again, a more straightforward methodology is better, and there are many projects that utilize pictures and designs. My World: My World 3 and its broad scope of asset packs offers exercises utilizing designs that cover numerous educational programme regions, ages, and capacity levels.

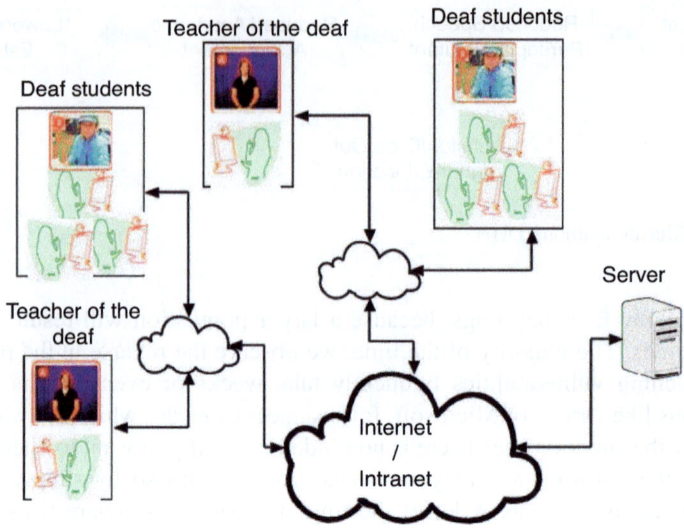

Fig. 37.5 ICT learning for DHH

37.8.1 IntelliTools

IntelliTools programming can be utilized to make language and graphical exercises reasonable for a wide age and capacity range.

37.8.2 Language Advancement

First Keys 2 purposes pictures, liveliness, discourse, and sound to build up effective finishing of errands. Action screens can be printed to follow-up work away from the PC. At the point when an action is finished, a basic record sheet can be shown or printed to use as a prize or to assist with observing advancement.

37.8.3 Image Software

Programs that have been intended to involve images for language and correspondence purposes can be utilized to make picture and image exercises on-screen and are likewise valuable for making paper-based assets. Boardmaker has been intended to make correspondence diagrams and overlays utilizing broad image libraries.

37.8.4 *Marking CD-ROM*

The Sign Now – BSL CD ROM (Forest Bookshop) gives a broad library of signs and addresses the capability of interactive media for the introduction of learning and available material for the hard of hearing.

37.8.5 *E-Learning*

A helpful instrument that has helped facilitate education for individuals all around the world is e-learning. Deaf persons need to have access to e-learning since they have trouble studying in traditional classroom settings. For instance, when lecturers demonstrate on the board, they often face the wall, making lip-reading impossible. Additionally, students will not be able to take notes and listen to the lecturer, interpreter, or lip-speaker at the same time if they do not have a note-taker. Jordan has a large population of deaf youngsters. Due to the absence of educational infrastructure, resources, and specialized services, they confront even greater difficulties. Inequalities in education and impediments to effective learning and teaching are targeted by contemporary inclusive educational practices. Due to this, it is essential to diversify instructional tools and content utilizing ICT in order to ensure that all students, including those with disabilities, have access to education. The purpose of this essay is to outline several cutting-edge interactive tools for teaching deaf and hard-of-hearing (DHH) pupils (Fig. 37.6).

DHH kids' education is becoming more and more reliant on technology. This chapter examines two ways that technology is utilized for the education of these students as well as two ways that it is used to enable communication access for DHH students (real-time captioning in classrooms and messaging and associated technologies to allow conversation in small groups) (multimedia materials for the development of literacy and online tutoring). Real-time captioning and multimedia resources are effective in the instruction of DHH pupils, according to a number of studies. The scant research to date on online tutoring and messaging to enhance group communication with DHH and hearing students shows that these topics have the potential to be significant since they meet the unmet requirements of DHH students.

37.9 Characteristics of Effective Instructors for ICT-Based Teaching for Mutants

The field of study known as "moral philosophy", or ethics, is concerned with what is morally good and evil as well as morally right and wrong. Ethics is founded on moral principles that may be justified as good and bad, and that suggest what people should do. Any idea or system of good values or principles can also be included under this umbrella phrase (Fig. 37.7).

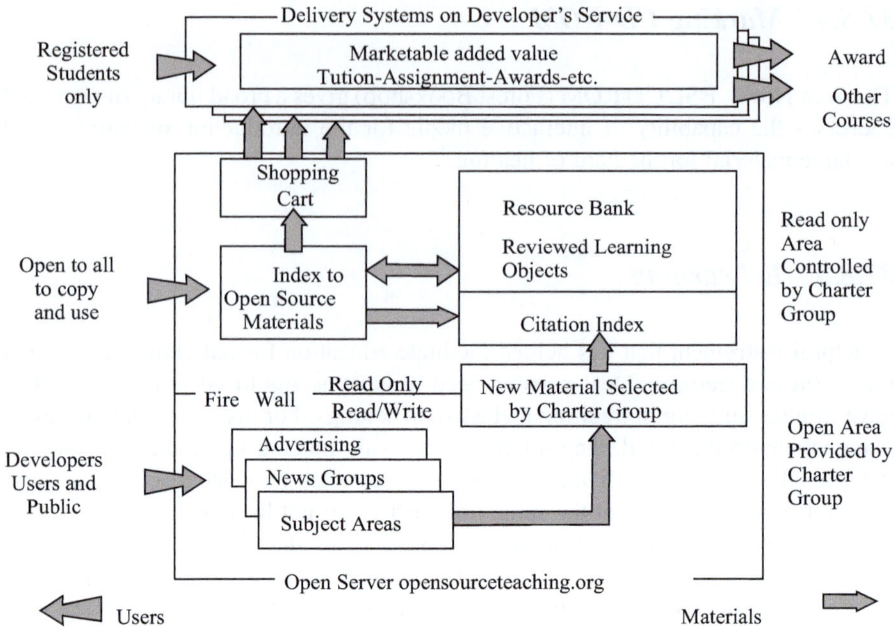

Fig. 37.6 Teaching methodology of open source DHH healthcare issues

Fig. 37.7 ICT teaching for DHH

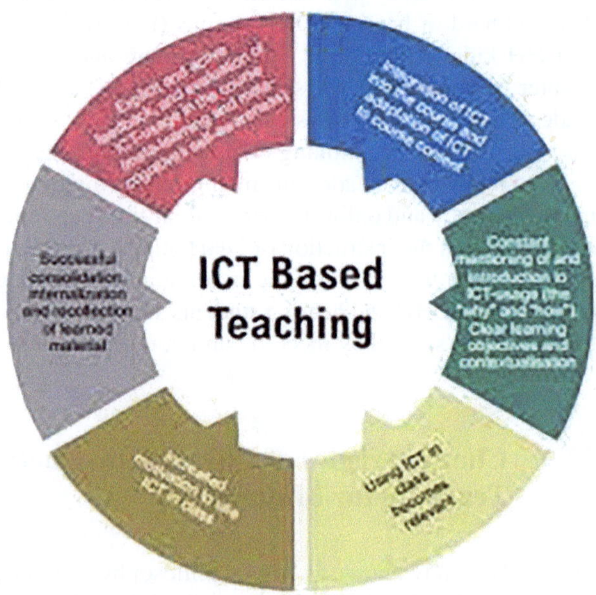

It is notable that these profoundly successful instructors can have an improving impact on the day-to-day routines as long-lasting instructive and vocation desires. Long periods of exploration on educator quality help the reality that viable instructors [12–14] not just cause understudies to feel great about learning. It has been confirmed that a variety of personal and professional characteristics are associated with greater degrees of understudy success. Important qualities of effective instructors:

- Have official teacher agreements prepared.
- Possess a certificate or equivalent (standard, elective, or temporary) and are qualified in their specialities
- Have at least three years of education.
- Show compassion, fairness, and awareness.
- Enhance instruction by using a variety of instructional strategies, assignments, and exercises.
- Pre- and post-assessments can be used to monitor how well students are progressing. Students who didn't achieve success can then receive more instruction.
- The availability of source code as a source of inspiration when creating complementary systems is one of the common advantages of all shared source applications.
- In addition, having access to the source code enables security inspection and review, which some big businesses and governments are now requiring.
- A few shared source licenses incorporate numerous open-source license advantages.
- Other shared source licenses are proprietary rather than open source, which typically entails the voluntary waiver of many of the author's rights. This allows the copyright holder to maintain tighter control over the usage of their work.

37.9.1 Assessment of Student Learning

The method used to assess learning is another concern with using understudy learning appraisals in the educator's [15, 16] assessment process.

- The precision of reviewing methodology.
- Arrangement of accomplishment tests with the educational programme.
- The demonstrative worth of one or the other methodologies for informative improvement.
- Single-moment nature of these pointers.

A much more precise proportion of what an understudy has realized would be reflected by an evaluation that is educational plan adjusted and directed both toward the start and year's end.

37.9.2 Meaningful Input for Informative Improvement

Input as appraisal information offers an important device for oversight [17, 18]. Assessment prompts proficient development, which expects instructors to genuinely look at their own assets and shortcoming. The motivation behind self-assessment is restricted because of the absence of objectivity. Essentially, criticism from associates in view of a couple of study hall visits is similarly restricted in light of the fact that it gives a thin inspection of conduct. Appraisal information and information technology of understudy learning over a period can give sufficient input on understudies' general comprehension of the subject. Additionally, more thorough testing of the educator's impact on students' in the mastery of the concepts and skills that are been taught. Information investigation has been utilized as a method of observing achievement and guaranteeing responsibility for distinguishing the objectives of the whole system. Review of the data revealed that for improved results and to understand the gaps in understudies' their routine observation is done to ensure their abilities and needs.

37.9.3 Teaching Techniques

Provide the student and interpreter with a list of any new words or terms that will be used while discussing unfamiliar technical vocabulary. It is challenging to understand unfamiliar terms. Students who need interpreters learn things a few seconds later than the rest of the class. Give the student adequate time to speak with the interpreter and obtain the necessary information before asking for assistance. Ask the students to raise their hands when they have an answer rather than just shouting it out. The pupil who has hearing loss will be able to participate as a result. Before answering, rephrase the class's first inquiries. A student utilizing an academic language development (ALD) should keep in mind that they can only hear what is coming from the microphone and will miss anything else. Do not read aloud so rapidly that the student who is hard of hearing or deaf and their interpreter cannot follow along with the rest of the class. Keep in mind that hearing-impaired and deaf pupils rely on visual signals such as body language and expressions that elicit data.

37.10 For Hard of Hearing

The instructive advantages of web-based entertainment might be most articulated when they sway gatherings of students who are in a difficult situation in traditional up close and personal settings. Among such impeded bunches are the DHH [19] understudies who might encounter new open doors with the assistance of virtual entertainment. The utilization of virtual entertainment has filled extensively lately, spreading to different everyday issues, like training. Despite the fact that the writing is later and gives important suggestions toward conquering these difficulties, because of the quick advancement of virtual entertainment they might change consistently. Therefore, partners may not know about the proper translation of these proposals. Subsequently, the section gives an extensive understanding of the utilization of online entertainment and technology [20] among the hard of hearing and nearly deaf, alongside the advantages and difficulties being used. Existing suggestions for conquering the difficulties are explored, and approaches for the plan of virtual entertainment and its productivity use are proposed.

37.11 Conclusion

Open-source programming is utilized as a significant instrument for instructing understudies as well as different members at no expense. For understudies and networks who are unaware of this asset, courses, talks, and workshops are necessary for a deeper grasp of the value of open-source understanding. Regarding the selection of various open-source programming sources, one should use caution. With the speed at which technology is developing, many educators are incorporating cutting-edge methods into their classrooms. These kids are required to follow the teacher's instructions only with their eyes. Interactive whiteboard (IWBs) and sound amplification equipment are being added to the classrooms created, especially for deaf pupils, in order to transfer knowledge more effectively. Anybody, at any time and wherever, appeared to be able to benefit from the market and technologies. Online education is not, however, completely inclusive. This is because one of the assumptions underlying online learning models conflicts with the hearing impairment of DHH pupils.

References

1. Murray, J. (2011, December 18). Cloud network architecture and ICT – modern network architecture. *IT Knowledge Exchange*. TechTarget. Retrieved 2013 August 18.
2. *Information and communication technology from*. FOLDOC. 2008 September 19.
3. Zuppo, C. M. Defining ICT in a boundary less world: The development of a working hierarchy (PDF). *International Journal of Managing Information Technology (IJMIT)*, 19(4). Retrieved 2016 February *13*.
4. ICT in Education. From Wikipedia, the free encyclopedia, Unesco. Unesco. Retrieved 10 March 2016.
5. "IT Costs – The Costs, Growth and Financial Risk of Software Assets". OMT-CO Operations Management Technology Consulting GmbH. Retrieved 26 June 2011.
6. Verts, William T. (2008, January 13). "Open source software". World Book Online Reference Center. Archived from the original on January 1, 2011.
7. Rothwell, R. (2008, August 05). "Creating wealth with free software". Free. *Software Magazine.*. Retrieved 2008-09-08.

8. "Standish Newsroom Open Source" (Press release). Boston. 2008-04-16. Retrieved 2008 September 08.
9. Casson, T., & Ryan, P. S., *Open standards, open source adoption in the public sector, and their relationship to Microsoft's market dominance by: SSRN*. Papers.ssrn.com. Retrieved 2015 March 30.
10. Eric S. (1998). *Raymond and Bruce Perens, open source initiative*, from Wikipedia – the free encyclopedia.
11. Darling-Hammond, L. (2000). Teacher quality and student achievement: A review of state policy evidence. *Education Policy Analysis Archives, 8*(1)., ISSN 1068-2341.
12. Mendro, R. L. (1998). Student achievement and school and teacher accountability. *Journal of Personnel Evaluation in Education, 12*(257–267), 262.
13. *ITU releases annual global ICT data and ICT development index country rankings*. www.itu.int. Retrieved 2015 September 01.
14. Marzano, R. J., Pickering, D. J., & Pollock, J. E. (2001). *Classroom instruction that works: Research based strategies for increasing student achievement*. Association for Supervision and Curriculum Development. International Journal of Computer Applications (097).
15. Wright, S. P., Horn, S. P., & Sanders, W. L. (1997). Teacher and classroom context effects on student achievement: Implications for teacher evaluation||. *Journal of Personnel Evaluation in Education, 11*(57–67), 63.
16. Schalock, H. D. (1998). Student progress in learning: Teacher responsibility, accountability and reality. *Journal of Personnel Evaluation in Education, 12*(3), 237–246.
17. Stronge, J. H., & Tucker, P. D. (2003). *Handbook on teacher evaluation: Assessing and improving performance*. Eye on Education.
18. Howard, B. B., & McColskey, W. H. (2001). Evaluating experienced teachers. *Educational Leadership, 58*(5), 48–51, p. 49.
19. Chang, C.-M. (2014). New media, new technologies and new communication opportunities for deaf/hard of hearing people. *Online Journal of Communication and Media Technologies*. Special Issue – October, *4*, 38.
20. Lersilp, T., & Lersilp, S. (2019). Use of information technology for communication and learning in secondary school students with a hearing disability. *MDPI, Education Sciences, 9*, 57.

Chapter 38
Clinical Intelligence for Cloud Services Resource Scheduling Using RNN

B. Aarthi, S. Sridevi, Pallavi Ashok, and Yusra Naeem

38.1 Introduction

Customers are increasingly using public cloud applications to efficiently process big data or extensive data, primarily from social media, e-commerce platforms, and search engines. In general, these data are unevenly distributed, that is, data provided by different customers have different sizes and processing times. Understanding and using complex, elevated, and diverse biological data continues to be a major obstacle in the transformation of health care. Digital health records, neuroimaging, −omics, sensor data, and text, all of which are complicated, heterogeneous, infrequently described, and generally disorganized, all have been growing in contemporary biomedical research. Feature engineering is often required in classical, big data, and statistically learning methods before building prediction or clustered models on top of the aspects to generate useful and so more robust attributes from the data.

Nevertheless, effectively training a deep learning model is a challenging undertaking because they usually involve a huge number of parameters. As a result, the Long Short-Term Memory Algorithm, which is considerably more effective than the current one, a deep learning network, is introduced in this project to show the workload. Deep learning excels at forecasting cloud workload for industrial processing, even though it is the most significant intelligence infrastructure in contemporary computation. One of the most significant areas to be focused on in distributed computing has been distributed storage management, data security, and workload prediction [1].

B. Aarthi (✉) · S. Sridevi · P. Ashok · Y. Naeem
Department of Computer Science and Engineering, SRM Institute of Science and Technology, Ramapuram, Chennai, India
e-mail: aarthib@srmist.edu.in; sridevis@srmist.edu.in; pa5830@srmist.edu.in; yn2063@srmist.edu.in

F. J. J. Joseph et al. (eds.), *Computational Intelligence for Clinical Diagnosis*, EAI/Springer Innovations in Communication and Computing,
https://doi.org/10.1007/978-3-031-23683-9_38

This chapter is structured as follows: Several literature reviews are discussed in Section 38.2. The description of the issue is illustrated in Sect. 38.3. The current system, its flaws, and the current algorithm are covered in Sect. 38.4, and the proposed method and algorithm, as well as their respective benefits, are covered in Sect. 38.5. The different modules utilized are detailed in Sect. 38.6. The outcome analysis which includes graphs, a system requirement diagram, and an architectural diagram is illustrated in Sect. 38.7 and conclusion is discussed in Sect. 38.8.

The development of the proposed system was aided by comparisons of existing models, approaches, surveys, and analyses of current methods [2–5]. To develop an efficient system, the prioritization approaches in various types of testing, and the various test case generation methods [2, 6, 7] were thoroughly understood. To understand the practical applications of testing, the various applications of software testing processes [2, 8–11] were also studied.

38.2 Related Works

Islam and his partners propose a Spark service allocation framework to provide an effective service allocation for any big data app to maximize efficiency and reduce costs. When the big data application is running on all nodes in the Spark collection, app crashes occur. To address this, dividing algorithms were developed by Gounaris and others. These algorithms mimic the performance of the Spark app during use in order to minimize app usage by rotating a small amount of operating time. Chen and colleagues have proposed a split algorithm in the Spark framework to reduce data communication costs and increase data usage training by improving data similarity and work compatibility. To address the problem of single machine-induced killings in a separate Spark collection, Yang and his colleagues predicted the remaining work time based on a variety of conditions, finding time-consuming jobs. Islam and its allies have investigated the Spark deadline-based distribution of large data requests. They have created a new resource allocation plan by showing the cost of employee requests and completion times. In their diagram, the value is determined by the number of builders and the time taken to complete the application. Wang and Khan's study predicted application time by collecting execution times from various stages of the application. Wang and colleagues used DAG-based memory analysis forums to model the application performance of the application. Spark confirmed their methods again. Gibilisco and its partners have many polynomial retrieval models based on in-app data to predict big data processing time with anonymous setup settings. Chen and Wang have introduced entropy-based online-based editing in the Spark collection to provide QoS confirmation of Spark's online analysis. Resources are sorted by entropy in their algorithm, and tasks are sent in the sequence of resources.

38.3 Problem Description

Job scheduling is the main factor in achieving the high-performance goal in extensive data analysis. Nominally clever planning strategies to achieve performance can be impacted by energy, regionality, equity, and synchronization issues. Processing data requires a lot of energy and sharing of resources among workers, and appropriate action is necessary when planning work. Another issue with considerable data planning is the locality of the data. Finally, we need to aim to reduce the cost of processing time for order planning in comprehensive data analysis. In other words, scheduling seeks to minimize the response time by using the best procedures for scheduling, with better resource utilization and to make jobs faster in processing. Big data processing runs on any framework cluster by separating a job into lesser tasks and classifying the load to the worker nodes, as shown in Fig. 38.1. The main point in analyzing big data is how these tasks are assigned to agent nodes with two different types of prioritization within the cluster. Usually, the controller node is responsible for distributing the charges to the agent nodes and making the best scheduling techniques execute.

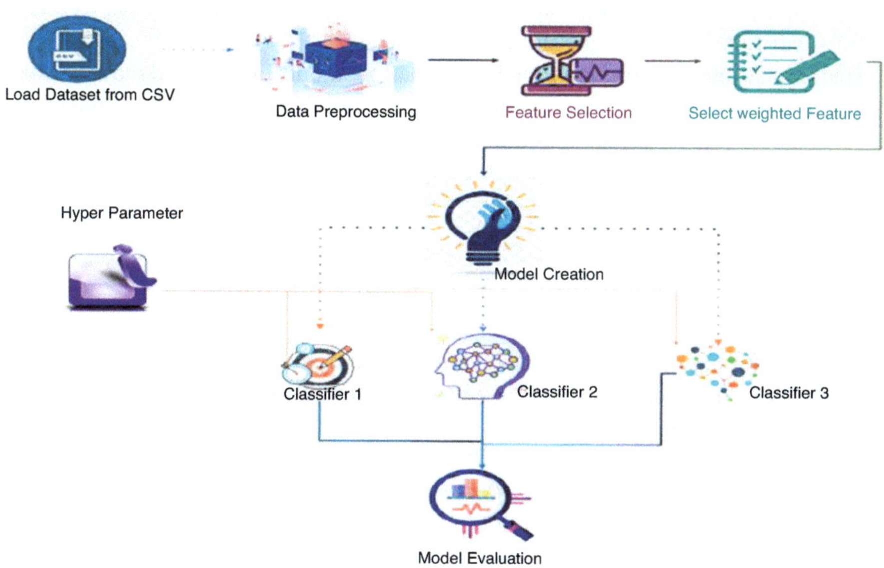

Fig. 38.1 Architecture diagram

38.4 Existing System

38.4.1 Apache Hadoop

Apache Hadoop is an open-source software program framework for keeping datasets in a cluster of commodity hardware for large-scale processing. A Hadoop cluster contains a primary node and various agent nodes. The primary node encompasses four units; a JobTracker, TaskTracker, Data node, and Name node. JobTracker's primary role is to control the task trackers and is a node that manages the execution of the job. TaskTracker also delivers the reports to JobTracker. MapReduce operates double functions: Map and Reduce operations. Scheduling mechanisms are being shared with Hadoop jobs.

38.4.1.1 Disadvantages of Apache Hadoop

- Hadoop will fail if you need to access small files in bulk. These tiny files surcharge the NameNode and make it difficult to work.
- Hadoop is a framework written in Java that makes it less secure because cyber criminals can easily abuse Java.
- By default, security features are not available in Hadoop. Hadoop uses Kerberos for security features that are not easy to manage.
- Hadoop has other restrictions, such as some constraints in Map and reduced steps when the significant data pipeline is executed. Hadoop is not efficient for performing extensive data pipelines. To overcome the shortcomings of Hadoop, Spark came out to do and expand the MapReduce framework.

38.4.2 Existing Algorithm: Deep Belief Network

The deep belief network (DBN) was invented as an answer to the troubles that occur when coaching usual neural networks with deep trust networks, such as it is sluggish to learn, poorly chosen parameters, and requires a lot of coaching datasets. Hence, it stays at a nearby minimum. This algorithm uses a layer-by-layer strategy to examine all top-down processes and key generative weights. These related weights decide how all variables in a layer rely on different variables in the layer above. Except for the first and remaining layers, every layer in the DBN serves two roles: a hidden layer for the preceding node and an enter layer for subsequent nodes. Some purposes in deep trust networks are image, video sequence, action capture information detection, clustering, and generation.

1. The architecture of DBN: DBN consists of a sequence of limited Boltzmann machines linked in sequence. Each layer of the Boltzmann desktop is educated to converge and then freeze. The effects of the machine's output layer are fed as

inputs to the subsequent Boltzmann system in the sequence and are skilled to converge on their very own till the whole section is deployed.

2. Disadvantages of using DBN: Despite being vastly less expressive than a deep neural network, DBNs impart significant restrictions on their weight connections, outperforming them on tasks for which sufficient input data is available. Even in their prime, DBNs were rarely used in direct application. Instead, they were used as a pre-training step: a DBN with the same overall architecture as a corresponding DBN is denied and trained. Its weights are then taken and placed into the connected deep neural network, then fine-tuned and applied. It eventually fell out of favor because they are just a particular case of autoencoders, which were more broadly flexible and helpful for pre-training and other applications.

For another thing, introducing more sophisticated optimizers, learning late schedulers, and dropout techniques have dramatically alleviated the vanishing gradient problem in practice. Increased data volumes and computing power have made direct deep neural network applications to problems more tractable.

38.5 Proposed System

38.5.1 Apache Spark

Apache Spark is an open-source processor that is used for many loads of facts. Dash analysis questions at points of any scale are the use of memory retention and prepared questionnaires. Provides advanced APIs in Java, Scala, Python, and R to help re-use code for a number of tasks such as bulk processing, responsive questions, real-time analysis, computer learning, and format processing. With Spark, performance is faster with just one step: uploading data to memory, performing the process, and writing back results. Spark also uses the memory repository to process data, which speeds up machine learning algorithms that cost tasks to the same database over and over again. Data re-use achieved through the Data frames and abbreviated over resilient distributed datasets (RDDs). A collection of archived material is re-used in all Spark operations, which greatly reduces delays, especially when it performs machine learning and interactive analysis.

38.5.1.1 Features of Apache Spark

Swift Processing: one can obtain about one hundred instances quicker facts processing velocity in reminiscence and ten more instantaneous statistics processing rates in a disk. This is feasible by lowering the range of examining/writing accesses to the challenging disk.

In-Memory Computation: one can use in-memory processing to pace up processing. This is where the records are cached, so you do not have to fetch the statistics from the disk every time. Therefore, it saves time. Spark is quicker because it has a DAG execution engine that allows in-memory computation and non-circular data. Supports a couple of languages – Spark offers a built-in Java, Scala, or Python API. Therefore, you can write functions in one-of-a-kind languages.

Advanced Analytics: Spark does more significant than help Map and Reduce. It additionally allows SQL queries, streaming data, desktop studying (ML), and layout algorithms.

Multilingual Support: Several languages such as Java, R, Scala, and Python are supported by Spark. Therefore, it presents dynamism and overcomes Hadoop's hindrance of being capable of constructing functions solely in Java.

Real-Time Stream Processing: Spark has a real-time move processing function. Previously, the trouble with Hadoop MapReduce was once the capacity to system and manner current data; however, instead of real-time data, you ought to use Spark Streaming.

38.5.1.2 Ecosystem of Apache Spark

SparkCore forms the basis of the platform. Spark SQL can connect to a data source and convert query results to RDDs in Java, Scala, and Python programs. This is because it contains the API responsible for these transformations. SQLContexts can create DataFrames to provide complex operations on datasets. DataFrame is considered a programming abstraction. Spark Streaming for real-time analysis is used to implement and process live data streams, such as sensor data that tracks weather conditions and log files.

Spark MLlib contains many techniques and algorithms used in the machine-learning process. It provides algorithms for building regression, clustering, and classification models, as well as multiple techniques for evaluating the resulting model, enabling MLlib to run faster with iterative calculations.

Spark GraphX is a library for performing parallel graph computation and manipulating graphs. GraphX is generated with a special RDD of vertices and edges. Supports a library of combined graph algorithms. Iterative graphing algorithms and the fastest graphing systems make GraphX more powerful while maintaining.

38.5.1.3 Advantages of Apache Spark

- Spark analytics software can also accelerate jobs on Hadoop data processing platforms.
- Spark provides jobs in short bursts of 5 s or less, excluding micro-batch as an alternative to MapReduce.
- Spark's library is designed to complement the types of processing jobs investigated more intensively in the latest commercially supported Hadoop deployments.
- Apache Spark provides a robust API that allows developers to interact with Spark through their applications.

38.5.2 Proposed Algorithm: Long Short-Term Memory Algorithm

38.5.2.1 Architecture of Long Short-Term Memory Algorithm

LSTM networks have special features. LSTMs have the ability to store data sequences. There is another section focused on deleting new information. Textual data always contains many details that LSTMs can eliminate to reduce computational time and cost. By removing unused information and saving sequences of data, LSTMs become a powerful tool for text classification and other text-based tasks.

38.5.2.2 Advantages of Long Short-Term Memory Algorithm

- Improved traceability
- Have well-understood formal properties
- Simple, fast, and less complex
- Minimizes the workload on infrastructures
- Effectiveness for distributed optimization
- Achieve a well-balanced tradeoff among various parameters

38.6 Modules

38.6.1 Module 1: Data Evaluation

Exploratory data analysis relies heavily on data visualization and graphical interpretation. Statistical modelling provides a simple low-dimensional representation of the relationships between variables but generally requires a high degree of knowledge of statistical methods and mathematical principles. Visualizations and charts tend to be much easier to interpret and create, so one can quickly explore various aspects of your dataset. The final goal is to create an easy data summary that informs the query. This is not the final destination in the pipeline but an important destination.

38.6.1.1 Characteristics of Exploratory Graphs

Charts generated by exploratory data analysis (EDA) are different from all charts. When you analyze a dataset, you usually create dozens, if not hundreds, of search charts. You can post one or two of these graphics in the final format. One of the purposes of EDA is to deepen a personal understanding of the data. Therefore, all code and graphics need to be tuned for that purpose. Exploratory graphics do not require any essential details that you might add when publishing your graphics. EDA is a method for analyzing data and its regularity based on the actual data distribution by using visual techniques. The human eye and brain have strong structural recognition capabilities and occupy an important position in data exploration. Visual analysis is also designed to reproduce different human models with the processing power of a unique way of displaying data. Analysts always recommend and suggest performing exploratory data analysis of the data. First, you need to select the structure size or stochastic size mode. Exploratory data analysis can also show unexpected deviations that are not possible with regular models.

38.6.2 Module 2: Feature Engineering

Information capture IG measures how much information is provided to make a classification decision for a class, with or without terminology. If the document belongs to each category and the time is on the paper, the IG will reach its maximum. The discriminator selection method assigns a more important score to the discriminator and lowers the score to an irrelevant trait. The ambiguity scale (AM) feature selection method gives high scores to items that are consistently displayed in a selected category. The AM score is calculated for the individual features. A threshold is specified, and based on the criteria set, the ability of the AM score to fall below this scale is modified, and the ability of the AM score to exceed this threshold is used during the learning phase. The feature information gain calculates the difference in whether entropy occurs in the text. The wider the information obtained, the more meaningful the contribution of the trait to the reader. Select a function with high information gain as a function. Dimensionality reduction is a widely used pre-processing in the analysis, visualization, and modelling of high-dimensional data. Feature selection is used to reduce dimensions. Only input dimensions are selected, which contain the pertinent information to resolve the problem at hand.

38.6.3 Module 3: Model Prediction and Evaluation

The algorithm uses gradient descent to build a backpropagation neighborhood for supervised read errors. This type of neural network (NN) is made up of neuron-like elements called nodes. The node is built into the layer. NN sends the input file to the secret layer node and the secret layer information to the output node using the activation properties between the layers and vice versa. The final result can be received at the output layer. The NN neighborhood consists of two parts: forward propagation and reverse propagation. The scaled data is sent to the input layer grid. At the start of training, the connection weights are initialized with a large amount of small random data. In previous propagation, the land of neurons in individual layers can completely affect subsequent connecting layers. There are no connections between neurons in the same layer. If the output layer no longer receives the intended output, then the tutorial reverses the backpropagation process in case of an error between the neighborhood output and the expected output. Evaluation of predictive models needs to predict unknown future energy consumption. Therefore, we used the data for 1 week as the training dataset and the records for the other week as the test dataset. View different training examples or examples. Also, choose to normalize the intervals before training the data.

38.7 Modules

38.7.1 Analysis

Various header files like Numpy, Pandas, Tensorflow, and Keras are used to work with the dataset. Here we are training an empty model and creating the empty model; Tensorflow and Keras are used. The data is then split for training and testing. Using the MinMaxScaler, the values are set, like 1 s and 0 s. To read the data set, we run the following command (Tables 38.1, 38.2, and 38.3),

```
train = pd.read_csv('train_1.csv').fillna(0)
page = train['Page']
train.head()
train.tail()
train.sample(9)
```

We also check for null values in the dataset and sum the number of null values. We drop to page 1, which contains the country names and different languages, using the command below, since we just need the values in the dataset to train our algorithm.

```
train = train.drop('Page',axis = 1)
```

We use the following command to split the dataset. It is split into two: training and testing.

```
X_train, X_test, y_train, y_test = train_test_split(X, y, test_size =
0.3, random_state = 0
```

30% of the dataset is used for testing, and the remaining 70% is taken for training.

```
y_pred = model1.predict(inputs)
y_pred = sc.inverse_transform(y_pred)
```

Table 38.1 Using the head() method, the first five rows of the dataset are displayed

		2015-	2016-	2015-	2016-	2016-	2013-	2015•	2015-	2016.	2016-	2016-	2016-	2016-	2016–2016	
	Page	07–01	07–02	07–03	0744	0746	07–06	07–07	0746	0749	12–22	12–23	12–24	12–26	12–26	12.7
145068	utiderwodd_(setle_de oeliculas) es %%Aped's 0	00	00	00	00	0.0	0.0	00	00	00	0.0	00	0.0	00	130	121
145059	Res41ent Eva Caoituk) Fmal es seeinpFla org	00	00	00	00	00	00	00	00	00	00	00	00	00	00	01
145060	Enamoranckinefie_Flamtn_eS wylvedia org_ali-	00	00	00	00	00	0.0	00	00	00	00	00	0.0	00	00	01
	acc-															
145061	Hasta_el_Utimo .hombr_es wikipedia all ac	00	00	00	00	00	00	00	00	00	00	00	00	00	00	01
145062	Francisco elirtacemiacojsene_clejaysionj	00	00	00	00	00	00	00	00	00	00	00	00	00	00	0

Table 38.2 Using the tail() method, the last five rows of the dataset are displayed

PaCal	2015-07-01	2015.0742	2015-0743	2015.0744	2015.0745	2015-0746	2015-0747	2015.0748	2015.0749	2016.12.22	2016-12.23	2016.12.24	2016.12.25	2016.12.25	2016.12-27	2016.12.28	2016 12.21
0 2NI' rn wkceisa ×949	180	11.0	5.0	130	14.0	9.0	90	220	260	32.0	630	150	260	14.0	20.0	220	19.0
80 (055_48.0er)	110	140	15.0	180	110	130	220	110	100	170	420	280	150	90	300	620	45.0
I 2PM_SI tvOupeclu	10	00	10	10	00	40	00	30	40	30	10	10	70	40	40	60	3.0
org_l. acans_spicki	350	130	10.0	940	4.0	26.0	140	90	110	320	100	260	270	160	110	17.0	191
2 3C_Th witpede erg _all access_spoer 3 4rnmule_Th Allupe)a C49_81- access_spodel 52 Hz 1 Low You rh vutlopfla org_al. access_s	00	00	0.0	00	0.0	00	00	00	00	*480*	00	250	130	3.0	11.0	270	131

Table. 38.3 Using the sample(9) method, nine random rows of the dataset are displayed

100814	ParnaA_CCCP _ru wilopacha mg al acraas ail ag	70860	14160	14800	17760	1189 0	1798 0	13670	14330	1410 0	43250	36980
121184	X51133113ija 611upecta cotal-access_al-agents	0.0	0.0	0.0	0.0	0.0	00	0.0	00	0.0	3420	3620
22619	Hcipjalk Calegonc51b_www medsawlo org_mola	00	00	0.0	00	00	00	00	00	00	00	00
15907	Frevaaehru vakipecaa org_mobae web414agen1s	00	00	00	00	00	00	00	00	00	650	880
35219	lusxeLeanueinmiLen v41095081orta6acc	90	10.0	100	40	30	50	90	30	1.0	1200	1900
40200	Jenneler_Aarston_c6 wicipedc of9_411-access_a	179750	15723 0	16353 0	18003 0	1/ 1380	17051 0	16021 0	18947 0	17116.0	173570	17655 0
13302	6,11,64m Ka5.1.0lang en wiggeda erg e. . . .SktCp $_A$l	00	00	00	00	00	00	00	00	00	6740	5070
30193	+74iN[1]3.3154981n1111183&Th mlogedsa 449_411-acccatall.	830	7660	1000	570	590	500	450	1060	500	637 0	60 0
135829	WE ja •ak.pagia 0rg_a11-900455_spget	190	120	140	260	120	130	90	100	13.0	540	600

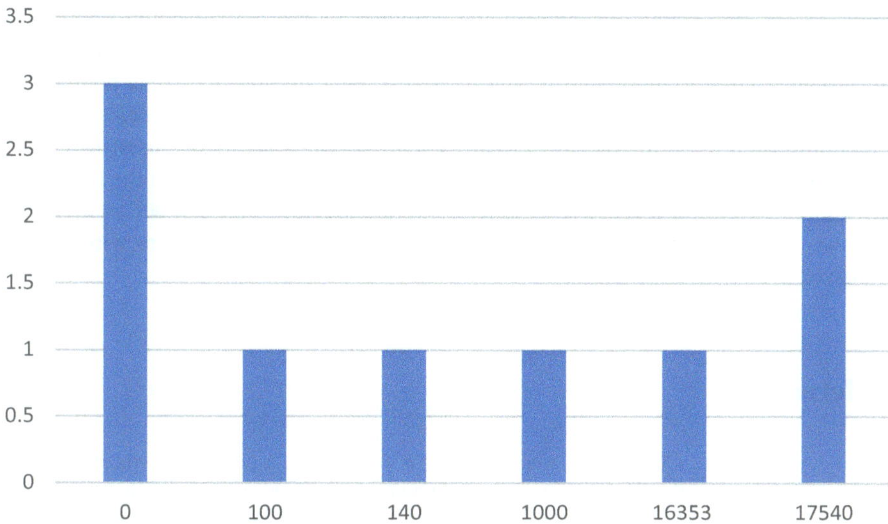

Fig. 38.2 Traffic workload prediction

Now that the training part is over, we predict the data next. Using the above command. We plot a graph using the command below for the predicted workload and the actual workload.

```
plt.figure
plt.plot(y_test, color = 'red', label = 'Real Cloud Traffic Workload
View')
plt.plot(y_pred, color = 'blue', label = 'Predicted Cloud Traffic
Workload View')
plt.title('Cloud Traffic Workload View Forecasting')
plt.xlabel('Number of Days from Start')
plt.ylabel('Cloud Traffic Workload View')
plt.legend()
plt.show()
```

In Fig. 38.2, the red line shows the Real Traffic Workload View Forecasting. At the same time, the blue line shows the Predicted Cloud Traffic Workload View Forecasting.

38.8 Conclusion and Future Work

Deep learning techniques are potent tools that enhance conventional machine learning and enable computers to gain knowledge from the data in order to find ways to develop smarter applications as well as for healthcare. Many industries, particularly in natural language and computer vision interpretation, have already exploited these methods. In this paper, we present the structure of the hybrid cloud computing model. Structured workload management technology allows users to build a new design with a hybrid cloud computing model. A dedicated service arena handles the primary service load, while a separate and shared service platform deals with the maximum amount from the ash crowd. Cloud services are being used to extend existing infrastructure due to the expansion of the cloud foundation. In the future, we have planned to add a reactive engine to the architecture that can act as a second defense against degraded QoS by compensating for prediction errors with ad hoc dynamic deployment decisions.

References

1. Vijayalakshmi, T., Chelliah, B., Alagumani, S., & Jagadeesan, J. (2014). An efficient security based multi owner data sharing for un-trusted groups using broadcast encryption techniques in cloud. *International Journal of Application or Innovation in Engineering & Management, 3*(3), 15–21.
2. Li, H., Wang, H., Xiong, A., Lai, J., & Tian, W. (2018). Comparative analysis of energy-efficient scheduling algorithms for big data applications. *IEEE Access, 6*, 40073–40084.
3. Zaharia, M., Borthakur, D., Sen Sarma, J., Elmeleegy, K., Shenker, S., & Stoica, I. (2010, April). Delay scheduling: A simple technique for achieving locality and fairness in cluster scheduling. In *Proceedings of the 5th European Conference on Computer Systems* (pp. 265–278).
4. Acharjya, D. P., & Ahmed, K. (2016). A survey on big data analytics: Challenges, open research issues and tools. *International Journal of Advanced Computer Science and Applications, 7*(2), 511–518.
5. Ho, L. Y., Wu, J. J., & Liu, P. (2011, July). Optimal algorithms for cross-rack communication optimization in mapreduce framework. In *2011 IEEE 4th International Conference on Cloud Computing* (pp. 420–427). IEEE.
6. Schintler, L. A., & McNeely, C. L. (Eds.). (2019). *Encyclopedia of big data*. Springer International Publishing.
7. Khalil, W. A., Torkey, H., & Attiya, G. (2020). Survey of apache spark optimized job scheduling in big data. *International Journal of Industry and Sustainable Development, 1*(1), 39–48.
8. Sabzevari, M., Toosizadeh, S., Quchani, S. R., & Abrishami, V. (2010, August). A fast and accurate facial expression synthesis system for colour face images using face graph and deep belief network. In *2010 International Conference on Electronics and Information Engineering* (Vol. 2, pp. V2–354). IEEE.
9. Agana, N. A., Oleka, E., Awogbami, G., & Homaifar, A. (2018, April). Short-term load forecasting based on a hybrid deep learning model. In *SoutheastCon 2018* (pp. 1–6). IEEE.
10. Patel, J., Jindal, V., Yen, I. L., Bastani, F., Xu, J., & Garraghan, P. (2015, March). Workload estimation for improving resource management decisions in the cloud. In *2015 IEEE Twelfth International Symposium on Autonomous Decentralized Systems* (pp. 25–32). IEEE.
11. Gu, H., Li, X., & Lu, Z. (2020). Scheduling spark tasks with data skew and deadline constraints. *IEEE Access, 9*, 2793–2804.

Chapter 39
The Capability of Observing Performance in Healthcare Systems

Vivek Basavegowda Ramu and Ajay Reddy Yeruva

39.1 Introduction

Healthcare systems have to be designed more robustly as they host customer PHI (protected/personal health information) data. Similar to other sectors, customers in healthcare also expect seamless service and a website loading experience. In fact, it becomes even more crucial for the healthcare system to be performance efficient as someone could be accessing it to find the nearest medical facility, medication, or doctor, and someone's life could be dependent on it. With this responsibility comes the added pressure of architecture designing and performance reliability so that healthcare systems are accessible at any time of the day. Initially, not many healthcare applications adopted cloud technology because of concerns over data and security. With time, as cloud computing matured and hybrid-cloud and multi-cloud became more reliable, healthcare systems have slowly adopted cloud computing. Like cloud computing, many technological advancements have happened in recent years, like microservice architecture, containerization, container orchestration, etc.; along with this comes the challenge of monitoring the different components at once and more. Most importantly, they monitor the most important aspects of the healthcare system to ensure performance is maintained at an optimal level. Reasons to implement and enforce full stack observability in healthcare are also discussed.

V. Basavegowda Ramu (✉)
Independent Researcher, Hartford, CT, USA
e-mail: vivekgowda.br@gmail.com

A. R. Yeruva
Independent Researcher, Pleasanton, CA, USA
e-mail: ajayr.yeruva@gmail.com

F. J. J. Joseph et al. (eds.), *Computational Intelligence for Clinical Diagnosis*,
EAI/Springer Innovations in Communication and Computing,
https://doi.org/10.1007/978-3-031-23683-9_39

39.1.1 Background and Key Issues

39.1.1.1 Increased Use of Healthcare Systems

As the population grows day by day, healthcare subscriptions are bound to increase, and especially after the pandemic, more users are interested in knowing about healthcare options and coverage. With access to smartphones and high-speed Internet users accessing healthcare provider applications more frequently, high application processing power is required to meet the demand and to serve all customers. In the event of any issue with the application, it should be fixed and ready to serve within the blink of an eye to avoid any impact on reputation and revenue.

39.1.1.2 Raise of IoT Devices

IOT is one of the emerging technologies that has seen maximum growth in recent years, and as shown in Fig. 39.1, 18% growth is expected in the year 2022 for IoT devices, which will result in 14.4 billion active connections [1]. It is more relevant in healthcare because of the smartwatches, smart devices, and smart monitors that can track vital human health measurements and automatically trigger help requests in medical emergencies. Additional overhead is added by these devices for healthcare systems to process requests and maintain application uptime.

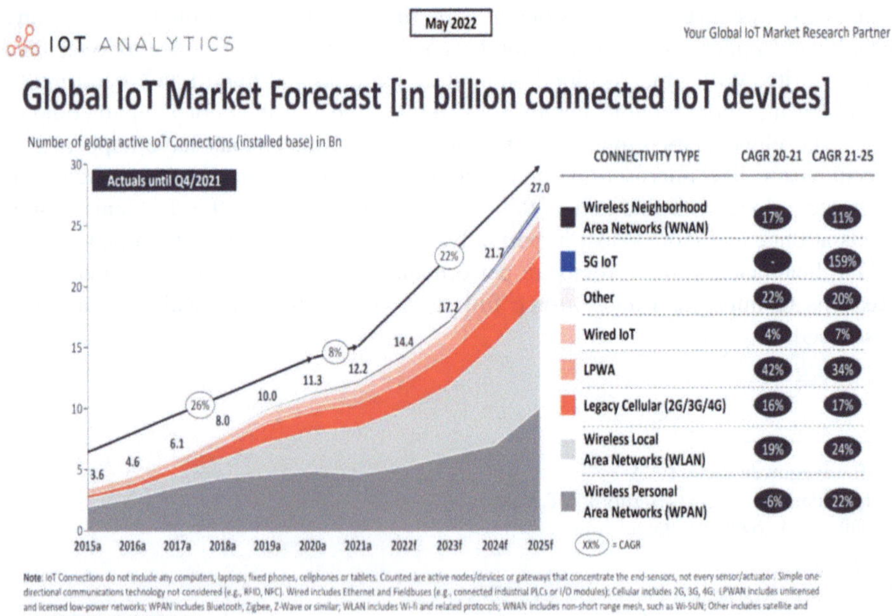

Fig. 39.1 Number of global active IoT connections in billion

39.1.1.3 Forecasting Trends to Meet Demand

Healthcare trends are one of the hardest to predict. As an example, the recent COVID-19 pandemic could not have been forecasted, resulting in a worldwide shutdown and the need for new vaccines to be developed and clinical trials conducted, manufactured, distributed, and implemented. Even without a pandemic, the forecasting for vaccine supplies, staffing, the spread of viruses, etc., is a mammoth task [2].

39.2 How Healthcare Systems Differ from Non-healthcare Systems

39.2.1 Sensitive Data

Unlike other fields, healthcare data is highly sensitive in nature as it keeps account of patient information along with address, phone number, SSN, bank/payment details, medical history, medications, etc. This data should be very securely stored and processed. Any breach in security or if anyone hacks the system, then it will be a disaster. Healthcare data is also challenged by:

- Data stored in multiple locations and devices
- Structured and unstructured data
- Different formats of data
- The constant change in regulatory requirements for data

39.2.2 Architectural and Functional Complexities

Healthcare systems are typically equipped with multiple functionalities ranging from subscriber data storage, bill processing, data encryption/decryption, applying discounts, membership ID generation, and claims processing; each will have one or many frontend and backend calls triggered to fulfil the requests. The architecture should be robust to handle the load and also account for future technology changes, user increases, and year-end processing to scale the infrastructure accordingly.

39.2.3 Multiple Components

Healthcare systems have many components to maintain, and each of them works in its own ecosystem, infrastructure, application development process, communication complexities, etc. Some of the major components are as follows:

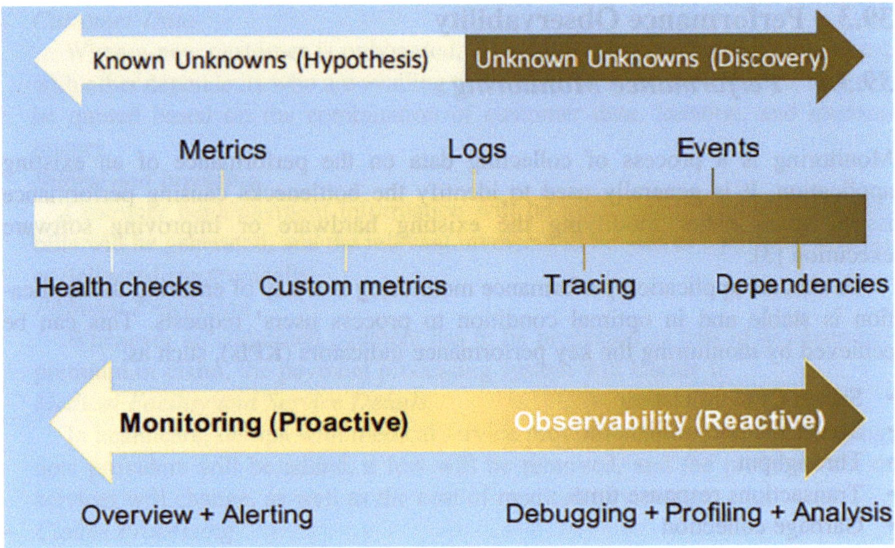

Fig. 39.3 Observability vs monitoring [5]

39.3.3 Reasons to Implement Full Stack Performance Observability in Healthcare

- Physical and mental health is now tied closely with apps, consumer expectations are at a peak, and with this, performance has become even more critical.
- For healthcare apps, issues such as slow page response, website crashes, and bad connectivity are all causes for concern. This is because an issue with a healthcare app could result in a patient not receiving the necessary care.
- Patients must be able to connect to the website information, required medication, full service, or nearby physician that they require; it is no longer sufficient to simply maintain a positive user experience in order to prevent customers from switching to a different healthcare provider; rather, this must now be a primary concern.
- Observability, with a particular emphasis on the complete stack, needs to be placed front and center in terms of IT strategy in healthcare and hospital settings because the flawless operation of applications is of the utmost importance.
- The IT department is able to identify the source of the problem and mitigate it even before the user is even aware that there is a problem because of full-stack observability. This enables patients to obtain the care they need faster and more efficiently in the short term, but in the long run, it has the potential to develop profound trust between doctors and patients by removing additional barriers to a process that is already stressful.

- The observability of the full stack has a natural tie to security. Security is essential in the healthcare industry, where HIPAA compliance and the privacy of the patient are of the utmost significance. This makes the need for security in the healthcare industry extremely pressing. Full-stack observability inherently requires the collaboration between CIOs and CISOs to ensure that applications have the highest level of security possible, starting with the applications themselves and extending to the network.

39.4 Healthcare System Performance Observability

39.4.1 KPIs

Healthcare system observability should be set up to view components at a minute level and also from different areas. Observability helps in eliminating some key existing issues in the application, like data silos, high velocity of raw data, and high troubleshooting time. Some of the metrics which will help with the full-stack performance observability of the system are as follows:

- Log analysis
- Distributed tracing – End-to-end request tracking across multiple components and services
- End-user experience metrics

39.4.2 Solution Providers

Many traditional monitoring and profiling tools like Dynatrace, Splunk, and New Relic have come up with observability options. Dashboards can be built for the system with observability metrics to view holistic application performance.

39.4.3 AI Model to Boost Observability

Observability coupled with an AI model can do wonders for healthcare systems. Instead of relying on humans to analyze and take steps to mitigate risk, an AI model can learn from past experience and analyze the raw/collected data, predict the occurrence probability, and also take proactive steps to resolve the issues.

39.4.4 Future Directions

Despite the increasing complexity in the healthcare infrastructure, companies are yet to adopt observability, and some are in very early stages. Further awareness and study are required to create a standard observability approach along with AI models so that a system can be developed that can be deployed and co-exist with observability practice to mitigate issues. The healthcare system should maintain 99.9% uptime to create a better healthcare environment.

39.5 Conclusion

The article has argued the rationale for performance observability needed in the healthcare system, and how it can help to analyze the issues proactively and take measures to mitigate them to ensure healthcare application uptime is maintained at the highest level. With the current healthcare infrastructure evolution and technology in modernization, just by monitoring the system, it is impossible to ensure high availability for the end users. As healthcare infrastructure is expected to become even more complex and high volume processed in coming years, full-stack observability should be implemented as a standard practice, and further relevant AI models should be developed to take a proactive approach.

References

1. Hasan, M. (2022, May 18). State of IoT 2022, *IOT Analytics*. https://iot-analytics.com/number-connected-iot-devices/
2. Ostrowski, G. (2021, October). *Regional CTO of AppDynamics, part of Cisco*. https://hitconsultant.net/2021/10/08/health-it-full-stack-observability/
3. Lucas, H. (1971). Performance evaluation and monitoring. *ACM Computing Surveys, 3*(3), 79–91. https://doi.org/10.1145/356589.356590
4. Usman, M., Ferlin, S., Brunstrom, A., & Taheri, J. (2022). A survey on observability of distributed edge & container-based microservices. *IEEE Access*. https://doi.org/10.1109/ACCESS.2022.3193102
5. Gartner. *Innovation insight for observability*. Refreshed March 9, 2022, Published September 28, 2020 - ID G00720189.

Chapter 40
Prediction of Lung Cancer from Electronic Health Records Using CNN Supported NLP

K. Jabir and A. Thirumurthi Raja

40.1 Introduction

Since the beginning of time, writing and speaking have been crucial tools for individuals in expressing and articulating their understanding of a wide range of complex abstract and real-world circumstances, and they continue to be so today. There is increasing agreement that written narratives are important sources of knowledge that may be used for decision-making in a wide range of sectors, and this consensus is developing. Due to the explosion of unstructured data from the origin of the Internet, data analytics using natural language processing (NLP) has hence appeared as a crucial technology to deal with experience and complex tasks, including machine translation, automated search, opinion mining, and question answering [1]. Natural language processing (NLP) is becoming increasingly important in a variety of fields, including healthcare, education, and government. The increasing use of electronic health records (EHRs) leads to increasing data volumes that contain numerous text documents that are found available over different healthcare networks. This has led to research and development of new clinical NLP solutions that can help improve patient outcomes and clinical care across the healthcare consortium [2].

Over the past few years, electronic medical records (EMR) have grown in popularity, and they are currently used to document patient treatment in the vast majority of developed countries. Except for the fact that EMRs ease the exchange of data between patient care and healthcare practitioners, this EMR data can thus be utilized as a piece of knowledge on real-world evidence and epidemiological research in the healthcare field. When it comes to electronic medical records, on

K. Jabir (✉) · A. Thirumurthi Raja
Department of Computer Science, School of Computing Sciences, Vels Institute of Science Technology and Advanced Studies (VISTAS), Chennai, India

F. J. J. Joseph et al. (eds.), *Computational Intelligence for Clinical Diagnosis*,
EAI/Springer Innovations in Communication and Computing,
https://doi.org/10.1007/978-3-031-23683-9_40

the other hand, they frequently only record a limited amount of information about patients in case notes or text fields in specified areas. Unstructured EMR data makes it hard to organize clinical research [3].

With enough application of advanced data analytics techniques, including text mining and machine learning (ML) methodologies [2–4], unstructured electronic medical record data can be more efficiently utilized for finding the relevance of disease in the case of medical research [2]. Modification of development of algorithm in relation to the classification of features from the EHR is found beneficial, and this is found to provide solutions or diagnosis of the disease [5].

Smoking status has been classified in the majority of research [5–7] using secondary data sources, which is common practice. Another study on oral health records conducted in the United States recently developed a model that is similar to the one described here, except that it was centered on tobacco use rather than alcohol consumption [8]. As a result, despite recent breakthroughs in the case of ML and NLP approaches, researchers are still having difficulty finding the unstructured data that exists from different EHRs, including smoking. The construction of a text mining model to categorize the smoking mannerism of individuals was accomplished through the use of machine or deep learning (DL) techniques, and the best ML model was evaluated in comparison to a rule-based model [9]. People read this paper to see how an ML model and a manual classification method compare [10].

DL techniques have been shown to be better than traditional ML techniques at things like language modelling, point-of-sale tagging, and paraphrase identification [11]. These unique clinical documents include the non-standard clinical jargon and acronyms by healthcare providers, the inconsistency of document structure and organization, the need to rigorously de-identify and anonymize patient data in order to keep it safe, and so on [12].

The more clinical research and development we do, the more useful clinical applications we can make, such as clinical text summarization, patient group identification, clinical decision support, engagement support, and pharmacovigilance, if we can get past these barriers.

In this study, lung cancer is retrieved and forecasted from input information using DL architecture and NLP. With this text mining approach, it is possible to predict cancer cases from input datasets in a fully automated fashion. Testing of the model is done in a number of contexts to confirm that DL and NLP are compatible with one another. When compared to the current approaches, there was a considerable increase in the accuracy of the predictions made. It can be good for research into lung cancer because the model is very durable, according to the results of the simulation.

40.2 Related Works

Examples of CNN applications include identifying cancer as in Araujo et al. [13], and this includes training the testing of the expression from the various representations of the text documents via the extraction of temporal relations. There are articles that relate to the relevance of modelling the search query, finding the interaction or relations between the protein–protein pairs, and interaction or extraction of drug–drug pairs from biomedical articles [14].

The application of CNN-based models to code radiological findings in accordance with the ICD-10 coding scheme has also been demonstrated [14], outperforming standard ML classifiers. A new semi-supervised CNN architecture for automatic ADE detection in social media has been proposed, which was motivated by the success of CNNs in a variety of clinical NLP applications, as previously described. In contrast to conventional systems, the proposed techniques utilize ML or lexicon approaches. These models rely entirely on expert annotations for the generation of the large volume of labelled data to train the supervised ML models for the detection of lung cancer. This model learns effectively from the increased volumes of data that consist of unlabelled data in association with labelled sets. They explored the utilization of CNN architecture for the classification and detection of clinical events, including treatments, disorders, adverse medication, and tests, from different text EHRs. These architectures have been shown to be effective for the detection of disease, tests, treatments, and medication events. Bidirectional RNNs and LSTMs can be used for a variety of tasks, including modelling contextual and relational similarities between the labelled entities to gain insights that can be used to make appropriate treatment recommendations, extracting clinical information or insights from EHR, and named entities, among others [15].

Recently, it was revealed that the use of knowledge graph embeddings in LSTM transducers to detect hazardous pharmaceutical reactions in social media data could be effective. Using word- and character-level embedding data, RNNs and CNNs are combined to create sickness name and recognition models. Because of these past investigations, we developed a bidirectional RNN architecture based on attention that can be used inside an encoder-decoder-based CNN framework for the detection of disease from the clinical text [16].

Unlike domain-specific clinical paraphrasing that had relied on several unsupervised or semi-supervised models with word embedding for the extraction of medical synonyms, the proposed method developed an architecture based on a neural network that is capable of modelling a character or word sequences for addressing essentially the issues raised earlier. To train medical image caption generation models that exceeded their contemporaries in a benchmark evaluation assignment, we use CNNs. The result was a model that outperformed its colleagues in the benchmark assessment test.

Memory network variants allow for greater versatility in using knowledge sources for NLP jobs requiring more complex reasoning and inference, such as answering questions, by exploiting information sources in a more flexible manner. A novel network architecture has been developed in order to infer clinical diagnoses from several clinical unstructured documents. The use of CNN-trained models on unstructured clinical documents is hence proposed for the classification and diagnostic purposes. This model was trained on unstructured clinical documents to find probable diagnoses.

Reinforcement learning-based CDS tasks are currently restricted to medical imaging and a small number of domain-dependent clinical investigations and use cases in the area. It has been demonstrated to be beneficial for a variety of tasks in the past. For example, playing games and extracting entities have both been found to benefit from deep reinforcement learning techniques in the past.

40.3 Proposed Method

Using EMRs and natural language processing, Fig. 40.1 demonstrates the workflow of CNN analysis in the diagnosis of lung cancer. It was decided to use the text format of the EMRs on lung illnesses, which was retrieved from the healthcare management system, to store the syndromes, symptoms, and other relevant data. The diagnosis and syndrome components are retrieved from the database and thereafter saved in accordance with the distinct code allocated to each patient and the related pattern diagnosis.

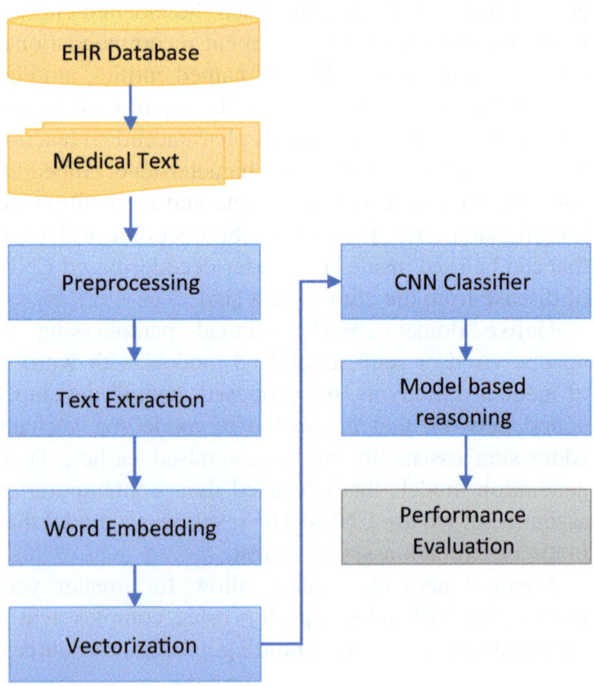

Fig. 40.1 Workflow of proposed CNN detection model

The mapping of syndrome and lung cancer sign content from the texts obtained from the computability vectors is developed via word embedding. CNN is used for the classification models, which are composed of syndrome vectors and lung cancer sign information, as well as elements or patterns of syndromes or patterns of syndromes.

40.3.1 Input Representation

Words, named objects, and fragments of speech are all examples of natural language inputs to consider. In some cases, it is feasible to express the words or text meaning by employing methodologies such as bag-of-words (BOW) modelling, which is described below. It is possible to generate a fixed-length vector representation using BOW modelling, which compares the word (i.e., presence or absence) in a phrase within a corpus.

The score from "Term Frequency-Inverse Document Frequency" (TF-IDF) is a method for producing vector representations of input text that can be used as an alternative to the TF-IDF score. Because each word in the corpus/vocabulary can be represented as an n-dimensional vector when encoded using one-hot vector encoding, it is possible to represent each word in the corpus/vocabulary as an n-dimensional vector in the corpus. In this method, the ten-word vocabulary is hence mathematically represented as an n-dimensional vector with a point set. A one-hot encoding method, like BOW, does not take word order into account, which makes the representation sparse because the dimension is based on vocabulary size.

Building a co-occurrence matrix for a corpus can help to reduce some of the limits stated above. Singular value decomposition (SVD) can be used to compress the dimensions even further, alleviating the size and sparsity issues that still exist. However, SVD has a higher computational cost and has a more difficult time absorbing new words and documents into the corpus that is being researched than the other two algorithms. Using a corpus of words to directly learn low-dimensional word vectors could be a viable method. Instead of counting co-occurrences between words, the primary idea behind this strategy is to either forecast the surrounding words (Skip-gram model) or each individual word (Continuous BoW or CBoW model) depending on the surrounding words (Continuous BoW or CBoW model that uses Word2Vec embedding). When you use stochastic gradient descent (SGD), you can use a feedforward neural network design that minimizes loss functions like hierarchical softmax and cross-entropy to learn representations of the corpus.

CNN architectures are used for learning the high-dimensional representations of the vector from the characters, phrases, words, documents, or sentences, as well as their associations (referred to as embeddings). A bag-of-words model is not very good at complex NLP mechanisms like dialogue generation and machine translation. This architecture is better because it can learn vector representations of fixed-length for different text structures of variable length through a CNN, which makes it easier to train for these tasks.

40.3.2 CNN Classifier

For example, in CNN, at least one of its levels employs convolution rather than matrix multiplication, instead of matrix multiplication. CNNs automatically learn the filter values based on the tasks they are given to perform (kernels). Each filter processes the input through the use of a sliding window function in order to encode lower-level information. When it comes to CNNs, there are two critical aspects that must be addressed in order for them to be effective: location invariance (considering the features rather than their specific location as important) and compositionality, (i.e., encoding of features at lower-level into the representations at higher-level when the data goes via higher layers).

When a linear activation is generated by the convolution layer, which applies numerous convolutions in parallel, the detector layer uses a nonlinear activation function. An output from one or more sublayers is transmitted up to a higher layer, which then uses the output as an input to do further processing. Later layers can utilize that value as an input to their own calculations. To make it simpler to view the model weights, W_1, W_2, and W_6 are all shown in the same color to make them stand out more.

CNNs can be used to perform classification tasks, including spam detection, sentiment analysis, and subject classification, since they operate in a manner that is similar to BOW principles in nature. Because location invariance is analogous to the absence of care for word order, we can say that data can be submitted to a number of filters and kernels, which can then be used to extract different features from the original data. Thus, each filter has the capability of encapsulating important characteristics of the words under consideration in an array that may be represented in two dimensions (also known as a channel).

By focusing on certain words within a range of window widths, a number of filters can be utilized to capture distinct parts of the corpus that would otherwise be missed. Using a sentiment analysis filter, it is possible to detect negative aspects in sentences, such as “not extraordinary” from the line “the product is not outstanding.” Because of their location invariance and local compositionality characteristics, CNNs, on the other hand, are unable to distinguish between “not amazing” and “amazing not.”

From Eq. (40.1), an input vector obtained from the word $w_i(t)$ that is extracted from a sentence s, a bias vector b, a weight matrix, and the activation function is hence formulated as:

$$\sigma(W \cdot x_i(t) + b) \tag{40.1}$$

It is possible for all neurons in a layer to use the model parameters W and b, which can be learned by practicing with a labelled data set. A nonlinear activation function such as

$$f(x) = \tan h(x) = \max(0, x) \tag{40.2}$$

This can be used to compute higher-layer abstractions in the same way that the hyperbolic tangent or tan$h(x)$ can be used to compute higher-layer abstractions. Finally, the output layer uses a linear classifier for the prediction of the label for any classification job based on the features that have been learned.

40.4 Results and Discussions

On the basis of an EHR and NLP data set, the study uses CNN techniques for the detection of lung disorders and further lung cancer diagnosis. The dataset is obtained from the MIMIC-III Clinical Database [17] that contains several EHR. The large volumes of real-world data from previous studies were used to train CNN in the field of integrative medicine. These researchers were able to construct models that could be used by a computer to interpret real numbers by using real-world medical records from clinical scenarios. In order to accurately diagnose lung disease, proposed approaches rely primarily on the high performance of CNN algorithms, which are capable of automatically extracting features from word vectors. The application of NLP and DL is to investigate the proposed methods for the diagnosis of lung cancer from large data sets. Such decision-making systems and integrated medicine diagnostic tools have a variety of applications. There may be substantial ramifications from this research for the incorporation of artificial intelligence into medical practice.

In the field of detection and diagnosis, the discovery of the high efficacy (Figs. 40.2, 40.3, 40.4, and 40.5) of proposed techniques for the diagnosis of syndrome patterns is a promising development. The best Word2Vec CNN proposed technique was utilized to find symptom patterns in the development and external data sets, with an accuracy score of 0.95 (Fig. 40.2), respectively. The use of word embedding and CNN has sincerely contributed to the system's increased efficiency.

The use of word embedding enables the mapping of words with computability vectors, and this makes it possible to conduct quantitative analysis of textual information. Using CNN, it is possible to automatically extract characteristics from medical literature in order to improve the CNN. Once a diagnosis in modern medicine has been determined, reasoning can be used to make a more accurate diagnosis of a syndrome pattern because the information related to diagnosis from modern medicine is hence added as a knowledge corpus.

In order to assess the accuracy of CNN algorithms, an association study was performed, in which the number of different syndrome pattern types was compared to the sample sizes of the various groups. A linear regression analysis with an accuracy of 0.95 was also carried out to evaluate the linear association between the syndrome pattern and the sample size found in each group of participants. There were just a few studies that looked at the statistical link between the two variables.

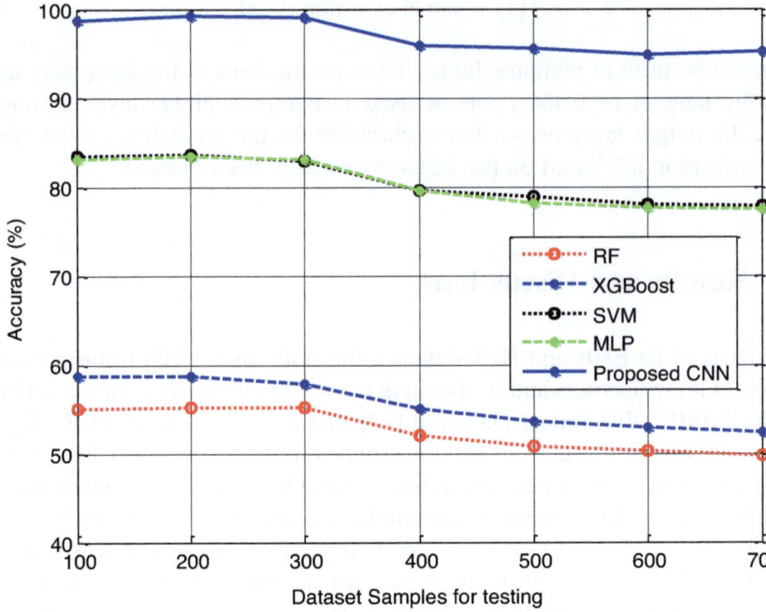

Fig. 40.2 Accuracy

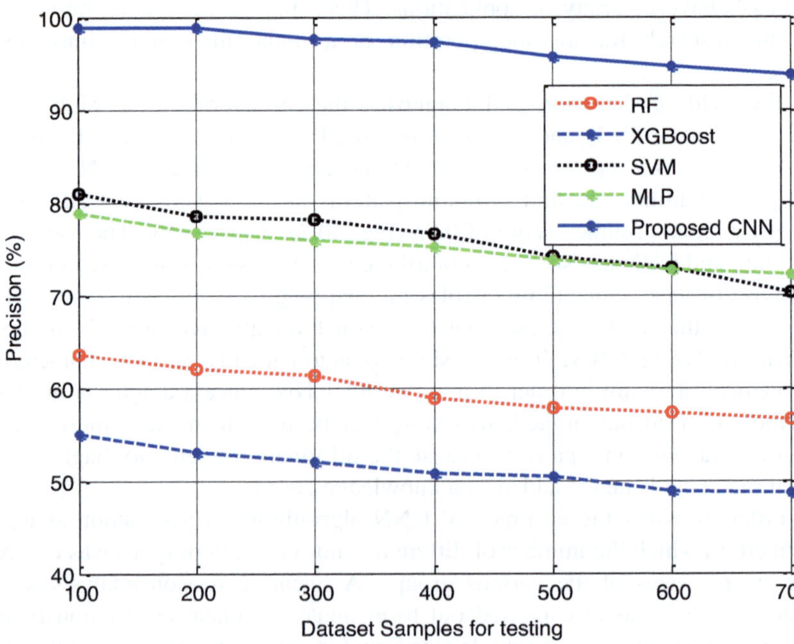

Fig. 40.3 Precision

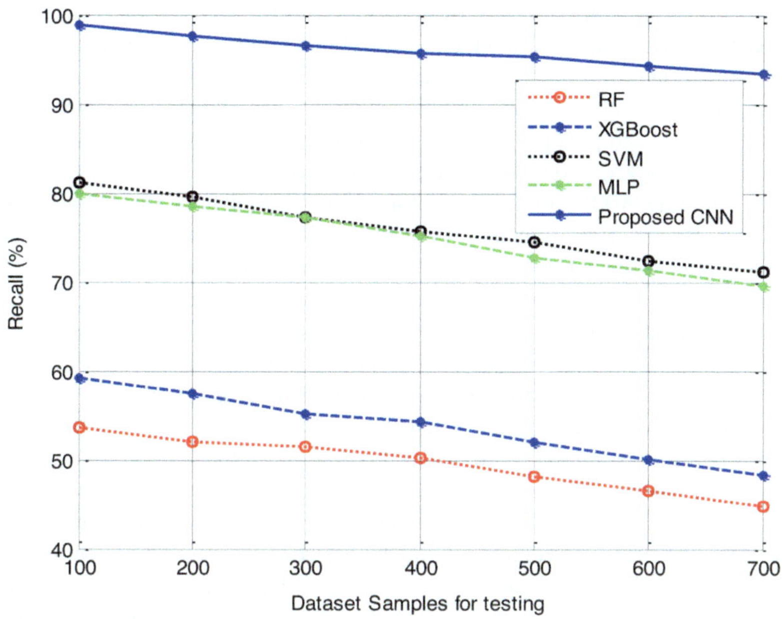

Fig. 40.4 Recall

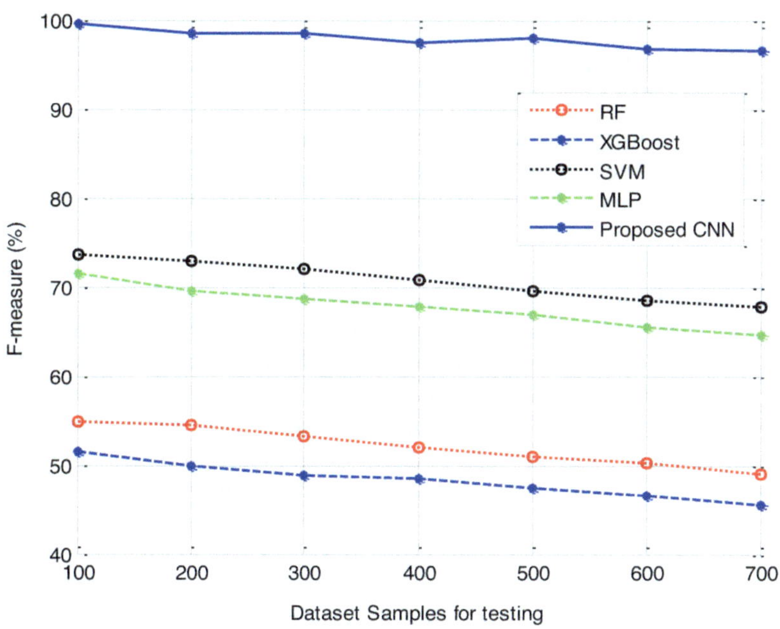

Fig. 40.5 F-measure

Only two syndrome pattern types were included in the CNN with Word2Vec, and hence each group is required to have at least 800 sample sizes in order to contain all ten syndrome pattern types. The Word2Vec CNN accuracy method was 0.95. Following the recommendations of a linear model, the Word2Vec CNN technique with at least 1200 samples per group outperformed the control group in a syndrome pattern with 20 types, as shown in the linear model. Systemic integrative internal medicine includes 400 common symptom patterns that have been classified into 20 systems. By incorporating the Word2Vec CNN algorithms into an integrative system, the algorithms were capable of satisfying a large volume of medical records that have an accuracy of 95% in the case of lung cancer cases.

The study finds that the proposed techniques perform remarkably well when utilized to diagnose symptom patterns in patients. Utilizing the Word2Vec CNN algorithms, along with information on current medical diagnoses, an accuracy of 0.9559 was achieved in corpus 2 using the Word2Vec CNN methods. When compared to the existing CNN methods, this reasoning method offered clinicians a more comprehensive understanding of lung disorders, according to the researchers. Furthermore, it was better suited to integrative medicine practitioners and their patients than the previous version. In healthcare contexts, hybrid reasoning is often preferred over traditional reasoning. Incorporating data and expertise into CNN has resulted in hybrid reasoning that poses sincere advantages of reasoning that is found understandable to physicians.

40.5 Conclusions

In this paper, we use CNN and NLP to extract and forecast lung cancer from the datasets. A relationship was discovered between the parameters associated with sample size, symptom pattern, and clinical symptoms. With this text mining approach, it is possible to predict cancer cases from input datasets in a fully automated fashion. Testing of the model is done in a number of contexts to confirm that DL and NLP are compatible with one another. When compared to the current approaches, there was a considerable increase in the accuracy of the predictions made. It can be good for research into lung cancer because the model is very durable, according to the results of the simulation. A novel methodology for the development of finding the patterns in EHR in finding lung cancer is hence used in this work, despite the fact that it has a few disadvantages. In part, we were able to reduce our search to only ten syndrome pattern categories because there were no clinical case records for the other ten syndrome pattern categories. Future research should make use of entire patterns of the syndrome in diseases of the lungs or other organ systems as a result of this discovery. Because it was too small, it could not include all of the Chinese words for lung disease or other special terms. This is because it was too small.

References

1. Li, I., Pan, J., Goldwasser, J., Verma, N., Wong, W. P., Nuzumlalı, M. Y., ... & Radev, D. (2021). Neural natural language processing for unstructured data in electronic health records: A review. *arXiv preprint arXiv:2107.02975.*
2. Patra, B. G., Sharma, M. M., Vekaria, V., Adekkanattu, P., Patterson, O. V., Glicksberg, B., et al. (2021). Extracting social determinants of health from electronic health records using natural language processing: A systematic review. *Journal of the American Medical Informatics Association, 28*(12), 2716–2727.
3. Rasmy, L., Xiang, Y., Xie, Z., Tao, C., & Zhi, D. (2021). Med-BERT: Pretrained contextualized embeddings on large-scale structured electronic health records for disease prediction. *NPJ Digital Medicine, 4*(1), 1–13.
4. Yuan, Q., Cai, T., Hong, C., Du, M., Johnson, B. E., Lanuti, M., et al. (2021). Performance of a machine learning algorithm using electronic health record data to identify and estimate survival in a longitudinal cohort of patients with lung cancer. *JAMA Network Open, 4*(7), e2114723–e2114723.
5. Morin, O., Vallières, M., Braunstein, S., Ginart, J. B., Upadhaya, T., Woodruff, H. C., et al. (2021). An artificial intelligence framework integrating longitudinal electronic health records with real-world data enables continuous pan-cancer prognostication. *Nature Cancer, 2*(7), 709–722.
6. Kehl, K. L., Xu, W., Gusev, A., Bakouny, Z., Choueiri, T. K., Riaz, I. B., et al. (2021). Artificial intelligence-aided clinical annotation of a large multi-cancer genomic dataset. *Nature Communications, 12*(1), 1–9.
7. Hao, T., Huang, Z., Liang, L., Weng, H., & Tang, B. (2021). Health natural language processing: Methodology development and applications. *JMIR Medical Informatics, 9*(10), e23898.
8. Choi, Y. C., Zhang, D., & Tyczynski, J. E. (2021). Comparison between health insurance claims and electronic health records (EHRs) for metastatic non-small-cell lung cancer (NSCLC) patient characteristics and treatment patterns: A retrospective cohort study. *Drugs-Real World Outcomes, 8*(4), 577–587.
9. Zeng, J., Gensheimer, M. F., Rubin, D. L., Athey, S., & Shachter, R. D. (2022). Uncovering interpretable potential confounders in electronic medical records. *Nature Communications, 13*(1), 1–14.
10. Montazeri, M., Afraz, A., Farimani, R. M., & Ghasemian, F. (2021). Natural language processing systems for diagnosing and determining level of lung cancer: A systematic review. *Frontiers in Health Informatics, 10*(1), 68.
11. Vaid, A., Jaladanki, S. K., Xu, J., Teng, S., Kumar, A., Lee, S., et al. (2021). Federated learning of electronic health records to improve mortality prediction in hospitalized patients with COVID-19: Machine learning approach. *JMIR Medical Informatics, 9*(1), e24207.
12. Nemesure, M. D., Heinz, M. V., Huang, R., & Jacobson, N. C. (2021). Predictive modeling of depression and anxiety using electronic health records and a novel machine learning approach with artificial intelligence. *Scientific Reports, 11*(1), 1–9.
13. Araujo, P., Astray, G., Ferrerio-Lage, J. A., Mejuto, J. C., Rodriguez-Suarez, J. A., & Soto, B. (2011). Multilayer perceptron neural network for flow prediction. *Journal of Environmental Monitoring, 13*(1), 35–41.

14. Zheng, T., Gao, Y., Wang, F., Fan, C., Fu, X., Li, M., et al. (2019). Detection of medical text semantic similarity based on convolutional neural network. *BMC Medical Informatics and Decision Making, 19*(1), 1–11.
15. Jang, B., Kim, I., & Kim, J. W. (2019). Word2vec convolutional neural networks for classification of news articles and tweets. *PLoS One, 14*(8), e0220976.
16. Turner, C. A., Jacobs, A. D., Marques, C. K., Oates, J. C., Kamen, D. L., Anderson, P. E., & Obeid, J. S. (2017). Word2Vec inversion and traditional text classifiers for phenotyping lupus. *BMC Medical Informatics and Decision Making, 17*(1), 1–11.
17. https://physionet.org/content/mimiciii/1.4/. Accessed 15 May 2022.

Chapter 41 Challenges and Opportunities for IoT Deployment in India's Healthcare Sector

Navaneethakumar V., Vinoth Kumar V., Ravishankar S. Ulle, and Yoganathan S.

41.1 Introduction

Internet of Things (IoT) has been a buzzword in the current technological era due to its presence in all devices that are getting used. Recently, the usage of many latest technologies, such as the Blockchain, enabled medical recording and monitoring systems, smart devices, watches, mobile applications, biosensors, virtual voice assistants, and other electronic-based wearables. These technologies are slowly penetrating the healthcare sector to bring a major impact on the industry in the form of easy access to personal health data. Using the various sensors, the data can be linked with a mobile application which can be used to read, monitor, and interpret according to various parameters. The information is sent straight to our persons as well as medical facilities to handle any urgent situations. According to a survey by Grand View Research Inc., the healthcare sector's IoT growth is presently estimated at $409.9 billion USD. Technavio forecasts a CAGR of almost 37% for the worldwide healthcare IoT industry. Patients with diabetes mellitus (diabetes) have a great need for smart medical devices that allow them to self-monitor their condition, and these reports detail some of the current efforts in this area. Other gadgets, including as digital pill containers, inhalers, and syringe pens, are likewise anticipated.

These smart devices can be used or implemented in healthcare through biosensors, which are a crucial part of IoT implementation in healthcare. A wide variety of biosensors are part of the continuing digital change in the healthcare industry and can wirelessly communicate medical data to smartphones and web apps. Thus, doctors or health consultants can monitor the patient's health and provide relevant treatment even from a remote location. The biosensors can help the users on a daily

Navaneethakumar V. (✉) · Vinoth Kumar V. · R. S. Ulle · Yoganathan S.
Department of Decision Science, Faculty of Management Studies, CMS Business School, Jain University, Bangalore, India

F. J. J. Joseph et al. (eds.), *Computational Intelligence for Clinical Diagnosis*, EAI/Springer Innovations in Communication and Computing,
https://doi.org/10.1007/978-3-031-23683-9_41

basis, gathering information about all activities starting from mobility, sleep, and any unusual symptoms. These biosensors help people in checking their heart rate, glucose levels, blood alcohol levels, arterial pressure, oxygen level, and pulse rate and thus transmit information in concurrent time and inform the consumers [1, 2].

The most advantageous concept of this technology is the effective communication part. These devices can communicate with each other by sharing the test results and monitoring the status of patients on a real-time basis. This adaptation will create drastic growth in the healthcare industry. There are developments in diverse types of patient health portals (PHP) that play a significant part in connecting the healthcare supply chain by providing real-time services for patients and improving patient satisfaction. Also, it is able to provide easy access to hospital employees and caregivers to follow the procedures needed immediately. The doctors and specialists can check their patients online and provide consultation for suggesting tests and prescribing medicine. This will also enable the patients to fix appointments with doctors, process their payments, enable health-related discussions with other patients through communication forums, chat, discussions, and advice about healthy lifestyles, and thus make it easier for them to satisfy the services provided by the healthcare providers. These changes will be very useful in reducing unnecessary occupancy in hospitals and resource utilization for basic requirements [1].

We have witnessed a constant increase in the introduction of new health monitoring applications in the past two decades. This is due to constant demand in the market for easy access to healthcare support. Many pharmacy and healthcare organizations are investing in new research and development of these health monitoring applications. Many projects have been developed and suggested for remote and personal health monitoring devices like wearables and implants. These projects are majorly based on sensors and wireless technologies that can link through IoT.

Projects have been developed with a lot of suggestions for remote personal health monitoring achieved through implantable wearables and other solutions that can be handled through wireless technologies and sensors at less cost. Wearable of ubiquitous monitoring environment and implantable sensors [2] is one kind of project that addresses people with arrhythmic heart disease. This project is intended to track heart operation securely through defined parameters of wearable, or portable sensor, mobile/wearable sensor systems. Their proposed system consists of a personal computer (PC), processor(s), web server(s), patient database(s), and body sensor network (BSN) nodes. Additional sensors, such as wireless-fidelity electrocardiogram (ECG) and pulse-oximetry (SpO2) sensors, can be added to the mix and mounted on dedicated Wi-Fi playing cards to complete the BSN loop. The warnings are received on a tiny flash card that can also act as a router between the BSN and the central server over a wireless-fidelity or cell community (Wi-Fi/GPRS) for PDAs, allowing for easier monitoring and analysis. The PC host interface can recognize and handle the patient sensor data as it arrives. Using the custom-built, all-encompassing software, relevant medical staff can be notified of any relevant updates immediately.

The transfer of ECG data information to a databank system is proposed [3]. ECG information can be transferred over ZigBee to a main Internet server. The central database lets health workers view data. In this setting, the ECG pulse oximeter needs more data [4]. The ZigBee-based system is also designed to track the patient's movement and gather ECG readings. The transmitter can be placed on the patient's neck, and the receiver on a PDA can be monitored by nurses/doctors using wireless and contact mics. In this setup, a ZigBee network collects ECG and pulse rate in a central database. The system uses triggered queries to the main databank, where the error rate is 5.97% or less.

Based on these types above, current implementation and innovation in IoT has enhanced the improvement of the far-off affected person monitoring functions and many features and extra complicated structures overlaying outsized ranges. The influence of IoT in the healthcare sector is going to change the way we are currently experiencing health care, like delivery of medication, precautionary diagnostic systems, early intimation of terminal disease, and emergency services to operate patients. Also, the integration of hospital management, like the availability of resources, inventory, maintenance, and medical equipment details, can all be tracked for efficient planning of the healthcare service. The Ege University hospital [5] has a comprehensive depiction and investigational outcomes of an application that was prototyped and tested the major components in the design of a medical IoT system.

41.2 IoT in the Healthcare Industry

Before the introduction of the IoT, patient–physician interactions were limited to visits, telecommunications, and texts. There was no way for doctors and hospitals to continuously monitor a patient's health and make recommendations accordingly.

Thinking of the IoT only as smart devices in homes/factories that communicate with each other to enable people to educate is a much narrower and simplistic definition. The idea is powerfully linked to the intrinsic capability of these components to function in refined ways via various communication technologies. IoT will bring innovation to all areas of modern society, not just homes and industries. Among them, the healthcare sector is the most likely candidate. IoT enables immediate and continuous real-time monitoring of patient conditions. This is especially important for many patients, such as those with chronic diseases [6].

Using the definitions provided in Gope and Hwang [1] and Catarinucci et al. [7], we can identify the following key areas in which IoT technologies are having an impact on the healthcare industry: peripheral healthcare and monitoring and surveillance services; assisted living and geriatric care; early detection and treatment of chronic diseases; patient-centric medicine; reduced emergency room wait times; monitoring of hospital resources, staff, equipment, and safety; guaranteed critical evaluations of medical devices.

IoT devices enables peripheral healthcare nursing, unlocking the potential for patient safety, wellness and empowering physicians to deliver superior care. It also improved patient engagement and satisfaction as interactions with doctors became easier and more efficient. In addition, remote monitoring of patient health can extend hospital stays and prevent readmissions. IoT will also have a significant influence on significantly declining healthcare costs and humanizing patient outcomes. The IoT is certainly changing the healthcare business, defining again the realm of components and how individuals interact in bringing healthcare resolutions. IoT has a medical implementation that benefits patients, people, medical practitioners, healthcare units, and indemnity organizations.

41.3 Review of Literature

IoT technology has recently advanced, making it possible for medical equipment to perform real-time analyses that were previously impossible for doctors to perform (Fig. 41.1). Additionally, it has helped healthcare facilities serve a larger population at once and do it at a low expense. The applications using cloud computing and Big data have also improved and streamlined doctor–patient communication, reducing the patient's financial burden while increasing the patient's engagement in the healing process. The development of healthcare IoT applications, which include health monitoring, disease detection, earlier detection of chronic disease, and personal care for young and senior citizens, is being aided by the significant influence of IoT that has been seen in recent years.

The author of the paper [8] has presented an activity identification system that incorporates wearable gadgets into a wireless sensor network for remote patient monitoring. Healthcare charting, which clinicians currently perform physically during the patient review, physical examinations, patient monitoring, and registration of patients' medical history and medicines, is a crucial activity.

Medical professionals may now concentrate more on patient care and other medical tasks thanks to Augmedix's IoT-based technology, which has helped them eliminate time-consuming and redundant tasks. With Augmedix, practitioners may

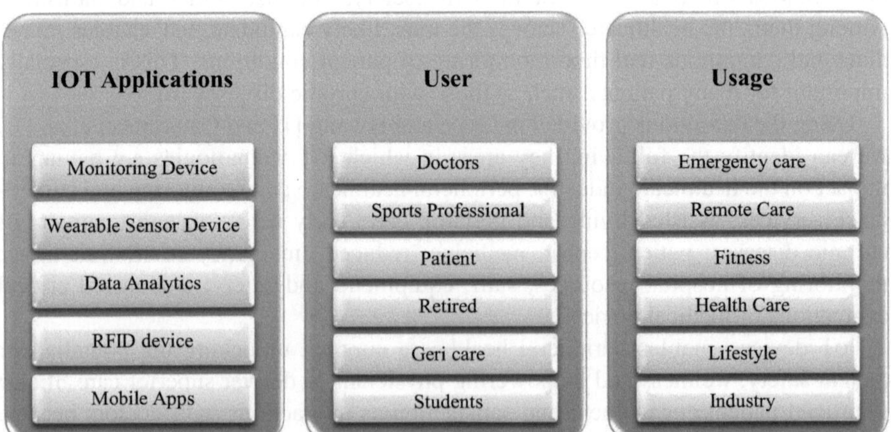

Fig. 41.1 IoT-based application, users, and their usage

record patients and input data into a hands-free platform using encrypted data that has been HIPAA-certified using smart glass technology similar to Google Glass. The technology eliminates the possibility of information leakage or misunderstanding by allowing for speedy data collection as well as safe transmission and storage of information. In a related study, the author [9] created an IoT-enabled health monitoring tool with embedded sensors for blood pressure, body temperature, and heart rate that enables remote health monitoring.

In order to extract the patient's essential information, biosignals like electrocardiogram (ECG) and electromyography (EMG) signals were also examined with the aid of IoT-enabled wearable systems [10]. A cooperative IoT-based medical network was established in Wang [11] to offer rural areas healthcare monitoring. Various procedures for authentication and permission were used to provide a secure connection between the networks.

In a household or other public service setting, this personalized customer approach system uses mobile apps to evaluate metabolic activity [12]. It is envisaged in the system that numerous users communicating with the same or separate healthcare facility use an IoT-based glucose meter. The glucose meter is registered in the IoT server using a personal mobile device. Once the glucose level has been measured using the glucose meter, the system recognizes a legitimate registered user and sends the data to the diabetes center at the medical center. The following uses of the same glucometer can take the measurement in a similar manner and send the information to a different medical facility. Consequently, even though the glucometer is used for personal measurement, the data can be shared with medical organizations for personalized healthcare with safe data transfer [13]. An algorithm that is constructed on the basis of a double moving average was used in the IoT architecture in another work for the detection of the blood glucose level. It is important to note that optical sensors, like near-infrared photodiodes and infrared LEDs, have also been used to assess glucose levels. Here Sunny and Kumar [14], the light signal received from the human body is utilized to calculate the body's glucose level.

41.4 Implementation of IoT for Patients

With implantable glucose monitoring systems, diabetics can have units with sensors implanted simply underneath the skin. Additionally, it also lets the subject by intimating the probability of getting hypoglycemia in the future and present.

41.4.1 Implementation of IoT for Physicians and Hospitals

41.4.1.1 Medical Alert Systems

Individuals may wear what appear to be ornaments – but are intended to caution people in situations of crisis. In the event of a fall, the person designated to respond to the emergency will be notified via smartphone that immediate assistance is required.

41.4.1.2 Consumable Sensors

People can now consume sensors like pills. Once the sensor is ingested, the information is relayed to the patient's mobile app to help maintain the correct dosage of medication. Most medications are not taken as recommended owing to absent-mindedness or the human tendency to forget due to stress and work conditions. This ingestible sensor ensures that patients are consuming the right medication at appropriate time durations and in the correct dosages. Few consumable sensors are additionally being used to extra precisely detect patients with stipulations such as colon cancer and also irritable bowel syndrome.

41.4.1.3 Medication Dispenser

The device can now be implanted in patients who are on regular doses of medication during the day. Patients are advised when their medication needs refilling. Medical practitioners can additionally remind you of neglected doses for the duration of regular check-ups.

41.4.1.4 Portable Sensor

Portable sensors are utilized in laboratories and in cold storage in healthcare units to confirm that samples of blood, refrigerated medicines, and additional biomedical materials are continuously at the appropriate temperature.

41.4.1.5 Identifiable/Trackable Inhaler

Trackable/identifiable inhalers inform patients about the situation or going through to cause an asthma attack, informing them on their smartphone or tablet. The data received can also be shared with a medical practitioner. An associated inhaler tells the patient appropriately about the medication.

41.4.1.6 Wearables for Anti-depression

Apple Inc. has developed an application for the Apple Watch that aids people with a tendency of anxiety/depression to cope with it. The application helps to track the patients' conduct, outdoor schedules, appointments, screen cognitive and temper functions.

41.4.1.7 Connectable Contacts

Connectable contacts now measure blood sugar levels in diabetics. But quickly, you will be in a position to fix your eye's focal point and enhance your vision.

41.4.1.8 Position Services

Things such as defibrillators, wheelchairs, nebulizers, scales, pumps, and observing devices are mapped and connected with IoT sensors so they can be easily found by healthcare workers. Physical devices are often out-of-place or difficult to find in time, but with the help of IoT sensors, staffs know where they are placed and where their position is.

41.4.1.9 Remote Monitoring

Medical professionals can use IoT devices to monitor people who have just undergone surgical procedures or are moving to outpatient care. The healthcare professional will be notified when a patient is in a serious condition that needs to be attended immediately. In the past 5 years, the innovation in IoT-based healthcare is increasing. There is much more application in the healthcare division that could be highlighted.

This capacitance takes into account all of the impacts from the touch screen components, such as the interactions between the sensor pad, overlay, and ground or the pin capacitance from the controller. Thus, CP represents the complex electric field produced by all of the components.

41.5 Data Analysis of IoT Implementation

The following category and area of applicants data were collected as listed in the table for further analysis, and the results were found as discussed in Table 41.1:

Table 41.1 Between-subjects factors

		Value label	N
Category of applicants	1.00	Student	4
	2.00	Doctor	4
	3.00	Industry	4
	4.00	Sports person	4
	5.00	Geri care	4
Area of applications	1.00	Fitness	5
	2.00	Health care	5
	3.00	Style	5
	4.00	Work-related	5

Table 41.2 Dependent variable: usage level of IoT

Source	Type III sum of squares	df	Mean square	F	Sig.
Model	12805.300	8	1600.663	1.281	0.337
Category of applicants	25.700	4	6.425	0.005	1.000
Area of applications	478.800	3	159.600	0.128	0.942
Error	14992.700	12	1249.392		
Total	27798.000	20			

41.5.1 Two Way ANOVA Table

The influence of IoT on the medical field is tested through this research by collecting data from different categories of applicants. Two-way Anova (Table 41.2) is employed with the following hypothesis.

41.5.2 Null Hypothesis

H01: All the categories are using the same level of IoT
H11: All the categories are not used equally

41.5.3 Alternative Hypothesis

H02: All the fields have an equal level of application
H12: All the fields are not equally applied

Accepted

H11: All the categories are not used equally
H12: All the fields are not equal

Table 41.3 Descriptive statistics table

Dependent variable: IoT usage level				
Category of applicants	Area of applications	Mean	Std. deviation	N
Student	Fitness	10.0000	.	1
	Health care	15.0000	.	1
	Style	70.0000	.	1
	Work-related	5.0000	.	1
	Total	25.0000	30.27650	4
Doctor	Fitness	15.0000	.	1
	Health care	45.0000	.	1
	Style	10.0000	.	1
	Work-related	30.0000	.	1
	Total	25.0000	15.81139	4
Industry	Fitness	10.0000	.	1
	Health care	5.0000	.	1
	Style	0.0000	.	1
	Work-related	90.0000	.	1
	Total	26.2500	42.69563	4
Sports person	Fitness	69.0000	.	1
	Health care	6.0000	.	1
	Style	5.0000	.	1
	Work-related	20.0000	.	1
	Total	25.0000	30.12197	4
Geri care	Fitness	15.0000	.	1
	Health care	75.0000	.	1
	Style	1.0000	.	1
	Work-related	0.0000	.	1
	Total	22.7500	35.50000	4
Total	Fitness	23.8000	25.39094	5
	Health care	29.2000	30.30182	5
	Style	17.2000	29.77751	5
	Work-related	29.0000	36.12478	5
	Total	24.8000	28.55945	20

This reveals the results that all the categories were not used IoT applications equally in all the fields. Further, to get clarity, the mean values and standard deviations were also calculated for the data collected in the study area and listed below.

Mean and standard are found for the study area data and listed in Table 41.3.

The above table reveals the mean and standard deviations of each category from others; the following results were observed:

1. Though students are using IoT applications, most are using them as fashion, and standard deviation also reveals high fluctuation.

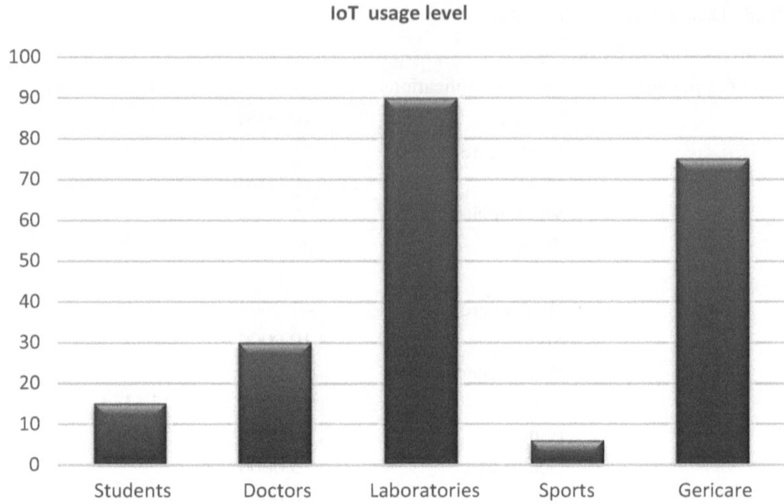

Fig. 41.2 Healthcare industry uses IoT applications

2. Doctors were using profession-related applications with fewer standard deviations than any other category.
3. Medical industry uses 90% of IoT applications.
4. Sports persons using fitness purpose with high fluctuations.
5. Geri people also use almost 75% of applications toward health.

The same result is shown in the chart (Fig. 41.2).

The chart reveals the fact that the healthcare industry uses IoT applications more than any other industry, considerably on the high side.

41.6 Conclusions and Future Work

The research paper is intended to identify the IoT implementation in the area of healthcare industry. It discusses thus projects and implementations carried over in the recent timeframe and focuses on their practical application. The scope of this research is based on the responses received from various profiles from Bangalore, India. The category of a profile is given as students, medical professionals, industry practitioners, sports, and Geri care. At the same time, the area of IoT applications is given as lifestyle, fitness, healthcare, and work-related. The impact of the IoT on the healthcare industry is examined in this article. It also discusses the opportunities and threats that IoT technology presents to the health industry. Furthermore, it identifies the area that needs more attention for further implementation of this kind of project. This will help both technology innovation and the healthcare industry to work together to increase the level of investment needed. Though the recent impact of healthy lifestyles among people has increased, this study denotes that the majority of the requirement comes from doctor professionals for healthcare requirements. Hence, the IoT application and implementation will be required more in this area in the near future, and it will lead to an efficient healthcare operation.

References

1. Gope, P., & Hwang, T. (2015). BSN-Care: A secure IoT-based modern healthcare system using body sensor network. *IEEE Sensors Journal, 16*(5), 1368–1137.
2. Ng, J. W. P., Lo, B. P. L., Wells, O., Sloman, M., Peters, N., Darzi, A., Toumazou, C., & Yang, G.-Z. (2004, September 7–14). Ubiquitous Monitoring Environment for Wearable and Implantable Sensors (UbiMon). In *Proceedings of 6th International Conference on Ubiquitous Computing (UbiComp'04)*, Nottingham.
3. Dagtas, S., Pekhteryev, G., & Sahinoglu, Z. (2007). *Multisreal-time time health monitoring via ZigBee in smart homes*. Mitsubishi Electric Research Laboratories.
4. Hong, J. H., Kim, N. J., Cha, E. J., & Lee, T. S. (2006). Development of ZigBee-based mobile healthcare system. *IFMBE Proceedings, 6*, JC27.
5. Sokullu, R., Akkaş, M., & Cetin, H. (2010). Wireless patient monitoring system. In *Fourth International Conference on Sensor Technologies and Applications* (pp.179–184).
6. Aktaş, F., Çeken, C., & Erdemli, Y. E. (2015). Transmission of physiological signals with quality of service support by using Wireless Body Area Networks. In *Medical Technologies National Conference, 2015* (pp. 1–4). IEEE.
7. Catarinucci, L., De Donno, D., Mainetti, L., Palano, L., Patrono, L., Stefanizzi, M. L., & Tarricone, L. (2015). An IoT-aware architecture for smart healthcare systems. *IEEE Internet of Things Journal, 2*(6), 515–526.
8. Castillejo, P., Martinez, J.-F., Rodriguez-Molina, J., & Cuerva, A. (2013). Integration of wearable devices in a wireless sensor network for an E-health application. *IEEE Wireless Communications, 20*(4), 38–49.
9. Wan, J., AAH Al-awlaqi, M., Li, M., O'Grady, M., Gu, X., Wang, J., & Cao, N. (2018). Wearable IoT enabled real-time health monitoring system. *EURASIP Journal on Wireless Communications and Networking, 2018*(1), 1–10.
10. Kelati, A. (2018, May). Biosignal monitoring platform using Wearable IoT. In *Proceedings of the 22nd Conference of Open Innovations Association FRUCT* (pp. 9–13). Petrozavodsk.
11. Wang, W. (2011, May). The internet of things for resident health information service platform research. In *Proceedings of the IET International Conference on Communication Technology and Application*, Beijing.
12. Lee, B. M. (2015). Personalized service model for sharing medical devices in IoT health-platform. *Advanced Science and Technology Letters, 99*, 180–182.
13. Valenzuela, F., García, A., Ruiz, E., Vazquez, M., Cortez, J., & Espinoza, A. (2020). An IoT-based glucose monitoring algorithm to prevent diabetes complications. *Applied Sciences, 10*(3), 921.
14. Sunny, S., & Kumar, S. S. (2018, January). Optical based non invasive glucometer with IoT. In *Proceedings of the 2018 International Conference on Power, Signals, Control and Computation* (pp. 1–3). Thrissur.

Chapter 42
WADET: A Novel Approach to Chronic Kidney Disease Detection and Analysis

S. Mohammed Imran and N. Prakash

42.1 Introduction

Chronic kidney diseases reflex the health condition of human kidneys in a timely basis. If the kidney cannot filter the bloodstream, it gets rid of metabolic activity because the waste stages are in the kidney. The infections inside the kidney take longer to reflect; hence one of the critical chronic diseases identified by the diagnosis is kidney disease. Large millions of people all over the world are affected by kidney diseases, including chronic kidney diseases. It requires previous healthcare records of the patients to analyze the chronic kidney diseases. Predictive healthcare analytics supports various healthcare segments of life, aiming to provide diagnostic steps more accurate and precise to the relevant disease criteria. In an effort to raise awareness on health transformation impacts of lifestyle habits on chronic diseases, various diseases hit humans with various new symptoms until the critical condition of the disease abstract the normal will be in people are not taking care of it. Chronic kidney disease is one of the most common diseases with a high-risk impact.

The kidney is the fundamental organ that purges the circulatory system and disposes of metabolic waste. Constant kidney sickness demonstrates the condition where the human kidney is versatilely harmed. Constant kidney sickness tainted organs by shifting the circulatory system and disposing of metabolic wastages. Constant kidney illness can be treated by examining the verifiable records of kidney

S. Mohammed Imran (✉)
Research Scholar, Department of computer applications, B.S Abdur Rahman Institute of Science and Technology, Vandalur, Chennai, Tamil Nadu, India

N. Prakash
Department of Information Technology, B.S Abdur Rahman Institute of Science and Technology, Vandalur, Chennai, Tamil Nadu, India
e-mail: prakash@crescent.education

F. J. Joseph et al. (eds.), *Computational Intelligence for Clinical Diagnosis*, EAI/Springer Innovations in Communication and Computing,
https://doi.org/10.1007/978-3-031-23683-9_42

disorders [1]. The strength of the kidney relies upon different factors, for example, a healthy way of life, food propensities, race, age, and sort of constant medical problems and so forth. If kidney sicknesses are not treated in the early phase, constant kidney illnesses smother the kidney's working in the long haul. Ineffective clinical treatment and untreated kidney problems lead absurdly to serious kidney give. Continuing mechanical development has made numerous strategies for diagnosing kidney problems in the beginning phases. Understanding the verifiable treatment and working boundaries of the kidney is useful for the individual to treat the issue successfully [2]. Chronic kidney diseases (CKD) analysis should be limited to several tests to cover the populace. CKD can be investigated through clinical well-being records, CT pictures, and determination tests [3].

Figure 42.1 shows the general process of healthcare data analysis using data analytics [5]. The computational intelligence of existing record analysis made doctors and technology experts decide on certain therapies. Several studies impact the usage of machine learning algorithms to analyze patients' clinical records regarding chronic kidney diseases to make relevant decisions.

- The proposed approach focuses on developing a robust methodology in which the feature extraction and classification processes are highlighted. In terms of handling the big dataset, the challenge in handling the multivariable nonlinear data is focused.

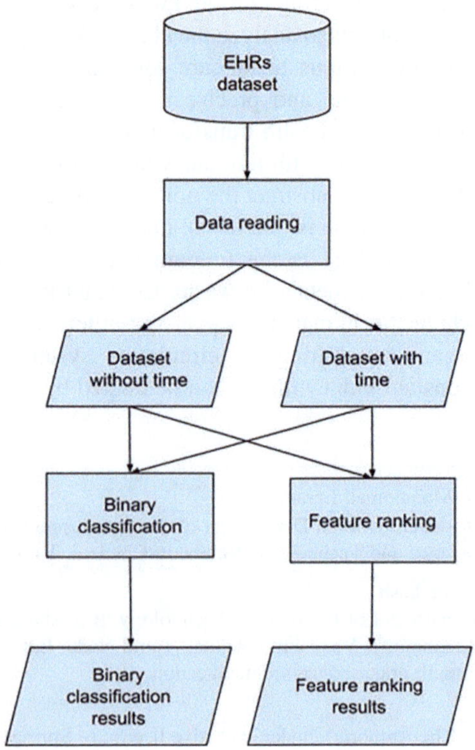

Fig. 42.1 General process involved in healthcare data analysis [6]

- Here multivariate feature extraction technique is utilized using an exploratory data analysis window. Further preprocessor data is split into training data on testing data to make a pattern verification process.
- A novel wide and deep ensemble technique is developed here in which three regression algorithms come together. Linear gradient regression (LGR), random forest regression (RFR), and sparse greedy regression (SGR) techniques are proposed to form ensemble techniques that capture the highest correlation factor.
- Utilizing the statistical evaluation based on correlation factors further system is a validator. The process validation is achieved using the K-fold cross-validation method using a deep aggressive network (DAN).

The performance of the overall system is validator using accuracy (ACC), precision (P), recall (R), sensitivity (S), and Matthew's correlation coefficient (MCC). The rest of the chapter is formulated as a detailed background study in Sect. 42.3. This is followed by system tool selection and problem identification of the existing system in Sect. 42.4. Further, in Sect. 42.4, the system design methodology is developed. Results and discussions are obtained with Sect. 42.5. Conclusion and future enhancement follow.

42.2 Background Study

D. Chicco et al. [6] presented a machine learning algorithm using medical records of chronic kidney disease–infected patients. The severe cases of chronic kidney diseases and the normal patients with chronic kidney data are combined to form a predictive analysis method. The presented approach achieves Mathew's correlation coefficient of 0.499, and in the formal cases, the main value achieved is 0.469. Due to various lifestyle habits, smoking, food habits, and lack of water intake, chronic kidney diseases are developed. Diabetes is also one of the reasons for chronic kidney diseases. The methodology is introduced in the presented system using the feature-based ranking method. Various parameters such as age, creatine, blood rate, and diabetics level are included to make the analysis.

Bhaskar et al. [7] have approached a new urea level discussed in the presented paper. The author collects various information on RAW signals, collects the urea level of saliva, and normalizes the data. Using one-dimensional convolutional neural network architecture, this process incorporated with support vector machine and ensemble approach is developed to make the classification. The proposed approach achieved the classification of 98.04%.

G. Chen et al. [8] utilization deep learning methods and adaptive deep learning mechanism for helping to make the early prediction of kidney diseases effectively. Any kind of classification methodology and its accuracy is based on the effective utilization of collector data. Most classification algorithms focus on feature extraction tricks to enhance the accuracy of the classification process and reduce the feature extraction time. The presented chapter developed the supervised tissue classifier methodology, which classifies the input features into two categories; hence the dimensionality is reduced.

A. Ogunleye et al. [9] presented an artificial intelligence algorithm for chronic kidney disease detection using the XGboost regression process. The model is created with optimal training inputs and achieves the highest feature extraction technique using CKD optimizers. The presented chapter achieves the highest accuracy of 100% for static data with the highest sensitivity of 1. The reduced model with few features is desirable until the highest performance is achieved.

J. McAllister et al. [10] presented a predictive control system is compared with the standard model in detecting kidney disorders. The predictive model approach iteratively adjusts the weight of the desired input to the training input. Computational prediction of that optimization for anemia in chronic kidney disease is discussed in which zone model predictive control is utilized.

Hoi et al. [11] presented a joint learning hidden algorithm for electronic healthcare records. The proposed approach transforms the given data into graphical convolutional data that combines various statistical measures to make a pattern comparison. The proposed approach consistently outperforms comparing with the previous approaches and achieves the accuracy of greater than 90% for general purpose representation of learning algorithms. The proposed approach analyzes various electronic health records based on classification.

S. M. M. Elkholy et al. [12] presented an artificial intelligence (AI) classification approach and a predictive analysis method using a deep belief network (DBN). In order to obtain the maximum information on kidney diseases for the given dataset, a categorical cross entropy method is used for the loss function. The proposed approach achieves the highest accuracy of 98.5% sensitivity of 87.5% and comfort with various data for approaches. As mentioned in the proposed paper, utilizing deep learning techniques in clinical data analysis provides early prediction of chronic kidney diseases. Early renal disease prediction helps to prevent the advancement of kidney illnesses and the life-shortening effects of kidney damage.

42.2.1 Summary of Findings

- The challenges existing frameworks face are complexity in multivariate data, handling the nonlinear dataset, and similarity issues. The false sensitive data need to be removed from the dataset. Data normalization needs to be focused on.
- The cumulative data on a single formulation creates more propagation delay in analysis; hence, the wise sparse approximation is recommended.

42.2.2 System Design

The proposed model is developed using Python IDE 3.8 35-level computing environment for complex numerical computations and scientific implementations. It consists of libraries that enable automated numerical operations and scientific computing key points within the integrated environment. The graphical representation of the presented method is evaluated with the Google collaborator window. It consists of recalling the Python libraries in an automated way that reduces the time of experimental setup.

42.2.3 Problem Identification

The current lifestyle changing habits, obesity, and hypertension act as one of the common criteria for people's problems. Numerous medical issues are the root kidney diseases because of family history, a hierarchical record of people having kidney transplantation problems, kidney disease medicines that cause severe kidney disorders, most of the pain killers, and age and race, such as old people and certain racial groups who have a high chance of developing kidney diseases. Kidney disease diagnosis of early stage helpful for the patients to save their life with the protocol provided by the health experts. The pattern of medical records, healthcare records, and habitual records are gathered and evaluated using multivariate exploratory data analysis in the promising field of study on chronic kidney disease. Chronic the major challenge in data analysis is handling a large amount of data that occurs in a nonlinear pattern. In order to make the early prediction and develop a prediction algorithm, handling the data set in the future extraction process is vital.

42.3 Methodology

42.3.1 System Architecture

Figure 42.2 shows the system architecture of the proposed chronic kidney disease detection system using the novel wide and deep ensemble tree (WADET) method.

42.3.2 Data Preparation

The data preprocessing enables the Kaggle datasets CKD dataset to read, resize into fixed frames of blocks, etc. These data are processed block-wise and further utilized for the multivariate feature extraction (MVFE) technique.

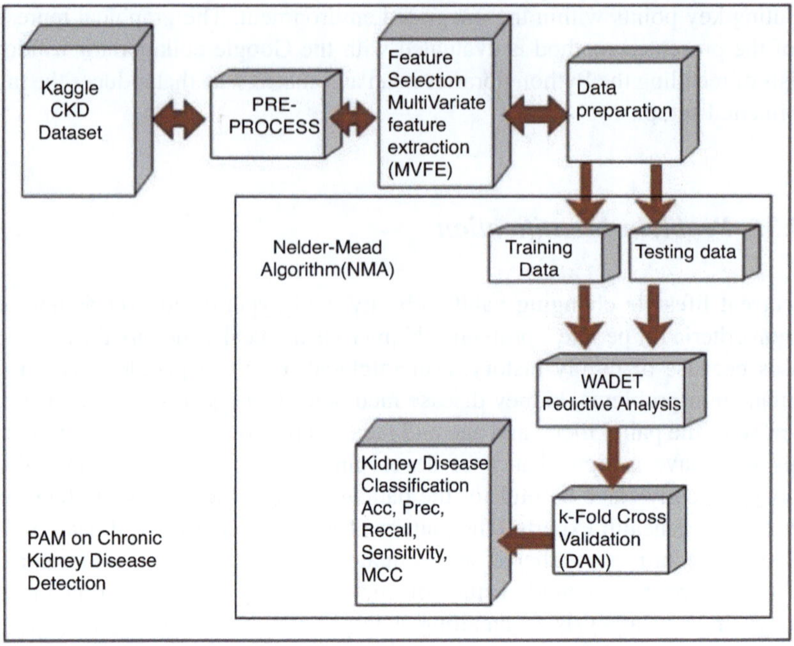

Fig. 42.2 System architecture

42.3.3 Feature Analysis

Data visualization is graphically visualizing the data to analyze the patterns, decide on repeated patterns, etc. Most of the data visualizations are divided into three types of categories. Univariate analysis is where the data type contains only one variable, and it looks like a simple analysis format that deals with one quantity change throughout the data. This version is simple, attaining your good pattern from the data within the existing graph. By various analyses, this type of data involves two different variables utilized to impact the data set. The relationship between the two impacts data is also important for the pattern process. In the case of multivariate analysis, the data have different pattern generation where the challenge is to make a unique pattern with a certain relationship between the data. This kind of multi-Manually checked notes for variance data not automated methods.

42.3.4 Proposed Novel WADET Model

In the LGR model, the target is to make the best fit to the regression line where the given data value of x is compared and trained with the database value of Y. Some statistics are behind the two data sets, such as root means the square error is utilized to make the true prediction value are false value. The lower the cost function then, the higher the correlation. To minimize the cost function, the model must be trained between higher iterations and randomly with recursive updates to the data. By order for the final update of the hypothesized equation for non-linear data, Data predictive score should be one according to the formula given below.

42.3.4.1 Linear Regression Cost Function

RFR is a supervised learning algorithm in which combined learning of regression methodologies has recently been utilized to make multiple decisions for a single model. These regression algorithms help make multiple decisions in a data tree where the aggregation focuses on the highest co-correlated decision. Using Multivariate data analysis techniques, different forms of data in algorithm End point. These data are split into blocks of frames, and each has a certain decision achieved by the random for a. The majority of voting is achieved if it has a major value related to the correlation date. The regression problem is further solved by making the decisions related and non-related to the zero value.

The greedy spas regression algorithm effectively approximates the multivariate data given by the chronic kidney disease data set (Fig. 42.3). Due to the scattered patterns of multivariate nonlinear data, it requires large titrations of learning to format the data to the best pattern. A set of features is selected from diversity. A feature extraction technique for selecting a subset of features for a learning mechanism has been created. A best-pass regression algorithm adjusts the weight of each frame It can be adjusted with a specific data frame to create a subset. In the case of no subset, the values match the existing subject, which are then modelled as a different subset. At the end of the result, the learning algorithm demonstrates the

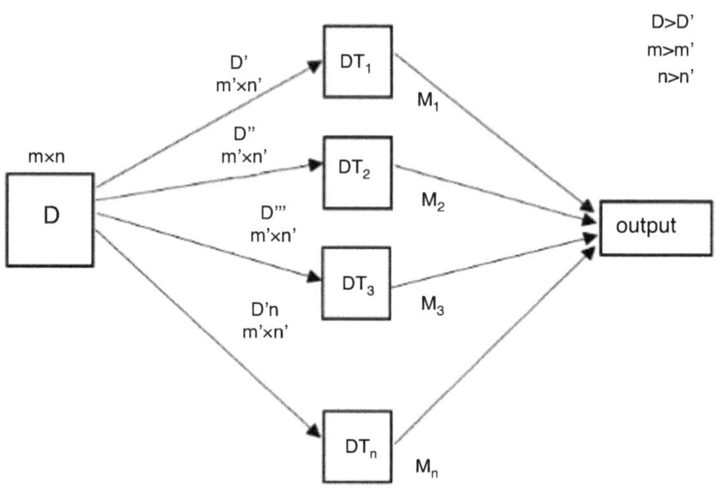

Fig. 42.3 Random forest regressions

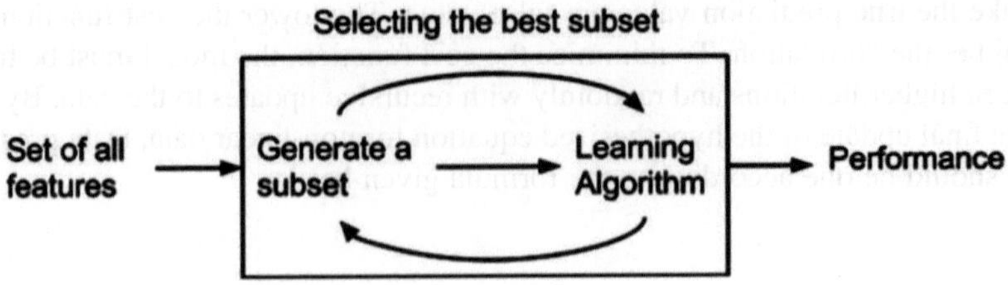

Fig. 42.4 SGR process

robustness of fat signal recovery using the cluster data of feature extracted chronic kidney values. The Nelder–Mead algorithm explains this step by step below. The sparse greedy algorithm works with finding the greedy solution of the probability weight p until the maximum iteration runs over time. The number of weights initiated to zero is further incremented to the next hydration, and the weights are incremented. The data is normalized, and the evaluation matrix is parallel calculated. If the accuracy means in the assessment matrix, such as the accuracy means calculated during the iteration, it should reach the maximum value. For example, the accuracy should be high, and the main square error should be low (Fig. 42.4).

42.3.5 WADET Pseudocode Using Nelder–Mead Algorithm

```
Input: Get dataset, make convergence thresholds
Output: W optimized weights of each column
Mm, d1 = number of rows
W = Null Vector, length d
P = Null vector of length Mm
S = 0; Initially
        While (Conv<0) do
    S = s + 1;
For j = 1:d1, perform
    X[j] = metric(y, (P + z(:,j)/s));
End
Max(j) = argmax(x(j));
P = p + x(:,jmax).
W(jmax) = wjmax+1;
End
Return process w/s;
```

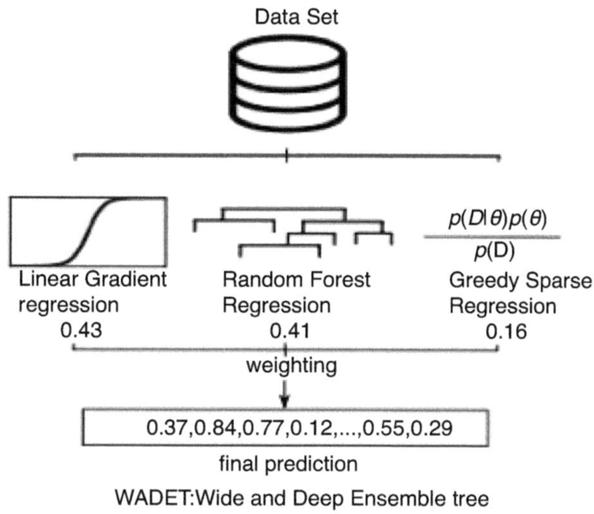

Fig. 42.5 Proposed WADET model

42.4 Formulation of WADET Model

Figure 42.5 shows the aggregate fusion of LGR, RFR, and SGR and their weights accumulation to enable the final prediction. Each model has a unique way of statistical analysis window to act on the prediction mechanism. The proposed model WADET is created to the aggregate result of each model.

42.5 Results and Discussion

42.5.1 MVFE for Feature Mapping

Figure 42.6 shows the MVFE process where various chronic kidney disease features are formulated as unique attributes. These attributes are manually encoded before fetching into the analysis models.

42.5.2 Classification Result

Figure 42.7 shows the classification result of CKD and non-CKD data from the data analysis. Further, the independent analysis is discussed in Fig. 42.8.

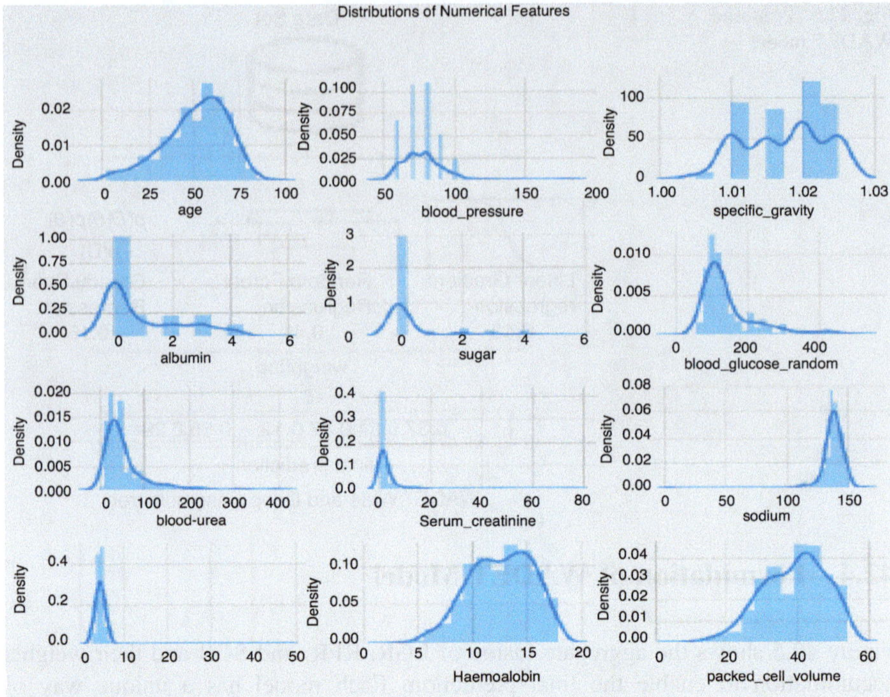

Fig. 42.6 MVFE model for feature mapping

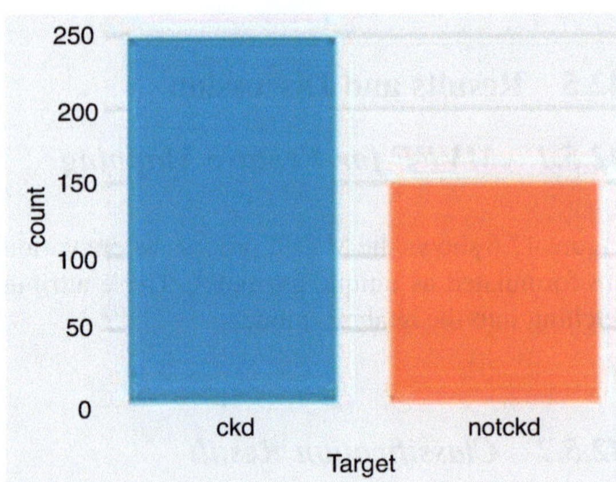

Fig. 42.7 CKD classification results

42.5.3 Performance of Independent Models

Figure 42.8 shows the accuracy of three independent models, LGR, RFR, and SGR, plotted as performance metrics.

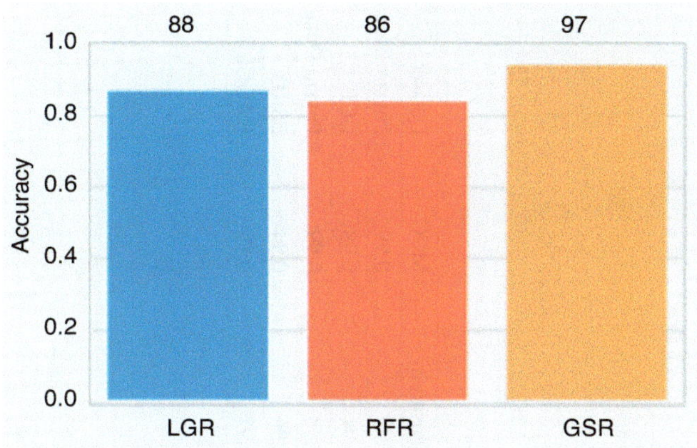

Fig. 42.8 Accuracy of LGR, RFR, GR models

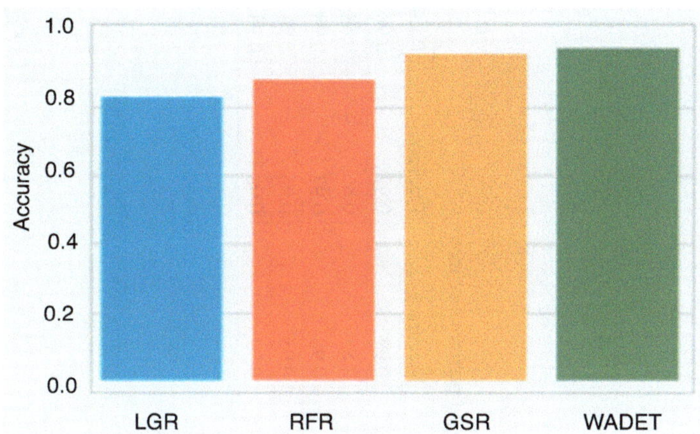

Fig. 42.9 Comparison of independent model with aggregate fusion model (WADET)

42.5.4 Comparison of Independent Model with Aggregate Fusion Model (WADET)

Figure 42.9 shows the comparison of independent models with an aggregate fusion model called WADET. The independent accuracy of LGR, RFR, and SGR is separately shown in Fig. 42.7. The fusion aggregated result combines the prediction benefit of each model and validates the result further to make an accurate decision on chronic kidney disease.

Table 42.1 shows the comparison of existing methods and the proposed WADET model.

Table 42.1 Comparative results on existing and proposed performance metrics

S no	Reference	Algorithms involved	Accuracy	Precision	Recall	Sensitivity	MCC	Dataset
1	[4]	CNN-SVM	0.99	0.97	0.98	0.99	0.99	Physio-Data
2	[6]	Random Forest	0.85	0.86	0.88	0.94	0.98	UCI
3	[2]	DBN	0.98	0.97	0.98	0.98	0.99	Physio-Data
4	[7]	XGBOOST	0.95	0.95	0.94	0.96	0.94	ESRD
5	Proposed	WADET + DAN	0.99	0.98	0.98	0.97	0.99	KAGGLE

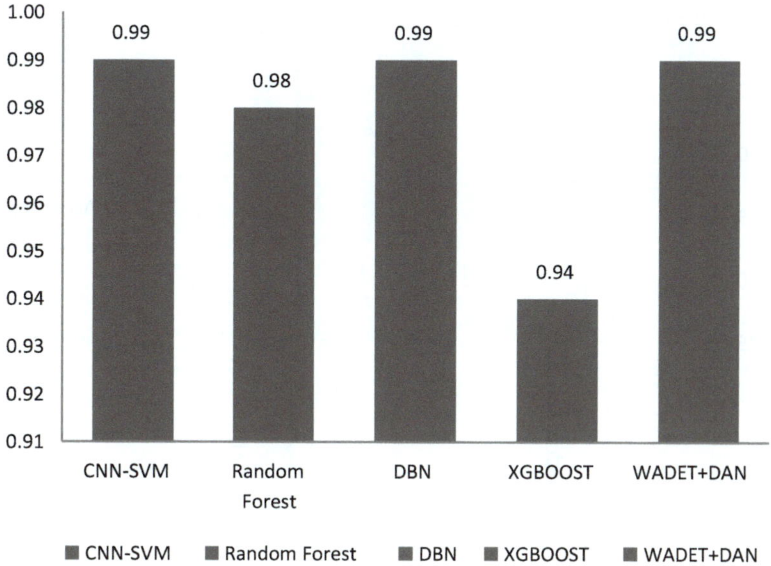

Fig. 42.10 Comparative metrics

Table 42.1 compares chronic kidney disease detection systems with various existing state of heart approaches discussed here. The author discusses the convolutional neural network with a support vector machine algorithm for the physiological data collected from the patients. The system achieves 98.04% using real-time data. The author utilized the random for our algorithm as a universe data in which the UCI dataset is combined. The random forest achieves the highest of 85.5%. A deep belief network is considered one of the robust methodologies for making complex decisions with complex input samples. The chronic kidney disease data of various patients combined with the physiological data. The author achieves an accuracy of 98.5% using the belief network with a low error rate.

Figure 42.10 shows the comparison results of various existing implementations on chronic kidney diseases to the proposed WADET model. The nonlinear data analysis is carried out with the MVFE process before fetching it into the aggregate fusion WADET model.

Using artificial intelligence algorithms and internal frameworks, chronic kidney disease detection and data analytics techniques are improved. Using the end-stage renal disease (ESRD) data set, the author presented an XGboost algorithm for making the classification of chronic kidney diseases (Fig. 42.11). The highest occurrence of 95% is achieved using the HG boost algorithm. The proposed framework on novel wide and deep model combines the benefit of the random forest algorithm, linear regression algorithm, and the SGR algorithm to form the highest correlation factor. The final decision-making on the proposed chronic kidney disease data set has arrived using the Nelson-made algorithm. The proposed approach is the highest circular of 99.3 percentage and compared with the existing state of the heart.

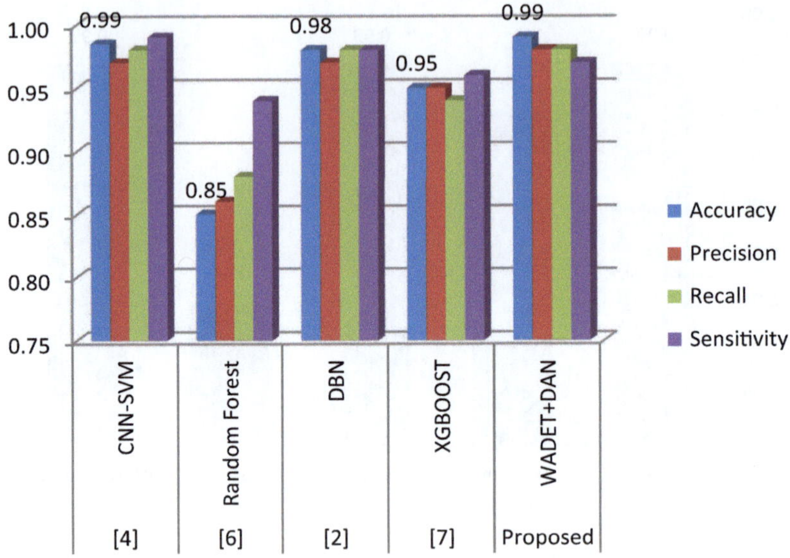

Fig. 42.11 Various comparative metrics

42.6 Conclusion

Currently, exploratory data mining of health records provides predictive estimates of essential diseases that cause life-altering difficulties. Due to various reasons, chronic kidney diseases are developing among millions of people around the globe, and they should be treated as early as possible. The proposed framework on novel wide and deep model combines the benefit of the random forest algorithm, linear regression algorithm, and the SGR algorithm to form the highest correlation factor. The final decision-making on the proposed chronic kidney disease data set has arrived using the Nelson-made algorithm. The proposed approach is the highest circular of 99.3 percentage and is compared with existing state-of-the-art approaches. Further, the system needs to be improved using a deep and generalized adversarial network to enhance the prediction performance to the next level.

References

1. Arjun, A. S., & Chandavarkar, B. R. (2021). Predictive analytics and data mining in healthcare. In *2021 12th International Conference on Computing Communication and Networking Technologies* (pp. 1–7).
2. Mangat, P. K., & Saini, K. S. (2021). Health CARE prediction using predictive analytics. In *2021 10th International Conference on System Modeling & Advancement in Research Trends (SMART)* (pp. 64–70).

3. Singh, S., Mukherjee, S., Dewan, R., & Ajala, J. A. (2019). Predictive analysis in health care. In *2019 International Conference on Computational Intelligence and Knowledge economy* (pp. 467–470).
4. Nithya, B., & Ilango, V. (2017). Predictive analytics in health care using machine learning tools and techniques. In *2017 International Conference on Intelligent Computing and Control Systems (ICICCS)* (pp. 492–499).
5. Antony, L., et al. (2021). A comprehensive unsupervised framework for chronic kidney disease prediction. *IEEE Access, 9*, 126481–126501.
6. Chicco, D., Lovejoy, C. A., & Oneto, L. (2021). A machine learning analysis of health records of patients with chronic kidney disease at risk of cardiovascular disease. *IEEE Access, 9*, 165132–165144.
7. Bhaskar, N., & Manikandan, S. (2019). A deep-learning-based system for automated sensing of chronic kidney disease. *IEEE Sensors Letters, 3*(10), 1–4.
8. Chen, G., et al. (2020). Prediction of chronic kidney disease using adaptive hybridized deep convolutional neural network on the internet of medical things platform. *IEEE Access, 8*, 100497–100508.
9. Ogunleye, A., & Wang, Q.-G. (2020). XGBoost model for chronic kidney disease diagnosis. *IEEE/ACM Trans Comput Biol Bioinf, 17*(6), 2131–2140.
10. McAllister, J., Li, Z., Liu, J., & Simonsmeier, U. (2019). Erythropoietin dose optimization for anemia in chronic kidney disease using recursive zone model predictive control. *IEEE Transactions on Control Systems Technology, 27*(3), 1181–1193.
11. Hoi, E., Xu, Z., Li, Y., Dusenberry, M., Flores, G., Xue, E., & Dai, A. (2020). Learning the graphical structure of electronic health records with graph convolutional transformer. *Proc AAAI Conf Artif Intell, 34*(01), 606–613.
12. Elkholy, S. M. M., Rezk, A., & Saleh, A. A. E. F. (2021). Early prediction of chronic kidney disease using deep belief network. *IEEE Access, 9*, 135542–135549.

Index

F. J. J. Joseph et al. (eds.), *Computational Intelligence for Clinical Diagnosis*,
EAI/Springer Innovations in Communication and Computing,
https://doi.org/10.1007/978-3-031-23683-9

MIX
Papier aus verantwortungsvollen Quellen
Paper from responsible sources
FSC® C105338

If you have any concerns about our products,
you can contact us on
ProductSafety@springernature.com

In case Publisher is established outside the EU,
the EU authorized representative is:
Springer Nature Customer Service Center GmbH
Europaplatz 3, 69115 Heidelberg, Germany

Printed by Libri Plureos GmbH
in Hamburg, Germany